Veterinary Pediatrics

Veterinary Pediatrics

Dogs and Cats from Birth to Six Months

3rd Edition

Johnny D. Hoskins, DVM, PhD
Professor Emeritus
Veterinary Clinical Medicine
Louisiana State University
School of Veterinary Medicine
Baton Rouge, Louisiana

W.B. SAUNDERS COMPANY
A Harcourt Health Sciences Company
Philadelphia London New York St. Louis Sydney Toronto

W.B. SAUNDERS COMPANY
A Harcourt Health Sciences Company

The Curtis Center
Independence Square West
Philadelphia, Pennsylvania 19106

Library of Congress Cataloging-in-Publication Data

Hoskins, Johnny D.
Veterinary pediatrics: dogs and cats from birth to six months / Johnny D. Hoskins.—3rd ed.

p.   cm.

ISBN 0–7216–7665–0

1. Puppies—Diseases.   2. Kittens—Diseases.   3. Veterinary
   pediatrics.   I. Title.

SF991.H594 2001
636.7′089892—dc21   00–050479

VETERINARY PEDIATRICS: ISBN 0–7216–7665–0
Dogs and Cats from Birth to Six Months

Printed in the United States of America

Last digit is the print number: 9   8   7   6   5   4   3   2   1

This textbook is dedicated to . . . those who nurture the concept that learning is a lifelong process.

Contributors

Dawn Merton Boothe, DVM, PhD, Dipl ACVIM
Associate Professor, Department of Veterinary Physiology and Pharmacology, Texas A&M University, College Station, Texas
Drug Therapy

Mary K. Boudreaux, DVM, PhD
Associate Professor, Department of Pathobiology, College of Veterinary Medicine, Auburn University, Auburn, Alabama
Disorders of Hemostasis

Janice McIntosh Bright, BSN, MS, DVM, Dipl ACVIM
Associate Professor of Cardiology, Colorado State University, College of Veterinary Medicine and Biomedical Sciences, Fort Collins, Colorado
The Cardiovascular System

Jorg Bucheler, DVM, PhD, Dipl ACVIM(IM), Dipl ECVIM-CA
Professor of Internal Medicine and Director of Clinical Operations, Ross University, West Farms, St. Kitts, West Indies
Blood Component Therapy

C. B. Chastain, DVM, MS, Dipl ACVIM
Professor of Small Animal Medicine, College of Veterinary Medicine, University of Missouri, Columbia, Missouri
The Metabolic System

Kenneth D. Clinkenbeard, PhD, DVM
Professor and Interim Head, Department of Veterinary Pathobiology, College of Veterinary Medicine, Oklahoma State University, Stillwater, Oklahoma
Hematology of Normal Dogs and Cats and Responses to Disease

Rick L. Cowell, DVM, MS, Dipl ACVP
Professor, Veterinary Clinical Pathology, Department of Pathobiology, College of Veterinary Medicine, Oklahoma State University; Director, Clinical Pathology Laboratory, College of Veterinary Medicine, Oklahoma State University, Stillwater, Oklahoma
Hematology of Normal Dogs and Cats and Responses to Disease

Lilli S. Decker, DVM, MS
Clinical Pathologist, Antech Diagnostics, Farmingdale, New York
Hematology of Normal Dogs and Cats and Responses to Disease

Scott D. Fitzgerald, DVM, PhD
Associate Professor of Veterinary Pathobiology, College of Veterinary Medicine, Michigan State University; Diagnostic Pathologist, Animal Health Diagnostic Laboratory, Michigan State University, East Lansing, Michigan
The Urinary System

Mary B. Glaze, DVM, MS, Dipl ACVO
Professor of Veterinary Ophthalmology, Louisiana State University; Veterinary Ophthalmologist, Veterinary Teaching Hospital and Clinics, Louisiana State University, Baton Rouge, Louisiana
The Eye

Deborah S. Greco, DVM, PhD
Associate Professor, Small Animal Internal Medicine, Department of Clinical Sciences, Colorado State University, Fort Collins, Colorado
The Endocrine System

B. Jean Hawkins, MS, DVM, Dipl AVDC
Director, Delta Dental Service for Pets, American Animal Hospital Association; Red Hill Animal Health Center, Carbondale, Colorado
Dental Disease and Care

Giselle Hosgood, BVSc, MS, FACVSc, Dipl ACVS
Professor, Veterinary Surgery, School of Veterinary Medicine, Louisiana State University, Baton Rouge, Louisiana
Anesthesia and Surgery

Johnny D. Hoskins, DVM, PhD, Dipl ACVIM
Professor Emeritus, Veterinary Clinical Medicine, Louisiana State University School of Veterinary Medicine, Baton Rouge, Louisiana
The Physical Examination; Puppy and Kitten Losses; Preventive Health-Care Programs and Heredity Tests; The Digestive System; The Liver and Pancreas; The Skin and Claws; The Eye; The Nervous System; Nutrition and Nutritional Problems; Toxicology

Lesley G. King, MVB, Dipl ACVECC, Dipl ACVIM
Associate Professor, Section of Critical Care, School of Veterinary Medicine, University of Pennsylvania, Philadelphia, Pennsylvania
Environmental Injuries

John M. Kruger, DVM, PhD, Dipl ACVIM
Associate Professor, Department of Small Animal Clinical Sciences, Michigan State University College of Veterinary Medicine, East Lansing, Michigan
The Urinary System

Gary Landsberg, BSc, DVM, Dipl ACVB
Doncaster Animal Clinic, Thornhill, Ontario, Canada
Behavior Development and Preventive Management

Jody P. Lulich, PhD, DVM, Dipl ACVIM
Associate Professor, Department of Small Animal Clinical Sciences, University of Minnesota, College of Veterinary Medicine, St. Paul, Minnesota
The Urinary System

Douglass K. Macintire, DVM, MS, Dipl ACVIM and ACVECC
Professor in Medicine, Department of Small Animal Surgery and Medicine, College of Veterinary Medicine, Auburn University, Auburn, Alabama
Intensive Care Management

James H. Meinkoth, DVM, MS, PhD
Associate Professor, Veterinary Pathobiology, Department of Veterinary Pathobiology, Oklahoma State University, Stillwater, Oklahoma
Hematology of Normal Dogs and Cats and Responses to Disease

Steven S. Nicholson, DVM, Dipl ABUT
Associate Professor of Veterinary Toxicology, School of Veterinary Medicine, Louisiana State University, Baton Rouge, Louisiana
Toxicology

Carl A. Osborne, DVM, PhD, Dipl ACVIM
Professor, Department of Small Animal Clinical Sciences, College of Veterinary Medicine, University of Minnesota, St. Paul, Minnesota
The Urinary System

Beth P. Partington, MS, DVM, Dipl ACVR
Associate Professor of Veterinary Radiology, School of Veterinary Medicine, Louisiana State University, Baton Rouge, Louisiana
Diagnostic Imaging Techniques

Augustine T. Peter, BVSc, MVSc, MSc, PhD
Associate Professor, Department of Veterinary Clinical Sciences, School of Veterinary Medicine, Purdue University, West Lafayette, Indiana
The Reproductive System

David P. Polzin, DVM, PhD, Dipl ACVIM
Professor of Internal Medicine, University of Minnesota, College of Veterinary Medicine, St. Paul, Minnesota
The Urinary System

Teresa M. Rieser, VMD, Dipl ACVECC
Director, Emergency Service, VCA Newark Animal Hospital, Newark, Delaware
Environmental Injuries

Kenita S. Rogers, DVM, MS, Dipl ACVIM

Associate Professor, Staff Oncologist, Department of Small Animal Medicine and Surgery, College of Veterinary Medicine, Texas A&M University, College Station, Texas
The Lymphoid System

Kurt S. Schulz, DVM, MS, Dipl ACVS

Assistant Professor, Small Animal Surgery, Department of Surgical and Radiological Sciences, University of California, Davis, California
The Skeletal System

G. Diane Shelton, DVM, PhD, Dipl ACVIM

Associate Adjunct Professor, Department of Pathology, School of Medicine, University of California, San Diego; Director, Comparative Neuromuscular Laboratory, Department of Pathology, University of California, San Diego, La Jolla, California
The Neuromuscular System

Peter K. Shires, BVSc, MS, Dipl ACVS

Professor of Small Animal Surgery, Virginia–Maryland Regional College of Veterinary Medicine; Director, Veterinary Educational Technology and Coordinator, Biological Sciences Initiative, Virginia Tech and University of Maryland, Blacksburg, Virginia
The Skeletal System

Joseph Taboada, DVM, Dipl ACVIM

Professor of Small Animal Internal Medicine and Director of Professional Instruction, Department of Veterinary Clinical Sciences, School of Veterinary Medicine, Louisiana State University, Baton Rouge, Louisiana
The Respiratory System

Grant H. Turnwald, BVSc, MS, Dipl ACVIM

Associate Dean of Academic Affairs, Virginia–Maryland Regional College of Veterinary Medicine, Virginia Tech and University of Maryland, Blacksburg, Virginia
The Respiratory System

A. J. Venker-van Haagen, DVM, PhD

Associate Professor, Ear, Nose, and Throat Diseases, Utrecht University, Faculty of Veterinary Medicine, Department of Clinical Sciences of Companion Animals, Utrecht, The Netherlands
The Ear

Preface

Welcome to the third edition of *Veterinary Pediatrics: Dogs and Cats from Birth to Six Months*. In keeping with the previous edition's style and format, this edition is a unique combination of state-of-the-art information from the first and second editions and new information from the latest developments in clinical veterinary medicine. Each subject is described again in a concise manner so that the textbook can serve as a quick reference and resource for those treating dogs and cats from birth to six months of age, whether they are healthy or afflicted with a congenital or acquired illness.

The purpose of the third edition is to provide interested readers with health-related information that is applicable to their field and quickly retrievable. For those readers who are already accustomed to the presentation of previous editions, it should not take long to feel comfortable with the third edition. Approximately one third of the original authors have returned to revise

their information. Thirteen new authors have been chosen to provide new state-of-the-art information.

I am indeed grateful to all of the contributors to this third edition. Thank you for sharing your expertise with colleagues. A very special thanks goes to Ms. Debra Adleman of Montrose, Pennsylvania, for her editorial assistance and genuine interest in the success of the project. I have also been privileged to work with a most supportive and enthusiastic team at the W.B. Saunders Company. Mr. Raymond R. Kersey provided invaluable guidance.

Ever since the first edition was published, colleagues have told me at meetings around the world how often they use *Veterinary Pediatrics: Dogs and Cats from Birth to Six Months* in their practices. Nothing gives an author more satisfaction than to receive positive feedback of this nature. It is, therefore, my sincere hope that this third edition will live up to your high expectations.

JOHNNY D. HOSKINS

NOTICE

Veterinary medicine is an ever-changing field. Standard safety precautions must be followed, but as new research and clinical experience broaden our knowledge, changes in treatment and drug therapy may become necessary or appropriate. Readers are advised to check the most current product information provided by the manufacturer of each drug to be administered to verify the recommended dose, the method and duration of administration, and contraindications. It is the responsibility of the treating veterinarian, relying on experience and knowledge of the animal, to determine dosages and the best treatment for the animal. Neither the publisher nor the editor assumes any responsibility for any injury and/or damage to animals or property arising from this publication.

THE PUBLISHER

Contents

Physical Examination and Diagnostic Imaging Procedures

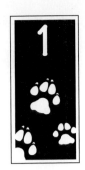

Johnny D. Hoskins and Beth P. Partington

The Physical Examination

Johnny D. Hoskins

Diagnosis of health status in any puppy or kitten is based on the assiduous collection of facts obtained through observation and ancillary diagnostic procedures, followed by the meticulous recording of these facts. The most important step, and sometimes the most difficult step, is the efficient and expert collection of facts in the history and physical examination (Hardy, 1981).

The physical examination should be conducted systematically; a systematic approach helps avoid confusion and apprehension on the part of the animal, owner, and veterinarian. The physical examination is most easily conducted by proceeding from head to tail; however, observations should be recorded according to the body system affected. As illustrated in Figure 1–1, most physical examination recording sheets are organized according to body systems. The most common errors committed during physical examination are those of omission or in technique, detection, interpretation, or recording (Wiener and Nathanson, 1976). A systematic approach to performing the examination and recording findings prevents most of these errors.

Restraint of puppies and kittens requires gentleness and patience. Puppies and kittens younger than 4 weeks of age are usually examined with their mother. The examiner should approach the mother cautiously because many otherwise gentle animals may become fractious when strangers approach their young. The mother may have to be removed from the examination room if she is uncooperative.

Equipment used to examine the puppy and kitten includes a small digital thermometer, an otoscope with infant-sized cones, a penlight and hand-held lens or an indirect ophthalmoscope, a small accurate gram scale for recording body weights, and a stethoscope equipped with a pediatric-sized or infant-sized bell (2 cm) and diaphragm (3 cm). In addition, a pediatric pleximeter for testing neurologic reflexes may be helpful.

PUPPIES AND KITTENS YOUNGER THAN FOUR WEEKS

Newborn puppies and kittens are fat and sleek; they sleep contentedly and nurse frequently. Body weight is one of the most important aspects of the physical examination of very young animals. Body weights should be recorded carefully with an accurate gram scale at birth, at 12

PHYSICAL EXAMINATION

REFERRING VETERINARIAN

NAME:

ADDRESS:

PHONE:

ADMISSION DATE:

SMALL ANIMAL CLINIC ☐	LARGE ANIMAL CLINIC ☐	HERDS/LITTERS TOTAL # SEEN

OUTLINE	NAF	
GEN—General		DATE:________ TIME:________ A.M. P.M.
Eyes, Ears, EENT—Nose Throat		Temp.______ C F Wt.______ KG Lbs Hydration______
		Pulse = ______/min;______(Rhythm)______(Character)
SKIN—Integument		Resp. = ______/min &______(Character)
MS–Musculoskeletal		PERMANENT MARKINGS:
CV—Cardiovascular		
RESP—Respiratory		DESCRIPTION OF ABNORMAL FINDINGS:
GI—Digestive		
UROL—Urinary		
REPRO—Genital		
NEURO—Neurologic		
LYMPH—Lymphatics		
OTHER—		
NAF = No Abnormal Findings		

Student____________ Clinician____________
Signature Signature

PHYSICAL EXAMINATION

FORM NO. VTH-04 (8-86)

COPY—MEDICAL RECORD

Figure 1–1. Record sheet for physical examination.

hours after birth, and then daily for the first 2 weeks of life. Newborn puppies and kittens may be identified by characteristic coloring or markings or by using colored collars made of ribbon or tape. The breeder or owner of each puppy or kitten should keep a growth chart so that weight-gain abnormalities may be quickly identified. Failure of weight gain often is the first sign of illness in a newborn animal.

Normal birth weight in puppies varies by breed, with toy breeds weighing approximately 100 to 400 g. Medium-sized breeds weigh 200 to 300 g at birth and large breeds approximately 400 to 500 g. Giant breeds often weigh in excess of 700 g at birth. The birth weights of puppies generally double by 10 to 12 days of age (Johnson and Grace, 1987; Mosier, 1978). Most kittens weigh about 100 ± 10 g at birth. Birth weight of kittens is doubled by 2 weeks of age (Johnson and Grace, 1987; Mosier, 1978).

After accurate assessment of body weight, vital signs (such as temperature, capillary refill time, pulse rate, and respiratory rate) are obtained. The heart rate is above 200 beats per minute, and the respiratory rate is from 15 to 35 breaths per minute in puppies and kittens younger than 2 weeks of age (Mosier, 1978; Small, 1980). Normal body temperature for newborn puppies and kittens is about 96° to 97° F. After 1 to 2 weeks, body temperature gradually increases to 100° F by 4 weeks of age (Mosier, 1978). Temperature should be recorded with a small pediatric rectal thermometer to minimize discomfort. Newborn puppies and kittens should never be left unattended or warmed on electric heating pads, because their neuromuscular reflexes are not present until 7 days of age; severe burns can easily result from electric pads (Johnson and Grace, 1987). Warm-water heating blankets, warm-rice bags, hot water bottles, or small cardboard boxes lined with blankets and infant diapers are better choices for maintaining warmth or for warming cold puppies and kittens when the mother is not available. Because normal body temperature is lower in newborn puppies and kittens, they should not be warmed to adult body temperature, or at least not above 99° to 100° F.

Upper and lower eyelids separate about 5 to 14 days after birth in most puppies and kittens (Johnson and Grace, 1987; Mosier, 1978). The iris is blue-gray in color and will change to the adult color in future weeks. Vision is not normal until 3 to 4 weeks of age (Johnson and Grace, 1987). Flexor tone predominates during the first 4 days of life, resulting in the characteristic comma shape of most newborns. After 4 days, extensor tone becomes dominant, and the puppies and kittens lie on their side or thorax with the head extended (Breazile, 1978). Pain perception is present at birth; however, withdrawal reflexes are not well developed until about 7 days of age. Puppies and kittens begin to crawl at 7 to 14 days of age. By 16 days of age, walking begins, and by 21 days of age, puppies and kittens exhibit a relatively normal gait (Johnson and Grace, 1987).

Puppies and kittens should be examined soon after birth. The physical examination should never be done on a nonwarmed examination table. The body weight of each puppy and kitten should be carefully recorded, and each animal should be examined individually. Puppies and kittens should be plump and round with no gross abnormalities of size or shape. Congenital abnormalities should be looked for specifically. The head should be mobile, and the puppy or kitten should exhibit a rooting reflex. The skull should be inspected for evidence of open fontanelle or harelip. The ears are checked for size and position and the nose for presence of fluid accumulation in the nostrils. The mouth should be inspected for evidence of cleft palate, presence of cyanosis, evidence of dehydration, and sucking reflex. The skin is examined for wounds, state of hydration, completeness of hair cover, and condition of foot pads. The haircoat should be shiny and free of debris.

Breathing should be regular and unlabored in a healthy puppy or kitten. The thoracic area may be inspected for symmetry, wounds, rib fractures, and congenital sternal and spinal abnormalities. Because of their very rapid heart rate, newborn puppies and kittens are difficult to auscultate. An infant-sized bell (2 cm) and diaphragm (3 cm) fitted to a standard stethoscope maximizes the possibility of hearing a heart murmur or altered lung sounds. If auscultation is unrewarding, the rate and depth of respiration, the heart rate, muscle tone, and activity are evaluated as indirect indicators of cardiopulmonary condition. The mucous membranes should be pink and moist.

Muscle tone should be strong, but newborns cannot support their own weight until about 16 days of age (Breazile, 1978; Johnson and Grace, 1987). The limbs are inspected for position, deformities or absence of long bones, number and position of toes and foot pads, tendon contracture, and joint mobility. Examination of the nervous system of puppies and kittens is difficult and generally requires serial evaluations (Breazile, 1978).

Following nursing, the abdomen is enlarged, and the puppy or kitten should be in a restful state. Enlargement of the abdomen with restlessness, weakness, and vocalization or complete silence may indicate illness (Bebiak et al, 1987). The umbilicus is carefully inspected for evidence of infection or abnormalities of the abdominal wall. The umbilical cord normally drops off by 2 to 3 days after birth (Bebiak et al, 1987). Rubbing the perineum with a moist, warm cloth or soft tissue paper stimulates micturition and defecation. Evidence of hematuria, abnormal micturition, or diarrhea is sought. The anus is checked for patency, swelling, and redness.

PUPPIES AND KITTENS FOUR WEEKS TO SIX MONTHS OF AGE

The first step in the physical examination of the 4-week-old to 6-month-old puppy or kitten is to observe the animal at rest and at play. Careful observations begin when the animal enters the room and is placed on the examination table or rests on the floor. One should look for obvious abnormalities of gait or orientation. Does the animal react appropriately to the strange environment, or does it appear disinterested? Is the animal withdrawn or friendly? Does it come when called by the owner or the examiner? Valuable information may be gained from carefully observing the animal's reaction to its environment. Careful note should be made of the animal's body condition, mentation, posture, locomotion, and breathing pattern.

Puppies and kittens should be allowed to approach the examiner rather than being seized and examined immediately. Friendly coaxing and rewards, in the form of treats, may be helpful in gaining the animal's trust. One must remember to keep this experience as positive as possible for the animal. Gentle handling ensures that the puppy or kitten will become a cooperative adult. Uncomfortable procedures, such as otoscopic examination or insertion of a rectal thermometer, should be performed in the middle of or at the completion of the examination. A treat or a "pat" may be offered after an unpleasant procedure has been performed.

HEAD AND NECK

When beginning the physical examination, approach the animal from the front, offer your hand for the puppy or kitten to smell and become accustomed to, and then grasp the animal gently behind the head and neck with one hand while gently holding the nose with the other. This serves two purposes—first, it prevents the examiner from being bitten, and second, it immobilizes the puppy's or kitten's head for inspection. The head and face should be examined for symmetry.

The eyes should be examined with a penlight. Look at the eyelids first, examining for cilia and evidence of accumulative discharge along the eyelid margins. Note the clarity of the cornea and the color of the sclera, which should be eggshell white with minimal blood vessel injection. The anterior chamber should be clear and of uniform thickness throughout. Note the color and texture of the iris, which is often blue-gray in young puppies and kittens. Look for irregular margins in the iris (colobomas) and persistent pupillary membranes, which appear as spidery strands of pigmented epithelium adhering to either the cornea or the lens. The fundus should be examined especially in those breeds with known heritable eye diseases. A penlight and hand-held lens often provide more information than a direct ophthalmoscope; however, the fundus should be examined

with the equipment available. Darken the room and look for a tapetal reflection when the penlight beam is directed into the animal's eyes. Place the hand-held lens between the eye and the light source. An inverse image of the retina should be visible in the lens. Move the lens toward or away from the eye to focus the image. It is often helpful to steady one's hand on the animal's nose. Again, in puppies and kittens, it is important to look for congenital abnormalities such as colobomas, lens opacity, or retinal dysplasia. The optic disc, vessels, and retina should be observed, and any abnormalities should be recorded.

Check the nares for obstruction, stenosis, discharge, or abnormal shape. The patency of the airways may be determined by closing the animal's mouth and allowing the puppy or kitten to breathe on a glass slide or metal table. Palpate the muzzle for any swellings or abnormalities. The skin around the nose, eyes, and muzzle should be examined carefully for papules, pustules, or alopecia that may be indicative of dermatophytosis or mange.

The pinnae should be examined for evidence of crusting or papular/pustular eruptions. Examine the external ear canals by pulling the pinnae vertically and caudally. Smell and visually inspect each ear canal for exudate. In particular, black crusty exudate is suggestive of ear mite infestation. Yeast infections of the ears typically cause a brown soupy exudate, and bacterial exudates are usually white, yellow, or green with a foul odor. If the external ear canal is clean and nonirritated, an otoscopic examination is probably not warranted. If the external ear canal appears abnormal or if neurologic disorders are suspected, the ear canal should be examined carefully to the level of the tympanic membrane. Obtain a swab for cytologic examination, and then insert the otoscope while holding the pinna vertically. Gently apply traction to the pinna and rotate the otoscopic cone into the horizontal canal. This can be an uncomfortable procedure, so be careful and gentle! The tympanic membrane should appear as a translucent oval membrane. Look for signs of irritation in the horizontal canal or bulging of the tympanic membrane that might indicate middle ear infection.

The mouth is examined by placing the fingers of the left hand over the muzzle at the level of the maxillary canines. The right hand is used to insert a finger into the mouth in front of the incisors, and the mandible is pushed downward by pressure on the lower lip or incisors. The maxilla is grasped by pushing the lips over the maxillary canines. The animal's head is elevated to a 45° angle while the mandible is held stationary, allowing complete inspection of the oral cavity. A young animal should be examined for congenital abnormalities such as anomalies of the tongue and cleft palate. Pressing the thumb between the rami of the mandible may elevate the tongue. Look for evidence of string or other foreign objects, especially in kittens. The color of the gingiva and hard palate should be examined for cyanosis or pallor. Capillary refill time, which should normally be less than 2 seconds, may be determined by applying digital pressure to the gingiva and timing the return of color to the blanched area. The pattern of eruption of the teeth should be noted. The tongue and sublingual area should be examined carefully for evidence of electrical cord burns or foreign objects. The tonsillar crypts and caudal region of the pharynx are examined for exudates or swelling that may be indicative of infectious disease. The larynx and soft palate should be examined for congenital abnormalities and for approximate length.

A cursory neurologic examination of the cranial nerves may be done by testing for menace reflex, which is not well developed until 2 to 3 months of age (Averill, 1981), pupillary light reflex, jaw tone, facial sensation, and swallowing reflex. The neck is examined for swelling. Pay particular attention to the left side of the neck, palpating carefully for swelling or other evidence of megaesophagus. The mandibular lymph nodes are located just cranial and dorsal to the mandibular salivary glands, which are larger and firmer. The lymph nodes should be examined for swelling, localized temperature increase, or ulceration.

FOREQUARTERS AND THORAX

The forequarters and thorax are examined next. Palpate the prescapular lymph nodes, which lie in a groove created by the supraspinous and longus colli muscles. The lymph nodes should be symmetric and barely discernible. In very small or very young animals, they may not be palpable.

The forelimbs should be examined joint by joint, beginning at the toes and proceeding to the shoulder. Each portion of the limb should be gently palpated and flexed to determine joint mobility or to detect the presence of pain and clicking suggestive of a joint mouse or a piece of loose articular cartilage. The long bones of the limbs should be firmly grasped and pressure applied to the center of the bone. This detects

pain resulting from panosteitis, an inflammatory disorder frequently observed in young dogs. Young dogs may also suffer from developmental disorders that affect the epiphyses; therefore, the distal radial and ulnar epiphyses and metaphyses should be carefully palpated. A complete orthopedic examination should be performed on large breed dogs between the ages of 2 and 6 months.

The thorax should be visually inspected for respiratory rate, breathing pattern, and evidence of respiratory distress. Palpate the thorax for abnormal rib and sternal conformation. Carefully inspect the thorax for evidence of fistulous tracts or other abnormalities that might indicate an underlying problem in the thorax. Auscultation is an important part of the thoracic examination. Listen to as many puppies and kittens as possible to obtain an appreciation for the "normal" sounds of the heart and lungs of animals of varying ages and breeds. Take the time to listen carefully, and shut out the sounds of the external world in order to concentrate. A good-quality stethoscope with an infant-sized or pediatric-sized bell (2 cm) and diaphragm (3 cm) is required for auscultating the small thorax of most puppies and kittens. Choose earpieces that are soft and comfortable for the listener and that fit tightly in the examiner's external ear canals.

Thoracic auscultation requires a systematic approach. This can be achieved by dividing the thorax into right and left sides, upper and lower lung fields, and cranial and caudal lung fields. Proceeding clockwise on the right side, examine the cranial upper quadrant, then the caudal upper quadrant, followed by the caudal lower quadrant, and finally the cranial lower quadrant. Repeat the same procedure on the left side. Hold the stethoscope tight to the animal's haircoat to avoid the sound of fur rubbing on the stethoscope head. With practice, the examiner will learn to "tune out" extraneous sounds and recognize the characteristic sounds of the lung and upper airway. Listen to respiratory sounds first and then to cardiac sounds. Abnormal respiratory sounds include stridor, wheezes, crackles, and pleural rubs. Listen for the absence of sounds that may indicate fluid or air accumulation within the thorax. Take particular note of audible asymmetry, which generally indicates disease.

Examination of the cardiovascular system includes visual inspection of the peripheral veins and estimation of capillary refill time. The jugular veins should be observed for distention or the presence of a prominent pulse. The heart rate should be determined by listening to the heart with a stethoscope while palpating the femoral pulse with the free hand. Normally, there is a 1:1 ratio of pulse to cardiac impulse. The character of the pulse is also important, especially in reference to congenital cardiac abnormalities. A "water-hammer" pulse characterizes patent ductus arteriosus, which is a strong pulse that fades quickly. A slow rising pulse is suggestive of aortic stenosis, whereas a weak thready pulse is characteristic of shock, hypovolemia, or congestive heart failure.

The heart is auscultated in the left and right sides of the thorax. Again, it is very important to be systematic in cardiac auscultation. The small size of most young dogs and cats makes it difficult to define the exact anatomic locations of heart sounds. Generally, heart sounds can be localized to the left cardiac apex, the left cardiac base, or the right cardiac apex. In addition, the great vessels should be auscultated where they exit the thorax at the thoracic inlet. Again, it is important to listen for normal sounds before attempting to identify abnormal sounds. The first heart sound, which signals closure of the atrioventricular valves, is longer, louder, and lower pitched than the second heart sound. The systolic interval occurs between the first and second heart sounds and is shorter than the diastolic interval (Hardy, 1981).

Heart murmurs in puppies and kittens may be pathologic or physiologic. Thorough auscultation, follow-up examination, and complete cardiac evaluations are indicated for most murmurs that persist in the puppy or kitten. Murmurs are systolic, diastolic, or continuous. Continuous murmurs are almost always associated with patent ductus arteriosus. The differential diagnosis for systolic or diastolic murmurs is a little more complicated; however, localization of the point of maximum intensity of the murmur, the characteristics of the murmur, and the history and signalment should suggest the most likely cause of the murmur.

ABDOMEN

A rapid superficial examination of the skin and musculature of the abdomen should be performed. In the female, the mammae and vulva should be examined, and, in the male, the prepuce should be observed for position and presence of an opening. Look carefully for evidence of umbilical herniation. If a hernia is detected, it should be palpated for size and the presence of a falciform ligament or intestine.

The abdomen may be palpated beginning at the cranial aspect and proceeding caudally. It is easier to palpate with both hands. The examiner stands behind the animal and uses both hands to press gently inward until the fingers of both hands are touching in the cranial region of the abdomen. The hands are then drawn ventrally, tracing any structures encountered, until the body wall is reached. The procedure is repeated throughout the abdomen until all areas have been covered. Most animals resist abdominal palpation by tensing the abdominal wall. Constant gentle pressure allows relaxation of the abdominal musculature so that an organ may be palpated. It is often helpful to conjure up a mental image of the structure being examined.

Palpate for changes in size, shape, and texture. Palpate as many abdominal organs as possible. Parts of the liver may be palpated in the younger puppies and kittens. The spleen may be palpable depending on its size and location. Sometimes, in older puppies, a spleen may be palpated by elevating the animal's forelimbs, which allows the abdominal organs to drop caudally in the abdominal cavity. The kidneys can be palpated in some dogs and in all cats. The left kidney is more caudal and more mobile than the right kidney, which lies in the renal fossa directly behind the liver. The kidney is cupped in one hand, while its outline is traced with the other hand. The ureters are not palpable, but the urinary bladder is easily palpable in the caudal abdomen. In most animals, the urinary bladder is freely movable and should be palpated for changes in texture and size. Gently squeeze the urinary bladder to determine resistance to urine outflow and the presence of urine drops at the umbilicus.

Palpation of the small and large intestines is a very important part of the physical examination of a puppy or kitten. The normal intestine is a soft, slightly fluid-filled or gas-filled structure that is freely movable and nonpainful. The stomach may feel like a large, fluid-filled sac if it is full or firm and painful to the animal if it contains a foreign object; however, in most cases, it feels similar to the rest of the intestinal tract. The small intestine is palpated in the cranial to middle abdominal area. The small intestinal loops are easily movable among themselves because of the increased amount of free fluid in the abdominal cavity. The cecum is palpated in the cranial abdomen, and the colon runs the length of the abdomen from cranial boundary to the caudal boundary of the abdominal cavity. Feces are often palpated in the colon and may be confused with a mass when palpated by an inexperienced examiner. Generally, a thumb or index finger may deform feces, whereas a mass lesion will not deform and may be painful to the animal.

HINDQUARTERS

Finally, the hindlimbs, genitals, and perineum are examined. The thermometer may be removed at this point and the body temperature recorded. Remember that excitement, high environmental temperature, and activity can affect the body temperature. Interpret body temperature elevations in light of the condition of the animal and its recent environmental history. Any feces or debris that may adhere to the thermometer should be examined visually and perhaps microscopically for parasites or cytologic abnormalities. In extremely small puppies and kittens, this may be the only available method of obtaining a stool sample. The hindlimbs should be given a rapid dermatologic and musculoskeletal examination. Examine the hindlimbs, pausing to palpate the popliteal lymph nodes, which lie just caudal and dorsal to the stifle joint. The femoral pulses should be palpated for symmetry, quality, and pulse rate. A cursory orthopedic examination of the hindlimbs should be performed similar to that performed on the forelimbs.

The perineal region and the genitals should be examined for congenital defects or intersexual characteristics. The testicles in the male puppy or kitten should be descended by 4 to 8 weeks of age; however, if both testes have not descended into the scrotum by 16 weeks of age, cryptorchidism should be suspected (Feldman and Nelson, 1987). If the animal is cryptorchid, the owner should be advised not to use it as a breeding animal because of the hereditary nature of the disorder. Female puppies or kittens should be examined for evidence of vaginal inflammation (puppy vaginitis) and congenital abnormalities. The rectum and anus should be examined for evidence of inflammation or congenital defects, such as imperforate anus. Rectal palpation is an important part of the physical examination in older, large-breed puppies. The pelvic canal, including the rectum, bony pelvis, prostate gland, uterus, vagina, urethra, and anal sacs, should be examined.

Diagnostic Imaging Techniques

Beth P. Partington

Puppies and kittens pose a special problem for the imager in both the technical aspects of diagnostic imaging studies and their interpretation. Puppies and kittens are more vocal and generally more mobile than adult dogs and cats. They are unaccustomed to restraint and become easily stressed during positioning. Puppies and kittens are also nonresponsive to voice commands that may calm or help immobilize a mature animal. Because of the small size of puppies and kittens, most of the radiographic studies are performed with tabletop techniques. It is imperative that the radiographic studies include proper positioning, correct exposures, and careful development of the film. Radiographs of poor technical quality are generally not helpful to the veterinarian and may even lead to misinterpretation or misdiagnosis of an animal's condition. One needs to accept that diagnostic imaging studies of puppies and kittens require increased time and patience.

Because of the small animal size, proper restraint and good radiation safety practices are sometimes difficult to combine. Holding on to puppy and kitten extremities while wearing lead gloves is almost impossible. Use of slipknot gauze-tie extenders on all limbs for positioning of radiographic studies is very helpful (Figs. 1–2 and 1–3). The gauze ties allow the imager to immobilize all four limbs while keeping lead-gloved hands out of the primary x-ray beam. Sponges can also be used to hold down the head and other mobile areas to extend the distance between the gloved fingers and the area of x-ray exposure. The use of very careful x-ray beam collimation to just cover the area of interest is critical. Correct close collimation decreases scatter radiation, which improves radiographic image quality and decreases radiation exposure to the imager.

Manual restraint is the only form of restraint used for radiographic positioning in puppies

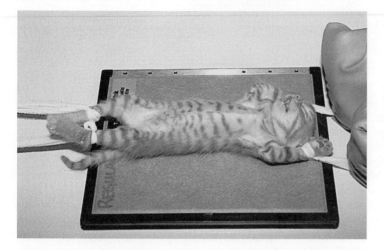

Figure 1–2. Tabletop positioning of a 4-week-old kitten for a ventrodorsal thoracic or abdominal radiograph. Gauze leg ties provide a firm grip of the limbs and allow the holder to keep gloved hands out of the primary x-ray beam.

and kittens younger than 2 weeks of age and for most radiographic studies. There are, however, some puppies and kittens that resist restraint so strongly that a diagnostic radiograph cannot be obtained without injury, excessive stress, or exposure of the imager to the primary x-ray beam. For these animals and for skull, spine, and some contrast studies, chemical sedation is necessary to prevent motion artifacts and achieve accurate positioning.

CHEMICAL RESTRAINT

For puppies and kittens younger than 6 weeks, mask induction and maintenance with isoflurane is the safest method for immobilization (see Chapter 24). Gas anesthesia restraint also avoids the problem of excessive motion due to opioid-induced panting. If isoflurane is not available in the practice, injectable anesthetic agents can be safely used for chemical restraint.

For puppies 6 weeks of age and older, opioids (oxymorphone and butorphanol) may be given for sedation. An anticholinergic agent should be administered simultaneously to prevent opioid-induced bradycardia. Oxymorphone is administered at a dosage of 0.1 mg/kg intramuscularly or subcutaneously, whereas butorphanol is given at a dosage of 0.1 to 0.2 mg/kg intramuscularly or subcutaneously. If more profound sedation is needed, diazepam (0.1 to 0.2 mg/kg intravenously) or midazolam (0.1 to 0.2 mg/kg intravenously or intramuscularly) can be given after the opioid has been administered. Midazolam has the advantage of being more rapidly absorbed and less irritating to tissue following intramuscular injection and has a shorter duration of action. The opioid antagonist naloxone should be available at all times during opioid sedation. Naloxone may be given intravenously, intramuscularly, or subcutaneously at a dosage of 0.03 mg/kg.

Complete immobilization for approximately 15 minutes can also be achieved with a 50:50

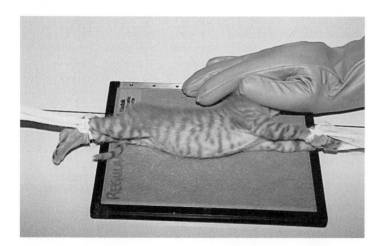

Figure 1–3. Lateral positioning for a thoracic or abdominal tabletop radiograph. Careful x-ray beam collimation is used to prevent exposure of the holder's gloved hand. Positioning sponges to restrain the animal's head will further separate the holder's hands from the x-ray beam.

solution of diazepam and ketamine given intravenously at a dosage of 0.1 ml/kg. Propofol can be used intravenously at a dose of 2 to 6 mg/kg with excellent results. Problems include the difficulty of intravenous access in the small puppy and apnea; thus, endotracheal tubes should be readily available.

Kittens 6 weeks of age and older may be sedated with butorphanol at 0.2 mg/kg subcutaneously. Midazolam (0.1 mg/kg intramuscularly) or diazepam (0.1 mg/kg intravenously) may be given after butorphanol if more profound sedation is required. Midazolam (0.1 mg/kg) plus ketamine (2 to 4 mg/kg) given intramuscularly may also be used for excellent immobilization.

RADIOGRAPHIC TECHNIQUES

Exposure Factors

Most technique charts list the milliamperage (mA), time (in fractions of seconds), and kilovoltage peak (kVp) settings that will produce diagnostic radiographs of specific body parts at measured thicknesses. Milliamperage X seconds (mAs) can be thought of as the quantity of radiation or number of x-ray photons produced during an exposure. A specific mAs can be produced in a number of ways, depending on the machine and timer. A 100-mA machine will produce 5 mAs with 100 mA set for 1/20 second. A 300-mA machine will produce 5 mAs with 300 mA set at 1/60 second. Both settings allow the same amount of radiation to reach the animal, but the 300-mA machine produces the radiation in a shorter period of time, thus decreasing the chance that animal motion will blur the radiograph.

The kVp setting establishes the peak energy level or penetrating power of the x-ray beam. Kilovoltage must be greatly reduced for radiography of puppies and kittens because of decreased absorption by undermineralized bones and thin body parts. Extrapolations to thinner animals can be made based on the fact that each 1 cm of soft tissue is the equivalent of 2 kVp at settings equal to or less than 80 kVp. The kVp setting affects not only x-ray beam penetration but also radiograph contrast. Lower kVp settings increase contrast, whereas higher kVp settings increase radiograph latitude or the number of shades of gray. Remember that one can increase radiograph blackness (overall radiograph density) by increasing the kVp or the mAs.

Most technique charts are variable-kVp charts that leave the mAs at one setting and increase the kVp with increasing body part thickness. Most radiographic studies of puppies and kittens are performed in the 40- to 60-kVp range. In this range, a change of 4 to 6 kVp will double or halve the film exposure. Technique charts need to be established for the veterinary practice and depend on what kind of intensifying screens are being used in the radiograph cassettes, the type of film, temperature of film development, focal film distance, and x-ray machine characteristics. It is necessary to have an accurate technique chart if good-quality radiographs are to be produced for all body parts of different-sized animals. It is especially important with the puppy and kitten that precise thickness measurements are made with a set of calipers. After the technique chart is established, it is also important to measure each body part in the same location in all animals. Very seldom can a technique chart designed for one machine be used for another machine with any degree of success. The abdominal radiography technique chart in Table 1–1 is an example of the establishment and fine-tuning of the practice's technique chart.

Thoracic Radiography

Thoracic radiographs are a very effective method for the evaluation of esophageal, car-

Table 1–1	Variable-kVp Technique Chart for Abdominal Radiography		
BODY PART THICKNESS (cm)	**kVp**	**mAs**	**GRID**
4	48	5	No
5	50	5	No
6	52	5	No
7	54	5	No
8	56	5	No
9	58	5	No
10	60	5	No
11	62	10	Yes
12	64	10	Yes
13	66	10	Yes
14	68	10	Yes
15	70	10	Yes
16	72	10	Yes
17	74	10	Yes
18	76	10	Yes
19	78	10	Yes
20	80	10	Yes

Technique chart established with a system using Kodak Lanex Regular screens, Kodak TML film, 100 cm focal film distance, and automatic processing. This is a 400-speed system.

diovascular, and pulmonary diseases. One cannot, however, produce and evaluate puppy and kitten radiographs as if the animals (and their images) were just smaller versions of the adult. Adult thoracic radiographs are taken with a high-kVp technique. High-kVp techniques increase film latitude to allow the imager to separate vascular, interstitial, and bronchial structures. High-kVp thoracic techniques require very low mAs settings to avoid radiographic overexposure. Unfortunately, because of the limitations of the timers in most x-ray machines, very low mAs settings (0.6 to 2.0 mAs) are not generally achievable. Therefore, most thoracic exposure settings for puppies and kittens are the same kVp as that for the equivalent abdomen thickness at one half the abdominal mAs. Table 1–2 is an example of a thoracic radiography technique chart based on Kodak Lanex Regular screens, Kodak TML film, a 100-cm focal film distance, and automatic processing.

Puppies and kittens 2 weeks or younger have one-third the alveolar surface area of an adult. As a result, younger animals have an increased respiratory rate to increase their minute volume. The rapid respiratory rate combined with their greater chest wall motion increases the difficulty of obtaining thoracic radiographs without motion. It is critical to time the radiographic exposure for the slight pause at the end of peak inspiration. This helps decrease radiographic blurring caused by motion and increases inherent thoracic contrast because of the increased volume of air.

Thoracic radiographs have a generalized increased interstitial opacity because of the decreased alveolar air volume present. The veterinarian should not be too quick to interpret a mildly increased interstitial opacity as a sign of disease. This is sometimes difficult, because early viral pneumonias appear as an increased interstitial opacity. It may be helpful to take a short series of thoracic radiographs of normal (healthy) animals using the equipment in the practice for comparison with radiographs of diseased animals. Keeping a separate radiograph log for puppies and kittens of different ages helps establish a comparison file.

One technique to increase the effectiveness and ease of interpretation of pulmonary disease is to place the affected lung up. If the kitten or puppy has increased respiratory noise on one side of the thorax, the opposite side should be laid against the radiographic cassette during exposure. By placing the affected side up, one increases the inflation of the more diseased hemithorax and increases the contrast between the affected and unaffected lung. Another tip to bear in mind is the presence of a larger thymus in the young animal. The cranial mediastinum will appear thicker and more opaque in the puppy and kitten, and the thymus may appear as an opaque triangle (sail sign) in the cranial left hemithorax in the dorsoventral or ventrodorsal view (Fig. 1–4).

One of the most common indications for thoracic radiographs is for evaluation of a heart murmur first detected on routine physical examination. Because of the decreased alveolar volume in the puppy's or kitten's thorax, the heart appears larger within the thoracic cavity. As the animal ages, the normal (adult) relationship of heart size to thorax size is gradually achieved. Remember the rough generalization that the smaller the breed of dog, the larger the heart size compared with the overall thorax size.

When taking thoracic radiographs for the evaluation of a congenital heart abnormality, it is critical to position the puppy or kitten in a perfectly straight line. Slight obliquity on the dorsoventral, ventrodorsal, or lateral exposure may cause misinterpretation of cardiac abnormalities. Figure 1–5 shows how an oblique ventrodorsal view of the thorax prevents the imager from making a diagnosis of a patent ductus arteriosus. On the oblique view, the dilation of

Table 1–2	Variable-kVp Technique Chart for Thoracic Radiography		
BODY PART THICKNESS (cm)	**kVp**	**mAs**	**GRID**
4	48	2.5	No
5	50	2.5	No
6	52	2.5	No
7	54	2.5	No
8	56	2.5	No
9	58	2.5	No
10	60	2.5	No
11	62	5	Yes
12	64	5	Yes
13	66	5	Yes
14	68	5	Yes
15	70	5	Yes
16	72	5	Yes
17	74	5	Yes
18	76	5	Yes
19	78	5	Yes
20	80	5	Yes

Technique chart established with a system using Kodak Lanex Regular screens, Kodak TML film, 100 cm focal film distance, and automatic processing. This is a 400-speed system.

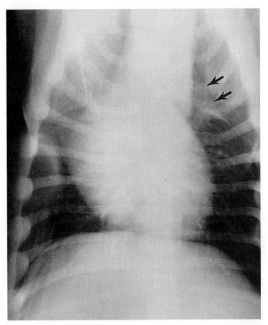

Figure 1–4. Ventrodorsal thoracic radiograph of a 6-week-old puppy. The normal thymus is seen as a triangle of soft tissue in the cranial mediastinum just to the left of midline (arrows).

the proximal descending aorta (ductus bump) and enlarged pulmonary artery trunk are not visible, whereas they are clearly seen on the correctly positioned radiograph.

It is a good idea to evaluate the pulmonary vascularity as the first step when interpreting thoracic radiographs of a possible congenital heart defect. Check pulmonary artery and vein size, and try to determine if the veins are enlarged (venous congestion), arteries are enlarged (pulmonary hypertension), both arteries and veins are small (pulmonary undercirculation), or both arteries and veins are large (pulmonary overcirculation). Once the circulatory status of the lungs is determined, look at the heart for chamber size alterations. One is often tempted to change one's assessment of vascularity after viewing the heart. Imagers must not fall into the trap of seeing a vascular change that does not exist because they want the radiographs to fit their clinical assessment.

Skeletal Radiography

Perhaps the most common radiographic procedure performed in puppies and kittens is radiography of extremities. Puppies and kittens differ from adults in that their bones have generalized decreased mineralization, flared metaphyseal

growth areas, open physes, thick articular cartilage, and numerous secondary centers of ossification that to the untrained observer can mimic disease. The bones of the very immature animal (younger than 60 days) have a nonlamellated structure and are described as woven bone. The flared irregular metaphysis is an area of active remodeling where the wide distal metaphysis decreases in diameter to form tubular bone. This area is called the "cutback zone" and has a very rough and irregular periosteal surface.

Open physes start out as very wide radiolucent bands between the metaphysis and epiphysis and can mimic fracture lines and joint spaces. The physes narrow as the animal ages, and finally the metaphysis and epiphysis fuse to form a radiopaque physeal scar in the adult. Joint spaces appear very wide in radiographs of the young animal because cartilage is the same soft tissue opacity as a joint fluid (synovial) and joint capsule. The pseudowidened joint spaces are formed from the cartilage model of the epiphyseal and cuboidal bones. The juvenile joint space is not appreciably wider than that of the adult. Figure 1–6 shows a dorsopalmar view of the carpus in a 6-week-old puppy. Note the presence of a radiolucent distal radial physis, flared metaphysis, thick cartilage model mimicking a widened joint space, and three separate centers of ossification (radial, central, and intermediate) forming the radial carpal bone.

Because of incomplete bone mineralization, technique charts for radiography of extremities in puppies and kittens have kVp ranges 5% to 7% lower than those of the corresponding adult charts. This prevents overexposure and increases visualization of soft tissue structures that can be important. Remember that if one finds an area of soft tissue swelling on the radiograph, one will find the area of trauma or disease. This is especially true in the puppy and kitten because trauma and infection are the most common lesions seen in the young skeleton. Just because there is no change in the radiographic appearance of the bone does not mean a lesion is not present. Damage to the cartilage model, early septic arthritis, and osteomyelitis may first appear as an increase in soft tissue opacity from joint effusion or soft tissue swelling. When in doubt, take a radiograph of the opposite limb for comparison.

No one can memorize the age of appearance of secondary ossification centers and the age of radiographic physeal closure for all anatomic locations. Tables 1–3 to 1–5 are a ready reference for the age of appearance and radiographic closure of the ossification centers in the puppy.

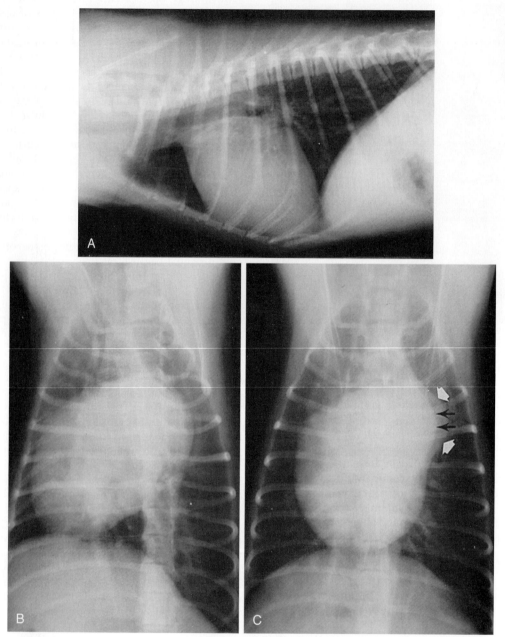

Figure 1–5. Radiography of a 10-week-old puppy with a holosystolic heart murmur. **A,** Lateral thoracic radiographic findings include moderate biventricular and left atrial enlargement. These radiographic findings are nonspecific and could be seen with ventricular septal defect, patent ductus arteriosus, or mitral valve insufficiency. **B,** Poorly positioned ventrodorsal radiograph. Puppy's obliquity prevents accurate assessment of the radiographic findings in the ventrodorsal view. Radiographic findings include generalized cardiomegaly and mild pulmonary overcirculation. The final diagnosis cannot be made from this radiograph. **C,** Properly positioned ventrodorsal radiograph. A straight ventrodorsal view allows the interpreter to identify the bulge in the proximal descending aorta (black arrows) and the enlarged main pulmonary segment (white arrows). These radiographic findings, combined with biventricular and left atrial enlargement and mild pulmonary overcirculation, correlate with the diagnosis of patent ductus arteriosus.

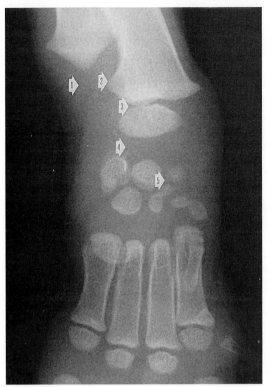

Figure 1–6. Dorsopalmar radiograph of a 6-week-old puppy's carpus. Note: (1) the absence of ossification of the ulnar styloid process or distal ulnar epiphysis, (2) the flared metaphysis or cut-back zone, (3) the radiolucent physis separating the distal radial metaphysis from the epiphysis, (4) the pseudowidened joint space due to epiphyseal and cuboidal cartilage, and (5) the center of the future radial carpal bone surrounded by its precursors the central, intermediate, and radial carpal ossification centers.

Because of breed variability and even variability between litters of the same breed, a reference chart may not answer all questions. For extremities, the best way to determine what is normal for the age and breed is to take a corresponding radiograph of an unaffected littermate or of the opposite limb if the puppy or kitten is unilaterally affected. Again, keeping a separate radiograph log for puppies and kittens at various ages allows quick reference to other similar radiographic studies if a littermate is not available.

One technique that can be helpful in the very small animal is magnification radiography. If the distance between the x-ray tube and film remains constant, magnification of the image of a body part will increase as the part is moved away from the film and closer to the x-ray tube. If the body part is placed halfway between the x-ray tube and film cassette, the x-ray image will be twice as large as the actual body part. Exposure techniques do not change if the film, screens, focal film distance, and development remain the same. Figure 1–7 shows an example of the technical setup for a magnified view of a carpus. The standard focal film distance is 100 cm, so the x-ray tube is lowered to 50 cm from the table and the cassette is placed 50 cm below the table. The carpus is positioned in between. Figure 1–8A shows a regular lateral view of a tibia and fibula, and Figure 1–8B shows a magnified view of the same animal. The magnified image is twice as large but has lost the edge sharpness of the nonmagnified image. Magnification radiography will only assist in the diagnosis if the original image is too small to be seen clearly; it does not increase detail or image sharpness. Magnification radiographs need to be made with an x-ray tube focal spot of 0.3 mm or less, and the animal must be completely motionless. Because of the loss of edge sharpness, any motion will severely degrade the image.

Abdominal Radiography

Positioning for abdominal radiographs in the puppy and kitten is the same as for the adult. The cranial margin of the lateral view is midway between the dorsal portion of the last rib and the xiphoid process. The caudal margin should include the ischiadic tuberosities. Ventrodorsal views are used in place of dorsoventral positioning, and the exposures should be made during expiration for maximum expansion of the abdominal cavity. Radiographic techniques for abdominal radiography can be extrapolated from the adult technique chart using tabletop techniques until the abdomen exceeds 10 cm in width. For abdominal widths over 10 cm, a grid is used on top of the cassette, or the cassette is placed beneath the table in a sliding grid tray.

The major problem with abdominal radiography in the puppy or kitten is the very poor abdominal detail (Fig. 1–9). This lack of radiographic detail is attributable to the lack of intraabdominal fat, greater amount of peritoneal fluid, and higher proportion of total body water (80% of body weight is water in puppies and kittens versus 60% in adults). This normal lack of detail decreases the value of abdominal radiographs for the evaluation of abdominal organ size, shape, and position. This also makes the detection of small volumes of abdominal fluid difficult. Gas and heterogenous ingesta aid in the evaluation of the gastrointestinal tract. Radiopaque foreign bodies and complete intestinal

Table 1–3	Ossification Center Appearance and Closure of the Pectoral Limb in the Dog	
	APPEARANCE (WEEKS)	CLOSURE (MONTHS)
Supraglenoid tubercle	6–9	4–7
Humerus		
Proximal epiphysis	1–2	10–13
Distal epiphysis	2–4	5–8
Medial epicondyle	6–9	4–8
Medial and lateral condyle of the distal epiphysis fuse at 6–9 weeks		
Radius		
Proximal epiphysis	3–5	6–11
Distal epiphysis	2–4	8–10
Ulna		
Olecranon	7–9	7–9
Distal epiphysis	7–8	8–10
Carpal bones		
Accessory	2	
Secondary center	7–11	3–5
Radial		
Radial	3	3–4
Intermediate	2–3	3–4
Central	4–6	3–4
Ulnar	4–6	
First	3	
Second	3–4	
Third	3–4	
Fourth	3	
Metacarpal bones		
Proximal epiphysis (1)	3–5	5–6
Distal epiphysis (2–5)	3–4	6–7
Phalanges		
Proximal		
Proximal epiphysis (1)	5–6	4–7
Proximal epiphysis (2–5)	4	4–7
Middle		
Proximal epiphysis (2, 5)	5–7	4–6
Proximal epiphysis (3, 4)	5–7	5–7

Sesamoid bones in the dorsal digits and the abductor pollicis longus appear at 4 months. The palmar digital sesamoid bones appear at 2 months.

obstruction are still identifiable, even with a lack of abdominal detail, because of gas distention of the intestine.

The liver is comparatively larger in the puppy and kitten and occupies a considerable portion of the abdominal cavity. The ratio of liver weight to body weight decreases as the animal ages. The liver occupies 40 to 50 g/kg body weight in the young animal versus 20 g/kg in the adult. In addition, the liver appears even larger radiographically, partially because of the lack of calcification of the costal cartilage, which makes the liver appear to extend further beyond the rib margins. Even with a lack of abdominal detail, the liver size can be estimated by the position of the stomach. If the pylorus is displaced dorsally and caudally, the liver is enlarged. If the pylorus is displaced cranially toward the diaphragm, the liver will be small, which is commonly seen with congenital portosystemic shunts.

Because of the lack of inherent abdominal detail, contrast agents may be used to further evaluate the gastrointestinal and urogenital systems. Barium sulfate suspensions can be used orally for examination of the upper gastrointestinal tract even in the very young animal. Barium is inert and nonirritating. If precautions are taken to prevent constipation, there should be no side effects with barium sulfate given orally. A 30% micropulverized suspension can be given via an orogastric tube at a dose of 7 to 10 ml/kg. For the evaluation of rectal anomalies, a 15% barium sulfate suspension can be gently

Table 1–4	Ossification Center Appearance and Closure of the Pelvic Limb in the Dog	
	APPEARANCE (WEEKS)	CLOSURE (MONTHS)
Femur		
Femoral head	2–3	6–10
Greater trochanter	4–10	8–11
Distal epiphysis	3–4	9–11

The medial and lateral condyles of the distal femur fuse at 3–4 months. The patella appears at 8–9 weeks. The fabellae appear at 12 weeks.

Tibia		
Proximal epiphysis	2–5	10–13
Tibial tuberosity	7–9	6–8
Distal epiphysis	2–6	8–9
Medial malleolus	12	8–9

The tibial tuberosity fuses to the proximal epiphysis (8 months), and then the entire proximal tibia fuses to the diaphysis at 10–13 months.

Fibula		
Proximal epiphysis	9–10	8–11
Distal epiphysis	2–6	8–9
Tarsal bones		
Talus and calcaneus	1	
Calcaneal tuberosity	5–6	5–7
Central and fourth	2	
First and second	5–6	
Third	3–4	

The proximal epiphysis of the first metatarsal and the distal epiphysis of metatarsals 2–5 appear at 4 weeks and close at 6 months.

The epiphyses of the first phalanges appear at 4 weeks and fuse at 6–7 months. The proximal epiphyses of the second phalanges appear at 6 weeks and fuse at 6–7 months.

The hindlimb dorsal sesamoid bones appear at 5 months. The plantar sesamoid bones appear at 2 months.

injected into the rectum via a soft-tipped Foley catheter.

Do not use barium sulfate USP powder mixed with water. The powder will not go into suspension well, and as it precipitates out along the gastrointestinal tract it mimics ulcerative disease and excessive mucus or protein on the surface of the mucosa.

Use of oral organic iodines is not recommended in puppies or kittens younger than 4 weeks. Oral iodines are irritating to the mucosa and are hyperosmotic. The hyperosmolality causes fluid to accumulate within the bowel lumen, resulting in diarrhea and dehydration. Because puppies and kittens have lower intracellular fluid reserves and a higher water turnover rate, oral iodines may put them at greater risk.

If perforation in the esophagus, stomach, or bowel is highly suspected in a puppy or kitten younger than 4 weeks, oral nonionic contrast

Table 1–5	Ossification Center Appearance and Closure in the Pelvis of the Dog	
	APPEARANCE	CLOSURE
Ilium	Birth	4–6 mo
Iliac crest	4–7 mo	12–30 mo
Pubis	Birth	4–6 mo
Ischium	Birth	4–5 mo
Ischiadic tuberosity	3–5 mo	8–10 mo
Ischial arch	6–10 mo	8–13 mo
Acetabulum	1–2 mo	3–5 mo
Pelvic symphysis		3–13 y

The vertebral physes close at 7–8 months.

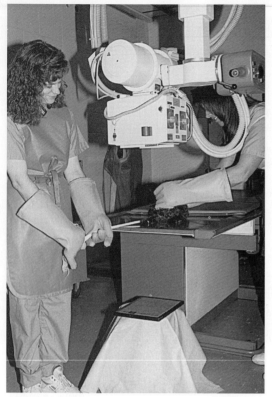

Figure 1–7. Technical setup to produce a magnified view of a puppy's carpus. Focal film distance remains at 100 cm. The film cassette is placed 50 cm below the puppy, and the x-ray tube is 50 cm above the carpus. Exposure and development factors are the same as those for standard carpal radiography. The resulting image will be twice as large as the actual anatomic structure.

such as iohexol or iopamidol may prove safer and be as effective. A diluted iohexol solution (this solution is prepared by mixing one part iohexol to two parts normal saline solution) can be given via orogastric tube at a dose of 5 to 10 ml/kg. The amount of diluted iohexol solution to be administered at a study time will vary according to the amount of liquid present in the gastrointestinal tract. The radiographic exposure should be at 0, 15, and 45 minutes.

Intravesicular contrast agents introduced into the urethra or urinary bladder for evaluation of the lower urinary tract should be relatively safe at any age. A more important concern in very young animals is avoiding trauma during catheterization.

Intravenous and intraarterial contrast agents administered for purposes of excretory urography, portography, and angiocardiography should be safe after 6 weeks of age. Unnecessary or excessive use of intravascular contrast agents should be avoided because of the puppy's or kitten's immature renal function and inability to conserve fluids. Maximum intravascular iodine dosage should not exceed 1500 mg iodine per kg body weight. Most special contrast procedures are postponed until 6 weeks of age or older to increase animal size for easier vascular access and to decrease animal problems with anesthesia. Nonionic iodine contrast may be safer in the puppy or kitten for both intraarterial and intravenous procedures.

ULTRASONOGRAPHY

Real-time, gray-scale ultrasound is an invaluable diagnostic tool in the puppy and kitten. It is especially useful in the diagnosis of abdominal and cardiac diseases. Ultrasonography is generally tolerated better than diagnostic radiology because absolute immobilization is rarely necessary. It is safer than radiology for the imager and holder because of the lack of ionizing radiation.

For accurate ultrasonography in puppies and kittens, an ultrasound transducer of at least 5 MHz is needed; a 7.5- to 10-MHz transducer is preferred. The higher the transducer frequency, the better the image resolution but the greater the ultrasound beam attenuation within soft tissue. This increased attenuation decreases the depth of ultrasound beam penetration, but because of the small animal size, attenuation is rarely a concern. The footprint or contact area of the transducer should be as small as possible. This will allow better access intercostally for cardiac imaging and subcostally for cranial abdominal imaging (Fig. 1–10). Linear array transducers commonly used transrectally for reproductive examination are inadequate for imaging puppies and kittens.

Ultrasonography is ideally suited for abdominal examination of puppies and kittens, especially in light of the limited information and poor detail present on abdominal radiographs. Gently restrain the animal in dorsal recumbency on a soft-padded warm surface. A well-padded surgical V-trough or V-trough table works well. It is important to carefully clip all hair, especially the short down coat present on the younger animal. Hair traps air and prevents the ultrasound beam from penetrating into the abdomen. Nearly 100% of the ultrasound beam is reflected back to the transducer at a soft tissue–air interface. The use of a generous volume of transducer coupling gel will assist in ultrasound beam penetration.

Many transducers have a specific focal zone

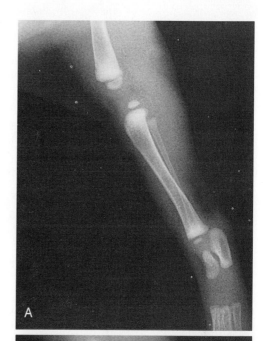

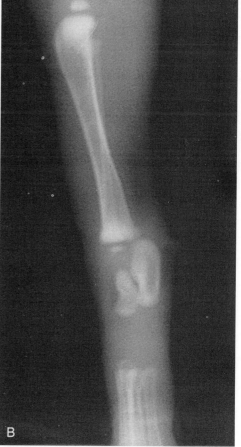

Figure 1–8. **A,** Standard mediolateral view of a 4-week-old kitten's tibia, fibula, and tarsus. **B,** Magnified mediolateral view of the kitten's hindlimb. The image is twice as large as the kitten's actual limb. Magnification simply enlarges the image; it does not increase image detail or margin sharpness.

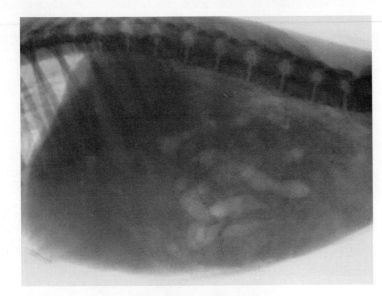

Figure 1–9. Lateral abdominal view of a puppy demonstrating the typical lack of abdominal detail.

or distance from the transducer surface where the image is sharpest. In the very small animal, the focal zone may be deeper than the animal is wide, dramatically decreasing the quality of the ultrasound examination. In addition, the bright band at the top of the ultrasound image or near-field artifact may obscure superficial structures. The use of an ultrasound standoff pad may help with both of these problems. An ultrasound standoff pad (Fig. 1–11) is a gelatin-like disk or cube that has the ultrasound characteristics of soft tissue. Ultrasound gel is placed on both sides of the standoff pad, and the pad is placed between the transducer and the animal. This will place the near-field artifact in the standoff pad and place the animal deeper into the transducer's focal zone. Newer ultrasound machines that support electronically focused transducers eliminate the need for standoff pads and are excellent for small animals. These machines do not produce a big band near-field artifact and allow examination of very superficial structures.

Abdominal ultrasonography can be used to identify peritoneal fluid; intestinal obstructions; inflammatory bowel disease; foreign bodies; tumors; hepatic, splenic, renal, and urinary bladder disease; and vascular anomalies such as congenital portosystemic shunts. Because ultrasonography is noninvasive and does not require the use of contrast agents to identify internal organ architecture, it is much less stressful to the puppy or kitten than is contrast radiology. Figure 1–12B shows an ultrasound image from a puppy with an intussusception that had caused complete intestinal obstruction but was difficult to define on abdominal radiographs.

A report from the United Kingdom described some important differences between the neonatal and adult ultrasonographic appearances of the canine abdomen (England, 1996). There are increased renal cortical echogenicity

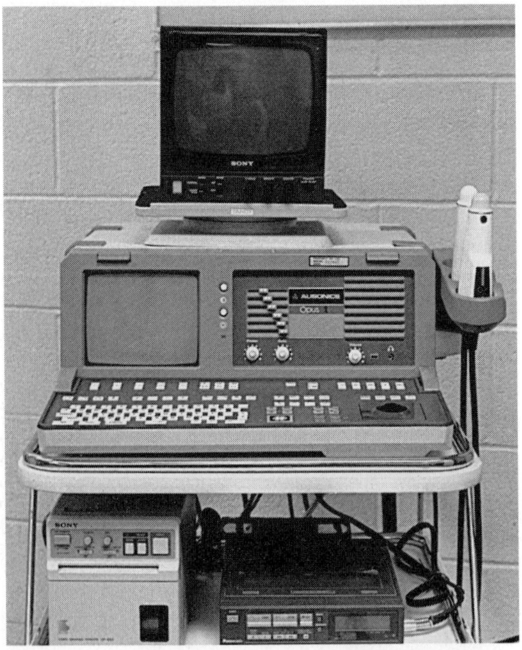

Figure 1–10. Real-time, gray-scale veterinary ultrasound unit with small-footprint sector transducers that are well suited to imaging puppies and kittens. This unit is capable of a brightness mode for abdominal imaging as well as time motion mode for echocardiography.

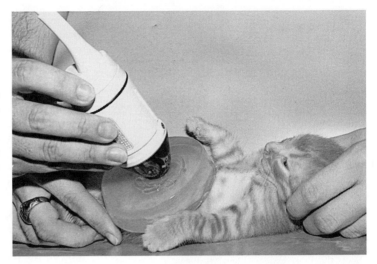

Figure 1–11. Ultrasound standoff pads may be necessary for the very small puppy or kitten to keep the transducer focal zone within the animal's body. The pad also moves the bright near-field artifact out of the superficial abdominal image.

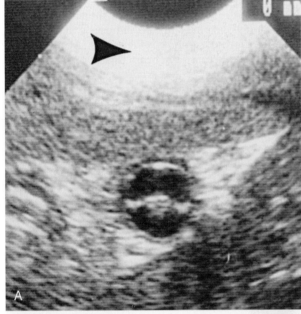

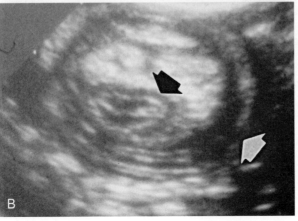

Figure 1–12. A, Abdominal ultrasonography of the cross section of a normal small intestine. The arrowhead identifies the bright band of echoes at the transducer–body wall junction known as the *near-field artifact*. **B,** Abdominal ultrasonography of the cross section of an intussusception in an 8-week-old puppy. The normal-appearing small intestinal loop (black arrow) is the intussusceptum surrounded by the dilated intussuscipiens (white arrow).

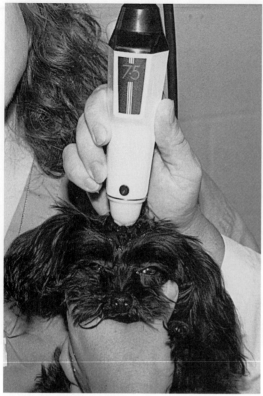

Figure 1–13. Transducer position for an intracranial ultrasonographic examination through an open fontanelle.

the liver and echogenic portal veins are less pronounced in the first 8 weeks of life.

The second most common use of ultrasonography in the puppy or kitten is for the evaluation of congenital heart defects. A small-footprint 7.5-MHz transducer and a special echocardiography table are very helpful in producing an echocardiogram that is maximally effective for diagnostic purposes. The echocardiography table can be easily made from plywood. It consists of a flat top approximately 50 by 24 inches with two circular holes cut in the middle 20 inches from each end. One hole, for older dogs, is 8 inches in diameter; the other hole, for puppies and kittens and older cats, is 4 inches in diameter. The legs are 18 to 24 inches long so the table can set on a regular ultrasound table when the V-trough is flat. The animal is held generally in right lateral recumbency with the cranial ventral thorax positioned over the appropriate-sized hole. The imager can then place the transducer beneath the table onto the animal's cardiac notch and use gravity to increase ultrasonographic access. Access is increased because the heart falls to the recumbent side, closer to the transducer, and the lungs become partially atelectatic during recumbency, increasing the size of the cardiac notch. Echocardiology of puppies and kittens is more comprehensively discussed in Chapter 8.

Ultrasonography can also be used for intracranial examination through an open fontanelle. The hair is clipped over the open fontanelle, a liberal volume of coupling gel is placed on top of the animal's head, and the transducer is placed on top of the head with the center of

and a poorly defined renal capsule from birth to 2 weeks. The kidneys appear larger ultrasonographically for the first 3 months of life. The normal coarse parenchymal stippling of

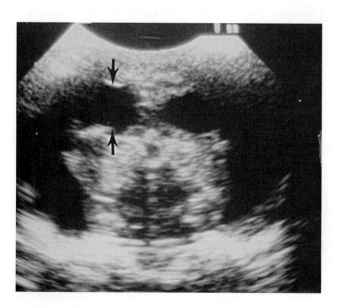

Figure 1–14. Intracranial cross-sectional ultrasonographic examination of a puppy with hydrocephalus. Lateral ventricular height is measured between the arrows and should not exceed 3.5 mm in the normal puppy. This puppy's lateral ventricular height was 7 mm.

the transducer placed directly over the skull depression of the open fontanelle (Fig. 1–13). Hydrocephalus is diagnosed by a lateral ventricular height of greater than 3.5 mm (Fig. 1–14).

References and Supplemental Reading

The Physical Examination

Averill DR Jr: The neurologic examination. Vet Clin North Am 11:511, 1981.

Bebiak DM, Lawler DF, Reutzel LF: Nutrition and management of the dog. Vet Clin North Am 17:527, 1987.

Breazile JE: Neurologic and behavioral development in the puppy. Vet Clin North Am 8:31, 1978.

Feldman EC, Nelson RW: Disorders of the canine male reproductive tract. In Feldman EC, Nelson RW (eds): Canine and Feline Endocrinology and Reproduction. Philadelphia, WB Saunders, 1987, p 482.

Hardy RM: General physical examination of the canine patient. Vet Clin North Am 11:453, 1981.

Hoskins JD: Clinical evaluation of the kitten: From birth to eight weeks of age. Compend Contin Educ Pract Vet 12:1215, 1990.

Johnson CA, Grace JA: Care of newborn puppies and kittens. Kal Kan Forum 6:9, 1987.

Mosier JE: The puppy from birth to six weeks. Vet Clin North Am 8:79, 1978.

Small E: Pediatrics. In Kirk RW (ed): Current Veterinary Therapy VII. Philadelphia, WB Saunders, 1980, p 77.

Wiener S, Nathanson M: Physical examination: Frequently observed errors. JAMA 236:852, 1976.

Diagnostic Imaging Techniques

Ackerman N: Radiology and Ultrasound of Urogenital Diseases in the Dog and Cat. Ames, Iowa State University Press, 1991.

Biller DS, Meyer W: Case examples demonstrating the clinical utility of obtaining both right and left lateral thoracic radiographs in small animals. J Am Anim Hosp Assoc 23:381, 1987.

Biller DS, Meyer W: Ultrasound scanning of superficial structures using an ultrasound standoff pad. Vet Radiol 29:3, 1988.

Boyd JS: Radiographic appearance of the bones in the feline foetus. Br Vet J 124:365, 1968.

Chapman WL: Appearance of ossification centers and epiphyseal closures as determined by radiographic technique. J Am Vet Med Assoc 147:138, 1965.

Curry TS, Dowdey JE, Murray RC: Christensen's Introduction to the Physics of Diagnostic Radiology, 4th ed. Philadelphia, Lea & Febiger, 1990.

England GCW: Renal and hepatic ultrasonography in the neonatal dog. Vet Radiol 37:374, 1996.

Hare WCD: Radiographic anatomy of the canine pectoral limb. Part III. The developing limb. J Am Vet Med Assoc 135:305, 1959.

Hare WCD: Radiographic anatomy of the canine pelvic limb. Part II. The developing limb. J Am Vet Med Assoc 136:603, 1960.

Hare WCD: Radiographic anatomy of the cervical region of the canine vertebral column. Part II. The developing vertebra. J Am Vet Med Assoc 139:217, 1961.

Herring DS: Symposium on diagnostic ultrasound. Vet Clin North Am (Small Anim Pract) 15:1105, 1985.

Hudson J: Ultrasound diagnosis of hydrocephalus in the dog. Vet Radiol 31:50, 1990.

Morgan JP: Radiology of Skeletal Disease. Ames, IA, Iowa State Univ Press, 1981.

Morgan JP, Silverman S: Techniques of Veterinary Radiography, 4th ed. Ames, Iowa State University Press, 1987.

Muir WW, Hubbell JAE: Handbook of Veterinary Anesthesia. St Louis, CV Mosby, 1989.

O'Brien T: Radiographic Diagnosis of Abdominal Disorders in the Dog and Cat. Davis, CA, Covell Park Vet Comp, 1981.

Pennick DG, Myland TG, Kerr LY, et al: Ultrasonographic evaluation of gastrointestinal diseases in small animals. Vet Radiol 31:134, 1990.

Poffenbarger EM, Ralston SL, Chandler ML, et al: Canine neonatology. Part I. Physiologic differences between puppies and adults. Compend Contin Educ Pract Vet 12:1601, 1990.

Poffenbarger EM, Ralston SL, Chandler ML, et al: Canine neonatology. Part II. Disorders of the neonate. Compend Contin Educ Pract Vet 13:25, 1991.

Robinson EP: Anesthesia of pediatric patients. Compend Contin Educ Pract Vet 12:1004, 1983.

Sumner-Smith G: Observations on epiphyseal fusion of the canine appendicular skeleton. J Small Anim Pract 7:303, 1966.

Suter PF: Thoracic Radiography—A Text Atlas of Thoracic Diseases of the Dog and Cat. Selbstuerlag, Wattwil, Switzerland, 1984.

Ticer JW: Radiographic Technique in Veterinary Practice, 2nd ed. Philadelphia, WB Saunders, 1984.

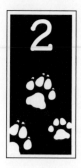

2

Behavior Development and Preventive Management

Gary Landsberg

CANINE DEVELOPMENT

Five developmental stages have been described in puppies: the neonatal stage (birth to 13 days), the transitional stage (13 to 19 days), the socialization period (19 days to approximately 13 weeks), the juvenile period (to sexual maturity), and the adult stage (from sexual maturity). There is a great deal of overlap between stages among the breeds and individuals within a breed.

During the neonatal period, the puppy spends most of its time nursing or sleeping. Puppies have limited motor ability, and until about 5 days movement is on the belly with stroking of the limbs. By 6 to 10 days, the forelimbs are capable of supporting weight, and by 11 to 15 days the hindlimbs can support weight and walking begins (Fox, 1965). From birth, if puppies are held by the neck they exhibit flexor dominance and this then changes to extensor dominance after 4 to 5 days (Fox, 1965). The rooting reflex is present from birth and begins to wane after about 14 days (Thorne, 1992). A slow and sustained pain response to toe pinch is present from birth, but withdrawal and escape from pain develops early in the transition period (Fox, 1968). Eyes and ear canals are closed at birth and open by 10 to 14 days, at which time the palpebral reflex to touch and light and the pupillary responses are already developed (Thorne, 1992). Defecation and urination are reflexes that are elicited by the mother's licking and cleaning of the perineal region (Thorne, 1992). Temperature regulation is poor at birth, and puppies huddle together. By 4 weeks of age, puppies tend to sleep in groups, and at 6 weeks they sleep alone (Thorne, 1992).

Important considerations during development are the effects of handling and strong stimuli on the behavioral and physical development of the puppy. Puppies that have been exposed to short periods of handling from birth to 5 weeks of age are more confident, exploratory, and socially dominant than controls (Fox, 1968). Handled puppies have increased nervous system maturation, rapid hair growth and weight gain, earlier opening of the eyes, and enhanced motor development. Thus, early handling may lead to improved learning ability and a more emotionally stable puppy. It has been suggested that early handling affects the pituitary-adrenocortical system in a way that helps the puppy better cope with stress later in life (Levine, 1967).

During the transitional period, the puppy begins to walk rather than crawl, both forward and backward (Thorne, 1992). Startle responses to auditory stimuli begin to develop at about 18 days, and the puppy begins to respond to light and moving stimuli (Serpell and Jagoe, 1995; Thorne, 1992). The puppy is still not capable of visual and auditory orientation until about 25 days (Fox, 1968). A puppy's performance on classic and operant conditioning reaches adult levels at about 4 to 5 weeks (Scott and Fuller, 1965), but vision and brain wave function do not reach adult levels until about 8 weeks (Fox, 1968). During the transitional period, puppies begin to exhibit voluntary control of elimination, but the mother still continues to clean the excretions (Fox, 1968; Houpt, 1991). Play mouthing by puppies begins to develop, and by 4 weeks of age nipping can be quite painful (Houpt, 1991). Weaning begins around 4 to 6 weeks of age. At this time, the puppy begins to show an interest in food, and the mother will begin to decrease nursing contact and may regurgitate food to her young (Houpt, 1991). This is a good time to begin offering canned or moistened food to puppies.

The socialization period is an important time for puppy development. The puppy develops attachments to its own and to other species that it encounters socially. At the end of the transition period, the puppy has developed enough that it can begin to interact with other individuals. It is also a time that the puppy begins to become familiar with and make attachments to places (localization or site attachment) and adapts to many of the stimuli around it (habituation). Because the socialization period is the time when social relationships are established, it is essential that puppies have contact with all potential social partners. Neither reward nor punishment needs to be involved, although excessive stimuli, whether positive or negative, appear to increase attachments. Fear postures begin to emerge at about 8 weeks of age (Houpt, 1991), and by 12 weeks the puppies' sociability lessens and they become increasingly fearful of novel situations and people (Serpell and Jagoe, 1995).

Although the puppy can support itself and becomes more mobile during the transition period, normal sitting and standing develop by about 28 days (Houpt, 1991). During the socialization period, social play and exploration become increasingly important (Fox, 1968). Play between puppies not only aids in physical development but also appears to be a form of exercise as well as an important step in the development of adult behaviors, including communication, predation, and sexual relationships. Although solitary play does occur, most play is social, with biting, barking, chasing, pouncing, and mounting (especially in male puppies) being the most frequent components. Puppies begin to eat solid food and are generally weaned by about 60 days of age (Houpt, 1991).

The juvenile period extends from the end of the socialization period to sexual maturity. It is a time of avoidance, so few if any new social contacts are likely to develop. The speed of learning begins to slow by about 4 months, likely because previous learning begins to interfere with new learning (Thorne, 1992). Object and environmental exploration increase during this period. By 4 to 6 months, males begin to show greater attraction to females showing signs of estrus (Houpt, 1991). The final period, adulthood, begins at puberty, that is, around 7

months or older in males and 6 months or older in females. Puppies are generally considered to be socially mature at about 18 months of age and behaviorally mature by about 2 years (Houpt, 1991).

Preventive Management
SOCIALIZATION AND HABITUATION

Socialization is the process by which an animal develops social relationships or bonds with members of its own or another species. The primary period of socialization in puppies is from 3 weeks to approximately 13 weeks (Freedman et al, 1961). Puppies should be kept with their mother and littermates until 6 to 8 weeks of age in order to develop healthy social relationships with other puppies. Puppies should be socialized to people and new environments well before 13 weeks of age; the peak of sensitivity is considered to be 6 to 8 weeks (Scott and Fuller, 1965). This can best be accomplished if prospective owners obtain their puppies at around 7 to 8 weeks of age and expose them to all of the types of people and animals that they might be required to interact with in their lives. For example, if there are no children in the family, socialization toward a variety of ages of children of both sexes should be a priority. An excellent way to introduce the puppy to new people and novel situations is to provide the owner with a package of puppy biscuits and advise the owner that the biscuits are only to be given by new people that the puppy meets (Landsberg et al, 1997). Periodic social reinforcement should then continue up until at least 6 to 8 months, or the puppy may regress. Continued socialization with other puppies is also essential if the puppy is to maintain healthy social relationships. One way to ensure continued socialization with other puppies as well as with a variety of people is to take the puppy to training classes before the end of the primary socialization period.

EXERCISE/PLAY

Insufficient exercise can contribute to a variety of problem behaviors, including destructiveness (chewing and digging), investigative behavior (garbage raiding), hyperactivity, unruliness, excitability, attention-getting behaviors, and even some forms of barking. Most puppies and some adult dogs, particularly those from breeds that have been bred for their stamina, have increased exercise requirements. The type and amount of exercise that each puppy requires will vary depending on its inherent instincts (e.g., retrieve and herd) and its personality. A puppy with sufficient training and exercise should be able to quiet down and relax (or even "nap") several times throughout the day. Playing "fly ball," playing "fetch," pulling carts, or jogging are often adequate substitutes for work.

LEADERSHIP AND CONTROL

Dogs are a social "pack" species. When puppies enter the home of the family effectively, the family becomes a new surrogate pack. Puppies adapt well to this artificial pack as long as the members of the family take a position of leadership, in much the same way as the mother or a more dominant pack member would assume control. If a pushy puppy does not receive direction and guidance and is allowed to get its own way, it will become increasingly difficult to control as it matures. Some trainers advocate a physical approach to control. For example, it has been suggested that grabbing a puppy around the muzzle or by the scruff of the neck and pinning it to the ground or rolling it over will teach it to submit. Handling exercises, however, are intended to acquaint the puppy with all forms of human contact so that it learns to accept and enjoy physical contact and handling. If the puppy displays any fear or defensive responses, these exercises should immediately be discontinued and a gradual shaping, handling, and reward program instituted.

Overall control should be achieved utilizing actions, attitude, training, and handling that demonstrate leadership (without confrontation). Compliance and a willingness to obey should earn rewards. Punishment during training is not only unnecessary but could lead to retaliation, aggression, fear, anxiety, or a weakening of the animal–owner bond. A very important concept for owners to embrace is that the human hand should always be positive—"a friend."

During all routine encounters the owner should be the initiator and leader and the puppy taught to obey and follow. This program, often referred to as "nothing in life is free" or "no free lunch," is intended to ensure that the puppy receive rewards only when they are earned and can never gain them on demand (Voith and Borchelt, 1982). In other words, before the puppy receives food, treats, play, toys, walks, or attention of any type, the puppy should be taught to obey an appropriate command (e.g., sit, stay, or down). Should the owner accede to any of the puppy's demands, this would actually reward the behavior and give away an otherwise valuable reward. During play and exercise the owner should always take a position of leadership. Games and play sessions should be initiated and terminated by the owner.

Obedience training, where the puppy is taught the correct responses to a variety of commands, is essential. Initial training should be focused on teaching the puppy to sit, stay, come, and lie down on command. Once the puppy responds to these basic commands, training should progress to quicker and longer responses in a variety of environments (shaping). It can also be invaluable to train the puppy to give up objects on command (give it or drop it), to cease barking on command (hush or quiet), and to associate a command with elimination. The owner should teach the puppy to heel and follow on walks from the moment the puppy steps out the front door of the home. It is essential that training be consistent and that the owner have sufficient control to ensure compliance if the puppy does not immediately obey. Inappropriate responses should be corrected in the act (never after), and correct responses should be encouraged and rewarded. Difficult, pushy, and hard to control puppies might be more easily managed with a head halter. In fact, whenever the puppy is out of its confinement area, the owners can easily supervise, prevent undesirable behavior, and ensure immediate control by leaving a long leash attached to the puppy's head halter.

It is also essential that the puppy learn to accept and enjoy handling from each family member. Handling exercises should include muzzle handling (including teeth brushing), brushing the coat, and touching the puppy around its face, ears, feet, and collar. Provided there are no signs of aggression, the owner should gradually proceed to lifting, nail trimming, grasping the muzzle and neck, and holding the puppy in place on its belly or on its side. Any attempts by the puppy to grasp, stand over, mount, or otherwise control the owners should not be tolerated. The puppy should also be taught to tolerate all approaches and handling by family members while it is eating or playing with a toy. This can usually be accomplished by training the puppy to drop toys and leave its food bowl for tasty food rewards.

TRAINING AND LEARNING

A few minutes is all that is required to teach a puppy to come and sit on command using the principles of food lure–reward training. Stand 2 feet away from the puppy, show it a piece of food held between your thumb and forefinger, and wiggle your fingers. As the puppy begins to approach, say the word "come." When the puppy reaches the food, slowly and deliberately move it over the top of its head. As the puppy moves its head back to follow the food, it will move into a sitting position. As it does this, say "sit." This can easily be demonstrated during one of the puppy's vaccination visits. If the puppy learns to obey even one simple command at a very early age, it will help the owner gain control of the puppy and serve as a tool for socializing. Teaching the "come–sit" command decreases jumping-up behaviors because the puppy learns to approach and greet by sitting. It also decreases hand shyness by associating an outstretched hand with a food reward. In addition to lure–reward training, puppies can be trained by rewarding and shaping desired responses and through prompting and reward (where a prompt is utilized to get the desired response so that rewards can be given).

The principle of halter training is to gain control over the puppy and encourage or shape appropriate behaviors so that it can be rewarded. With halter training, the puppy can be taught (or directed) to perform the desired response so that positive reinforcement (in the form of praise, affection, or food rewards) can be given. The halter also teaches the puppy that performing the desired behavior (sit, stay, heel, and quiet) leads to removal of the restraint (negative reinforcement). This is accomplished by pulling up and forward on the leash to achieve the desired response and releasing as soon as the puppy complies. Because the puppy's reaction is to pull backward, the mouth closes and the puppy retreats or begins to sit, at which point the behavior should be reinforced by first releasing and then providing positive reinforcement. Because the halter is attached to the puppy's muzzle, a pull on the leash immediately interrupts most common behavior problems (e.g., nipping, barking, jumping up, pulling, and stealing food). The Gentle Header Halter also allows the owner to leave a leash attached for remote correction. Although choke collars are intended to be used similar to halters, they are far more subject to abuse as they can choke the puppy and injure the trachea. Because choke collars are fitted around the puppy's neck, they also provide far less control, particularly of a large puppy with powerful neck muscles and forelegs. Pinch and prong collars should be avoided as they cause unnecessary discomfort and can raise the puppy's level of fear or anxiety.

SAFETY AND PUPPY-PROOFING PROCEDURES

Training should be designed to set up the puppy to succeed, providing no opportunity to fail. Keeping a puppy indoors or in a run will prevent digging, predation, and chase. Chewing, garbage raiding, destructiveness, food stealing, and jumping up on people or furniture can also be prevented by denying the puppy access to the areas where problems might occur. Whenever the owner is not available to supervise, the puppy should be kept in a puppy-proof room, a pen, puppy run, barricaded area, or a crate.

Confinement training not only prevents many behavior problems but also provides a secure home or den for the puppy. A common misconception is that confinement is cruel or unfair. On the contrary, leaving the puppy unsupervised to wander, investigate, destroy, and perhaps get injured is inappropriate and potentially dangerous. If the puppy learns from the outset that a pen or crate is its bed or sleeping area, it should soon enter voluntarily. Providing food rewards and toys each time the puppy enters the crate and ensuring that the crate is not used for punishment can also help the puppy adapt quickly. As long as the puppy has been recently exercised, allowed to eliminate, and has bedding and toys and perhaps food and water in its crate, the crate is a safe, humane area for housing the puppy when it cannot be supervised. The puppy should not be confined to its crate any longer than it can go without eliminating, and the owner should provide sufficient play and exercise sessions to meet the puppy's needs before crating.

Special problem areas can also be protected with booby traps. Booby traps teach the puppy that an area is aversive in much the same way that the puppy might learn to avoid other unpleasant stimuli in the environment (e.g., cactus plants or train tracks). Commonly used booby traps include motion detectors, aversive odors or tastes, or uncomfortable stimuli (e.g., double-sided tape, motion detectors, and electronic mats) (Landsberg, 1994).

HOUSE-TRAINING

Puppies should be well supervised so that they can be taught the proper area in which to eliminate and interrupted immediately any time elimination is attempted in an inappropriate area. Most puppies eliminate shortly after play, eating, drinking, and sleeping. The puppy should be taken outside to an appropriate elimination area and rewarded with praise, play, or food rewards when it eliminates. By pairing the elimination–reward sequence with a few key words, many puppies soon learn to associate these words with elimination. If the location is kept consistent, the odor and location will attract the puppy back for future elimination. When the puppy cannot be supervised, it should be prevented from eliminating in inappropriate locations by keeping it in its crate, in a paper-lined room, or in an outdoor run. Although it may be helpful and necessary to immediately disrupt indoor elimination as it begins and to take the puppy to its proper elimination area (if the problem is observed by the owners), punishment after elimination has ceased is useless.

Emerging Behavior Problems

DESTRUCTIVE CHEWING AND DIGGING

Chewing and destructiveness in puppies is often a result of insufficient stimulation as well as exploration, investigation, scavenging, teething, and attempts at escape from confinement. To prevent chewing, the puppy should receive adequate stimulation in the form of play, training, and exercise sessions and an ample opportunity to chew and explore. Once chewing problems emerge, the owner should first ensure that the puppy has adequate mental and physical stimulation and appropriate opportunities and outlets for chewing. Begin by offering a variety of toys and determine a few select toys that the puppy prefers. Then rotate the toys, leaving only a few out each day so that the toys remain novel and interesting. Encourage and reward the puppy each time it chews its toys. Toys made of sheet rawhide, nylon, and durable rubber are the most practical. Cheese or meat spreads can be coated on the toys to stimulate interest, or small pieces of food can be wedged into some toys. Some toys require manipulation for the food to be released. Frozen treats can also be used to keep the puppy occupied for an extended period of time. Until the owner can trust the puppy, it should be under constant supervision or confined to a safe area. As the puppy is allowed more freedom, it can be taught to avoid previously chewed objects by making them taste bad with a small amount of cayenne pepper, oil of citronella, or antichew spray. Booby traps may also be successful because they are an immediate deterrent and do not require the owner's presence. The Gentle Header Halter with a 10-foot remote leash can also be used to immediately interrupt chewing.

Digging is another form of "destructive" behavior. Some breeds, such as the northern dog breeds (Siberian husky and Malamute), dig cooling holes and lie in them, while other breeds, such as the terriers, have been purposely bred to flush out prey or dig for rodents. It is likely that many puppies dig as a direct result of odors or sounds from beneath the ground that attract the puppy. Some puppies dig to bury or retrieve bones. Puppies also dig to escape from confinement. Digging may also be an activity similar to destructive chewing that occurs when puppies are left alone with insufficient stimulation. Digging can be suppressed in the owner's presence. Unless the cause is identified and dealt with, however, the digging will continue in the owner's absence. Remote punishment (turning on a sprinkler or pulling on an extended leash) or booby traps (placing a motion detector, chicken wire, rocks, or water in the area where the puppy digs) might teach the puppy to avoid the digging site but does not deter the puppy from digging at new sites. In many cases, the preferred solution is to confine the puppy to a pen where it cannot dig or to provide an acceptable digging area.

UNRULINESS AND DISOBEDIENCE

Overexuberant play, jumping up, mounting, and play biting are just a few of the puppy problems that owners should control. It is first important to ensure that these puppies are receiving adequate exercise, play, and attention to meet their needs. In addition, the puppy should be receiving regular reward-based training. Teach the puppy first to respond briefly to commands in nondistracting environments and gradually progress to longer responses and more challenging environments. If the puppy acts excitedly, rambunctiously, or demands play or attention, it is essential that these actions not be rewarded. Many owners provide attention when the puppy is acting inappropriately (whining, jumping up, nipping, exploring, and garbage raiding) yet ignore the puppy when it is calm and quiet. In fact, it is the quiet, calm, and nondemanding behavior that needs to be rewarded. Whenever the inappropriate or undesirable behavior is displayed, the owner can either ignore the behavior and walk away (ensuring that no reward or attention has been given) or train the puppy to cease. This can be accomplished using a previously trained obedience command (sit or down) or with a prompt using a leash or head halter. Another option is to interrupt the behavior with a disruption/

punishment device (shake can, horn, or ultrasonic trainer). Disruption should be applied instantaneously as the problem begins, and once the puppy ceases it should be encouraged to perform an acceptable behavior and be rewarded. Physical punishment should be avoided.

VOCALIZATION

Puppies vocalize for a variety of reasons, but most puppy vocalization is an attempt to solicit attention, affection, food, or play. Territorial alerting toward novel sounds and the approach of strangers or other dogs begins to emerge between 3 and 6 months of age. Training puppies to bark on cue and cease on command is the best way to gain control over barking. Many owners inadvertently encourage (reward) barking by giving attention, food, or play to the puppy. The only acceptable responses are ignoring the barking, employing successful interruption techniques, or teaching the puppy to be quiet on command. Quiet training can be accomplished using food-lure training and gradually delaying the reward for longer periods of quiet. Owners who cannot quiet their puppies for training can use a leash and halter technique to ensure an immediate and correct response. The puppy can then be released and rewarded for being quiet. Interruption devices such as a shake can, audible alarm, ultrasonic device, or squirt from a water container may also be successful at interrupting the behavior. The puppy's attention should then be maintained by having it perform an alternative desirable behavior (e.g., playing with a favored toy or getting a tummy rub). Puppies that continue to bark in the owner's absence might be successfully controlled with a sonic or ultrasonic bark-activated device, a bark-activated citronella spray collar, or, if all else fails, a bark-activated electronic shock collar (Landsberg, 1994).

FOOD BOWL AND OBJECT GUARDING

The puppy that guards its food bowl or favored objects is generally an unacceptable and potentially dangerous puppy. A number of techniques can help to reduce the possibility of food bowl guarding and at the same time reaffirm the owner's leadership. Using obedience commands and food as a reward, the owner should teach the puppy to sit and stay before each meal. The bowl can be filled and placed in place and then the puppy can be released from the stay or commanded to come to its food bowl. Numer-

ous small feedings can be provided so that the puppy can be trained for many commands at each meal. The owner can also split the meal into numerous portions, stay nearby, and then command the puppy to sit and stay while the food bowl is empty and until it is refilled. Provided that the puppy shows no anxiety or threats, the owner can pat and handle the puppy during feeding and remove the food bowl before all of the food is gone. As long as the puppy shows no resistance, it should be rewarded with verbal encouragement and the food bowl should be returned with a little more food and perhaps even a special treat inside. The owner can then proceed to approach and handle the puppy during feeding, using treats or toys to reward acceptable behavior.

These techniques are intended to make handling and approaches a normal part of the feeding regimen and should teach the puppy that highly appealing rewards may be given whenever the feeding is disrupted and that the puppy's food will indeed be returned. If any growling or threats are displayed, immediate attention to the problem is essential. Having the puppy wear a leash and halter while feeding provides an opportunity for the owners to safely and successfully deal with some of these problems. Emerging threats cannot be tolerated and may be safely dealt with using the attached halter and remote leash. Hand feeding the entire meal as the puppy responds to a variety of commands can also be a useful technique until the puppy learns to tolerate the handler's presence during feeding.

Some puppies will allow approach and handling at the food bowl but refuse to drop objects or will exhibit aggression when in possession of objects such as a favored chew toy or selected "treasures" that have been stolen from the garbage. Again, obedience training and preventive techniques are essential. Household objects and garbage cans should be kept out of reach until the puppy learns that these are out of bounds. This can be accomplished with a combination of supervision (with a halter and remote leash, if necessary) and booby traps or remote punishment techniques. To teach the "drop" or "out" command, begin by having the puppy retrieve or pick up an object of minimal appeal. Then, with the command, teach the puppy to drop the object using an object of higher appeal (such as hot dog slice). Food-lure training may be useful to ensure success at the start, but food should be hidden in the hand and used intermittently once the puppy complies. If necessary, a leash and halter should be left attached to the puppy during initial training to prevent running away with the object.

UNDESIRABLE INGESTIVE BEHAVIORS

It is not unusual for puppies to steal and ingest a variety of objects and substances that are objectionable to the owners. Many of these problems are a result of exploratory and scavenging behavior. Garbage raiding and the ingestion of food-related items are also likely a form of scavenging, and the owner who chases after the puppy and tries to take these objects away may further aggravate the problem. Puppies that eat grass may be attracted to the fresh vegetation that is lacking in the diet. Because carnivores cannot digest cellulose, it is likely to irritate the stomach and cause vomiting. It has been suggested that puppies may eat grass when they feel the need to vomit, but it is uncertain whether this is a learned or an innate response to gastric irritation. Providing increased fiber in the form of cooked vegetables or diced raw vegetables added to the diet may help to satisfy the puppy's desire in much the same way as a human might be attracted to salads (Beaver, 1981).

Puppies may also ingest numerous other foreign objects, such as rocks, balls, toys, or cloth material, as a form of play or scavenging. In general, this must be prevented, although in rare cases it may be due to underlying medical (e.g., gastrointestinal) problems.

Coprophagia is another common complaint of puppy owners that usually resolves by adulthood. Puppies may eat their own stools, the stools of other puppies, or the stools of other species. When puppies eat kitten feces, the problem may simply be an appealing odor and perhaps taste in the stool even after it passes through the kitten's system, perhaps related to the high palatability of cat foods. Puppies that eat the stool of horses or cattle may be attracted to the digested nutrients from vegetation, which the puppy's system is not capable of digesting (Beaver, 1981). There have been many explanations suggested for why a puppy would eat its own or another puppy's stools. In general, puppies are attracted to the odors of other puppies, such as those found in the sexual discharge, stools, urine, and even infections of other puppies. Mothers are innately programmed to consume the feces of puppies in the nest. When left unsupervised, puppies may simply begin to investigate, play with, and even eat stools as a playful or investigative activity. Because coprophagia may attract a great deal of owner attention, the behavior may be further reinforced.

Supervision of the puppy when outdoors until it eliminates and thorough cleaning of the puppy's property before allowing the puppy to stay indoors can best correct coprophagia. At the first indication of stool sniffing or investigation, the puppy should be interrupted with a firm command or a quick pull on the leash; this is particularly effective for puppies wearing halters. Puppies with coprophagia should be tested for any medical problems that might lead to incomplete digestion of the food, such as pancreatic insufficiency and malabsorption. Overfeeding and nutritional deficiencies might also lead to coprophagia, although these are quite rare. Similarly, puppies on calorie-restricted diets may develop coprophagia. Increasing bulk in the diet, discontinuing the diet, or adding a vitamin or enzyme supplement may be helpful. Taste aversion is not usually successful because in many cases the stools are more appealing than the aversive substance and stools treated with the substance may ultimately have increased appeal. Even when taste aversion or booby traps are successful, the puppy soon learns to test each stool and only eat those that are not booby trapped. Scientific studies have shown that only a product that causes nausea is likely to be an effective deterrent (Gustafson, 1996). Occasionally, changing to a diet of higher digestibility or adding products such as meat tenderizers, papaya, or yogurt have been used to reduce the desirability of the stool. Adding stool softeners or bulk laxatives to the food may deter puppies that prefer the shape or texture of a well-formed stool.

FELINE DEVELOPMENT

Kittens go through the same development stages as puppies, although the periods may be shorter and more difficult to define (Overall, 1988). The neonatal period is a time primarily of nursing and sleep in which the kitten is fully dependent on its mother. The transitional period, when locomotion and sensory development emerge, begins in the second week, and the socialization period begins in the third week and extends to 7 to 9 weeks of age. The juvenile stage ends between about 6 and 12 months of age at sexual maturity (Martin and Bateson, 1988), although social maturity is not reached until 2.5 to 4 years of age (Overall, 1988).

During the neonatal period, the kitten is predominantly guided by tactile and olfactory stimuli (Martin and Bateson, 1988). Olfaction is present at birth and is mature by 3 weeks. Hearing is present by the fifth day, and the kitten begins to orient to sounds by 2 weeks, with adult development present by 4 weeks. The eyes remain closed until 7 to 10 days, and visual orienting and following develop by 25 days. At birth, kittens move toward warmth but do not begin to regulate their body temperature until 3 weeks and are capable of adult-like thermoregulation and sleep patterns at around 7 weeks. During the first 2 weeks the kittens are fairly immobile, with walking beginning around 3 weeks. Body righting, although present at birth, is not well developed until 1 month, and air righting develops at around 5 weeks (Beaver, 1992).

Within the socialization period, social attachments are formed most easily and rapidly (Karsh and Turner, 1988). Attachments can be formed at other times, but the process is much slower and involves extensive exposure. Socializing kittens to other species, including humans, may begin as early as 2 weeks of age and may only extend to 7 weeks of age (Overall, 1988). Kittens that were reared with rats did not kill their cage mates or similar rats even as adults (Kuo, 1930), while kittens raised with puppies did not show fear toward adult dogs (Fox, 1969). Kittens raised with no exposure to puppies before 12 weeks, however, showed avoidance and defensive responses when exposed to them.

Good maternal behavior is also essential for healthy kitten development. Kittens that were separated from their mother and hand raised from 2 weeks of age were more fearful of kittens and people, more sensitive to novel stimuli, and learned poorly (Seitz, 1979). Kittens that are hand raised may eventually develop social attachments to other kittens, although much more slowly (Overall, 1988). Kittens from undernourished mothers had growth stunting, behavioral abnormalities, and delays in the development of crawling, eyes opening, walking, playing, and climbing (Martin and Bateson, 1988). If these kittens were properly nourished after 6 weeks of age, they did grow to normal body size but had growth deficits in the cerebrum, cerebellum, and brain stem (Simonson, 1979). They had poorer learning ability, antisocial behavior toward other kittens, and abnormal levels of aggression and fear (Martin and Bateson, 1988; Smith and Jansen, 1977). Prematurely weaned kittens developed predatory behavior earlier and showed an earlier increase in object play, whereas normally weaned kittens were less likely to become predators and had a later onset of object play (Robinson, 1992).

Effects of Early Handling

Early handling of kittens by humans is not only beneficial for improving social relationships between kittens and humans but also leads to accelerated physical and central nervous system development. Kittens that were handled daily for the first 30 days of life opened their eyes earlier, began to explore earlier, and were less fearful of humans (Martin and Bateson, 1988). Kittens that were handled for 5 minutes daily from birth to 45 days approached and contacted people more frequently than nonhandled kittens (Karsh and Turner, 1988). In a study in which 5.5- to 9.5-week-old kittens were handled by no, one, or five people, the five-person kittens exhibited the least fear of strangers, whereas the one-person kittens showed the most play and social behavior to a familiar person (Collard, 1967). In another study, kittens that were handled between 3 and 14 weeks of age would accept holding for longer and would approach humans faster than either the kittens handled from 7 to 14 weeks of age or the kittens that had received no handling (Martin and Bateson, 1988). These studies thus indicate that the most receptive time for socializing kittens to people is up to 7 weeks of age.

Preventive Management

SOCIALIZATION

Socialization is the process in which an animal develops a social relationship or bond with members of its own or another species. Studies have shown that the most receptive period for kitten socialization is up to 7 weeks of age (Martin and Bateson, 1988). Kittens that begin to develop social relationships during the socialization period are often capable of maintaining these relationships for life. To reduce fearful or aggressive behavior toward people and other species of animals, kittens should receive as much exposure and contact as possible with other species before 7 weeks of age. The earlier and more frequent the handling, the more sociable the kitten is likely to be. Because there is such diversity in ages, physical appearances, and personalities in people, a wide variety of exposure experiences for the kitten are recommended. In some veterinary practices, kitty kindergarten sessions have proved to be a popular and practical method of educating new kitten owners, socializing the new kitten to a variety of people, and exposing the kitten to a number of different stimuli and environments while it is still young, playful, and exploratory. How sociable a kitten becomes is not solely dependent on early socialization but also on the kitten's inherited personality type.

HOUSING KITTENS INDOORS

Kittens that are housed exclusively indoors generally live long and healthy lives, free from the diseases, parasites, and potential injuries that are a serious risk to kittens if they are allowed to go outdoors in exclusively housed urban environments. Although indoor housing is obviously desirable for the kitten's physical health and longevity, can a kitten be housed indoors without any detrimental effects on its behavior? Certainly some kittens seem to have a strong desire to go outdoors, and frustrating these attempts could be difficult on both the owner and the kitten. Even with severe space constraints, however, most kittens that are neutered and provided with all of the "amenities" of outdoor living in their indoor environment can live their entire lives indoors and be free of behavioral problems.

KITTEN-PROOFING THE HOME

Some kittens may need to have their access to certain areas restricted to ensure safety and to prevent undesirable behaviors. Owners must be prepared for the kitten's ability to jump, climb, and get into problem areas, as well as its desire to chew on just about everything from thread to electric cords. Although crate training can work well for kittens, kitten-proofed rooms are usually sufficient as long as there is nothing that the kitten might damage and nothing dangerous to chew on, swallow, scratch, or climb onto. The room should contain appropriate play toys and a scratching post or an activity area, along with the kitten's litter box and provision of a soft resting area (Crowse et al, 1995).

Under no circumstances should the owner use physical punishment on a kitten. In fact, physical and verbal punishment by the owner could cause fear of the owner and increased anxiety or stress for the kitten. Even when punishment is effective at stopping a behavior like climbing the living room drapes, the kitten will likely continue to climb the drapes when the owner is not supervising, as there are no unpleasant consequences to the act.

The best way to keep the kitten away from selected areas is either to prevent access to the area or to use booby traps. Closing a few doors, putting up barricades, and using childproof containers and child locks are sometimes effective at keeping kittens away from potential problem areas. Booby traps are intended to teach the kitten that an area is aversive or out of bounds in much the same way that a kitten might learn to avoid chewing on certain plants or avoiding certain locations (e.g., swimming pools and train tracks) in their environment. Commonly used booby traps include motion detectors, aversive odors or tastes, or uncomfortable stimuli (such as double-sided tape, plastic carpet runners with nubs up, or electronic mats).

If the kitten begins to perform an undesirable action in the presence of the owner, the behavior could be immediately interrupted with a disruptive device such as an air horn, battery-operated alarm, ultrasonic kitten trainer, water rifle, can of compressed air, or a pair of rolled up socks tossed at the kitten. The use of a disruptive or "punishment" device reduces the chance that the kitten will retaliate or become fearful of the owner. In addition, if the owner can remain out of sight while administering the "punishment," the kitten may learn to associate the unpleasant consequence with the behavior and not the presence of the owner. Some more technically inclined owners may want to consider plugging an alarm, hair dryer, water pic, or tape recording into a remote control switch and placing it in the area where the kitten misbehaves. Then, as soon as the kitten enters the area or begins the inappropriate behavior, the aversive device is triggered by remote control while the owner remains out of sight.

PLAY AND EXPLORATION

Kitten play may be categorized as social, object, or locomotive play. Social play with the mother or littermates begins around 4 weeks of age, peaks at about 7 to 9 weeks of age, and begins to decline around 12 to 14 weeks of age (Collard, 1967; Martin and Bateson, 1988). Social play may include wrestling, bouts of biting, and play fighting. During the third month, social play becomes more predatory and agonistic (Martin and Bateson, 1988). Sexual components of play such as mounting and biting the scruff of females may begin in the male around 4.5 months (Houpt, 1991). Kittens that are weaned too early and those that do not have the opportunity to play with cospecies may not learn to control the intensity of their attacks and may play more aggressively with people. Object and locomotor play begin around 6 weeks of age and peak around 18 weeks of age (Collard, 1967). Locomotor play can be social or solitary and includes running, jumping, and climbing. Object play includes pawing, stalking, pouncing, and biting objects and may also be directed at adult cats, people, prey, or imaginary objects. Although object play is associated with many of the motor patterns associated with prey catching and killing, play experience does not appear to be necessary for the development of predation.

Understimulation, an excess of unused energy, and lack of appropriate opportunities for play can contribute to play aggression, destructiveness, exploratory behavior, or excessive nocturnal activity. Interactive play and exercise sessions provide the kitten with attention from the owner and an outlet for exploration and play. Although play is exhibited more by kittens, it often persists through adulthood (Houpt, 1991). Kittens are most stimulated by moving objects that can be stalked, chased, swatted, or pounced on. Some successful interactive toys might include wiggling ropes, wands, dangling toys, and those that are thrown or rolled for the kitten to chase. For self-play, the kitten can be provided with toys that roll such as ping pong balls or walnuts, toys that dangle, battery-operated and spring-mounted toys, scratching posts, and toys within containers that can be "batted" and manipulated. Many kittens explore novel items and areas, so allowing the kitten the opportunity to explore a kitten-proofed room or providing the kitten with some empty boxes, paper bags, or an activity center can be useful. Some kittens enjoy and are adept at climbing and perching, so for these kittens it is recommended that opportunities to climb and perch be provided. Catnip-treated toys and toys with food or treats inside them can help to stimulate play and exploration. Kittens with a strong desire for social play might benefit from the addition of a second kitten to act as a playmate, provided that both kittens have been adequately socialized to other cats.

LITTER BOX TRAINING

Although kittens begin to voluntarily eliminate at about 3 weeks of age, the anogenital reflex by which the mother's cleaning of the genital and rectal areas stimulates elimination persists for 5 to 6 weeks (Beaver, 1992). At 5 to 6 weeks, the kittens begin to seek out appropriate substrates in which they can eliminate, generally in an area where they can perform earth raking. Exploration including ingestion of litter is also common around this time. Following elimination, kittens perform an almost reflexive burying, which may be a form of hygiene because it is practiced more frequently near the center of the kitten's territory and is less likely to be performed away from the core of the territory. Lack of burying may be a form of marking, may

be related to the type of substrate, or may be due to the lack of the genetic and/or learned components necessary for the behavior to develop. Generally, if the kitten is going to cover, it will have begun to do so by 7 weeks (Overall, 1988). Because the odor of fecal matter seems to stimulate burying, some fastidious kittens may cover their own feces as well as other kitten's feces and may go through the motions of burying even when they eliminate on a solid surface (Beaver, 1992). Some kittens are stimulated to bury by the odor of food.

Because most kittens instinctively eliminate in loose dirt, litter box training is relatively simple as long as the kitten is provided with an appropriate litter box and litter material in an appealing and easily accessible location, and the litter is cleaned regularly. Access to all other potential targets, such as plant soil and fireplace hearths, should be prevented. Kittens should be taken to their litter box when first obtained and allowed to investigate. Owners should be advised that a small kitten should be housed or confined near its litter at first so that it does not wander too far from its litter when it has to eliminate. It might also be helpful to take the kitten to its litter after waking and eating or to confine the kitten in a room with its litter when it cannot be supervised.

If the kitten eliminates outside its litter box, the owner should immediately reassess the litter box location, including whether it is readily accessible, whether there are any deterrents in the area (e.g., a furnace, washing machine, or noxious cleansers), the type of litter being used, and whether it has been sufficiently cleaned. Sandy, clumping litter is often preferred by kittens over conventional clay litter (Borchelt, 1991). Next, the owner should either prevent access to the problem areas or reduce the appeal of the new area. For example, kittens that eliminate in plant containers may prefer the texture or odor of soil. The simplest solution may be to keep the kitten away from the plants or the plants away from the kitten. Placing a layer of decorative rocks over the soil may help. Other options are to add some soil to the litter to make it more desirable or to place booby traps in or around the plants. Kittens that eliminate in one or two inappropriate locations may desist if the function of the area is changed by placing food, a scratching post, or play center in the area. All areas of inappropriate elimination should be thoroughly cleaned with a commercial odor remover, and when the area cannot be made inaccessible it should be made less desirable with deterrents or booby traps. If the kitten persists at one particular location, a second litter box can be placed at that location and gradually relocated to a more appropriate area.

Emerging Behavior Problems

NOCTURNAL ACTIVITY

A number of feline behavior problems are due to the kitten's crepuscular nature. Typical complaints are kittens that nibble or even attack the owner's ears or toes in bed, walk across the sleeping owners, vocalize, or entertain themselves with explosive, uncontrollable play sessions across the furniture and/or owners during the night or early morning. By providing activity, attention, and play periods throughout the early evening, the kitten may sleep better through the night. Injuries can be prevented by confining the kitten away from the owner by closing the bedroom door or confining it to a separate room or crate with play toys. Alternatively, punishment devices such as a water sprayer, ultrasonic alarm, or compressed air may be helpful to deter nighttime play.

EXCESSIVE VOCALIZATION

Occasionally, kitten vocalization may be loud enough to generate complaints of excessive noise, but generally it is the persistent or nocturnal nature of the vocalization that is of concern to the owner. Kittens may also vocalize as a threat, as sexual behavior, or in an attempt to solicit resources, such as social contact, food, or attention. Some cat breeds, such as the Siamese, may have an increased genetic predisposition toward vocalization (Mendl and Harcourt, 1988). Vocalization should never be rewarded (e.g., by providing food, attention, or play on demand). Vocalization can be interrupted with a water gun, compressed air, a loud verbal "no," or an alarm device, and the kitten should be ignored until it is calm and quiet. Spaying and castration eliminate most vocalizations associated with sexual behavior.

INGESTIVE BEHAVIORS

Kittens often begin eating solid food by following the mother to the food bowl or by walking through the food (Beaver, 1992). Dirt and litter eating may precede the eating of solid food. For most kittens, especially those that scavenge, novel foods are most appealing (Church et al, 1994). Kittens may, however, develop taste and food preferences related to the flavors, textures, and ingredients that they have been exposed to during the first 6 months. At weaning, kittens tend to imitate their mother's food choice, so those kittens may become less "finicky" if both the mother and the kitten are exposed to a variety of foods at the time of weaning. Similarly, prey preferences and the skill of catching and killing that particular prey are also dictated in part by early experience (Martin and Bateson, 1988).

The mother starts to bring prey to the kittens as early as 4 weeks of age, and kittens may be able to kill prey as early as 5 weeks of age (Martin and Bateson, 1988). Over the next 3 to 4 weeks, the kittens begin to join the mother on hunts. Learning to kill prey develops between the fifth and twentieth weeks; it is much more difficult for kittens to learn to hunt after that age (Beaver, 1992). Most kittens kill the same type of prey as their mother killed when they were young. For example, adult cats may not be able to catch fish unless they learn to do so when young, and kittens raised as vegetarians have a reduced desire to eat prey (Collard, 1967). Competition between littermates for prey and hunger also increase predatory behavior (Overall, 1988). A combination of hunger and exposure to prey when young is most likely to produce a predatory adult (Martin and Bateson, 1988). Kittens that are weaned early and exposed to prey will develop predatory skills earlier and will be more likely to be predators. Although trying to reduce a kitten's predatory drive when it becomes an adult is often futile, avoiding early weaning, rearing kittens in an environment where they are not exposed to predation, and keeping the kittens well fed may reduce predation.

Kittens that chew on plants may benefit from a high bulk diet (perhaps with some added raw or cooked vegetables) or a safe kitty herb garden to chew. By providing small meals in a variety of locations or requiring some form of manipulation to obtain food (cat scratch feeders, toys, or entertainment centers with food inside), feeding can become a much more active and productive part of the kitten's day. Some kittens, many of which are the Oriental cat breeds, have an overly strong desire to suck and chew material, particularly wool (Bradshaw et al, 1997). Providing alternative oral stimulation in the form of dog chew toys, bulky, dry, or chewy foods, tough chunks of meat, or large bones with bits of meat or sinew attached might satisfy the desires of some kittens. Providing an acceptable fabric to suck on such as an old sweater or sock may be successful when combined with booby traps and taste deterrents on the chewed objects such as menthol or oil of eucalyptus to keep the kitten away from objects.

DESTRUCTIVE AND EXPLORATORY BEHAVIORS

Kittens that climb drapes, jump onto counters, or chew on household objects (e.g., string and electric cords) are usually exhibiting playful and exploratory behaviors. Exploration and investigation should not be curtailed but should be channeled into acceptable locations. Providing high places for perching, play areas for climbing and scratching, and toys and interactive play sessions for play predation hunting help keep the kitten occupied and satisfy some of its innate needs. It is also essential that exploration not be rewarded, as this would further encourage the behavior. For example, kittens that jump on countertops or tables and find even a few morsels of food will keep coming back, and some kittens will jump onto counters and furniture to play with their owner's personal possessions. Supervising the kitten will usually stop these problems in the owner's presence, but most kittens will continue when the owner is not supervising. When owners are out of the home or cannot supervise, problems can be prevented by confining the kitten to a kitten-proofed area where there is no opportunity to get into "mischief" or by booby-trapping areas.

SCRATCHING

Scratching is a normal behavior that conditions the claws, serves as a visual and scent mark, and is a means of stretching. When scratching is directed at furniture or members of the family, however, it is unacceptable. Inappropriate scratching can be prevented by keeping the kitten away from problem areas, trimming the nails regularly, and providing a proper scratching post. Should the kitten continue to scratch in an inappropriate area, the post could be moved to that area and the scratched furniture could be covered with a less appealing material, such as plastic or a loosely draped piece of material. Remote and environmental punishment can be used to deter further scratching of an area. Some owners may want to consider plastic nail coverings that can be glued over the kitten's claws and replaced monthly.

For those owners with destructive kittens who cannot train them to use a scratching post, declawing is another alternative. The primary reasons for declawing are property damage and the risk of injury to people or other kittens. Occasionally, declawing the family kitten may best protect the welfare of a family member. Declawing allows the family to keep the kitten and enjoy the rewards of kitten ownership. Declawing means that fewer kittens need to be placed in another home or destroyed and that more kittens can be placed. In numerous studies, declawing has been shown to cause no increase in behavior problems (Landsberg, 1991; Bennett et al, 1988; Borchelt and Voith, 1987; Morgan and Houpt, 1989). In fact, many kittens continue to scratch furniture after declawing but cause no significant damage.

References and Supplemental Reading

Beaver BV: Grass eating by carnivores. Vet Med Small Anim Clinician 76:968, 1981.

Beaver BV: Feline Behavior: A Guide for Veterinarians. Philadelphia, WB Saunders, 1992.

Bennett M, Houpt KA, Erb HN: Effects of declawing on feline behavior. Comp Anim Pract 2:7, 1988.

Borchelt PL: Cat elimination problems. Vet Clin North Am Small Anim Pract 21:254, 1991.

Borchelt PL, Voith VL: Aggressive behavior in cats. Compend Contin Educ Pract Vet 1:49, 1987.

Bradshaw JWS, Neville PF, Sawyer D: Factors affecting pica in the domestic cat. J Appl Anim Behav Sci 52:373, 1997.

Church SC, Allen JA, Bradshaw JWS: Anti-apostatic food selection by the domestic cat. Anim Behav 48:747, 1994.

Collard RR: Fear of strangers and play behavior in kittens varied with social experience. Child Dev 38:877, 1967.

Crowse SJ, Atwill ER, Lagana M, et al: Soft surfaces—A factor in feline psychological well-being. Contemp Top Lab Anim Sci 34:94, 1995.

Fox MW: Canine Behavior. Springfield, IL, Charles C Thomas, 1965.

Fox MW: Socialization, environmental factors, and abnormal behavioral development in animals. *In* Fox MW (ed): Abnormal Behavior in Animals. Philadelphia, WB Saunders, 1968, p 332.

Fox MW: Behavioral effects of rearing dogs with cats during the "critical period of socialization." Behaviour 35:273, 1969.

Freedman DG, King JA, Elliot O: Critical period in the social development of dogs. Science 133:1016, 1961.

Gustafson CR: Taste aversion conditioning versus conditioning using aversive peripheral stimuli. *In* Voith VL, Borchelt PL (eds): Readings in Companion Animal Behavior. Trenton, NJ, Veterinary Learning Systems, 1996, p 89.

Houpt K: Domestic Animal Behavior for Veterinarians and Animal Scientists, 2nd ed. Ames, Iowa State University Press, 1991.

Karsh E, Turner DC: The human–cat relationship.

In Turner D, Bateson P (eds): The Domestic Cat: The Biology of Its Behavior. New York, Cambridge University Press, 1988, p 159.

Kuo ZY: The genesis of the cat's response to the rat. J Comp Psychol 11:1, 1930.

Landsberg G: Cat owners' attitudes toward declawing. Anthrozoos 4:192, 1991.

Landsberg GM: Products for preventing or controlling undesirable behavior. Vet Med Oct:970, 1994.

Landsberg GM, Hunthausen W, Ackerman L: Handbook of Behaviour Problems of the Dog and Cat. Oxford, England, Butterworth-Heinemann, 1997.

Levine S: Maternal and environmental influences on the adrenocortical response to stress in weanling rats. Science 156:258, 1967.

Martin P, Bateson P: Behavioural development in the cat. *In* Turner D, Bateson P (eds): The Domestic Cat: The Biology of Its Behavior. New York, Cambridge University Press, 1988, p 9.

Mendl M, Harcourt R: Individuality in the domestic cat. *In* Turner D, Bateson P (eds): The Domestic Cat: The Biology of Its Behavior. New York, Cambridge University Press, 1988, p 41.

Morgan M, Houpt KA: Feline behavior problems. The influence of declawing. Anthrozoos 3:50, 1989.

Overall KL: How understanding normal cat behavior can help prevent behavior problems. Vet Med Feb:160, 1988.

Robinson I: Behavioural development of the cat. *In* Thorne C (ed): The Waltham Book of Dog and Cat Behaviour. Pergamon, New York, 1992, p 79.

Scott JP, Fuller JL: Genetics and the Social Behavior of the Dog. Chicago, Chicago University Press, 1965.

Seitz PFD: Infantile experience in adult behavior in animal subjects, II. Age of separation from the mother and adult behavior in the cat. Psychosom Med 21:353, 1979.

Serpell J, Jagoe JA: Early experience and the development of behavior. *In* Serpell J (ed): The Domestic Dog: Its Evolution, Behavior, and Interaction with People. Cambridge, Cambridge University Press, 1995, p 79.

Simonson M: Effects of maternal malnourishment, development and behavior in successive generations in the rat and cat. *In* Levitsky DA (ed): Malnutrition, Environment and Behavior. Ithaca, NY, Cornell University Press, 1979.

Smith BA, Jansen GR: Maternal undernutrition in the feline: Behavioral sequelae. Nutr Rep Int 16:513, 1977.

Thorne C: The Waltham Book of Dog and Cat Behaviour. Pergamon Press, New York, 1992.

Voith VL, Borchelt PL: Diagnosis of dominance aggression in dogs. Vet Clin North Am Small Anim Pract 12:655, 1982.

Drug and Blood Component Therapy and Neonatal Isoerythrolysis

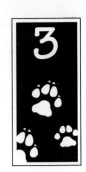

Dawn Merton Boothe and Jorg Bucheler

Drug Therapy

Dawn Merton Boothe

Current drug and fluid therapy for puppies and kittens is largely based on information extrapolated from other species. Normal maturation changes in puppies and kittens from birth to 6 months will cause accompanying changes in drug disposition, thus rendering the puppies and kittens more susceptible to drug-induced adverse reactions.

DRUG DISPOSITION

Puppies and kittens can be exposed to drugs through three sources: the mother, either just before or during parturition (placental transfer); the mother's milk during nursing; and direct administration. It is beyond the scope of this paper to describe the factors determining drug disposition in normal, healthy adults (Riviere, 1988a, b). A working knowledge of these factors is, however, crucial in predicting the effects of age-induced differences in drug disposition. Only through an appreciation of these differences can drug and fluid therapy be individualized and the incidence of adverse drug reactions reduced in young animals. Generally, adverse drug reactions reflect plasma drug concentrations that have reached the toxic range. Occasionally, therapeutic failure results from genera-tion of plasma concentrations that are subtherapeutic. All four determinants of drug disposition (i.e., absorption, distribution, metabolism, and excretion) undergo dramatic changes as the puppy and kitten mature. The clinical significance of these sequelae varies (Table 3–1).

After oral administration, most drugs are absorbed from the small intestine. Because the surface area of the small intestine is large even in young animals, the extent of drug absorption probably does not differ clinically between young animals and adults. The rate of drug absorption tends to be slower in young animals, however, probably due to decreased gastric emptying and irregular intestinal motility. As a result, peak plasma drug concentrations may be lower. The decreased rate of absorption might actually protect against toxic drug concentrations (Heimann, 1980; Rane and Wilson, 1989). These protective mechanisms may not, however, be present in puppies and kittens before absorption of colostrum. During this period, permeability of the intestinal mucosa is increased along with the rate and extent of drug absorption. Occasionally, drugs that normally are not absorbed from the gastrointestinal tract (such as aminoglycosides, carbenicillin and

35

Table 3–1	Differences in Drug Disposition in Puppies and Kittens Compared with Adults		
	DIFFERENCE	**SEQUELAE**	**POSSIBLE CLINICAL SIGNIFICANCE**
	Decreased gastric emptying and irregular peristalsis	Slower absorption and lower PDC	Therapeutic failure; dose increase may be indicated
	Increased intestinal permeability	Increased rate of oral absorption and higher peak PDC	Toxic concentrations
	Increased gastric pH	Increased oral absorption of acid-labile or weakly basic drugs; higher peak PDC and longer duration of PDC	Toxic concentrations
	Increased absorption of volatile gases	Higher PDC	Increased sensitivity
	Increased absorption of topically applied drugs	Higher peak PDC and longer duration of PDC	Toxicity to topically applied drugs or drug/toxins in environment
	Greater total body water with a greater proportion located extracellularly	Increased distribution of drugs; lower peak PDC but longer drug half-life	Therapeutic failure; dose increase may be indicated; however, longer dosing interval may be indicated
	Lower concentrations of serum proteins	Decreased binding of significantly protein-bound drugs; increased active drug accumulation; longer drug half-life?	Toxicity; increased drug accumulation may necessitate longer dosing intervals
	Decreased body fat	Decreased accumulation of lipid-soluble drugs; higher peak PDC	Toxicity to drugs distributed to fat

PDC = plasma drug concentration.

other acid-sensitive β-lactams, and enteric sulfonamides) can reach systemic circulation. Intestinal permeability decreases rapidly following the ingestion of colostrum (Gillette and Filkins, 1966) possibly due to endogenous release of hydrocortisone or adrenocorticotropic hormone. Exogenous supplementation of either of these hormones in the mother 24 hours before her giving birth prevents increased permeability and colostrum absorption in the neonate (Gillette and Filkins, 1966).

A number of other factors may alter drug absorption from the small intestine in puppies and kittens. Gastric pH is neutral in the newborn; adult levels are not reached until some time after birth, depending on the species (Gillette and Filkins, 1966; Heimann, 1980). Increased gastric pH (achlorhydria) may decrease the absorption of many drugs that require disintegration and dissolution or are ionized in a less acidic environment (e.g., weak acids such as β-lactam antimicrobials) (Gillette and Filkins, 1966; Rane and Wilson, 1989). On the other hand, increased pH may facilitate absorption of weak bases that are generally not absorbed in adult animals (e.g., aminoglycosides). Milk diets can reduce absorption of some drugs by either decreasing gastric emptying or directly interacting with drugs. The "unstirred water layer" adjacent to the surface area of the mucosal cells is thicker in the neonate than the older animal and may limit the rate of absorption of some drugs (Heimann, 1980). Until biliary function matures, the absorption of fat-soluble drugs (e.g., griseofulvin and fat-soluble vitamins) may be impaired. Microbial colonization of the gastrointestinal tract may alter response to antimicrobial drugs undergoing intestinal metabolism or enterohepatic circulation (Jones, 1987; Morselli et al, 1983).

Absorption in puppies and kittens of parenterally administered drugs also varies from that in adults. The rate of absorption after intramuscular administration will increase with age as muscle mass and its accompanying blood flow increase and as vasomotor responses mature (Morselli et al, 1983). Because muscle mass is small in young animals, subcutaneous administration is frequently used. Again, variability in subcutaneous absorption rates can be anticipated with age. Less fat but more water may result in faster absorption in puppies and kittens compared with adults. Environmental temperature probably influences subcutaneous absorption, particularly in newborns whose thermoregulatory mechanisms are not fully functional

(Shifrine et al, 1973). Cold environments are likely to reduce subcutaneous drug absorption if the neonate is not provided warmth. The same is true for the animal in a state of hypothermia. Subcutaneous and intramuscular drug absorption may be impaired until body temperature approximates the norm.

Several nontraditional routes of administration can be used in puppies and kittens. Intraperitoneal administration can be a lifesaving method of blood and fluid administration, particularly in the newborn with inaccessible central veins. Isotonic fluid solutions are absorbed rapidly, and up to 70% of red blood cells is absorbed within 48 to 72 hours (Authement et al, 1987). Blood and fluid solutions can also be administered into the medullary cavity of large bones (Authement et al, 1987; Fiser, 1990). Flow is the rate-limiting factor in intraosseous absorption. Factors such as the size of the medullary space, vascular tortuosity, sinusoidal pressure, and total venous cross-sectional area determine flow rate (Fiser, 1990; Schoffstall et al, 1989). Absorption of volatile anesthetic agents from the respiratory tract is rapid because minute ventilation is greater (Robinson, 1983). Thus, young animals are more sensitive to the effects of gas anesthetic agents. Although percutaneous routes are not commonly used in drug administration, percutaneous absorption of drugs is likely to be greater in young animals. Percutaneous absorption is related directly to skin hydration, which is greatest in neonates. Topical administration of potentially toxic lipid-soluble drugs (e.g., hexachlorophene and organophosphates) should be avoided.

Absorption from the rectal mucosa is rapid in all ages. Thus rectal administration of drugs or fluids can be used. Limited data gathered from human infants indicate that peak plasma concentrations after rectal administration may be higher than those obtained by other routes (Morselli et al, 1983). The following situations are among those that indicate this route of administration: when venous catheterization is difficult; when there is need to reduce complications associated with intravenous administration (as with sedation or anesthesia); or when oral administration is undesirable (as with antiemetic agents). Several pediatric drugs intended for systemic effects are available as rectal suppositories.

DRUG DISTRIBUTION

The most important factors contributing to differences in drug distribution in puppies and kittens are differences in body fluid compartments and binding of drug to serum proteins. Body fluid compartments undergo profound changes with the growth of the neonate. Both the percentage of total body water and the ratio of compartmental volumes change with maturation. The percentage of total body water decreases with age, but the decrease is more substantial in the extracellular than the intracellular compartment (Table 3–2) (Sheng and Huggins, 1972). Daily fluid requirements are greater in puppies and kittens in part because a larger proportion of their body weight is represented by water. The sequelae of these body compartment differences depend on the normal distribution of the drug. Most water-soluble drugs are distributed to extracellular fluids. As a result, in puppies and kittens, the volume of fluid to which these drugs are distributed is increased compared with adults; plasma drug concentrations will decrease correspondingly. A similar pattern would be expected for unbound lipid-soluble drugs because they tend to be dis-

Table 3–2	Proportion of Body Weight Represented by Body Compartments in the Maturing Neonatal Puppy			
AGE	TOTAL BODY WATER*	EXTRACELLULAR FLUID*	INTRACELLULAR FLUID*	RATIO OF EXTRACELLULAR FLUID TO INTRACELLULAR FLUID
0 days	84	53	33	1.6
14 days	77	48	29	1.7
42 days	70	47	24	2.0
90 days	68	37	31	1.2
180 days	63	32	30	1.0
1 year	59	27	32	0.84
2–5 years	50	23	27	0.85

*Values represent percentages of total body weight.

tributed to total body water. Changes in the half-life of each drug will parallel changes in distribution. Although decreased plasma drug concentrations resulting from increased distribution may protect the young animal from potentially toxic drug concentrations (Davis et al, 1973), a poor therapeutic response may result from failure to generate therapeutic drug concentrations.

The proportion of body fat is smaller in puppies and kittens. Thus the distribution of lipid-soluble drugs that accumulate in fat (such as organophosphates, chlorinated hydrocarbons, and ultrashort thiobarbiturates) may be decreased proportionately. Although drug half-life decreases with the volume of tissues to which a drug is distributed, plasma drug concentrations may initially be toxic. Many lipid-soluble drugs have a high affinity for and are bound by plasma proteins, thus facilitating their movement through the body. Binding, however, limits their distribution from plasma to tissue. Predicting the distribution of highly protein-bound drugs is complicated. Serum concentrations of both serum albumin (the protein to which most drugs are bound) and α-glycoproteins (to which basic drugs preferentially bind) are decreased in the younger animals (Poffenbarger et al, 1990; Short, 1984). Protein binding of drugs also may be reduced because of differences in albumin structure or because drugs compete with endogenous substrates (such as bilirubin) for binding sites (Ehrnebo et al, 1971; Rane and Wilson, 1989). As drugs are displaced, the concentration of free, pharmacologically active drugs and the risk of adverse reactions increase. However, these changes are significant only if the drug is highly (i.e., more than 80%) protein bound and characterized by a small therapeutic index. While the concentration of free drug increases, that of total drug in the plasma tends to decrease since unbound drug is free to distribute into tissue (Ehrnebo et al, 1971). Consequently, drug half-life may increase, and longer dosing intervals may be indicated for potentially toxic drugs.

Differences in regional blood flow to the organs might cause clinically important changes in drug disposition in puppies and kittens. Differences in intraorgan distribution (e.g., renal blood flow) may cause clinically important differences in drug disposition (Horster et al, 1971; Horster and Valtin, 1971). Blood flow to vessel-rich tissues of the body (i.e., the heart and brain) is greater and faster (Robinson, 1983); the puppy and kitten are, thus, more susceptible to drug-induced cardiac and central nervous system toxic conditions. The potential for central nervous system poisoning is increased further because the blood-brain barrier is poorly developed immediately after birth. Increased permeability is a protective mechanism to the brain. Deficiency of nutritional fuels in stressful states (e.g., hypoglycemia, hypoxia, and acidosis) is prevented by allowing the movement of oxidizable substrates such as lactate into brain cells (Hellmann et al, 1982). Drugs normally incapable of reaching the adult brain are also, however, able to reach brain cells that are very susceptible to their effects.

DRUG METABOLISM

Drug elimination is limited in puppies and kittens (Green and Mirkin, 1984; Rane and Wilson, 1989; Short, 1984). In contrast to that in infants, hepatic metabolism of drugs is incompetent in the near-term and neonatal puppy (Inman and Yeary, 1971; Reiche, 1983). Both phase I (e.g., oxidative) and phase II (e.g., glucuronidation) reactions are reduced. The various pathways of metabolism mature at different rates. Progressive increases in phase I activity do not occur until day 25, and adult levels are not attained until 135 days postpartum. Generally, decreased hepatic drug metabolism is reflected in decreased plasma clearance, increased plasma half-life, and potentially toxic plasma drug concentrations. Dose reduction or prolongation of intervals may be indicated for some drugs (Table 3–3). Oral bioavailability of drugs characterized by significant first-pass metabolism in adults (e.g., propranolol) will probably be greater in puppies and kittens. Response to prodrugs—such as primidone, prednisone, and, potentially, methylprednisolone—may be reduced because of decreased formation of active drug products. Hepatic drug-metabolizing enzymes can be induced by phenobarbital and other drugs (Peters et al, 1971; Rane and Wilson, 1989). Phenobarbital has been used therapeutically to stimulate drug elimination in fetal or neonatal human infants (Sjoqvist, 1985). Nonhepatic drug metabolism, which also tends to be deficient in puppies and kittens, is important for the elimination of some drugs. Lower plasma cholinesterase levels can result in increased sensitivity to organophosphates, succinylcholine, and procaine (Robinson, 1983).

DRUG EXCRETION

Reduced renal excretion, characteristic of the puppy, results in decreased clearance of renally

Table 3–3	Drug Classes Affected by Decreased Hepatic Metabolism in Pediatric Animals

Antimicrobial agents*, †, ‡	Methylxanthines
Chloramphenicol	Caffeine*
Sulfonamides	Theophylline‡
Tetracyclines	Nonsteroidal antiinflammatory drugs*, ‡
Trimethoprim	Opiates*
Metronidazole	Phenothiazines*, ‡
Anticonvulsants*, ‡	Chlorpromazine
Phenobarbital	Salicylates*, ‡
Diazepam	
Primidone	
Barbiturates*, ‡	
Hexobarbital	
Sodium pentobarbital	
Central depressants*	
Local anesthetics*	
Procaine	

*Canine.
† Feline.
‡ Human.

excreted parent drugs and products of phase II drug metabolism. Glomerular filtration rate and tubular secretion increase sevenfold and fourfold, respectively, from day 2 to day 77 in puppies. These increases presumably reflect an increase in the permeability of the filtration apparatus. In human infants, renal clearance of a 15,000-molecular weight dextran is essentially zero compared with a 90% clearance in adults (Dorrestein et al, 1986). Changes in renal blood flow parallel those of nephron maturation (Cowan et al, 1980). Although the number of glomeruli remains constant throughout development, both glomerular filtration and renal tubular function progressively increase (Cowan et al, 1980; Horster and Valtin, 1971). The distribution of maturing nephrons also changes with age in the puppy (Horster et al, 1971). Morphologically, renal maturation follows a centrifugal pattern such that the most mature nephrons are located at the corticomedullary junction and the youngest in the subcapsular layer. Neither renal blood flow nor glomerular filtration rate increases appreciably until blood flow is redistributed to the cortices at 2 weeks of age (Cowan et al, 1980). As kidneys mature in the puppy, the rate of tubular growth appears to exceed glomerular growth (Horster et al, 1971). Glomerular-tubular balance of sodium and water is poorly developed in the neonate (Horster and Valtin, 1971). In contrast to filtration and secretion, renal tubular resorption appears to be similar to that in adults as long

as body fluids and electrolytes are maintained (Kleinman, 1978; Silva et al, 1987).

The sequelae of developmental changes in pediatric renal function include decreased clearance and prolonged half-life of drugs (primarily water-soluble drugs) excreted by the kidneys. Such a pattern has been shown for several drugs (Table 3–4). The effects of renal maturation on drug disposition can be complex. For example, serum gentamicin half-life was twice as long in 10-day-old puppies (80 minutes) as in 20-day-old puppies (45 minutes). Tubular damage does not, however, begin to occur until 20 days of age despite tubular accumulation of gentamicin,

Table 3–4	Drug Classes Affected by Decreased Renal Excretion in Pediatric Animals

Antimicrobial agents*, †, ‡	Antiarrhythmics‡
Aminoglycosides	Digoxin
Cephalosporins	Anesthetics*, ‡
Penicillins	Ketamine
Tetracyclines	
Sulfonamides	
Trimethoprim	
Anticonvulsants‡	
Diazepam	

*Canine.
†Feline.
‡Human.

which is similar to that in adults. The site of accumulation is primarily the inner cortex for the first 10 days of life and then the outer cortex as the cortical nephrons mature. A centrifugal pattern of nephron maturation in puppies appears to protect against gentamicin nephrotoxicity by ensuring that the outer cortical nephrons are probably protected from damage until maturation. Another difference in aminoglycoside toxicity in puppies and kittens is the lack of clinical indicators. Pathologic damage induced by gentamicin appears to be evidenced solely by histologic lesions. Plasma creatinine is normally decreased in pediatric individuals (Cowan et al, 1980) and thus does not increase above normal in the presence of gentamicin nephrotoxicity. Changes in urine sediment, osmolarity, glucose, and protein are not evident even when tubular damage is marked at 30 days (Cowan et al, 1980). Renal damage can occur in puppies and kittens treated with gentamicin at trough concentrations (0.21 μg/ml) that are well below those recommended to avoid nephrotoxicity (2 μg/ml). This fact, and the observation that peak plasma gentamicin concentrations (4.92 μg/ml) are much lower in young animals at a dose of 7.5 mg/kg once daily compared with the recommended targets (10 μg/ml) generally achieved in adult dogs at lower doses (4 mg/kg daily), suggest that a different dosing regimen should be used for aminoglycosides. Compared with current recommendations for adults, puppies may require a higher dose and longer interval for gentamicin administration. The gentamicin-dosing regimen for unhealthy puppies probably should be further modified because they are likely to be suffering from conditions that increase the potential for aminoglycosides-induced nephrotoxicity (e.g., dehydration). Further investigations are needed to establish safe yet effective doses of aminoglycosides for the puppy and kitten.

PLACENTAL TRANSFER OF DRUGS

Unique differences in drug disposition predispose the near-term fetus and neonate to adverse drug reactions. The idea of absolute placental selectivity has been replaced with the realization that essentially all drugs administered to a pregnant animal will be transferred across the placenta regardless of the degree of intimacy between fetal and placental membranes (Levy, 1981; Welsch, 1982). The response of the fetus and newborn to the individual drugs, however, varies for several reasons. Even the simplest

pharmacokinetic representation of the maternal-fetal system is complex, being composed of at least three compartments: maternal, placental, and fetal. The pharmacokinetics of each compartment is determined, in turn, by its own rates of absorption, distribution, metabolism, and elimination (Krauer and Krauer, 1991; Welsch, 1982). Furthermore, pregnancy is a dynamic state characterized by dramatic changes in placental and fetal growth and in the physiology of the pregnant animal. All pharmacokinetic processes change in concert with the progression of pregnancy. In addition, specific differences in placental drug transfer preclude extrapolation of information among species. Finally, the route of administration is also likely to determine the amount of placental transfer; routes that result in higher plasma peak concentrations (i.e., intravenous, intravenous infusion, and multiple dosing routes) are likely to expose the fetus to higher drug concentrations.

Although many factors determine the rate and extent of drug transfer across the placenta, lipid solubility of the drug and a steep maternal-fetal drug concentration gradient are probably the most important (Welsch, 1982). In general, nonionized compounds with high lipid solubility cross rapidly, whereas drugs with little lipid solubility cross slowly (Malkinson and Gehlmann, 1977). A number of drugs that are polar at physiologic pH can, however, cross the placenta rapidly. Differences in drug disposition compared with both pediatric animals and adults can lead to adverse reactions in the near-term fetus receiving drugs through the placenta. Thus higher concentrations of unbound and pharmacologically active drugs can be anticipated because fetal protein is generally less than that in more mature animals. The anatomic peculiarities of fetal circulation—that is, bypasses of the fetal liver and lungs—result in higher concentrations of drugs reaching the heart and brain. Although fetal metabolism of drugs can contribute to the ultimate elimination of drugs in the human neonate, the amount of drug-metabolizing enzymes present in near-term animals is negligible (Malkinson and Gehlmann, 1977).

Examples of drugs that have been shown to reach detectable and potentially clinically important concentrations in the human fetus include β-lactam antimicrobial agents, salicylates and other nonsteroidal antiinflammatory drugs, anticonvulsants (phenytoin and diazepam), local anesthetics such as lidocaine, gentamicin (in some species), and narcotic analgesic agents. Although drugs administered to pregnant animals may be detectable in the fetus, they may not produce clinically important effects.

DRUG THERAPY FOR THE NURSING ANIMAL

As is the fetus, the nursing animal is an inadvertent recipient of drugs administered to the mother. Most of the pertinent information in the veterinary literature is concerned with excretion of drugs in the milk of food animals; there appears to be no information for small animals. Studies in humans indicate that drugs diffuse into the milk from maternal circulation. Low molecular weight (less than 200), nonionized, highly lipid-soluble drugs that are minimally protein bound diffuse into the lactating mammary gland rapidly, whereas water-soluble drugs diffuse more slowly (Berlin, 1981). The pK$_a$ of a drug will largely determine its concentration in milk. Animal milk tends to be acidic compared with plasma pH. Thus, although a weakly basic drug may be nonionized in the plasma and thus more likely to diffuse into milk, it may become ionized and nondiffusible once in the milk. Such "ion trapping" can concentrate drugs in milk. The ratio of drug in milk to drug in plasma is predictable, being greater for weak bases and weak acids whose pK$_a$s differ from the pH of milk by 2 pH units (minus 2 for acids and plus 2 for bases) (Rasmussen, 1971). Generally, the amount of drug excreted in milk is less than 2% of the maternal dose (Berlin, 1981). Greater concentrations can, however, be expected if a drug is administered to the mother intravenously, as an intravenous infusion or in multiple doses.

Not all drugs ingested with milk during nursing will be absorbed from the gastrointestinal tract of the nursing animal. For example, milk may decrease the absorption of some drugs, and the pharmacokinetic properties of other drugs (i.e., aminoglycosides) preclude their absorption except in the very young. Not all drugs must, however, be absorbed to cause clinically important adverse effects. For example, antimicrobial agents can potentially alter the developing flora of the puppy's or kitten's alimentary tract (Jones, 1987; Smith, 1965). Thus it is prudent to avoid administration of potentially toxic drugs to the lactating mothers (Table 3–5).

OTHER EFFECTS OF DRUGS

Hematologic changes (polychromasia, anisocytosis, and target cells) occur in 8- to 12-week-old puppies treated with chloramphenicol at a

Table 3–5	Drugs to Avoid in the Preterm and Lactating Animal	
PRETERM	**LACTATING**
Glucocorticoids	Aminoglycosides
Aminoglycosides	Anticancer drugs
Anticancer drugs	Chloramphenicol
Organophosphates	Tetracyclines
Chlorinated hydrocarbons	
Tetracyclines	

dosage of 50 mg/kg given three times daily (Nara et al, 1982). Changes in white blood cells include basophilic granulation. Chloramphenicol does not, however, appear to affect in vitro or in vivo immune response (Nara et al, 1982). Puppies and kittens are more susceptible to hemolytic anemia after administration of drugs capable of oxidizing hemoglobin (Gross et al, 1967). Red blood cells are predisposed to methemoglobinemia, Heinz body formation, and in vitro hemolysis. Several mechanisms have been proposed, including decreased intracellular concentrations of antioxidants and radical scavengers.

Necrotic enterocolitis can be a complication of orally administered solutions (see "Enteral Hyperalimentation," later) and intravenously administered hypertonic solutions (e.g., sodium bicarbonate). Clinical signs reflect gastric distention and gastrointestinal hemorrhage. Vomitus may be bile stained; intestinal perforation can be a sequela.

Puppies and kittens cannot accommodate a large shift in osmolality as well as adults. Administration of hypertonic solutions to young animals can result in a variety of adverse effects. Intraventricular hemorrhage and necrotizing enterocolitis have occurred after intravenous administration of sodium bicarbonate and radiocontrast materials (Arant and Gooch, 1979; Turberville et al, 1976). Drug additives can contribute significantly to the osmolality of intravenous preparations (Ernst et al, 1983). Hyperosmolarity can also be a sequela of oral drug or fluid administration.

RESPONSE TO DRUGS

Just as pharmacokinetic differences in drug disposition can lead to adverse drug reactions due to increased or decreased plasma drug concentrations in puppies and kittens, pharmacodynamic differences can result in toxic or subtherapeutic responses, particularly by the cardiovascular system. Cardiovascular responses to anticholinergic and inotropic drugs are likely to be attenuated in the neonate. For example, increased heart rate after administration of β-adrenergic drugs (isoproterenol, dopamine, or dobutamine) does not reach adult levels until 9 to 10 weeks of age (Driscoll et al, 1979; Poffenbarger et al, 1990). Immaturity of innervation has been cited as a cause of decreased response to atropine (Robinson, 1983). The different components of the immune system mature at various ages (Poffenbarger et al, 1990; Shifrine et al, 1971). The thymus undergoes a 200-fold increase in size during the first 12 weeks of life in puppies and is probably a major determinant of immunocompetence. Although a humoral response is evident at birth, only IgM is produced. Neonatal puppies generally respond poorly to strong antigens (Shifrine et al, 1971). Thus, although puppies and kittens should not be expected to develop drug allergies, response to immunomodulators should be attenuated. In addition, immunoincompetence necessitates the use of bactericidal drugs.

SPECIFIC THERAPIES
Fluid Therapy

Puppies and kittens are predisposed to dehydration because extracellular fluid is increased, renal capacity to conserve water is decreased, the ratio of surface area to body weight is large, and fluid loss through immature skin is greater (Kerner and Sunshine, 1979). Brain volume normally decreases during the first 2 days of life in puppies and kittens; hypovolemic hypotension at this age predisposes the neonate to intracranial hemorrhage, particularly if followed by rapid volume replacement (Coulter et al, 1985; Turberville et al, 1976). Hyperosmolarity increases the risk of intracranial hemorrhage due to water loss in the brain (Arant and Gooch, 1979; Coulter et al, 1985; Turberville et al, 1976).

Fluid requirements are greater for puppies and kittens than for adults. Rates recommended for daily maintenance vary from 60 to 180 ml/kg/day (Mosier, 1981). Puppies and kittens cannot accommodate volume overload as efficiently as adults can. Although larger fluid amounts are indicated, care must be taken with both the amount and rate of fluid administration. Fluids can be administered by several routes. Crystalloids administered rectally should be isotonic; rapid rectal absorption of hyperosmotic solu-

tions can lead to life-threatening hyperosmolarity. Subcutaneous administration may be an acceptable route if small volumes of isotonic fluids are administered to puppies and kittens with normal hydration. Despite a less than ideal flow rate, intraosseous drug and fluid infusion can be lifesaving in hypovolemic, hypothermic, or very small animals whose central veins are not initially accessible for catheterization (Fiser, 1990; Schoffstall et al, 1989). The femur and humerus are preferred sites.

An 18- to 25-gauge hypodermic needle or an 18- to 22-gauge spinal needle can be used as an intraosseous catheter, depending on the size of the animal (Otto et al, 1989). In larger animals, a second catheter can be placed in a second medullary cavity to facilitate rapid fluid administration. Gravity flow can be used in smaller animals; for larger animals, multiple catheters and pressure-assisted flow may be necessary to administer sufficient volumes rapidly (Otto et al, 1989). Potential complications, which are uncommon in human patients, include infection (resulting in cellulitis, subcutaneous abscess, or osteomyelitis) and extravasation of fluid around the puncture site. Factors contributing to therapeutic failure with intraosseous administration include misplacement of the needle or catheter, bending of the needle or clotting of its contents, puncture throughout the bone, and replacement of the marrow cavity with fat or fibrous tissue (Fiser, 1990; Schoffstall et al, 1989).

Intravenous administration via an indwelling cephalic or jugular catheter is preferred for continuous fluid or drug administration in dehydrated, hypovolemic, and hypotensive animals. Fluids should be accurately measured before administration, and a pediatric minidrip set designed to deliver 60 drops per ml should be used. Infusion pumps will facilitate accurate administration. Fluids should be administered to the surgical pediatric animal weighing less than 10 kg at a rate of 4 ml/kg per hour; fluids lost during surgery are added to this volume (Robinson, 1983). Hypoglycemia can be prevented by the administration of 10% dextrose solution or of 5% dextrose in 0.25% normal saline solution (Robinson, 1983). Alternatively, dextrose sufficient to make a 5% (50 mg/ml) solution can be added to lactated Ringer's solution, although the resulting hypertonic solution should be administered cautiously. All fluid solutions and blood or blood components should be warmed to 37° C before administration.

Monitoring fluid therapy is critical; overhydration can lead to cardiovascular overload. Signs of vascular overload are difficult to detect.

Cardiomegaly, hepatic enlargement, and pulmonary edema are not generally conspicuous until respiratory distress occurs. In human infants, volume overload can lead to congestive heart failure associated with opening of the ductus arteriosus and intracranial hemorrhage (Rowe et al, 1986). Texture of body skin, moistness of mucous membranes, and degree of anophthalmia are relatively insensitive methods used to assess hydration status in puppies and kittens. Serial measurements of urinary output and urine concentration are used to assess fluid therapy in human infants (Rowe et al, 1986). Weighing the animal every 12 hours can also help establish hydration status if accurate gram scales are available; generally, puppies and kittens should gain 1 to 1.5 g for each pound of anticipated adult weight per day (Mosier, 1981).

Oral rehydration is recommended as the preferred therapy for dehydration caused by diarrhea in human pediatric patients (Greenwood and Davison, 1987; Hirschhorn, 1982). Sodium is cotransported with several substrates actively transported across the epithelium of the small intestine. Oral administration of sodium, potassium, bicarbonate, chloride, and glucose in a single solution is the sole method of hydration needed to maintain normal blood volume and electrolyte concentrations in human patients with cholera. The World Health Organization has formulated a solution consisting of (in mM per liter) 90 Na^+, 20 K^+, 30 HCO_3^-, 80 Cl^-, and 111 glucose (total osmolarity of 331) (Hirschhorn, 1982). The solution is suitable for most cases of diarrhea in human patients regardless of cause, electrolyte status, hydration status (short of shock), or patient age. The only requirement is that the patient be sufficiently conscious to drink. If vomiting occurs, the patient is allowed to rest, and administration is reinstituted more slowly. Recent modifications of this recipe include the addition of organic nonelectrolytes, such as amino acids, particularly for secretory diarrhea (Wapnir et al, 1988, 1990).

Parenteral Hyperalimentation

Nutritional maintenance is critical for the puppy and kitten. Studies performed with newborn puppies have shown that a 9-hour fast is accompanied by reduced hepatic adenosine 5'-triphosphate levels, suggesting that endogenous fuels are not capable of maintaining hepatic energy production. With a 24-hour fast, other oxidizable energy stores are depleted, total body metabolism decreases (Kliegman and Morton,

1987), and fuels available for cerebral metabolism are restricted (Kliegman et al, 1983). Cerebral hypoglycemia is considered (along with hypoxia, seizures, and acidosis) to be a major metabolic stress leading to the loss of autoregulation of cerebral blood flow (Anwar and Vannucci, 1988). Although parenteral hyperalimentation is a well-described therapeutic means of maintaining nutrition in adult dogs and cats, little information is available regarding its application to the puppy and kitten. Pediatric humans require 80 to 130 calories/kg per day (Kerner and Sunshine, 1979). Studies in humans have, however, shown that weight is gained if 60 to 88 calories/kg per day is provided in the form of glucose, amino acid, and lipid infusion (Kerner and Sunshine, 1979). Caloric requirements of the puppy and kitten increase with age, ranging from 120 kcal/kg at 1 week to 180 kcal/kg at 4 weeks (Mosier, 1981).

Glucose intolerance can occur in neonates after infusion of 10% dextrose solution. Hyperglycemia will result in osmotic diuresis and electrolyte loss. In human infants, an infusion rate of 6 to 8 mg/kg per minute should not be exceeded, particularly in low-birth-weight infants (Kerner and Sunshine, 1979). Rebound hypoglycemia can occur if a glucose infusion is stopped suddenly; infusion should be reinitiated as soon as possible. As the infant develops a tolerance for glucose, amino acids can be added. The recommended amount of enteral amino acid supplementation for optimal growth in human infants is 2 to 9 g/kg per day; a parenteral dose of 2 to 3 g/kg per day can be well tolerated. Free amino acids are preferred to casein hydrolysates and are generally infused as 2.0% to 2.5% solutions (Ernst et al, 1983). As with glucose infusion, amino acid infusions should be initiated at a low concentration (1%) and gradually increased as the patient develops tolerance to 2.5 g/kg per day (Ernst et al, 1983). The optimal amino acid mixture varies with the age of the human pediatric patient; it is likely that a similar variation exists for the puppy and kitten as hepatic enzymes mature. Hyperchloremia metabolic acidosis is recognized as a possible complication of amino acid infusion in human pediatric patients, particularly if synthetic preparations are administered. Although infusion of fat emulsion appears to be safe in human infants, decreased tolerance may occur in the premature infant as evidenced by increased serum triglycerides and free fatty acids. Term infants tolerate infusion much better. If the rate of infusion surpasses clearance, however, potential complications include altered pulmonary function and "overload" characterized by hyperlipemia, fever, lethargy, liver damage, and coagulopathy. Visual inspection of plasma turbidity and measurement of serum triglycerides can be used to monitor the development of overload (Ernst et al, 1983). Maintenance of sodium and potassium in human infants requires 2 to 3 mEq/kg per day (Ernst et al, 1983). Requirements may be even greater in the neonate. Daily requirements of calcium, phosphorus, and magnesium on a kg basis are 14 mEq, 2mM, and 0.25 to 0.50 mEq, respectively. Vitamins generally can be supplemented by the administration of 1 ml of a multivitamin infusion product with the addition of folate (50 μg), vitamin B_{12} (50 μg), and vitamin K_1 (0.25 to 0.5 mg) (Ernst et al, 1983).

Total parenteral nutrition must be monitored closely. Evaluation of serum chemistries can help determine success in meeting metabolic needs (Ernst et al, 1983). The growth of an animal can be evaluated by weight; in humans, measurements of subcutaneous fat and muscle mass (made with the aid of calipers) and skinfold thickness are indirect indicators of caloric and protein reserves (Ernst et al, 1983).

Enteral Hyperalimentation

Adverse effects may limit the use of enteral hyperalimentation in puppies and kittens. Necrotizing enterocolitis is a common complication of alimentary infusion of solutions in human infants. Direct mucosal irritation by hypertonic solutions has been cited as the primary cause. Formulas administered to 1- and 9-day-old puppies, however, resulted in hypertonic intestinal contents regardless of the tonicity of the infusion (Goldblum et al, 1981). Delayed gastric emptying and interference with absorption of nutrients may also contribute to the pathophysiology. Although the cause of necrotizing enterocolitis is not clear, administration of hypertonic solutions should be avoided in the neonate.

Antimicrobial Therapy

Just as in the adult, an appreciation of the chemotherapeutic triangle (i.e., the relationship between host, drug, and microorganism) is necessary for the appropriate use of antimicrobial agents in puppies and kittens. Several antimicrobial agents should be avoided. The use of chloramphenicol in neonates was discussed earlier. In addition to its effects on the hematopoietic system, chloramphenicol causes acute myocardial depression in humans (gray baby syndrome), possibly due to inhibition of protein synthesis or mitochondrial oxidation (Werner et al, 1985). Chloramphenicol should be avoided in puppies and kittens. Although tetracyclines may not be overtly toxic to puppies and kittens, chelation to calcium in growing bones can inhibit growth or cause deformities. Chelation in teeth results in enamel dysplasia and discoloration. A major consideration with the puppies and kittens receiving oral antimicrobial agents is the effect on colonization of the alimentary tract (Jones, 1987). Tetracycline (and particularly doxycycline) and other drugs that undergo enterohepatic circulation are more likely to disrupt the normal colonization of the alimentary tract.

β-Lactam antimicrobial agents are generally the drugs of choice for puppies and kittens, whenever possible. Although their half-lives are likely to be prolonged, these drugs tend to be safe because they are characterized by a wide therapeutic index. Higher doses may be necessary to achieve desired peak plasma drug concentrations because their distribution will be greater. Time interval of administration can be prolonged to compensate for the longer half-life. Parenteral absorption is preferred because bioavailability of oral preparations is not predictable. Caution is indicated when using high doses. β-Lactam antimicrobial agents can cause bleeding tendencies in animals with risk factors for bleeding (Babiak and Rybak, 1986). Although undocumented, bleeding tendencies have been noted in puppies receiving β-lactam antimicrobial agents. Caution is indicated when administering these drugs, particularly at high doses, to the very young.

The risks of giving aminoglycosides to puppies and kittens may outweigh the benefits of these drugs. The information necessary for appropriate dosing regimens for this age group simply is not available. Therapeutic drug monitoring should be used when possible to guide therapy. Higher doses and longer intervals may be necessary to achieve recommended peak and trough concentrations. Amikacin, which is less nephrotoxic (and more effective against *Pseudomonas* species) than gentamicin, should be used whenever possible. Quinolones are very effective and, for most animals, safe antimicrobial agents. They are characterized by excellent tissue distribution. These drugs should, however, be avoided in large- to giant-breed puppies younger than 18 months because of destructive lesions in the cartilage of long bones. Thus the author does not recommend these drugs as first choice for any puppy or kitten. The combination of a sulfonamide with trimethoprim or ormetoprim tends to be safe and effective for puppies and kittens. Doses may, however, need to be reduced for neonatal puppies because the half-life of some sulfonamides is very prolonged in this age group (Inman and Yeary, 1971). Potentiated sulfonamides should be avoided in animals with anemia.

Therapeutic indications for lincosamides and macrolides are limited for puppies and kittens. Because both groups of drugs undergo extensive

biliary secretion and enterohepatic circulation, they should not be used as first-choice antimicrobial agents. An exception can be made for *Mycoplasma* infections for which tylosin is the drug of choice. Metronidazole is a drug of choice for the treatment of anaerobic infections. Decreased clearance and prolonged half-life should be anticipated in puppies and kittens; lower doses and longer intervals may be necessary to avoid central nervous system toxicity.

Blood Component Therapy

Jorg Bucheler

Transfusion of blood components is a frequent necessity in the adjunctive treatment of puppies and kittens. Blood components commonly used are fresh whole blood, packed red blood cells, and plasma (Authement et al, 1987; Bucheler and Cotter, 1993). An indication for fresh whole blood is hemorrhagic shock with ongoing bleeding (simultaneous loss of red cells and plasma). Most other anemias require only erythrocytes and may be treated with transfusions of packed red cells (Cotter, 1988b). Bleeding disorders secondary to congenital coagulopathies are treated with plasma transfusions. Some veterinarians also believe that hypoproteinemic or septic puppies and kittens that were colostrum deprived benefit from plasma infusions.

PREREQUISITES FOR BLOOD DONORS

Donor dogs are usually large dogs that have a packed cell volume (PCV) over 40%, should not be on medication with the exception of heartworm-preventive and flea/tick-preventive medications in heartworm-infested and flea/tick-infested areas, and should not have been sensitized by prior transfusions or pregnancies (Cotter, 1988a; Pichler and Turnwald, 1985). Donors should be blood typed and be negative for dog erythrocyte antigens 1.1 and 1.2 (DEA 1.1 and 1.2) loci (Table 3–6) unless the recipient is to be typed as well (Bull, 1982; Dodds, 1984). Cat blood donors are usually large domestic short-haired cats of either gender. Their weight

should be more than 5 kg and their age optimally between 2 and 5 years. Donor cats must be kept strictly indoors because of the risk of viral infections. Cats should have a PCV over 35% (Pichler and Turnwald, 1985). Donors should be blood typed and have type A blood (see Table 3–6). Simple blood typing kits for dogs and cats are now commercially available.

Blood donors should have periodic examinations (e.g., complete blood counts, serum chemistry profiles, urinalyses, and fecal examinations). Donor dogs should be serologically negative for *Dirofilaria immitis*, *Ehrlichia* species, Rocky Mountain spotted fever, Lyme disease, *Babesia canis*, *Haemobartonella canis*, and *Brucella*

Table 3–6	Blood Groups of Dogs and Cats	
DOG BLOOD GROUPS	**CAT BLOOD GROUPS**
DEA 1.1*	Type A
DEA 1.2*	Type B
DEA 3	Type AB
DEA 4	
DEA 5	
DEA 6	
DEA 7*	

*All blood group antigens are capable of stimulating formation of specific antibodies; however, these antigens have the greatest potential for antigenic stimulation. Cats have naturally occurring antibodies, rendering them susceptible to transfusion reactions even during the first one.

DEA = dog erythrocyte antigen.

canis (Authement et al, 1987; Cotter, 1988b; Pichler and Turnwald, 1985). Donor cats should be serologically negative for *Toxoplasma gondii*, *Haemobartonella felis* via polymerase chain reaction, *Ehrlichia* species, dirofilariasis, feline coronavirus titers (risk for feline infectious peritonitis), feline leukemia virus infection, and feline immunodeficiency virus infection (Bucheler and Cotter, 1993; Cotter, 1988b; Pichler and Turnwald, 1985). Donors should be well vaccinated, maintained on a good nutritional feeding program, and kept free of fleas, ticks, and intestinal parasites, particularly hookworms and *Giardia* and *Cryptosporidium* species.

BLOOD COLLECTION PROCEDURE

There are various sites available from which to draw blood from dog and cat donors. The safest and most accessible site for blood collection is the external jugular vein. The amount of blood that can be safely withdrawn via the external jugular vein from a donor dog or cat is up to 22 ml/kg (10 ml/lb) body weight every 2 to 3 weeks (Authement et al, 1987; Greene, 1980; Potkay and Zinn, 1969). This usually amounts to approximately 450 ml of blood taken from a large canine donor and 50 ml taken from a cat. Donors may be minimally restrained or sedated (Cotter, 1988a) and the venipuncture site surgically prepared. A hemostat is placed over the tubing of the plastic blood-collecting bag and is removed only after the external jugular vein has been entered. Venipuncture should be clean with rapid blood flow to minimize activation of platelets and clotting factors and to minimize tissue thromboplastin contamination (Authement et al, 1987). When the full blood volume is collected, the collecting tube is reclamped before the needle is removed from the external jugular vein. Direct pressure should be applied over the collection site for 5 to 10 minutes after collection of blood for hemostasis.

Some cats appear pale after blood collection, probably as a result of a combination of hypovolemia and sedation (Cotter, 1988a). For this reason, an intravenous infusion of 100 ml of lactated Ringer's solution is given to donor cats immediately after blood is drawn (Bucheler and Cotter, 1993). This infusion is usually not necessary for most donor dogs.

Fresh Whole Blood Collection

Blood collected should be anticoagulated with citrate-phosphate-adenine (CPD-A$_1$) solution or, less preferably, acid-citrate-dextrose (ACD) solution (Authement et al, 1987; Pichler and Turnwald, 1985). The ratio of the volume of CPD-A$_1$ or ACD anticoagulant to blood is 1:7 for storage of blood components (canine blood in CPD-A$_1$ has a storage life of 35 days versus 21 days for ACD at 1° to 6° C) (Authement et al, 1987; Bucheler and Cotter, 1994; Greene, 1980; Smith et al, 1978). If blood is given immediately after collection, a more diluted ratio of 1:10 of anticoagulant to blood can be used. If heparin is used, 625 units is used per 50 ml of blood collected (Authement et al, 1987). Citrate is preferred because citrate is metabolized more quickly and platelet function is preserved. Heparin is not recommended as an anticoagulant because red blood cells cannot be stored and platelet function is abnormal.

Procedurally, whole blood is collected in 450-ml CPD-A$_1$ or ACD plastic blood-collecting bags to appropriate volume, with swirling of blood during collection to ensure adequate mixing with anticoagulant. To monitor the volume of blood being withdrawn, a triple beam balance scale or digital electronic scale may be used. One milliliter of blood weighs approximately 1 g, so a unit containing 450 ml of blood should weigh 450 g plus the weight of the container with the anticoagulant (Widmann, 1985). After collection, the collecting tube is tied off at the needle end and blood left in the tube is stripped using a tube stripper twice, allowing the collected blood to be mixed with anticoagulant in the collecting bag. The unit of collected blood is then used immediately or stored at appropriate temperature for later use.

If a small volume of whole blood is needed for immediate use, 7 ml of CPD-A$_1$ or ACD anticoagulant may be drawn into a 50-ml plastic syringe and the rest filled with blood (Cotter, 1988a). Any open system such as a plastic syringe or bag entered with a needle should be used within 24 hours.

Packed Red Blood Cells and Plasma Collection

After whole blood collection, one can proceed with separating the fresh whole blood into packed red cells and plasma. The best way to have these blood components available, in most veterinary practices, is to work cooperatively with a local human blood bank facility. Blood collected in plastic blood-collecting bags with CPD-A$_1$ or ACD anticoagulant is transported directly to the local blood bank facility in a ice-filled cooler; the blood should not be allowed to come in contact with the ice (Authement et al, 1987). At the blood bank facility, the blood-filled CPD-A$_1$ or ACD bags will be centrifuged at 1° to 6° C in a centrifuge at a speed (rpm) of 3000 to 5000 g for 5 to 40 minutes (methodology varies with the protocol used by the local blood bank). After centrifugation, extracted plasma is transferred into a satellite storage container. The red blood cells remaining after extraction of the plasma are then labeled as packed red blood cells and can be stored for later use.

Some clinicians freeze plasma in individual boxes (available at local blood banks) because the plastic blood-collecting bags are fragile at cold temperatures and may crack with manipulation (Authement et al, 1987). Fresh-frozen plasma is plasma that is frozen within 6 hours from the time of blood collection and is used primarily to supply clotting factors (for treatment of hemophilia A, von Willebrand's disease, rodenticide toxicity, and disseminated intravascular coagulation). It should be frozen (stored) at −19° to −70° C for optimal preservation of clotting factors for 1 year or in a household freezer for 3 months. Frozen plasma is plasma that is frozen more than 6 hours from the time of collection or is fresh-frozen plasma that is older than 1 year. It is not used for supplying more labile factors such as for the treatment of hemophilia A, von Willebrand's disease, and disseminated intravascular coagulation, although it can be used in the treatment of hemophilia B (factor IX required) or rodenticide toxicity (factors II, VII, IX, and X required) and has a shelf life of up to 5 years if stored in a similar manner as fresh-frozen plasma.

CROSSMATCHING PROCEDURES

The best alternative to typing the blood of in-house donors for recipient animals is crossmatching donor and recipient blood (Dodds, 1978). Incompatibilities revealed by crossmatching indicate earlier sensitization of the recipient or naturally occurring isoantibodies. Puppies and kittens needing repeated transfusions should be given blood from donors with which they are blood-type and crossmatch compatible.

Crossmatching is performed for major or minor compatibilities (Turnwald and Pichler, 1985). The major crossmatch, performed with donor cells and recipient serum, determines whether the recipient has antibodies against donor cells. The minor crossmatch, using recipient cells and donor serum, detects antibodies in donor serum against recipient cells. Both tests are performed on fresh blood.

Blood samples (approximately 3 ml) are collected from donor and recipient animals and allowed to clot. After centrifugation, the serum is withdrawn and placed in separate tubes. The clots are then gently broken down, and 0.3 ml of cells is aspirated from each sample and added to separate tubes, each containing 9.7 ml of normal saline solution. Alternatively, one can collect 3 ml of blood in ethylenediamine tetraacetic acid tubes and separate red cells after centrifugation.

Cells should be washed at least once with the normal saline solution to remove plasma and prevent formation of small fibrin clots (Widmann, 1985). After cell washing, supernatant fluid is discarded and cells are resuspended to a dilution of 0.3 ml of cells to 9.7 ml of normal saline solution.

The major crossmatch is performed by adding 0.1 ml of recipient serum to 0.1 ml of donor red cell suspension. The minor crossmatch is performed by adding 0.1 ml of donor serum to 0.1 ml of recipient red cell suspension. A control reaction test is performed using recipient serum and washed cells. Optimally, each test is done in triplicate and incubated for 15 minutes—one set at 37° C (98.6° F), one set at room temperature, and one set at 4° C (39.2° F). Incubation at various temperatures may be beneficial because incompatibility reactions can occur over a range of temperatures (Turnwald and Pichler, 1985). Canine blood group antibodies are often more hemolytic than agglutinating, and some clinicians believe it beneficial to add a drop of rabbit complement to the crossmatch tubes.

After incubation, each tube is centrifuged for 1 minute at 280 g, and the supernatant fluid is examined for hemolysis. The tubes are then gently tapped to check for agglutination. Compatible crossmatches do not show agglutination or hemolysis. If overt agglutination is not noted, a small amount of the suspended material is transferred to a clean glass slide and microscopically examined at low power. Any degree of agglutination or hemolysis in the major crossmatch is considered evidence of incompatibility, indicating that transfusion should not be performed. If slight agglutination or hemolysis is detected in the minor crossmatch, transfusion can be performed on an emergency basis (Turnwald and Pichler, 1985).

BLOOD COMPONENTS ADMINISTRATION

Stored blood components should be warmed to room temperature before administration to prevent inducing hypothermia in the recipient. To be warmed, blood components can be passed through coils of transfusion tubing immersed in a water bath maintained at 37° to 38° C. Alternatively, a blood component container can be placed in a water bath or dry incubator maintained at that temperature, and frozen plasma can be warmed slowly in a microwave oven (Dula et al, 1981; Hurst et al, 1987). Excessive heat should not be used to accelerate warming of blood components because fibrinogen precipitates at 50° C (122° F) and autoagglutination occurs when temperatures exceed 45° C (113° F).

If blood component containers have been opened or entered with a needle or warmed to 10° C (50° F) or more, the contents should be given within 4 hours to reduce the possibility of bacterial growth (Cotter, 1988a). Warmed blood components should not be returned to storage.

For microwave thawing of frozen plasma, the plasma containers are placed in a water bath (37° C) for 60 seconds (Hurst et al, 1987). The plasma containers are then dried with a towel, enclosed in an outer plastic bag, and placed in the center of a microwave oven. The oven is set at its highest setting (700 W). The plasma containers are irradiated with microwaves for intervals of 10 seconds. Between exposures to microwaves, the plasma containers are agitated by hand for approximately 3 to 5 seconds. This procedure is continued until single pieces of ice less than 1 cm long remain. The containers are then removed from the microwave oven and inverted several times until no frozen particles remain (approximately 30 seconds).

Appropriate filters and administration sets should be used when blood components are transfused. Filters are designed to retain blood clots and leukocyte/platelet aggregates because pulmonary microembolism is a potential complication after transfusion of blood components (Authement et al, 1987). Most transfusions of blood components require the 170-μm-size filter. Blood in a syringe also can be given through a standard blood transfusion set or an infusion set with a side-arm Luer connector for a syringe.

Blood components can be given intravenously to large dogs by the cephalic or external jugular veins through a 20-gauge indwelling catheter. Smaller dogs and large cats can be infused by cephalic or external jugular veins through a 22-gauge indwelling catheter. Young puppies and kittens can be transfused by cephalic or external jugular veins with 23-gauge infusion sets. To reduce viscosity when a small-bore needle is used, blood components can be mixed with normal saline solution before and during infusion. The use of fluid solutions other than normal saline is not recommended (Greene, 1982).

Hypothermic, dehydrated puppies and kittens (younger than 4 months), in which venipuncture is often impossible, can be transfused by an intraosseous route, which is considered better than the intraperitoneal route (Turnwald and Pichler, 1985). Blood components may be given into the intramedullary space of the femur or humerus through a 20-gauge 1.5-inch, 20-gauge 2.5-inch, or 18-gauge 3.5-inch spinal needle; appropriate needle size and length vary with the size and age of the animal transfused. The spinal needle is inserted aseptically parallel to the long axis of the bone, through the trochanteric fossa of the femur or the greater tubercle of the humerus, and into the respective medullary space (Fig. 3–1). The stylet within the needle should not be withdrawn until immediately before the infusion of blood components (Turnwald and Pichler, 1985). Absorption of the infused blood components is rapid (Clark and Woodley, 1959; Corley, 1963). The spinal needle within the intramedullary space should be removed after infusion or left in place for up to 72 hours if needed further. The intraperitoneal route results in approximately 50% absorption of blood components into the systemic circulation within 24 hours and 70% within 48 to 72 hours (Clark and Woodley, 1959). Because of this inefficient rate of absorption, the intraperitoneal route is discouraged.

Before the infusion of blood components, baseline values for such variables as body weight and temperature, pulse and respiratory rate, mucous membrane color, PCV, and total plasma protein concentration should be obtained from

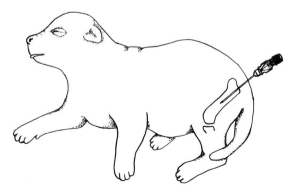

Figure 3–1. Spinal needle placement for intraosseous infusion of blood components into the medullary space of the femur of a recipient puppy. The needle placement would be similar for a recipient kitten.

the recipient. A slow infusion rate of 1 ml/kg body weight is used for a 15- to 30-minute period, during which the recipient should be watched carefully for transfusion reactions (Turnwald and Pichler, 1985). With a slow initial infusion rate, a minimal amount of incompatible blood component is administered in the event that a recipient displays an immediate reaction. If the recipient has no problems after the initial period, the rate of infusion can be increased. After the transfusion, one should check a blood sample for PCV increases and possible presence of hemoglobinemia.

The recommended infusion rate of whole blood in dogs and cats is 22 ml/kg per day (Greene, 1982). This guideline should be flexible because the infusion rate depends on the physical condition and hydration status of the recipient. With a hypovolemic recipient, up to 22 ml/kg per hour is acceptable (Greene, 1982). Circulatory overload, a continuing problem in normovolemic recipients, may be compounded in a recipient with cardiac or renal failure, as evidenced by urticaria, coughing, vomiting, prominent jugular veins, and signs of pulmonary edema. Dogs or cats in cardiac failure may not tolerate infusion rates exceeding 4 ml/kg per hour and therefore require careful monitoring of central venous pressure (Authement et al, 1987; Greene, 1982). Circulatory overload also can be induced easily in transfusing anemic cats, especially young kittens (Cotter, 1988b).

The amount of whole blood necessary for infusion can be estimated by using the donor's and recipient's hematocrits and the recipient's body weight in kilograms, as follows (Greene, 1982):

$$\text{ml of donor blood in anticoagulant} = 2.2 \times \text{recipient weight in kg} \times 40 \text{ (dog) or } 30 \text{ (cat)} \times \frac{\text{hematocrit desired minus hematocrit of recipient}}{\text{hematocrit of donor blood in anticoagulant}}$$

Alternatively, a simple guideline is that 2.2 ml/kg of whole blood and 1.1 ml/kg of packed red cells raises the PCV by 1% when the PCV of the transfused blood is 40% (Greene, 1982).

Packed red blood cells (PCV of 60% to 80%) are infused into the recipient in the same manner as whole blood (Masouredis, 1983). A disadvantage in their use is the slower infusion rate, which can be a problem when a large volume of blood must be infused at a rapid rate. The slower rate of infusion can be overcome by diluting the packed red blood cells with normal saline solution immediately before infusion. When dilution is required, normal saline solu-

tion can be added at a ratio of 0.5 to 1.0 ml of saline solution to 1 ml of packed red blood cells (Turnwald and Pichler, 1985). The amount of normal saline solution to be added for infusion varies with the recipient's circulatory function and hydration status (Cotter, 1988b).

If fresh plasma, fresh-frozen plasma, or frozen plasma is being administered for active bleeding owing to clotting factor deficiencies, a suggested dose is 6 to 10 ml/kg body weight 2 or 3 times a day for 3 to 5 days or until bleeding is controlled (Authement et al, 1987; Dodds, 1978).

COMPLICATIONS OF BLOOD COMPONENT THERAPY

Although complications of blood component transfusions are relatively rare in puppies and kittens, they do occur. Hemolytic reactions result from incompatible red blood cells given to a recipient that has developed antibodies from prior sensitization or transfusion. Type B cats generally have strong preformed anti-A antibodies and can react by hemolysis to the first transfusion (Cotter, 1988b; Bucheler, 1997). Most hemolytic reactions in dogs are delayed and are evident only because of shorter red blood cell survival after transfusion and the development of a positive result to a direct Coombs' test (Tangner, 1982). These reactions can be prevented by blood typing donor dogs, using donors that are negative for DEA 1.1 and DEA 1.2, and performing crossmatching for recipients that have received prior transfusions (Authement et al, 1987). Hemolysis can also occur as a result of overheating or freezing of blood components; concurrent administration of hypotonic solutions; mechanical damage of red blood cells caused by use of faulty equipment during collection, storage, and administration; or infusion under pressure through a small-bore needle or catheter or a plugged filter (Cotter, 1988b).

Adverse effects of leukocyte, platelet, and plasma protein incompatibilities include fever, neurologic signs, vomiting, and urticaria (Greene, 1980). Pretreatment with diphenhydramine hydrochloride at a dosage of 2 to 4 mg/kg body weight and prednisolone at 2 to 4 mg/kg 20 to 40 minutes before transfusion may reduce these reactions (Tangner, 1982). If these reactions become evident during the transfusion, the infusion rate should be slowed, and diphenhydramine hydrochloride and prednisolone should be administered intravenously (Turnwald and Pichler, 1985).

Febrile reactions to infused blood components occur occasionally and are usually mild. These reactions must be differentiated from sepsis caused by contaminated blood components, resulting in severe shock-like reaction (Cotter, 1988b). If the latter occurs, the infusion is stopped, a Gram's stain and culture are performed on the transfused blood component, and supportive care and antimicrobial agents are given. Septic reactions are very rare if aseptic collection, proper storage, and administration are used.

Hypocalcemia can occur as a result of rapid administration of whole blood or, especially, plasma (Cotter, 1988b). Signs associated with the hypocalcemia include restlessness, vomiting, tremors, seizures, and cardiac arrhythmias. Hypocalcemia is most likely to occur in small animals with severe hepatic disease or hypothermia or when excess citrate anticoagulant is present in the plasma administered (Wintrobe et al, 1981). The transfusion should be stopped temporarily; the signs of hypocalcemia usually subside quickly so that intravenous calcium is rarely needed (Cotter, 1988b). Other rare adverse reactions include hypothermia (rapid transfusion of cold blood products), neurologic signs (young animals with hepatopathies may not be able to rapidly detoxify the often increased ammonia levels in stored blood), circulatory overload, and acidosis (stored blood may have a pH of <6.5) (Bucheler, 1997).

NEONATAL ISOERYTHROLYSIS

Neonatal isoerythrolysis is an immunogenetic disorder resulting from damage to a kitten's red blood cells by maternal colostrally acquired antibodies (Cain and Suzuki, 1985; Gandolfi, 1988; Hubler et al, 1987; Jonsson et al, 1990; McClain et al, 1988). The overall incidence of neonatal isoerythrolysis in feline populations is unknown. It is probably low among domestic short-haired cats but may be responsible for up to 50% of neonatal deaths in certain purebred catteries where the parents have not been blood typed (Giger, 1990, 1991; Giger et al, 1997). Neonatal isoerythrolysis is a disorder that occurs in the first days of life primarily because this is the only time that significant amounts of exogenous antibody can gain access to the body in natural situations. Ingestion of colostral antibody directed against surface antigens on neonatal red blood cells results in accelerated removal or destruction of circulating red blood cells, leading to anemia and other secondary problems.

Feline Blood Groups

Much knowledge about feline blood groups and transfusion medicine has been gained over the last 10 years (Andrews et al, 1992; Bucheler, 1990; Bucheler and Giger, 1990, 1993; Griot-Wenk et al, 1993; Griot-Wenk and Giger, 1995). Blood types, also known as blood groups, are species-specific simply inherited antigenic epitopes on the surface of erythrocytes (see Table 3–6) (Giger et al, 1991b). The antigens produced by a group of allelic genes form a blood group system. Individuals that lack a blood type may have naturally occurring antibodies or may generate antibodies on exposure to the antigens. Since the early 1950s, researchers have described two major feline blood types known as A and B. The blood type predominantly found is type A (Auer and Bell, 1981; Eyquem et al, 1962; Giger et al, 1991a). A few cats were found to carry both antigens on their erythrocytes (blood type AB) (Griot-Wenk et al, 1996).

Recent surveys of feline blood type frequencies in the United States demonstrate a low frequency of type B blood in domestic short-haired cats (on average, 1.7% but reaching 4.7% in some regions) (Giger and Casal, 1997; Giger et al, 1991a,b). Siamese cats, those related to the Siamese (Tonkinese, Oriental short-haired, Burmese), and American short-haired cats (related to the domestic short-haired) have only type A blood. In contrast, breeds such as the Persian, British short-haired, Abyssinian, Birman, Devon Rex, Himalayan, and Somali breeds have type B frequencies ranging from 15% to 59% (Table 3–7). Subsequently, a few type AB cats were found, but their frequency is considered extremely low (Griot-Wenk and Giger, 1995; Griot-Wenk et al, 1996).

Genetic Profile

Feline blood types A and B are red blood cell phenotypes due to the action of two different alleles at the same autosomal gene locus. A is completely dominant over B; therefore, cats with type A blood have the genotype AA or AB (Giger et al, 1991a). The rare blood type AB could be explained by the action of a third allele at the same gene locus that is recessive to A and dominant over B (Griot-Wenk et al, 1996). Only homozygous BB cats express blood type B. The gene frequencies for A and B alleles can be estimated in certain breeds using the Hardy-Weinberg law. Assuming random mating, the frequency of the B allele is estimated as the

Table 3–7	Frequencies of Types A and B Blood in Cats in the United States		
BREED	NO. OF CATS	TYPE A (%)	TYPE B (%)
Abyssinian	194	81	19
Birman	216	82	18
British short-haired	85	41	59
Devon Rex	100	57	43
Himalayan	35	80	20
Persian	170	76	24
Scottish fold	27	85	15
Somali	27	78	22
Others, group A*	41	80	20
Others, group B†	205	100	0
Domestic short-haired	1072	99	1

*Maine Coon, Norwegian Forest, Sphinx, Cornish Rex.

†American short-haired, Burmese, Oriental short-haired, Siamese, Tonkinese, Russian Blue.

Data from Bucheler J: Type A and B blood types and their clinical importance [doctoral thesis]. Berlin, Free University of Berlin, 1990.

square root of the frequency of type B cats. In Persians, 24% of which have type B blood, the gene frequency of B (0.49) is nearly equal to the frequency of A. In British short-haired cats, the frequency of the B allele is higher (0.77) (Bucheler, 1990). Because of breeding practices and chance events, the B allele frequency may vary greatly between catteries, purebred lines, and parts of the world.

Because all tested type B cats have strong naturally occurring alloantibodies, fatal neonatal isoerythrolysis can occur in type A offspring of type B queens bred to type A males (Bucheler and Giger, 1993). Matings of two type B cats will produce only type B offspring. If the father has the genotype AA, all of the offspring are heterozygous (AB) and at risk for developing neonatal isoerythrolysis. If the father has the genotype AB, one half of the offspring will have the genotype AB and are at risk for neonatal isoerythrolysis.

Assuming the equilibrium of the Hardy-Weinberg law, the proportion of incompatible matings can be estimated. In domestic short-haired cats, only 0.25% of matings at random would produce litters at risk. On the other hand, in purebred cats such as Persians or Abyssinians, the risk of incompatible matings ranges between 14% and 25% (Bucheler, 1990).

Neonatal Antibodies

All type B cats have strong hemagglutinin and hemolysin, with serum titers ranging from a 1:64 to 1:2064 ratio against type A cells, whereas type A cats have low anti-B antibody

titers (typically only a 1:2 ratio and rarely reaching a 1:32 ratio) (Bucheler and Giger, 1993). The antibodies are naturally occurring, which means that these antibodies are present without prior sensitization by transfusion or pregnancy, leaving even primiparous queens at risk of having litters with neonatal isoerythrolysis.

Neonatal kittens acquire maternal antibodies of the IgG class via colostrum during the first 2 days of life (Casal et al, 1996; Giger and Casal, 1997). Between 6 and 8 weeks of age, kittens begin to produce their own alloantibodies, and alloantibody titers reach their maximum level at a few months of age (Bucheler and Giger, 1993). In contrast to other species, no previous transfusion or pregnancy is required for the production of alloantibodies in cats.

The feline placenta is of the endotheliochorial type and only allows small and insignificant passage of maternal antibodies, which prevents the fetus from harm. If the kitten has type A or AB and the queen has type B, colostral antibodies will bind to and lyse red blood cells in the newborn (Bucheler, 1990). The hemolysis may occur intravascularly as well as extravascularly and may cause anemia, chromoproteinuric nephropathy, and other organ failure as well as disseminated intravascular coagulation (Giger, 1990, 1991).

Clinical Findings

Clinical signs of neonatal isoerythrolysis relate to the degree and rapidity of onset of anemia and hemolysis. The factors that determine the severity of hemolysis have not been identified, and large variations in clinical signs may be observed in the same litter, suggesting that differences in colostral antibody uptake are responsible for this high variability (Giger, 1990, 1991).

Kittens are born healthy and start nursing vigorously. As a result of colostrum intake, kittens start to show clinical signs of illness within hours to days. Some kittens die peracutely within the first few hours without showing any clinical signs. Other kittens may stop nursing during the first 3 days of life and fail to thrive (Giger, 1990, 1991). The key clinical finding is dark red-brown urine, indicating severe hemoglobinuria. Affected kittens may develop icterus and anemia, continue to fade, and die during the first week of life. Accompanying signs are pallor of the mucous membranes and those referable to decreased oxygenation such as lethargy, weakness, tachypnea, tachycardia, collapse, and death. Secondary problems may include metabolic acidosis and hypoglycemia resulting from altered nutrition (Giger, 1990, 1991).

Surviving kittens may develop a tail-tip necrosis with sloughing of the distal part of the tail between 3 days and 2 weeks of age (Bridle and Littlewood, 1998; Giger, 1990). It appears to be possible that cold-reacting IgM antibodies lead to hemagglutination in peripheral capillaries as well as localized thrombus formation and ischemic necrosis. Some kittens may suffer from a subclinical progression and continue to nurse, thrive, and show no obvious clinical signs but may exhibit some laboratory abnormalities such as a positive Coombs' test and mild to moderate anemia.

DIAGNOSIS

As the hallmark clinical finding of neonatal isoerythrolysis is hemoglobinuria, breeders and veterinarians are urged to collect urine manually from kittens that fade in order to determine the urine color and presence of hemoglobin. Urine may be obtained by gently stroking the perineal areas with a wet warm cloth or dry soft tissue paper, mimicking the queen's tongue (anogenital reflex) (Hoskins, 1990).

Pathologic findings in kittens with neonatal isoerythrolysis may vary depending on the time of death. The urinary bladder may be filled with dark red-brown urine and precipitated hemoglobin. The spleen may be enlarged, and the body may appear icteric. Marked erythrophagocytosis and extramedullary hematopoiesis are seen in liver and spleen, and there may be evidence of acute tubular necrosis in the kidneys.

The systemic effects of immune-mediated hemolysis, disseminated intravascular coagulation, acute renal failure, and anemia are likely causes of fatal neonatal isoerythrolysis.

Management

Kittens showing clinical signs of neonatal isoerythrolysis should be immediately removed from their mothers as soon as the first clinical signs are recognized in order to prevent any further absorption of maternal antibodies by the kitten. In kittens, the duration of transfer of maternal antibodies appears to be approximately 12 to 16 hours. Thus, kittens at risk for neonatal isoerythrolysis need only be removed from the queen during the first 16 to 24 hours of life to avoid incompatibility. They should be foster nursed either by tube-feeding a commercial milk replacer or by placing the kitten with another queen who has type A blood.

If anemia is severe and worsening, replacement red blood cells are necessary to provide oxygenation to the tissues. A key consideration with regard to transfusion is the necessity of identifying a red blood cell that is compatible with the type B queen's serum/colostral antibody as this is the only antibody that is circulating in the type A kitten. Transfusion of type A cells simply adds more vulnerable cells to the milieu that are destroyed by the maternal colostral antibodies, further compounding secondary complications. The ideal blood donor would be the queen as she obviously will not react with her own antibody. Severely anemic kittens may benefit from a transfusion of washed type B blood during the first 3 days of life, which may be administered by intraosseous transfusion (Giger, 1991). A total of 2 to 3 ml of the queen's blood should be collected in ethylenediamine tetraacetic acid or heparin and centrifuged at 1000 RPM for 1 minute; the supernatant should then be discarded. The blood is restored to its previous volume with normal saline solution and again centrifuged. After the supernatant is discarded the cells are diluted with an equal volume of normal saline solution, the blood can be transfused via a 22-gauge spinal needle into the trochanteric fossa of the femur.

After transfusion, the packed cell volume may again decline for several days as a result of continued destruction of the kitten's cells and shortened lifespan of the transfused cells. The kitten starts to form its own anti-B alloantibodies soon after birth. Therefore, if a kitten requires another transfusion after 5 days postpartum, one should consider administering washed type A blood. In addition to transfusions, kittens with neonatal isoerythrolysis should receive intensive supportive care to maintain fluid and electrolyte status, nutritional status, and normothermia. Despite removing the kittens as soon as the first clinical signs appear, mortality as a result of neonatal isoerythrolysis can be considerable.

Prevention

Neonatal isoerythrolysis is best prevented by avoiding incompatible matings between type B queens and type A toms. Blood typing of all cats in catteries is recommended to ensure blood compatibility. A simple in-practice blood typing card test is available from DMS Laboratories (2 Darts Mill Road, Flemington, NJ 08822; 1-800-567-4367). Placenta blood could be used to determine the kitten's blood type or to perform a crossmatch with serum from the queen. Because of the type B queen's high hemagglutinin titers, a Coombs' reagent is not required for crossmatching (Bucheler and Giger, 1993). A sample protocol for major crossmatching of feline blood types might include the following steps:

1. Label a small tube for donor cells and another tube for the control sample.
2. Fill both tubes 70% to 80% full with normal saline solution.
3. Add one drop of donor blood to each test tube.
4. Centrifuge the test tubes for 15 seconds at 3500 RPM and discard the supernatant.
5. Add two drops of the queen's plasma or serum to the donor test tube and two drops of normal saline solution to the control test tube.
6. Centrifuge the test tubes and discard the supernatant.
7. Check both test tubes for agglutination grossly and microscopically.

References and Supplemental Reading

Pharmacologic Considerations

Anwar M, Vannucci RC: Autoradiographic determination of regional cerebral blood flow during hypoglycemia in newborn dogs. Pediatr Res 24:41, 1988.

Arant BS Jr, Gooch WM: Effects of acute hyperglycemia on brains of neonatal puppies. Pediatr Res 13:488, 1979 (abstract).

Authement JM, Wolfsheimer KJ, Catchings S: Canine blood component therapy: Product preparation, storage, and administration. J Am Anim Hosp Assoc 23:483, 1987.

Babiak LM, Rybak MJ: Hematological effects associated with beta-lactam use. DICP Ann Pharmacother 20:833, 1986.

Berlin CM: Pharmacologic considerations of drug use in the lactating mother. Obstet Gynecol 58(suppl):17S, 1981.

Coulter DM, Lapine TR, Gooch WM: Treatment to prevent postnatal loss of brain water reduces the risk of intracranial hemorrhage in the beagle puppy. Pediatr Res 19:1322, 1985.

Cowan RH, Jukkola AF, Arant BS: Pathophysiologic evidence of gentamicin nephrotoxicity in neonatal puppies. Pediatr Res 14:1204, 1980.

Davis LE, Westfall BA, Short CR: Biotransformation and pharmacokinetics of salicylate in newborn animals. Am J Vet Res 34:1105, 1973.

Dorrestein GM, Van Gogh H, Rinzema JD, et al: Bioavailability and pharmacokinetics of ampicillin and amoxycillin from tablets, capsules and long-acting preparations in the homing pigeon. J Vet Pharmacol Ther 9:394, 1986.

Driscoll DJ, Gillette PC, Lewis RM: Comparative hemodynamic effects of isoproterenol, dopamine, and dobutamine in the newborn dog. Pediatr Res 13:1006, 1979.

Ehrnebo M, Agurell S, Jalling B, et al: Age differences in drug binding by plasma proteins: Studies on human fetuses, neonates and adults. Eur J Clin Pharmacol 3:189, 1971.

Ernst JA, Williams JM, Glick MR, et al: Osmolality of substances used in the intensive care nursery. Pediatrics 72:347, 1983.

Fiser DH: Intraosseous infusion. N Engl J Med 322:1579, 1990.

Gillette DD, Filkins M: Factors affecting antibody transfer in the newborn puppy. Am J Physiol 210:419, 1966.

Goldblum OM, Holman IR, Fisher SE: Intragastric feeding in the neonatal dog. Am J Dis Child 135:631, 1981.

Green TP, Mirkin BL: Clinical pharmacokinetics: Pediatric considerations. In Benet LZ (ed): Pharmacokinetic Basis for Drug Treatment. New York, Raven Press, 1984, p 269.

Greene CE, Hoskins JD, Authement JM: Drug and blood component therapy. In Hoskins JD (ed): Veterinary Pediatrics: Dogs and Cats from Birth to Six Months, 1st ed. Philadelphia, WB Saunders, 1990, p 29.

Greenwood B, Davison JS: The relationship between gastrointestinal motility and secretion. Am J Physiol 252:G1, 1987.

Gross RT, Bracci R, Rudolph N, et al: Hydrogen peroxide toxicity and detoxification in the erythrocytes of newborn infants. Blood 29:481, 1967.

Heimann G: Enteral absorption and bioavailability in children in relation to age. Eur J Clin Pharmacol 18:43, 1980.

Hellmann J, Vannucci RC, Nardis EE: Blood-brain barrier permeability to lactic acid in the newborn dog: Lactate as a cerebral metabolic fuel. Pediatr Res 16:40, 1982.

Hirschhorn N: Oral rehydration therapy for diarrhea in children: A basic primer. Nutr Rev 40:97, 1982.

Horster M, Kemler BJ, Valtin H: Intracortical distribution of number and volume of glomeruli during postnatal maturation in the dog. J Clin Invest 50:796, 1971.

Horster M, Valtin H: Postnatal development of renal function: Micropuncture and clearance studies in the dog. J Clin Invest 50:779, 1971.

Inman RC, Yeary RA: Sulfadimethoxine pharmacokinetics in neonatal and young dogs. Fed Proc Am Soc Biol 30:560, 1971 (abstract).

Jones RL: Special considerations for appropriate antimicrobial therapy in neonates. Vet Clin North Am Small Anim Pract 17:577, 1987.

Kerner JA, Sunshine P: Parenteral alimentation. Semin Perinatol 3:417, 1979.

Kleinman LI: Renal bicarbonate reabsorption in the newborn dog. J Physiol 281:487, 1978.

Kliegman RM, Miettinen EL, Morton SK: Hepatic and cerebral energy metabolism after neonatal canine alimentation. Pediatr Res 17:285, 1983.

Kliegman RM, Morton S: The metabolic response of the canine neonate to twenty-four hours of fasting. Metabolism 36:521, 1987.

Krauer B, Krauer F: Drug kinetics in pregnancy. In Gibaldi M, Prescott L (eds): Handbook of Clinical Pharmacokinetics. New York, ADIS Health Science Press, 1991, p 1.

Levy G: Pharmacokinetics of fetal and neonatal exposure to drugs. Obstet Gynecol 58(suppl):9, 1981.

Malkinson FD, Gehlmann L: Factors affecting percutaneous absorption. In Drill VA, Lazar P (eds): Cutaneous Toxicity. New York, Academic Press, 1977, p 63.

Morselli PL, Morselli RF, Bossi L: Clinical pharmacokinetics in newborns and infants: Age-related differences and therapeutic implications. In Gibaldi M, Prescott L (eds): Handbook of Clinical Pharmacokinetics. New York, ADIS Health Science Press, 1983, p 99.

Mosier JE: Canine pediatrics: The neonate. Proc Am Anim Hosp Assoc 48:339, 1981.

Nahata MC: Sedation in pediatric patients undergoing diagnostic procedures. DICP Ann Pharmacother 22 Sept:711, 1988.

Nara PL, Davis LE, Lauerman LH, et al: Effects of chloramphenicol on the development of immune responses to canine distemper virus in beagle pups. J Vet Pharmacol Ther 5:177, 1982.

Otto CM, Kaufman GM, Crowe DT: Intraosseous infusion of fluids and therapeutics. Compend Contin Educ Pract Vet 11:421, 1989.

Peters EL, Farber TM, Heider A, et al: The development of drug-metabolizing enzymes in the young dog. Fed Proc Am Soc Biol 30:560, 1971 (abstract).

Poffenbarger EM, Ralston SL, Chandler ML, et al: Canine neonatology. Part I. Physiological differences between puppies and adults. Compend Contin Educ Pract Vet 12:1601, 1990.

Rane A, Wilson JT: Clinical pharmacokinetics in infants and children. In Gibaldi M, Prescott L (eds): Handbook of Clinical Pharmacokinetics, 4th ed. New York, ADIS Health Science Press, 1989, p 142.

Rasmussen F: Excretion of drugs by milk. In Brodie BB, Gilette JR (eds): Handbook of Experimental Pharmacology, vol 28, Concepts in Biochemical Pharmacology, part I. New York, Springer-Verlag, 1971, p 390.

Reiche R: Drug disposition in the newborn. In Ruckesbusch P, Toutain P, Koritz D (eds): Veterinary Pharmacology and Toxicology. Westport, CT, AVI Publishing, 1983, p 49.

Riviere JE: Veterinary clinical pharmacokinetics. Part I. Fundamental concepts. Compend Contin Educ Pract Vet 10:241, 1988a.

Riviere JE: Veterinary clinical pharmacokinetics. Part II. Modeling. Compend Contin Educ Pract Vet 10:314, 1988b.

Robinson EP: Anesthesia of pediatric patients. Compend Contin Educ Pract Vet 5:1004, 1983.

Rowe MI, Lloyd DA, Lee M: Is the refractometer specific gravity a reliable index for pediatric fluid management? J Pediatr Surg 21:580, 1986.

Schoffstall JM, Spivey WH, Davidheiser S, et al: Intraosseous crystalloid and blood infusion in a swine model. J Trauma 29:384, 1989.

Sheng HP, Huggins RA: Growth of the beagle: Changes in the body fluid compartments. Proc Soc Exp Biol Med 139:330, 1972.

Shifrine M, Munn SL, Rosenblatt LS, et al: Hematologic changes to 60 days of age in clinically normal beagles. Lab Anim Sci 23:894, 1973.

Shifrine M, Smith JB, Bulgin MS, et al: Response of canine fetuses and neonates to antigenic stimulation. J Immunol 107:965, 1971.

Short CR: Drug disposition in neonatal animals. J Am Vet Med Assoc 184:1161, 1984.

Silva MD, Maujoks S, Guignard JP: Renal effects of tolazoline in newborn and adult rabbits. Dev Pharmacol Ther 10:301, 1987.

Sjoqvist F: Interindividual differences in drug responses: An overview. In Rowland M (ed): Variability in Drug Therapy, Description, Estimation and Control. New York, Raven Press, 1985, p 9.

Smith HW: The development of the flora of the alimentary tract in young animals. J Pathol Bacteriol 90:495, 1965.

Turberville DF, Bowen FW Jr, Killam AP: Intracranial hemorrhages in kittens: Hypernatremia versus hypoxia. J Pediatr 89:294, 1976.

Wapnir RA, Zdanowicz MM, Teichberg S: Oral hydration solutions in experimental osmotic diarrhea: Enhancement by alanine and other amino acids and oligopeptides. Am J Clin Nutr 48:84, 1988.

Wapnir RA, Zdanowicz MM, Teichberg S, et al: Alanine stimulation of water and sodium absorption in a model of secretory diarrhea. J Pediatr Gastroenterol Nutr 10:213, 1990.

Welsch F: Placental transfer and fetal uptake of drugs. J Vet Pharmacol Ther 5:91, 1982.

Werner JC, Whitman V, Schuler HG, et al: Acute myocardial effects of chloramphenicol in newborn pigs: A possible insight into the gray baby syndrome. J Infect Dis 152:344, 1985.

Blood Component Therapy

Authement JM, Wolfsheimer KJ, Catchings S: Canine blood component therapy: Product preparation, storage, and administration. J Am Anim Hosp Assoc 23:483, 1987.

Bucheler J: Blood transfusion reactions. *In* Tilley LP, Smith WK (eds): The Five Minute Veterinary Consult. Baltimore, Williams & Wilkins, 1997, p 398.

Bucheler J, Cotter SM: Setting up a feline blood donor program. Vet Med 88:838, 1993.

Bucheler J, Cotter SM: Storage of canine and feline erythrocytes in CPDA 1 and determination of the posttransfusion viability. J Vet Int Med 8:120, 1994.

Bull RW: Antigens, graft rejections, and transfusions. J Am Vet Med Assoc 181:1115, 1982.

Clark CH, Woodley CH: The absorption of red blood cells after parenteral injections at various sites. Am J Vet Res 20:1062, 1959.

Corley EA: Intramedullary transfusion in small animals. J Am Vet Med Assoc 142:1005, 1963.

Cotter SM: Blood banking I: Collection and storage. Proc Am Col Vet Intern Med Forum 6:45, 1988a.

Cotter SM: Blood banking II: Indications and side effects. Proc Am Col Vet Intern Med Forum 6:48, 1988b.

Dodds WJ: Management and therapy of bleeding disorders. Biweekly Small Anim Med Update Ser 20:1, 1978.

Dodds WJ: Bleeding disorders of small animals. Vet Ref Lab News 8(3):1, 1984.

Dula DJ, Mullar HA, Donovan JW: Flow rate variance of commonly used IV infusion techniques. J Trauma 21:480, 1981.

Greene CE: Practical considerations in blood transfusion therapy. Proc Ann Meet Am Anim Hosp Assoc 47:187, 1980.

Greene CE: Blood transfusion therapy: An updated review. Proc Ann Meet Am Anim Hosp Assoc 49:187, 1982.

Hurst TS, Turrentine MA, Johnson GS: Evaluation of microwave-thawed canine plasma for transfusion. J Am Vet Med Assoc 190:863, 1987.

Masouredis SP: Preservation and clinical use of erythrocytes and whole blood. *In* Williams WJ, Buetler E, Erslev AJ, Lichtman MA (eds): Hematology, 3rd ed. New York, McGraw-Hill, 1983, p 1529.

Pichler ME, Turnwald GH: Blood transfusion in the dog and cat. Part I. Physiology, collection, storage, and indications for whole blood therapy. Compend Contin Educ Pract Vet 7(1):64, 1985.

Potkay S, Zinn RD: Effect of collection material, body weight and season on the hemograms of canine blood donors. Lab Anim Care 19:192, 1969.

Smith JE, Mahaffey E, Board P: A new storage medium for canine blood. J Am Vet Med Assoc 172:701, 1978.

Tangner CH: Transfusion therapy for the dog and cat. Compend Contin Educ Pract Vet 4:521, 1982.

Turnwald GH, Pichler ME: Blood transfusion in dogs and cats. Part II. Administration, adverse effects, and component therapy. Compend Contin Educ Pract Vet 7(2):115, 1985.

Widmann FK (ed): Technical Manual of the American Association of Blood Banks, 9th ed. Arlington, VA, American Association of Blood Banks, 1985, pp 12, 202.

Wintrobe MH, Lee GR, Boggs DR, et al: Transfusion of blood and blood components. *In* Wintrobe MH, Lee GR, Boggs DR (eds): Clinical Hematology, 8th ed. Philadelphia, Lea & Febiger, 1981, p 491.

Neonatal Isoerythrolysis

Andrews GA, Chavey PS, Smith JE, et al: *N*-glycolylneuraminic acid and *N*-acetylneuraminic acid define feline blood group A and B antigens. Blood 79:2484, 1992.

Auer L, Bell K: The AB blood group system in cats. Anim Genet 12:287, 1981.

Bridle KH, Littlewood JD: Tail tip necrosis in two litters of Birman kittens. J Small Anim Pract 39:88, 1998.

Bucheler J: Typ A und B Blutgruppen der Katze und ihre klinische Bedeutung [doctoral dissertation]. Berlin, Free University of Berlin Press, 1990.

Bucheler J, Giger U: Transfusion of type A and B blood to cats. Proc Am Coll Vet Intern Med 8:687, 1990.

Bucheler J, Giger U: Alloantibodies against A and B blood types in cats. Vet Immunol Immunopathol 38:283, 1993.

Cain GR, Suzuki Y: Presumptive neonatal isoerythrolysis in cats. J Am Vet Med Assoc 187:46, 1985.

Casal ML, Jezyk PF, Giger U: Transfer of colostral antibodies from queens to their kittens. Am J Vet Res 57:1653, 1996.

Eyquem A, Podliachouk L, Milot P: Blood groups in chimpanzees, horses, sheep, pigs, and other mammals. Ann NY Acad Sci 97:320, 1962.

Gandolfi RC: Feline neonatal isoerythrolysis: A case report. Calif Vet 3:9, 1988.

Giger U: Feline blood groups and incompatibility reactions. Proc Am Coll Vet Intern Med 8:319, 1990.

Giger U: Feline neonatal isoerythrolysis: A major cause of the fading kitten syndrome. Proc Am Coll Vet Intern Med 9:347, 1991.

Giger U: The feline AB blood group system and incompatibility reactions. *In* Kirk RW (ed): Current Veterinary Therapy XI. Philadelphia, WB Saunders, 1992, p 470.

Giger U, Bucheler J: Transfusion of type A and type B blood to cats. J Am Vet Med Assoc 198:411, 1991.

Giger U, Bucheler J, Patterson DF: Frequency and inheritance of A and B blood types in feline breeds in the United States. J Hered 82:15, 1991a.

Giger U, Casal ML: Feline colostrum—Friend or foe: Maternal antibodies in queens and kittens. J Reprod Fertil 51:316, 1997.

Giger U, Casal ML, Niggemeier A: The fading kitten syndrome and neonatal isoerythrolysis. Proc Am Coll Vet Intern Med 15:208, 1997.

Giger U, Griot-Wenk ME, Bucheler J, et al: Geographical variation of the feline blood type frequencies in the United States. Feline Pract 19:21, 1991b.

Griot-Wenk ME, Callan MB, Casal ML, et al: Blood type AB in the feline AB blood group system. Am J Vet Res 57:1438, 1996.

Griot-Wenk ME, Giger U: Feline transfusion medicine; blood types and their clinical importance. Vet Clin North Am Small Anim Pract 25:1305, 1995.

Griot-Wenk ME, Pahlsson P, Chishol-Chait A, et al: Biochemical characterization of the feline AB blood group system. Anim Genet 24:401, 1993.

Holmes R: The occurrence of blood groups in cats. J Exp Biol 30:350, 1953.

Hoskins JD: Clinical evaluation of the kitten: From birth to eight weeks of age. Compend Contin Educ Pract Vet 12:1215, 1990.

Hubler M, Kaelin S, Hagen A, Ruesch P: Feline neonatal isoerythrolysis in two litters. J Small Anim Pract 28:833, 1987.

Jonsson NN, Pullen C, Watson ADJ: Neonatal isoerythrolysis in Himalayan kittens. Aust Vet J 67:416, 1990.

McClain J, et al: Presumptive neonatal isoerythrolysis: An unusual case of feline neonatal mortality. Texas Vet Med J:19, 1988.

Puppy and Kitten Losses

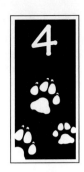

Johnny D. Hoskins

Puppy and kitten losses during the first 12 weeks of life usually approximate 15% to 40%, although exact figures may vary (Addie and Toth, 1993; Lawler and Monti, 1984; Norsworthy, 1979). Most puppy and kitten losses occur during specific times: in utero (as in abortions and fetal resorptions); at birth (stillbirths); immediately after birth (birth to 2 weeks of age); or immediately after weaning (5 to 12 weeks of age). Losses after 12 weeks of age are generally low.

Puppies and kittens that die immediately after birth are often referred to as part of the "fading puppy syndrome" or "fading kitten syndrome," a "fader" being a puppy or kitten apparently healthy at birth but failing to survive beyond 2 weeks of age. This age distinctness is arbitrary, however, and it might be considered more helpful to encompass the time from birth to 12 weeks of age.

CAUSES

Puppy and kitten losses between birth and 12 weeks of age usually result from problems acquired in utero, immediately after birth (birth to 2 weeks of age), or just after weaning (5 to 12 weeks of age) (Pedersen, 1991). Deaths during the postweaning period are primarily attributed to infectious diseases potentiated by weaning stress, exposure to pathogenic organisms in the immediate environment, and diminished local and/or systemic immunity. Puppy and kitten losses generally occur because of congenital anomalies, teratogenic effects, nutritional diseases resulting from improper diets fed to the mother or her young, abnormally low birth weights, traumatic insults during or after the birth process (i.e., dystocia, cannibalism, or maternal neglect), neonatal isoerythrolysis, infectious diseases, and other miscellaneous factors (Pedersen, 1991).

Congenital Anomalies

Congenital anomalies are those present at birth with their cause unspecified. In many situations, they are of genetic origin. Some congenital anomalies (particularly those involving the central nervous, cardiovascular, and respiratory systems) cause immediate threat to life, resulting in death at birth or within 2 weeks of a normal birth, whereas other anomalies might remain unnoticed until the animal is fully ambulatory. Often, these congenital anomalies are first diagnosed during the initial clinical examination before vaccination or as the result of obviously limited exercise tolerance or failure to grow. Anatomic anomalies include cleft palates, cranial deformities, agenesis of the small or large intestines, respiratory and cardiac anomalies, extensive umbilical or diaphragmatic hernias, anomalies of the kidneys and lower urinary tract, and musculoskeletal anomalies. Congenital anomalies of microanatomic or biochemical type probably account for an equal number of puppy and kitten losses (Pedersen, 1991). Such defects go unreported and are usually included under the general category of stillbirths, faders, or undetermined cause of death.

Teratogenic Effects

The proportion of puppy and kitten losses that may be attributed to teratogenic effects is unknown. There are known teratogenic potentials of a few drugs and chemicals that may contribute to congenital anomalies or faders. In general, it is always best to avoid the administration or application of any drug or chemical during the animal's pregnancy. Although specific information for dogs and cats of all ages may be lacking, it is certainly advisable to avoid the use of any drug or chemical, such as corticosteroids and griseofulvin, with known adverse teratologic effects in animals.

Poor Nutrition

Malnutrition of a puppy or kitten may occur as a result of severe maternal malnutrition or a lack of adequate maternal blood supply, possibly because of competition for placental space. Mothers fed poor-quality diets during pregnancy may produce diseased or weak puppies and kittens that become faders. For a puppy or kitten to survive after birth, it requires sufficient energy intake and adequate digestion, absorption, retention, and utilization of nutrients. An adequate amount of a good-quality palatable food of reasonable caloric density is required to obtain an optimum growth rate. If the owner is not aware of the animal's nutrition needs, consumption of a poor-quality food or insufficient calories to meet the requirements of the young growing animal can result in stunted growth or a fader. Deficiencies of dietary taurine are known to cause fetal resorptions, abortions, and stillbirths and inadequate growth in kittens (Sturman and Gargano, 1986).

Low Birth Weight

Low birth weights are associated with a higher probability of puppy and kitten losses. Sex, litter size, or weight of the mother (Festing and Bleby, 1970; Lawler and Monti, 1984) does not affect the birth weight of puppies and kittens. The causes of abnormally low birth weights have not been determined but probably involve several factors. Although low birth weight is often attributed to prematurity, most abnormally small puppies and kittens are born at term. Congenital anomalies or inadequate nutrition probably contributes to their small stature.

Not only is low birth weight associated with a greater likelihood of stillbirths and deaths during the first 6 weeks of life (Lawler and Monti, 1984) but there is a tendency for a disproportionate number of underweight puppies and kittens to do poorly in general and to die at a young age. Many faders that die in the first weeks of life are of normal size, but their growth is slow, and their weight is well below normal at the time of death; therefore, it is important to not only weigh puppies and kittens at birth but also to weigh at frequent intervals until they are at least 6 weeks of age or completely weaned.

Traumatic Insult

Puppy and kitten losses from traumatic insult during birth or the first 5 days of life are usually associated with dystocia, cannibalism, or maternal neglect. Cannibalism often occurs in nervous or high-strung mothers. In addition, cannibalism of sick puppies and kittens is common, so it is incorrect to always incriminate trauma as the primary cause of death. It is not always possible to differentiate maternal neglect of otherwise healthy puppies and kittens from maternal neglect of sick puppies and kittens, the latter being a programmed response of mothers that is akin to cannibalism.

Neonatal Isoerythrolysis

Neonatal isoerythrolysis is relatively common in certain purebred kittens (Giger, 1992). Unlike puppies, kittens have naturally occurring antibodies against the other blood types in their plasma. Kittens acquire maternal antibodies of the IgG class and to a lesser extent of the IgM class through colostrum ingestion. Kittens with blood type A have weak anti-B antibodies, whereas kittens with blood type B have strong anti-A antibodies. These antibodies, particularly anti-A antibodies, are responsible for the major incompatibility reactions: colostral anti-A antibodies from blood type B mothers may cause neonatal isoerythrolysis in blood type A (or blood type AB) kittens; blood type AB mismatched blood transfusions have a short half-life and are thus ineffective and cause life-threatening transfusion reactions in blood type B cats.

During the first 16 hours of life, maternal antibodies are normally transferred to the kitten through colostrum ingestion. If the kitten has blood type A (or blood type AB) and the mother has blood type B, these colostral antibodies will bind to and lyse red blood cells in the kitten. The hemolysis may be intravascular as well as extravascular and cause severe anemia, chromoproteinuric nephropathy, and other organ failures, as well as disseminated intravascular coagulopathy. Because all blood type B cats have high antibody titers, even primiparous mothers can have litters with neonatal isoerythrolysis.

Clinical signs of neonatal isoerythrolysis often develop in blood type A (or blood type AB) kittens born to blood type B mothers. Because the fetus is protected from maternal antibodies, kittens at risk are born healthy and usually start nursing vigorously; however, after colostrum intake (colostrum contains high titers of maternal antibodies), these kittens show the first clinical signs within hours to days. The clinical course may vary but often includes

- Kittens that suddenly die during the first day of life without showing any clinical signs
- Kittens that stop nursing during the first 3 days of life and fail to thrive (clinical findings include dark, brown-red urine caused by severe hemoglobinuria, and affected kittens may develop icterus and severe anemia, continue to fade, and may die during the first week of life; or, rarely, surviving kittens may develop a tail-tip necrosis between the first and second weeks of life as part of the syndrome)
- Kittens that continue to nurse, thrive, and show no obvious signs of clinical illness except for the tail-tip necrosis but that may exhibit laboratory abnormalities such as a positive direct Coombs' test and a moderately responsive anemia

Infectious Diseases

Infectious diseases account for a substantial proportion of puppy and kitten losses, especially bacterial and viral infections during and after weaning (5 to 12 weeks of age). During this time, most deaths are attributed to a primary infection of either the respiratory tract or the gastrointestinal tract and peritoneal cavity. When puppies and kittens are exposed to bacteria or viruses under nonstressful conditions, mild, self-limiting, or clinically inapparent infections usually occur. When host and environmental factors are unfavorable, immediate illnesses are more apt to be severe and puppy and kitten losses high. When bacterial or viral infections overpower the puppy's or kitten's defense mechanisms to protect against infectious agents, neonatal sepsis and/or viral disease occurs.

Neonatal sepsis is usually caused by common bacteria such as *Staphylococcus*, *Escherichia*, *Klebsiella*, *Streptococcus*, *Enterococcus*, *Pseudomonas*, *Clostridium*, *Bacteroides*, *Fusobacterium*, *Pasteurella*, *Brucella*, and *Salmonella* species; of these, gram-negative bacilli are the most common.

Sources from which gram-negative bacilli enter the bloodstream include the gastrointestinal tract and peritoneal cavity, respiratory tract, skin and associated wounds, and urinary tract.

Several viral groups (i.e., parvovirus, coronavirus, herpesvirus, adenovirus, calicivirus, retrovirus, and morbillivirus) are implicated in puppy and kitten losses. Clinical signs of viral infections vary according to the route and time of infection and the amount of passively derived antibody protection existent in the puppy or kitten. Even when there is a background of routine vaccinal immunization of breeding stock, situations exist in which passive immunity protection is not acquired, possibly because of colostral deprivation, and in which puppies and kittens are susceptible to viral infections normally considered to be well controlled.

Canine herpesvirus infection is a common cause of puppy losses (Carmichael and Greene, 1990). Most canine herpesvirus infections are acquired during the late stages of pregnancy and the first 3 weeks of life. The clinical signs manifested by puppies with canine herpesvirus infection may range from mild to severe, depending on the age of the puppy, the presence of maternal herpesvirus antibody, stress, and the presence of concurrent bacterial infections. If canine herpesvirus infection is acquired in utero, fetal death, mummification, abortion, or neonatal death can result. Most puppy losses occur between the ninth and fourteenth days of life. Severe clinical disease in a puppy older than 4 weeks of age is unlikely. Clinically, affected puppies show sudden onset and severe illness characterized by depression, anorexia, persistent crying, abdominal discomfort, bloating, rapid and shallow respiration, hypothermia, and profound weakness. Commonly, the clinical course ends in death in 18 to 24 hours.

Miscellaneous Factors

Roundworm, hookworm, coccidia, and *Giardia* infections have been implicated in puppy and kitten losses. No doubt, intestinal parasitism can be detrimental to the puppy's or kitten's growth and, in unusual situations, may also contribute to death. The severe infestation of puppies and kittens with ectoparasitism can also occur; deaths due to ectoparasitism are not common, however, although newly weaned puppies and kittens are not infrequently presented exhibiting well-established flea or tick burdens.

Fatty liver syndrome may cause puppies to languish at 4 to 16 weeks of age and mostly involves the toy breeds (van der Linde-Sipman et al, 1990). Clinically, affected puppies show sudden onset and severe illness characterized by depression, anorexia, persistent crying, diarrhea, rapid and shallow respiration, hypothermia, seizures, and profound weakness. The clinical course usually ends in death in 1 to 6 days.

Although they are poorly understood, other causes of kitten loss are known to exist. Kitten loss rates are lowest in fifth litters; first litters and litters after the fifth parity have higher kitten loss rates (Lawler and Monti, 1984). Medium-sized mothers tend to have fewer kitten losses than large or small mothers do. Kitten loss rates are twice as high in one-kitten litters as in larger litters; the fewest kitten losses occur in litters with five kittens.

DIAGNOSIS

Puppy and kitten losses are a common and often unavoidable problem within breeding establishments. Rates of preweaning puppy and kitten loss (liveborn deaths and stillbirths) of more than 20% and after weaning loss (from time of weaning to 7 months of age) of more than 10% are reasons for major concern (Pedersen, 1991). Higher percentages than these, or disproportionate losses to any one cause, such as congenital anomaly or specific infectious disease, are additional reasons for serious concern.

A complete history and physical examination should be performed on any puppy or kitten that is a potential fader (Hoskins, 1990). The owner should be questioned about the duration of the poor activity. Slow growth or activity since birth suggests the presence of a congenital anomaly, although acquired conditions should be considered when growth and activity are normal up to a certain point in time.

Questioning the owner regarding the amount and type of food fed and eaten by the animal as well as the presence or absence of other clinical signs may help to identify concurrent abnormalities (Table 4–1). The animal's breed, mental status, and general body condition should be assessed. An animal with stunted growth and poor body condition is likely to suffer from malnutrition or hepatic, renal, gastrointestinal, or cardiac disease. Most endocrinopathies that result in poor growth leave the animal in good physical condition compared with the effects of the metabolic diseases. Certain breeds or lines of dogs and cats may exhibit a higher than normal incidence of failure to thrive, which may be indicative of an underlying genetic disorder. Genetic testing and examina-

Table 4–1	Clinical Signs and Possible Associated Conditions
CLINICAL SIGNS	**POSSIBLE CONDITIONS**
Mental dullness	Hydrocephalus
	Hypothyroidism
	Growth hormone deficiency
	Hepatic encephalopathy
	Chronic renal failure
Inadequate food intake	Oral disease
	Pharyngeal disease
	Esophageal disease
	Gastrointestinal disease
	Renal disease
	Hepatic disease
	Hypoadrenocorticism
	Cardiac disease
	Inflammatory disease
Abnormal haircoat	Hypothyroidism
	Growth hormone deficiency
Regurgitation	Esophageal disease
Persistent vomiting	Gastrointestinal disease
	Renal failure
	Hepatic disease
	Neurologic disorders
	Hypoadrenocorticism
	Hypercalcemia
Diarrhea	Gastrointestinal disease
	Hypoadrenocorticism
	Exocrine pancreatic insufficiency
Cardiac murmur	Congenital heart disease
Cardiac arrhythmia	Congenital heart disease
Pale mucous membranes	Anemia
	Neonatal isoerythrolysis
	Cardiac disease
Polyuria and polydipsia	Diabetes mellitus
	Hypoadrenocorticism
	Hypercalcemia
	Renal disease
	Hepatic disease

tion of the pedigree may elucidate the genetic background for the observed changes.

In addition to the complete history and physical examination, a complete blood count, serum chemistry profile, and urinalysis should be performed. Specific laboratory tests (e.g., serum trypsin-like immunoreactivity, radiographs, electrocardiogram, cerebrospinal fluid analysis, computed tomography scan, hepatic function tests, biopsies of the affected organs, and hormonal tests) may also be indicated depending on the history and results of the physical examination and initial diagnostic tests.

Obtaining complete and accurate necropsy is the most expensive and crucial aspect of identifying the cause of faders in breeding establishments (Pedersen, 1991). It is preferable to sacrifice the puppy or kitten and perform a fresh necropsy as soon as it becomes apparent that death is inevitable. Puppies and kittens that die before they are euthanized should be immediately refrigerated; freezing ruins tissue for gross and histopathologic examination. Competent people must do the necropsy. Gross abnormalities are often subtle and may go unnoticed by untrained eyes. Representative tissue should be taken as aseptically as possible and frozen for microbiologic (i.e., viral, bacterial, and fungal cultures) or toxicologic studies, should they prove to be necessary. A wide sampling of tissue should also be preserved in formalin for histopathologic examination. Formalin-fixed tissue, along with detailed descriptions of gross lesions and clinical histories, should then be forwarded to veterinary pathologists for microscopic examination. If tissue indicates an infectious or toxic disease as the cause of death, samples of frozen tissue can then be submitted to competent microbiologists or toxicologists for further study.

MANAGEMENT

As previously indicated, a certain number of puppy and kitten losses is unavoidable; however, one may be able to identify the specific cause of a fader's illness and initiate the most appropriate management measures. A therapeutic trial of deworming and dietary modification can be started if the fader is still in fairly good condition and if parasitic infection or inadequate diet is a possible cause of the poor growth and activity. A concerted effort, if possible, must be made to eliminate the causative factors before the next breeding or purchase.

References and Supplemental Reading

Addie DD, Toth S: Feline coronavirus is not a major cause of neonatal kitten mortality. Feline Pract 21:13, 1993.

Carmichael LE, Greene CE: Canine herpesvirus infection. *In* Greene CE (ed): Infectious Diseases of the Dog and Cat. Philadelphia, WB Saunders, 1990, p 252.

Festing MFW, Bleby J: Breeding performance and growth of SPF cats (*Felis catus*). J Small Anim Pract 11:533, 1970.

Giger U: The feline AB blood group system and incompatibility reactions. *In* Kirk RW, Bonagura JD (eds): Current Veterinary Therapy XI. Philadelphia, WB Saunders, 1992, p 470.

Hoskins JD: Examination of the young dog and cat: Birth to four months. Proc Am Coll Vet Int Med 8:631, 1990.

Lawler DF, Monti KL: Morbidity and mortality in neonatal kittens. Am J Vet Res 45:1455, 1984.

Norsworthy GD: Kitten mortality complex. Feline Pract 9:57, 1979.

Pedersen NC: Common infectious diseases of multiple-cat environments. *In* Pedersen NC (ed): Feline Husbandry: Diseases and Management in the Multiple-Cat Environment. Goleta, CA, American Veterinary Publications, 1991, p 177.

Sturman JA, Gargano AD: Feline maternal taurine deficiency effects on mother and offspring. J Nutr 116:655, 1986.

van der Linde-Sipman JS, van den Ingh TSGAM, van Toor AJ: Fatty liver syndrome in puppies. J Am Anim Hosp Assoc 26:9, 1990.

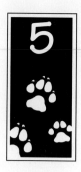

Intensive Care Management

Douglass K. Macintire

NEWBORN TO THREE-WEEK-OLD PUPPIES AND KITTENS

From birth to 3 weeks of age, a healthy puppy or kitten is firm, plump, and vigorous (Hoskins, 1990). Crying occurs in response to pain, coldness, failure to nurse (hunger), or loss of contact with the mother. It is abnormal for a healthy puppy or kitten to cry for longer than 20 minutes, whereas sickness commonly causes them to cry incessantly. A sick puppy or kitten is limp and relaxed, with poor muscle tone. They often have pale, gray, or cyanotic membranes and lack normal bowel sounds on abdominal auscultation. Diarrhea is present in approximately 60% of sick puppies and kittens.

GENERAL APPROACH TO SICKNESS

Regardless of the underlying cause, the approach to the sick puppy and kitten is similar and should address various concerns. If an animal is separated from its mother, external warming must be provided. A neonatal incubator can be used to provide an environmental temperature of 85° to 90° F and a humidity of 55% to 65%. A hot water blanket, rice bags, and hot water bottles can also be used, but the puppy or kitten should be able to crawl away from the heat source, and the source should be covered with a towel to prevent overheating and burns from direct exposure. A heat lamp can also be used to provide warmth. A pan of water can increase the humidity in the environment. A thermometer should be placed near the puppy or kitten to check ambient temperature.

Hypothermia (rectal temperature of 78° to 95° F) is common in sick puppies and kittens and is associated with depressed respiration, bradycardia, gastrointestinal paralysis, and coma. Until the hypothermic animal is rewarmed, oral feeding is not provided because digestion does not occur in the face of hypothermia and ileus. These animals must be rewarmed slowly over a 20-minute to 2-hour period. The most effective method is the use of warm inspired air because it warms the body's core as well as the external surface. This can be accomplished through an incubator or oxygen cage. Warm fluids can also be given by the intraosseous or intravenous route or as a warmwater enema.

Most sick puppies and kittens are hypoglycemic due to depletion of glycogen stores and immature hepatic function (Hoskins, 1990). A drop of blood should be placed on a glucose reagent stick and the immediate blood glucose level recorded. Glucose can be provided orally (initially, 1 to 2 ml of 5% to 15% dextrose solution) to animals that are not dehydrated or hypothermic. If mild dehydration is present, fluid solutions containing 2.5% dextrose and 0.45% sodium chloride can be given subcutaneously. Hypertonic dextrose solutions should never be given subcutaneously. Those animals exhibiting neurologic dysfunction, shock, or severe dehydration should receive glucose parenterally by the intravenous or intraosseous route at a dose of 0.25 ml per 25 g of 20% dextrose solution.

After dehydration and hypoglycemia are corrected, oral feeding can be initiated if a suckling reflex and bowel sounds are present. Puppy or kitten milk replacer can be fed with a bottle, dosing syringe, or feeding tube. If a feeding tube is used, care must be taken not to place it in the trachea. Improper placement is more likely in puppies and kittens because the gag reflex does not develop until 10 days of age. If diarrhea occurs, the milk replacer should be diluted at a 1:2 ratio with balanced multiple electrolyte solution until the diarrhea resolves.

Because of rapid total body water turnover, dehydration can occur acutely in puppies and kittens. Hydration status is difficult to assess in this age of animal. Skin turgor is not reliable due to the increased water and decreased fat content of the skin. Mucous membranes should be moist and not tacky. The color of the mucous membranes should be hyperemic for the first 4 to 7 days of life. Pale mucous membranes and slow capillary refill time in the absence of anemia indicate circulatory collapse and 12% to 15% dehydration. Warmed intravenous fluids can be given at an initial rate of 1 ml per 30 g over 5 to 10 minutes. Fluid loading is continued until color and capillary refill time have improved. The puppy or kitten is reassessed every 30 minutes until it is stable, and fluids are then administered at a maintenance level of 60 to 90 ml/lb per day.

Vitamin K_1 should be administered to any sick puppy or kitten that is less than 48 hours old or exhibits signs of hemorrhage (0.01 to 0.1 mg given subcutaneously or intramuscularly). At birth, puppies have decreased thrombin levels and are more prone to hemorrhage than adult dogs.

Weak puppies and kittens that are unable to nurse after parturition may have atelectatic lungs, aspiration of amniotic fluid, or hypoxemia from premature placental separation. They can also develop pulmonary contusions after trauma from the mother. Supplemental oxygen may be beneficial either from an oxygen cage (40%) or a nasal catheter.

SPECIFIC DISEASES

Poor sanitation can lead to infections of the skin, eyes, and umbilicus. Neonatal dermatitis results in crusting lesions on the head and neck at 4 to 10 days of age. Treatment involves gentle cleansing with a bactericidal shampoo and systemic antimicrobial agents. Neonatal conjunctivitis results when purulent exudate accumulates behind the eyelids before they completely open. Treatment involves gentle eyelid separation, drainage, cleansing, and topical antimicrobial agents.

Umbilical infections can occur in the first 4 days of life and are often due to a fecally derived bacterial or *Streptococcus* species infection. Treatment involves draining and flushing the abscess and providing fluids, antimicrobial agents, and other supportive care. Prevention can be accomplished by applying antiseptic solution to the newborn's umbilicus or by administering peripartum antimicrobial agents to mothers with known genital infections. Sanitation of the birthing quarters is also important.

Neonatal septicemia occurs when an infection becomes systemic. It may be secondary to lack of colostrum intake or to maternal infections such as mastitis or metritis. Causative organisms include *Staphylococcus* species, *Streptococcus* species, *Escherichia coli*, and *Pseudomonas* species. Affected animals should be isolated from the mother and treated with antimicrobial agents, fluids, and other supportive care (Table 5–1).

Canine herpesvirus and canine parvovirus type 1 infections cause a rapidly fatal syndrome in which the entire litter of puppies begins crying, develops lethargy and anorexia, and dies within 18 hours (Carmichael and Greene, 1998; Hoskins, 1998). Most canine herpesvirus infections are acquired during late pregnancy and the first 3 weeks of life. The signs shown by infected puppies with canine herpesvirus may vary from mild to severe depending on the age, presence of maternal herpesvirus antibody, stress, and presence of concurrent bacterial infections. If canine herpesvirus infection is acquired in utero, fetal death, mummification, abortion, or neonatal death can result. Most puppy losses occur between days 9 and 14 of life. Severe disease in a puppy older than 4 weeks of age is unlikely. Clinically, affected puppies present with a sudden onset of severe illness characterized by depression, anorexia, persistent crying, abdominal discomfort, bloating, rapid and shallow respiration, hypothermia, and profound weakness. Commonly, the clinical course ends in death in 18 to 24 hours. Canine herpesvirus replicates best at low core body temperatures (92° to 98° F); thus, medical treatment involves warmth and other supportive care. After one litter of puppies is lost, subsequent litters may be completely normal.

Before 1985, canine parvovirus type 1 was considered a nonpathogenic parvovirus of dogs; however, since 1985, clinical infections of canine parvovirus type 1 in neonatal puppies have been demonstrated. It appears to be widespread in the canine population and is restricted to causing clinical disease in puppies younger than

Table 5-1 Medical Management of a Septicemic Puppy or Kitten

I. Parenteral fluid therapy
    A. Use balanced multiple electrolyte solution supplemented with 5% dextrose solution
    B. Supplement the fluids with potassium chloride solution if plasma potassium concentration is less than 2.5 mEq/L
    C. Administer warm fluids slowly by intravenous or intraosseous route

II. Glucose replacement therapy
    A. Administer 5% dextrose solution intravenously or intraosseously to effect
    B. Administer 1 to 2 ml/kg of a 10% to 20% dextrose solution to the animal that is profoundly depressed or having seizures
    C. Maintain plasma glucose concentration at 80 to 200 mg/dl for euglycemia

III. Antimicrobial therapy
    A. Collect bacterial culture samples (whole blood, urine, exudate, and feces) before initiation of antimicrobial therapy
       1. For blood culture, collect 1 ml of whole blood aseptically and inoculate blood directly into enriched tryptic or trypticase soy broth, dilute the whole blood 1:5 to 1:10 in enriched broth, and examine broth for bacterial growth 6 to 18 hours later
       2. For urine culture, collect urine by cystocentesis and culture it by standard methods
       3. For exudate and fecal cultures, collect and culture by standard methods
    B. Empirical treatment with antimicrobial agent(s) begins immediately after collection of appropriate bacterial culture samples
    C. Adjust the dosage and dosing interval of antimicrobial agent(s) selected
    D. Administer antimicrobial agent(s) by the intravenous or intraosseous route

IV. External warming procedure
    A. Use circulating hot water blanket, rice bags, or hot water bottle
    B. Take at least 20 to 30 minutes for gradual warming of the animal
    C. Turn the animal every hour
    D. Record rectal temperature every hour

V. Provide oxygen and nutritional therapy
    A. Administer oxygen by mask or intranasal catheter to counteract tissue hypoxemia
    B. Encourage food intake once animal is normothermic and adequately hydrated

VI. Monitor the effectiveness of medical management
    A. Observe for improvement in the animal's general demeanor
    B. Regularly assess the cardiopulmonary status (it is extremely easy to overhydrate the ill puppy and kitten; thus, attentive monitoring of breathing pattern is helpful for early recognition of overhydration)
    C. Weigh the animal three to four times a day to record weight gain
    D. Observe for moistness and color of mucous membranes in assessing for adequate hydration

3 weeks. It is likely that the virus spread is similar to that of canine parvovirus type 2. Four to 6 days after oral exposure, canine parvovirus type 1 can be recovered from the small intestine and other organs. In addition, canine parvovirus type 1 is capable of crossing the placenta and producing early fetal deaths and birth defects. Affected puppies usually present with diarrhea, vomiting, dyspnea, constant crying, and sudden death—the same clinical signs as those seen in canine herpesvirus infection. Treatment of affected puppies is usually unrewarding because of the rapid progression of the disease. Mortality may be reduced by ensuring that the environmental temperature of newborn puppies is kept warm and that adequate nutrition and hydration are provided.

Toxic milk syndrome may cause bloating, green diarrhea, crying, and a red edematous rectum. Puppies should be removed from the mother and supplemented with milk replacer, and the mother should be evaluated for underlying diseases such as mastitis or metritis.

Puppies and kittens that die immediately after birth are often referred to as part of the "fading puppy syndrome" or "fading kitten syndrome," with a "fader" being a puppy or kitten apparently healthy at birth but failing to survive beyond 3 weeks of age. Faders generally occur because of congenital anomalies, teratogenic effects, nutritional diseases resulting from improper diets fed to the mother or her young, abnormally low birth weights, traumatic insults during or after the birth process (dystocia, cannibalism, or maternal neglect), neonatal isoerythrolysis, infectious diseases, and other miscellaneous factors.

Neonatal isoerythrolysis occurs infrequently among domestic kittens but may be relatively common in certain purebred kittens (Giger et al, 1997). Signs of neonatal isoerythrolysis often develop in blood type A (or blood type AB) kittens born to blood type B mothers. After colostrum intake, affected kittens show the first signs within hours to days. The clinical course may vary but often includes (1) kittens that suddenly die during the first day of life without showing any signs of illness; (2) kittens that stop nursing during the first 3 days of life and fail to thrive (clinical findings include dark brown-red urine caused by severe hemoglobinuria; affected kittens may develop icterus and severe anemia, continue to fade, and may die during the first week of life); and (3) kittens that continue to nurse, thrive, and show no obvious signs of illness except for a tail-tip necrosis between the first and second weeks of life as part of the syndrome and may exhibit laboratory abnormalities such as a positive direct Coombs' test and a moderately responsive anemia.

THREE- TO SIX-WEEK-OLD PUPPIES AND KITTENS

During the period between 3 and 6 weeks of age, the most life-threatening problems are internal and external parasites, juvenile hypoglycemia, dehydration from diarrhea, and traumatic insult. Renal function does not mature until 8 weeks of age; thus, these puppies and kittens remain prone to drug toxicity from decreased renal elimination and to dehydration from decreased ability to concentrate urine. Congenital defects such as megaesophagus may become evident with the change from a liquid to a solid food diet.

Internal parasites can result in a significant burden at 2 to 4 weeks of age. *Toxocara* species can be transmitted transplacentally from the mother, and *Ancylostoma* species are ingested through the mother's milk. Proper perinatal care of the mother should prevent severe parasitic infections in puppies and kittens of this age. In cases of poor husbandry, however, *Toxocara* species can cause weight loss, unthriftiness, abdominal distention, and diarrhea, whereas *Ancylostoma* species can cause life-threatening anemia. Puppies and kittens can be treated with pyrantel pamoate (5 to 10 mg/kg administered orally) as early as 2 to 3 weeks of age, and this can be repeated every 2 to 3 weeks until at least 12 weeks of age.

Severe anemia (pale mucous membranes, tachycardia, weakness, packed cell volume < 15) and hypoproteinemia may require a whole-blood transfusion. Whole blood is diluted at a 1:10 ratio with a citrate anticoagulant and is given through a millipore blood filter at a dosage of 10 ml/lb over 2 hours. Intraosseous or intravenous administration is preferred in critically ill puppies or kittens, but blood can be given by the intraperitoneal route as a last resort. Iron supplementation should be given after transfusion in anemias involving blood loss.

Protozoal parasites that may cause diarrhea in puppies and kittens include *Giardia* species and *Cystoisospora* species. Giardiasis is treated with metronidazole (30 mg/kg administered orally for 7 to 10 days), febantel (30 to 40 mg/kg administered orally once daily for 7 days), or fenbendazole (50 mg/kg administered orally once daily for 7 days) (Barr et al, 1994, 1998). Coccidiosis can be effectively managed with sulfadimethoxine at 50 mg/kg on the first day followed by a daily dose of 25 mg/kg until signs regress. External parasites may cause severe debilitation in young animals. Most flea and tick products should not be used in nursing animals. The mother should be treated, but her nipples should be avoided or rinsed. Bedding should be washed or discarded. The safest way to treat young puppies and kittens is to spray a towel with pyrethrin insecticide and wrap the animal's body in the towel, leaving the head out. A flea comb can be used to remove dead and dying fleas. If the puppy or kitten is bathed, extreme care must be taken to avoid hypothermia. In some cases, ectoparasite infestation is so severe that a blood transfusion is required.

Juvenile hypoglycemia can occur because of immature hepatic enzyme systems, lack of glycogen stores, and increased metabolic requirements for glucose. Signs include weakness, tremors, seizures, stupor, and coma. Treatment involves intravenous or intraosseous administration of glucose (0.5 to 1 g/kg) diluted to a 5% to 10% solution followed by other supportive care.

Fatty liver syndrome may cause failure to thrive in puppies 4 to 16 weeks of age and mostly involves the toy breeds (van der Linde-Sipman et al, 1990). Affected puppies present with a sudden onset of severe illness characterized by depression, anorexia, persistent crying, diarrhea, rapid and shallow respiration, hypothermia, seizures, and profound weakness. The clinical course usually ends in death in 1 to 6 days. Treatment involves intravenous or intraosseous administration of glucose (0.5 to 1 mL/kg) diluted to a 5% to 10% solution followed by other supportive care.

Dehydration is always a potential problem in young puppies and kittens that develop diarrhea. Severe consequences can be avoided by giving subcutaneous fluids at one to two times maintenance requirements while attempting to determine the cause of the diarrhea. Common reasons for diarrhea include overfeeding, lactose intolerance, excess solids, excess saturated fatty acids, parasites, infection, toxemia, or improper handling of milk replacement diet.

SIX- TO TWELVE-WEEK-OLD PUPPIES AND KITTENS

Puppies and kittens 6 to 12 weeks old are more similar to adults in terms of renal function, body temperature, and vital signs, but they still have an increased maintenance water requirement (60 to 90 ml/lb per day) and caloric requirement (378 kJ/lb per day). Because maternal antibody is lost during this period, they are susceptible to infectious diseases and should be isolated from other animals as much as possible until their vaccinations are completed by 12 to 16 weeks of age.

The most life-threatening diseases in 6- to 12-week-old puppies and kittens include infectious diseases (canine distemper and viral enteritis in puppies; feline leukemia virus infection, feline infectious peritonitis, and panleukopenia in kittens). General concerns regarding management of these sick puppies and kittens include prevention of hypoglycemia, dehydration, hypoproteinemia, and anemia.

Other emergencies that are common in 6- to 12-week-old puppies and kittens because of their inquisitive nature include foreign body ingestion and electric cord injury. Animals with foreign body ingestion will have a history of vomiting, and careful abdominal palpation may detect a mass and abdominal discomfort. Classic radiographic signs include distention of the bowel proximal to the obstruction.

Animals that bite into an electric cord may have burns on the lips, tongue, or oral mucous membranes. The life-threatening consequence to electric shock, however, is acute fulminant pulmonary edema, which progressively worsens for the first 24 hours after the electrical insult. The primary treatment includes cage rest, supplemental oxygen, and furosemide (2 mg/kg intravenously every 6 to 12 hours). Other treatments may include aminophylline (5 to 10 mg/kg administered intramuscularly) and a single dose of corticosteroids to help stabilize membranes. Other potential sequelae include cardiac arrhythmia, seizures, and secondary pneumonia. Most animals recover if they survive the initial 48 hours.

Juvenile cellulitis, sometimes referred to as "puppy strangles" or juvenile pyoderma, is an idiopathic skin disease occurring in 3- to 16-week-old puppies. No causative agent has been identified. The disease is characterized by facial swelling, lymphadenopathy, deep pyoderma of the head and face, fever, anorexia, and depression. Treatment involves topical therapy with antibacterial shampoos, systemic antimicrobial agents (cephalexin 20 mg/kg administered orally three times daily), and immunosuppressive doses of prednisolone (2.2 mg/kg administered once daily until signs resolve followed by alternate-day therapy for 2 to 3 weeks). There may be an immune-mediated cause for this disease, as the response to antimicrobial therapy alone is unrewarding and recrudescence can occur if corticosteroid therapy is withdrawn too early. Without treatment, the disease can be fatal.

BACTERIAL INFECTIONS

When bacterial infections overcome the ability of the puppy's or kitten's immune system to provide adequate protection, life-threatening illnesses occur (Table 5–2). The bacterial invasion of the bloodstream that regularly occurs in puppies and kittens after birth would rarely be of any consequence in healthy adults. When overwhelming bacteremia develops in puppies and kittens, however, the illness may be sufficiently severe to threaten survival. Factors predisposing puppies and kittens to natural microflora-induced bacterial infections include coexistence of inadequate nutrition and thermoregulation, viral infections, parasitism, and developmental and heritable defects of the immune system (Hoskins, 1991).

Bloodstream invasion usually occurs by the more common bacteria such as *Staphylococcus, Escherichia, Klebsiella, Enterobacter, Streptococcus, Enterococcus, Pseudomonas, Clostridium, Bacteroides, Fusobacterium,* and *Salmonella* species, and, of these, gram-negative bacilli occur most often (Dow et al, 1989). Sources from which gram-negative bacilli enter the bloodstream include the gastrointestinal tract and peritoneal infection ("navel ill"), respiratory tract infection, skin and wound infection, and urinary tract infection.

The clinical manifestations of bacterial infec-

Table 5-2	Bacterial Diseases of Puppies and Kittens
Infectious	Bacteremia, pneumonia, meningitis, omphalophlebitis ("naval ill"), septic arthritis, osteomyelitis, septic peritonitis
Gastrointestinal	Gastric and duodenal ulceration, enteritis, peritonitis, intraluminal obstruction, atresia coli, atresia recti, atresia ani
Respiratory	Respiratory distress complex, pneumonia, meconium aspiration
Cardiovascular	Endocarditis, thromboembolism
Musculoskeletal	Compound fracture, puncture wounds
Urogenital	Urinary tract infection, patent urachus
Immunologic	Failure of passive transfer, combined immunodeficiency

tions do not allow specific identification of the causative agent. Furthermore, many puppies and kittens have unusual clinical signs or a wide variety of clinical presentations that may not be immediately recognized as being associated with a bacterial infection. Death can occur so suddenly that noticeable signs are virtually absent. More typically, however, puppies and kittens will cry incessantly; will show signs of restlessness, weakness, hypothermia, diarrhea, altered respiration, hematuria, failure to thrive, and cyanosis; and in advanced stages may show sloughing of parts of their extremities (Hoskins, 1991).

The clinical diagnosis of bacterial infections is usually based on the history and physical examination findings. Ideally, a complete blood count, plasma chemistry profile, urinalysis, urine and/or blood culture, and culture of suspected sources of infection should also be obtained. It is imperative to conduct a thorough search for the primary source of bacterial infection and to collect appropriate bacterial culture samples before initiating antimicrobial therapy (see Table 5–1).

The hemograms of bacteremic animals are usually characterized by a normochromic, normocytic anemia. Thrombocytopenia and mild to moderate neutrophilia with a left shift may be present. Another laboratory finding that is consistent with, but by no means specific to, life-threatening bacteremia is hypoglycemia. The remaining laboratory values from the plasma chemistry profile and urinalysis may reflect a specific organ failure.

Because bacterial infections may cause sudden death, puppies and kittens suspected of having a severe bacteria-induced illness should be treated immediately. In most instances, initial antimicrobial therapy is selected empirically (Table 5–3). Puppies and kittens should also be given intravenous or intraosseous fluids for dehydration, oxygen to counter tissue hy-

poxemia, and glucose if hypoglycemia is present (see Table 5–1).

Meaningful advances in the treatment of bacterial infections have been made in recent years. Many of the new antimicrobial agents have either an increased spectrum of activity or a diminished toxicity in comparison with previously available antimicrobial agents (Dow and Papich, 1991). However, specific pharmacokinetic data for many of the new antimicrobial agents have not been obtained in puppies and kittens, and therefore, the veterinary use of these antimicrobial agents remains somewhat empiric (Boothe and Tannert, 1992).

Drug distribution in puppies and kittens, especially those younger than 5 weeks, differs from that in adults because of differences in body composition—that is, less total body fat, higher percentage of total body water, lower concentrations of albumin, and a poorly developed blood-brain barrier (Boothe and Tannert, 1992). Because of this, modifications of dosing amounts used for adult dogs and cats—as much as a 30% to 50% reduction of the adult dose—or changes in dosing frequency may be necessary when antimicrobial agents are administered to bacteremic puppies and kittens (Hoskins, 1991).

In addition, antimicrobial agents should be administered intravenously or intraosseously, because systemic absorption after oral, subcutaneous, or intramuscular administration may not be reliable. Most drugs ingested by the lactating mother appear in her milk; the amount generally is 1% to 2% of the mother's dose.

CANINE PARVOVIRUS TYPE 2 ENTERITIS

Without immediate treatment, canine parvovirus type 2 enteritis is often a rapidly fatal disease in puppies 6 weeks to 6 months old, ending in severe dehydration, endotoxic or septic shock,

Table 5-3	Summary of Products for Management of Bacterial Infection or Canine Parvoviral Enteritis

DRUG	DOSAGE AND ROUTE*
Antiemetic agents	
Chlorpromazine	0.5 mg/kg tid IM
	1.0 mg/kg tid rectal via plastic catheter (calculated dose diluted in 1 ml of normal saline solution)
	0.05 mg/kg tid IV
Metoclopramide	0.2–0.4 mg/kg tid SC
	1–2 mg/kg administered every 24 hours as a slow IV infusion for severe vomiting
Ondansetron	0.1–0.15 mg/kg bid–qid IV, IO
Prochlorperazine	0.1 mg/kg tid–qid IM
Antimicrobial agents	
Amikacin	10 mg/kg tid IM, SC
Ampicillin	10–20 mg/kg tid–qid IV, IM, SC, IO
Cefotaxime	25–50 mg/kg tid–qid IV, IM, IO
Cefazolin	22 mg/kg tid IV, IM, IO
Ceftiofur	2.2–4.4 mg/kg bid SC
Enrofloxacin	5 mg/kg bid IM, SC, IV, IO
Gentamicin	2.2 mg/kg tid IM, SC
Imipenem-cilastatin	5 mg/kg tid IM, IV, IO
Ticarcillin-clavulanate	20–30 mg/kg tid IV, IO
Adjunctive therapies	
Antiendotoxin	According to manufacturer's directions
Recombinant granulocyte colony–stimulating factor	5 μg/kg sid SC
Specific hyperimmune plasma	1.1–2.2 ml/kg IV, SC
Gastric protectants	
Cimetidine	5–10 mg/kg bid–tid IM, SC, IV, IO
Famotidine	0.5 mg/kg bid–tid IM, SC, IV, IO
Ranitidine	2–4 mg/kg bid–tid IM, SC, IV, IO
Sucralfate	1 g dissolved in 10 ml of warm water tid PO

*PO = oral administration; SC = subcutaneous administration; IV = intravenous administration; IM = intramuscular administration; IO = intraosseous administration; sid = once daily; bid = twice daily; tid = three times daily; qid = four times daily.

and multiple organ failure (Hoskins, 1997; Macintire and Smith-Carr, 1997). With aggressive therapy and supportive care, however, a survival rate of 85% to 95% can be achieved in most dog breeds, with the exception being the Rottweiler. A summary of various therapeutic products and management protocols for canine parvovirus type 2 enteritis is provided in Table 5–4 (see also Table 5–3) (Hoskins, 1997; Kirby, 1997).

Initial Evaluation

When a puppy is first presented to the veterinary facility with a history suggestive of canine parvovirus type 2 enteritis, a fecal parvovirus antigen test should be performed to confirm the diagnosis if possible (Hoskins et al, 1996; Macintire and Smith-Carr, 1997). If the fecal

antigen test is positive, the puppy should be isolated from other hospitalized animals and all contaminated surfaces cleaned with a household bleach solution diluted at a 1:30 ratio. Strict cleanliness should be observed to avoid spreading the disease to other animals. If the fecal antigen test is negative, other causes of acute vomiting and diarrhea, such as foreign body, pancreatitis, intestinal parasitism, toxicosis, or dietary indiscretion, should be ruled out. Because of the possibility of false-negative results on the fecal antigen test, animals with a compatible history should receive appropriate supportive care and be retested 48 hours later.

The severity of the disease should be assessed through evaluation of physical examination findings and blood drawn for an initial minimum database. Rapid screening tests that aid in the puppy's assessment and fluid choice include

| | Suggested Protocol for Optimal Care of Puppies with Canine Parvoviral Enteritis |

Initial Treatment Plan

1. Aseptically place an intravenous or intraosseous indwelling catheter.
2. Obtain a minimum database, including packed cell volume, total plasma solids, blood urea nitrogen, glucose, sodium, and potassium, or, even better, obtain a complete blood cell count and serum chemistry profile with electrolytes.
3. Provide adequate fluids for reperfusion of vital organs utilizing lactated Ringer's solution or Normosol-R at a volume and rate adequate to restore perfusion to the vital organ at a supranormal level. If perfusion is poor, rapidly infuse a bolus of hetastarch or dextran 70 at a rate of 20 ml/kg for initial resuscitation and provide supplemental oxygen by nasal catheter. Do not use hypertonic saline solution in this resuscitative process, as the puppy is usually severely dehydrated.
4. Rehydrate with lactated Ringer's solution or Normosol-R at a rate of 3 to 10 ml/kg/h initially until hydration is restored over 4 hours. The maintenance rate is 2 to 3 ml/kg/h. Using hetastarch or dextran 70, less fluid is lost into the gastrointestinal tract, and the total volume of fluid required for rehydration is approximately 50% of what is used when lactated Ringer's solution or Normosol-R is used alone.
5. Administer intravenous antimicrobial agents such as first-generation cephalosporins. If the puppy appears to be septic, consider cephalosporins, an aminoglycoside, and metronidazole once perfusion has improved.
6. Palpate the puppy's abdomen at least every 4 hours to detect intussusception.
7. Give nothing orally until vomiting is controlled.
8. Flush indwelling catheter with heparinized saline every 6 hours.
9. Warm or cool the puppy as deemed necessary once perfusion has been restored.
10. Listen for bowel sounds. If decreased or no bowel sounds are detected, administer metoclopramide via intravenous drip.
11. Control significant vomiting with metoclopramide or chlorpromazine. If vomiting is persistent, place a nasogastric tube and suction the gastric contents every 1 to 2 hours initially. Lessen the frequency of suctioning as directed by withdrawal of gastric fluid. Use the nasogastric tube to give microenteral nutrition.
12. Consider nutritional support early in the course of hospitalization. Once the vomiting has been controlled, begin the puppy on oral electrolyte solution supplemented with glucose. This can be done by giving 2 to 10 ml of an oral electrolyte solution by dosing syringe, or the oral electrolyte solution can be placed in a fluid bag and dripped continuously into the nasogastric tube at a rate of 2 to 10 ml/h. Once the puppy tolerates the oral electrolyte solution for at least 4 to 6 hours, begin liquid nutritional supplementation (such as Clinicare; Pet Ag Inc.).

Check Monitoring

1. Packed cell volume, total plasma solids, blood urea nitrogen, glucose, sodium, and potassium every 4 to 6 hours. Supplement and adjust fluid rate as deemed necessary.
2. Check perfusion parameters (mucous membrane color, pulse rate and intensity, capillary refill time, blood pressure, central venous pressure) every 2 to 4 hours, and resuscitate with fluids ± hetastarch or dextran 70 as necessary.
3. Estimate quantity of vomiting, diarrhea, and urine output, and record observations every 2 hours.
4. Monitor rectal temperature every 4 to 6 hours.

Maintenance

1. Anticipate the problems of poor perfusion, severe dehydration, hypokalemia, hypoglycemia, hypoproteinemia, aspiration pneumonia, sepsis and septic shock, intussusception, hyperthermia or hypothermia, and massive fluid replacement requirements.
2. Maintain the albumin concentration above 2 mg/dl, which likely needs to be done with fresh-frozen plasma on hospital days 2 to 4.
3. Administer hetastarch or dextran 70 at a rate of 20 ml/kg over 4 hours, decreasing lactated Ringer's solution or Normosol-R during this time interval, on hospital days 2 and 3.

the packed cell volume, total plasma solids, serum electrolytes, and reagent sticks for blood glucose and blood urea nitrogen levels. A complete blood count or blood smear also aids in the assessment, because leukopenia is generally associated with more severe disease and a more guarded prognosis. The percentage of dehydra-

tion should be estimated through physical examination findings.

Initial Fluid Therapy

Fluid replacement for losses incurred through vomiting and diarrhea is the immediate treatment for puppies with canine parvovirus type 2 enteritis and should be continued until oral intake is resumed. The initial fluid of choice is a balanced multiple electrolyte solution (lactated Ringer's solution or Normosol-R). The route and rate of initial fluid therapy vary. If canine parvovirus type 2 infection has resulted in hypovolemic shock, a rapid intravenous fluid bolus of up to 90 ml/kg per hour may be necessary to restore perfusion.

Puppies in shock have pale or muddy mucous membranes and a slow capillary refill time. Fluid therapy should be administered at a fairly rapid rate until mucous membrane color becomes pinker and capillary refill time is restored to 1.0 to 1.5 seconds. If circulatory collapse prevents venous access, warm fluid solutions can be administered initially via a 20-gauge 1.5-inch spinal needle placed aseptically in the intraosseous space in the shaft of the femur or humerus. Once circulation has improved with intraosseous fluids, an intravenous catheter can be placed for continued fluid therapy. It is important to note that puppies with severe dehydration or circulatory collapse because of peripheral vasoconstriction do not absorb subcutaneous fluids. In addition, hypertonic solutions should be avoided in dehydrated animals.

Puppies that are dehydrated but not in shock should be rehydrated over 4 hours. The amount of fluid given is estimated by the following formula: % dehydration × body weight (kg) = number of liters required to replace deficit. Maintenance requirements (2 to 3 ml/kg per hour) as well as continuing losses from vomiting and diarrhea must also be taken into consideration during initial fluid therapy.

Maintenance Fluid Therapy

Once perfusion has been restored, the fluid rate can be decreased to 4 to 6 ml/kg per hour in most puppies. Hydration should be monitored by evaluating mucous membrane color, capillary refill time, pulse quality, packed cell volume and total plasma solids, urine output (which should approximate 1 to 2 ml/kg per hour), and urine specific gravity (which should range from 1.015 to 1.020). Fluid therapy should be adjusted to replace continuing losses through vomiting and diarrhea. As fluid losses subside, the fluid rate is gradually tapered.

Many puppies, especially the toy breeds or septic puppies, are more prone to hypoglycemia with canine parvovirus type 2 enteritis. After rehydration, 2.5% to 5% dextrose solution can

be added to lactated Ringer's solution or Normosol-R (100 ml of 50% dextrose added to 1 liter of lactated Ringer's solution or Normosol-R makes a 5% solution).

Puppies with anorexia and vomiting or diarrhea are also prone to hypokalemia, which can result in muscle weakness, ileus, polyuria, cardiac arrhythmia, and general malaise. Serum potassium levels should be monitored daily in these puppies. If low, potassium chloride should be added to the fluids—up to 40 mEq of potassium chloride is added to 500 ml lactated Ringer's solution or Normosol-R. If serum potassium is within its normal range, 14 to 20 mEq of potassium chloride should be added to each liter of lactated Ringer's solution or Normosol-R.

If the puppy is anemic because of parasitism or gastrointestinal blood loss, a transfusion of whole blood (preferably from a recovered animal with a high serum canine parvovirus type 2 antibody titer) is indicated. A dose of 10 to 20 ml/kg can safely be administered to most puppies over a 4-hour period. If the puppy is not anemic but is hypoproteinemic, a plasma transfusion (10 to 20 ml/kg intravenously) should be administered through an in-line filter over 2 to 4 hours. In addition to providing oncotic components, both whole blood and plasma contain antibodies and serum protease inhibitors that may be beneficial in neutralizing circulating viruses and controlling the systemic inflammatory response associated with the disease. Plasma and blood products are available through commercial blood banks.

Puppies with decreasing total protein and edema should receive a synthetic colloid such as hetastarch or dextran 70. To avoid potential volume overload, the dosage of 20 ml/kg per day should not be exceeded, but colloid infusions can be repeated after 24 hours if needed. Colloid solutions can be given rapidly to puppies in shock or as a continuous infusion over 24 hours to more stable puppies. General guidelines are to supply one third of fluid needs as a colloid and two thirds as lactated Ringer's solution or Normosol-R.

Systemic Antimicrobial Agents

Hemorrhagic diarrhea and mucosal sloughing are commonly seen in dogs with canine parvovirus type 2 enteritis and are indicators of breakdown of the gastrointestinal mucosal barrier that may contribute to bacterial translocation, endotoxemia, and sepsis. Severe neutropenia often coincides with severe enteritis and contributes to the risk of sepsis. For these reasons, intravenous, broad-spectrum, bactericidal antimicrobial agents are indicated for severely affected puppies. A combination of an aminoglycoside (2.2 mg/kg of gentamicin administered every 8 hours or 10 mg/kg of amikacin administered every 8 hours) with a β-lactam antimicrobial (22 mg/kg of ampicillin administered every 8 hours or 22 mg/kg of cefazolin administered every 8 hours) provides excellent therapy against gram-negative and anaerobic bacteria that originate from the gastrointestinal tract.

Aminoglycosides can cause acute renal failure and should only be administered after rehydration has been accomplished. Once-daily dosing of aminoglycosides may minimize renal damage while maximizing bacterial kill because of high peak and low trough antimicrobial concentrations, but the high dose should never be given to dehydrated puppies. Urine sediment should be monitored for the appearance of proteinuria or renal tubular casts, which would warrant discontinuation of aminoglycoside therapy.

Enrofloxacin (5 mg/kg administered every 12 hours) is an alternative choice to the aminoglycosides. It has excellent gram-negative activity but is not approved for intravenous use and may cause cartilage abnormalities in young growing puppies. The author has not encountered any problems with enrofloxacin when it is diluted at a 1:1 ratio with normal saline solution and administered slowly and intravenously for a relatively short-term basis (usually 3 to 5 days) in puppies with canine parvovirus type 2 enteritis. Rapid administration may cause vomiting.

Mildly affected puppies with an adequate neutrophil count generally do not require combination antimicrobial therapy. Appropriate antimicrobial choices might include ampicillin, cephalosporins, or a trimethoprim-sulfonamide combination.

Antiemetics

Vomiting often decreases when oral intake of food and water is discontinued, but in some puppies the problem persists and must be treated to reduce fluid losses and to increase the animal's comfort. The antiemetics most commonly used for puppies with canine parvovirus type 2 enteritis are metoclopramide and chlorpromazine. Metoclopramide is a gastric promotility drug that reduces vomiting by stimulating gastric emptying and inhibiting the chemoreceptor trigger zone. Metoclopramide can be added to the intravenous fluids or administered

in a separate drip at a dosage of 1 to 2 mg/kg given as a constant rate infusion over 24 hours.

If metoclopramide is ineffective in controlling vomiting, chlorpromazine can be used. This drug is a phenothiazine derivative and acts on the emetic center, chemoreceptor trigger zone, and peripheral receptors to reduce the vomiting reflex. The recommended dosage is 0.1 mg/kg administered intravenously every 4 to 6 hours or 0.2 to 0.5 mg/kg administered intramuscularly every 6 to 8 hours as needed. Phenothiazine derivatives can cause hypotension and systemic vasodilation via their α-adrenergic blocking effect and should only be given after the puppy is well hydrated.

For puppies with intractable vomiting, metoclopramide and chlorpromazine may be used together but only with caution, because the potential for side effects increases. Puppies should be monitored for restlessness, hyperactivity, bizarre behavior, or extreme drowsiness, and if any of these signs occur antiemetic therapy should be discontinued. Intractable vomiting may respond to treatment with the new serotonin antagonist ondansetron (Zofran, Cerenex Pharmaceuticals, Research Triangle Park, NC) administered intravenously at the rate of 0.1 to 0.15 mg/kg every 6 to 12 hours. Although the drug is highly effective and safe, it is also expensive.

Anticholinergic drugs should not be administered to dogs with canine parvovirus type 2 enteritis, as they increase the potential for gastric atony, ileus, and intussusception of an irritated bowel segment. Dogs with intractable vomiting should always be evaluated for foreign body obstruction or intussusception. Other causes of continued vomiting include reflux esophagitis and acute pancreatitis. Reflux esophagitis may be manifested by signs of drooling, nausea, and exaggerated swallowing motions. Treatment involves administration of a systemic antacid (0.5 mg/kg of famotidine given intravenously or 5 mg/kg of ranitidine given intravenously every 12 hours) and an oral suspension of sucralfate (1 g dissolved in 10 ml warm water given every 8 hours). Ideally, the antacid should be administered 1 to 2 hours after the sucralfate.

Immunotherapy

Bacterial endotoxemia is believed to be an important factor in the terminal acute shock that occurs in severe cases of canine parvovirus type 2 enteritis. A polyvalent antiserum of equine origin directed against lipopolysaccharide endotoxin is available for use in small animals

(SEPTI-Serum; Immvac Inc., Columbia, MO). It is recommended that the product be administered over 30 to 60 minutes at a rate of 4.4 ml/kg and diluted at a 1:1 ratio with intravenous crystalloid fluids (Dimmitt, 1991).

Antiendotoxin should be most effective if it is administered before antimicrobial therapy, because circulating plasma lipopolysaccharide concentrations can increase dramatically after antimicrobial kill-off of gram-negative bacteria. Puppies receiving the antiserum of equine origin must be observed closely during administration for signs of anaphylaxis. If a second administration of antiserum is deemed necessary, it should be given within 5 to 7 days after the initial treatment. After that time, a severe immunologic reaction is more likely to occur.

Anecdotal reports describe the use of convalescent serum (1.1 to 2.2 ml/kg administered intravenously or subcutaneously) collected from canine parvovirus type 2–recovered dogs in an effort to provide passive immunity to exposed or infected dogs. Research is needed to determine the efficacy and safety of this practice.

Aggressive Adjunctive Treatments

Corticosteroids and flunixin meglumine (Banamine, Schering-Plough Animal Health, Union, NJ) have shown beneficial effects in animal models of septic and endotoxic shock if administered early in the shock state. Potential beneficial effects of corticosteroids include improved tissue perfusion, decreased leukocyte margination, enhanced membrane stabilization, and reduced absorption of endotoxins. Flunixin meglumine is a potent nonsteroidal antiinflammatory analgesic agent that has antidiarrheal and antipyretic effects and may reduce the severity of the intestinal inflammation associated with canine parvovirus type 2 enteritis.

Both corticosteroids and flunixin meglumine can cause severe gastrointestinal ulceration as an unwanted side effect. Because of this possibility, the author reserves the use of these agents for puppies exhibiting early signs of sepsis or endotoxemia, specifically fever, tachycardia, injected or muddy mucous membranes, and evidence of gastrointestinal mucosal barrier breakdown. These agents should not be administered until after the initial fluid bolus has been given. In select cases, the author uses dexamethasone sodium phosphate (2 to 4 mg/kg administered intravenously) or flunixin meglumine (1 mg/kg administered intravenously). Repeated doses are not recommended, as they increase the likelihood of deleterious side effects.

Recombinant granulocyte colony-stimulating factor has been used in puppies with severe leukopenia secondary to canine parvovirus type 2 enteritis (Rewerts et al, 1996). The recommended dosage is 5 to 10 μg/kg per day administered subcutaneously. Puppies that respond generally show an increase in white blood cell count within 24 hours. Unfortunately, preliminary findings do not show an increased rate of survival with the use of this product, and it is expensive.

Intestinal Parasites

The presence of intestinal parasites has been identified as a factor that can exacerbate canine parvovirus type 2 enteritis by enhancing intestinal cell turnover and subsequent viral replication. Fecal samples should be evaluated to identify coccidia, *Giardia* species, hookworms, roundworms, or whipworms. Appropriate oral therapy can be initiated as soon as vomiting ceases or ivermectin (250 μg/kg administered subcutaneously) can be given to non–Collie mix dogs.

Nutritional Support

Puppies with severe canine parvovirus type 2 enteritis may have an extended course of hospitalization and may require nutritional support to prevent catabolism and immune dysfunction associated with negative nitrogen balance. Partial parenteral nutrition does not supply the puppy's entire nutrient needs but may provide short-term support for puppies that are expected to recover soon. The advantage of partial parenteral nutrition solutions is that they can be delivered through a peripheral vein rather than through a large central vein. Partial parenteral nutrition solutions are usually given at a maintenance dosage (60 ml/kg per day), and additional fluid needs are met with lactated Ringer's solution or Normosol-R as described earlier.

ProcalAmine (McGaw, Inc.) is a commercial product that contains 3% amino acids, 3% glycerol, and electrolytes (Kirby, 1997). A "homemade" partial parenteral nutrition solution can be made by adding 300 ml of 8.5% amino acid solution (Travenol, Baxter, Inc.) to 700 ml lactated Ringer's solution with 5% dextrose. The addition of lipid emulsions is controversial. Although lipids are rich in caloric content, they have been associated with immunosuppression through impairment of reticuloendothelial function and reduction in white blood cell phagocytosis. A common complication of partial parenteral nutrition solutions is catheter phlebitis, because the solutions are hypertonic. Catheters must be placed aseptically and the site monitored carefully for redness, swelling, or pain. Solutions containing dextrose should be tapered off gradually to prevent rebound hypoglycemia.

Most veterinarians offer water after vomiting has been absent for 12 to 24 hours. Early enteral nutrition is important to promote intestinal regeneration. A liquid nutritional supplementation can be offered initially, or gruel can be made with an easily digestible high-carbohydrate low-fat diet. The addition of glutamine powder (0.5 g/kg divided and administered every 12 hours) to drinking water may promote gastrointestinal healing in puppies recovering from canine parvovirus type 2 enteritis. Various veterinary recovery diets are available for post-hospital care. The puppy may have temporary intestinal malabsorption and protein-losing enteropathy until intestinal villi are repaired. Complete repair may require as long as 6 weeks. Initial feeding should consist of small amounts of an easily digestible low-fat diet fed frequently. The normal diet is gradually reintroduced after appetite and stools are returned to normal. After recovery, immunity to canine parvovirus type 2 enteritis lasts at least 2 years and may even be lifelong.

References and Supplemental Reading

Barr SC, Bowman DD, Heller RL: Efficacy of fenbendazole against giardiasis in dogs. Am J Vet Res 55:988, 1994.

Barr SC, Bowman DD, Frongillo MF, et al: Efficacy of a drug combination of praziquantel, pyrantel pamoate, and febantel against giardiasis in dogs. Am J Vet Res 59:1134, 1998.

Boothe DM, Tannert K: Special considerations for drug and fluid therapy in the pediatric patient. Compend Contin Educ Pract Vet 14:313, 1992.

Carmichael LE, Greene CE: Canine herpesvirus infection. *In* Greene CE (ed): Infectious Diseases of the Dog and Cat, ed 2. Philadelphia, WB Saunders, 1998, p 28.

Dimmitt R: Clinical experience with cross-protective antiendotoxin antiserum in dogs with parvoviral enteritis. Canine Pract 16:23, 1991.

Dow SW, Curtis CR, Jones RL, et al: Results of blood culture from critically-ill dogs and cats: 100 cases (1985–1987). J Am Vet Med Assoc 195:113, 1989.

Dow SW, Papich MG: Keeping current on developments in antimicrobial therapy. Vet Med 86:600, 1991.

Giger U, Casal ML, Niggemeier A: The fading kitten syndrome and neonatal isoerythrolysis. Proc Am Coll Vet Intern Med 15:208, 1997.

Hoskins JD: Examination of the young dog and cat: Birth to four months. Proc Am Coll Vet Intern Med 8:631, 1990.

Hoskins JD: Special problems in the pediatric patient. Proc Am Coll Vet Intern Med Forum 9:351, 1991.

Hoskins JD: Update on canine parvoviral enteritis. Vet Med 92:694, 1997.

Hoskins JD: Canine viral enteritis. *In* Greene CE (ed): Infectious Diseases of the Dog and Cat, ed 2. Philadelphia, WB Saunders, 1998, p 40.

Hoskins JD, Mirza T, Taylor HW: Evaluation of a fecal antigen ELISA test for the diagnosis of canine parvovirus. J Am Coll Vet Intern Med 10:159, 1996.

Kirby R: Cases, protocols, techniques, and procedures. Proc Central Vet Conf 9:104, 1997.

Macintire DK, Smith-Carr S: Canine parvovirus. Part II. Clinical signs, diagnosis, and treatment. Compend Contin Educ Pract Vet 19:291, 1997.

Rewerts JM, Harrington DP, McCaw D, et al: Effect of rhG-CSF administration on the clinical outcome of neutropenic parvovirus-infected puppies. J Am Coll Vet Intern Med 10:178, 1996.

van der Linde-Sipman JS, van den Ingh TSGAM, van Toor AJ: Fatty liver syndrome in puppies. J Am Anim Hosp Assoc 26:9, 1990.

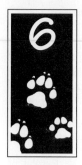

Preventive Health-Care Programs and Heredity Tests

Johnny D. Hoskins

In veterinary practice, pediatric health care is an integral part of providing for the general health needs of puppies and kittens from birth to 6 months of age. The time and effort invested in pediatric health care are rewarding not only to the animal but also to its owner(s) and those individuals attending to the animal's health-care needs.

PUPPY HEALTH CARE

Pediatric health care begins when the puppy is first presented to the veterinary hospital or clinic at 6 weeks of age or older (Hoskins, 1995). The general outline of a pediatric health-care program and its implementation for puppies is presented in Table 6–1. At each office visit, a complete physical examination is performed. Specific notes regarding the animal's general condition, mentation, posture, locomotion, and breathing pattern are made. Next, the body temperature, respiratory and heart rates, capillary refill time, and body weight (expressed in pounds, kilograms, or grams) of the puppy are noted. The thorax is then thoroughly auscultated and the abdomen palpated for evidence of physical abnormalities. Body weights are always recorded for a couple of reasons. First, body weight provides information needed for dispensing medication, and second, it is an immediate indicator of the growth rate of the puppy. The body weight of a growing puppy should steadily increase at each office visit and

is an indication that the puppy is receiving adequate nutrition.

Physical inspection begins by checking the head and oral cavity for evidence of malformation of the skull, cleft lip, stenotic nares, or cleft palate. The mucous membranes should be a pale pink and moist. The teeth should be examined for occlusion problems and periodontal disease. Frequent dental examinations and dental care are part of any pediatric health-care program, and this information should be conveyed to the owner. The importance of brushing even a young dog's teeth on a regular basis is discussed with the owner.

The skin and ears should be inspected for wounds, state of hydration, completeness of haircoat, and condition of foot pads. When necessary, the dermatologic examination may also require diagnostic procedures such as exfoliative cytology, bacterial culture and sensitivity testing, skin scrapings, and dermatophyte culture and identification of external parasites (ear mites, fleas, ticks, and chiggers).

Regularly scheduled vaccinations are a vital part of any pediatric health-care program, especially to provide for immunization of puppies against canine distemper, kennel cough complex, infectious canine hepatitis, canine parvovirus, and rabies. The initial vaccination series consists of one injection of a multivalent vaccine given at 6 weeks of age and two boosters given at 9 and 12 weeks of age. The rabies is usually given at 12 weeks of age or older. Intranasal

Table 6-1	Outline of a Pediatric Health-Care Program for a Puppy

I. First office visit for health program is usually at 6 weeks of age
   A. Conduct a general physical examination and record the body weight
   B. Check for external parasites and dermatophytes, and initiate appropriate therapy
      1. Fleas, ticks, and ear mites *(Otodectes cyanotis)*
      2. Mange mites, especially *Demodex canis* and *Sarcoptes scabiei*
      3. Dermatophytes, particularly *Microsporum* species and *Trichophyton mentagrophytes*
   C. Conduct fecal examination, including both direct smear and flotation
   D. Initiate administration of heartworm preventive management
   E. Administer an anthelmintic such as pyrantel pamoate for hookworms and roundworms; if tapeworms are present, administer praziquantel or epsiprantel
   F. Vaccinate with DA₂PL-PC* and possibly with kennel cough vaccine,† *Giardia* vaccine, and canine Lyme borreliosis vaccine‡
   G. Advise on nutrition and routine grooming
   H. Provide the owner with client education pamphlets on topics such as
      1. Identification, treatment, and control of fleas, ticks, and ear mites
      2. Benefits of preventive management for canine heartworm disease
      3. Management of normal and abnormal canine behaviors
      4. Skin, nail, and ear care
      5. "How to" on grooming and nutrition
   I. Fill in the puppy's health record for the owner

II. Second office visit for health program is usually at 9 weeks of age
   A. Conduct a general physical examination, and record the body weight
   B. Check for external parasites and dermatophytes, and initiate appropriate therapy
      1. Fleas, ticks, and ear mites *(Otodectes cyanotis)*
      2. Mange mites, especially *Demodex canis* and *Sarcoptes scabiei*
      3. Dermatophytes, particularly *Microsporum* species and *Trichophyton mentagrophytes*
   C. Conduct fecal examination, including both direct smear and flotation
   D. Adjust the dosage of heartworm preventive medication(s) according to body weight
   E. Administer an anthelmintic such as pyranel pamoate for hookworms and roundworms; if tapeworms are present, administer praziquantel or epsiprantel
   F. Vaccinate with DA₂PL-PC* and possibly with kennel cough vaccine,† *Giardia* vaccine, and canine Lyme borreliosis vaccine‡
   G. Adjust nutrition according to health needs, and if needed, change grooming procedures
   H. Provide the owner with client education pamphlets on topics such as
      1. Identification, treatment, and control of fleas, ticks, and ear mites
      2. Benefits of preventive management for canine heartworm disease
      3. Dental, skin, nail, and ear care
      4. "How to" on grooming and nutrition
      5. Management of normal and abnormal canine behaviors
      6. Exercise and its importance
   I. Fill in the puppy's health record for the owner

III. Third office visit for health program is usually at 12 weeks of age
   A. Conduct a general physical examination and record the body weight
   B. Check for external parasites and dermatophytes and initiate appropriate therapy
      1. Fleas, ticks, and ear mites *(Otodectes cyanotis)*
      2. Mange mites, especially *Demodex canis* and *Sarcoptes scabiei*
      3. Dermatophytes, particularly *Microsporum* species and *Trichophyton mentagrophytes*
   C. Conduct fecal examination, including both direct smear and flotation
   D. Adjust the dosage of heartworm preventive medication(s) according to body weight
   E. Administer an anthelmintic such as pyrantel pamoate for hookworms and roundworms; if tapeworms are present, administer praziquantel or epsiprantel
   F. Vaccinate with DA₂PL-PC* and rabies vaccines and possibly with kennel cough vaccine,† *Giardia* vaccine, and canine Lyme borreliosis vaccine‡
   G. Adjust nutrition according to health needs, and if needed, change the grooming procedures
   H. Provide the owner with client education pamphlets on topics such as
      1. Identification, treatment, and control of fleas, ticks, and ear mites
      2. Dental, skin, nail, and ear care
      3. "How to" on grooming and nutrition
      4. Management of normal and abnormal canine behaviors
      5. Recommendations for spaying and neutering
      6. Exercise and its importance
   I. Fill in the puppy's health record for the owner

IV. Subsequent visits for health program are usually annual visits

*This refers to the use of a vaccine to protect agianst D, canine distemper; A₂ (canine adenovirus type 2), infectious canine hepatitis; P, canine parainfluenza; L, leptospirosis; P, canine parvovirus type 2 disease; and C, canine coronavirus disease.

†This refers to the use of vaccine to protect against canine *Bordetella bronchiseptica*–induced disease. Puppies may be vaccinated with an intranasal vaccine as young as 2 to 4 weeks of age.

‡Lyme disease vaccine provides protection against canine Lyme disease. According to the manufacturer currently marketing canine *Borrelia burgdorferi* vaccine, puppies 12 weeks of age or older should receive two doses administered intramuscularly at 2- to 3-week intervals, and annual revaccination with a single dose is recommended.

vaccination provides rapid long-term protection against *Bordetella bronchiseptica*. Puppies can be vaccinated intranasally as early as 2 weeks of age without interference from maternal antibody. One dose is effective for a full year. Canine *Borrelia burgdorferi* vaccine, available as killed bacteria and recombinant products, provides protection against canine Lyme borreliosis disease. According to the manufacturers currently marketing canine *Borrelia burgdorferi* vaccines, puppies 9 weeks of age or older should receive two doses administered at 2- to 3-week intervals, and annual revaccination with a single dose is recommended. Some veterinarians do recommend vaccinations for canine coronavirus infection, giardiasis, and leptospirosis.

Puppies should be checked for gastrointestinal parasites at 3 weeks of age, and they require fecal rechecks when they return for their scheduled vaccinations. Monthly heartworm and flea preventive medications should be started at 6 to 8 weeks of age in those areas where heartworms and fleas are endemic. Heartworm preventive products of any type should be started in heartworm areas 1 months before the beginning of mosquito season and continued until 2 months after the season's end.

Owner education pamphlets on a variety of puppy-related topics can be sent home with the owner each time the puppy is seen for pediatric health care. Generally, only one or two well-written owner education pamphlets are given to the owner at the end of each office visit. By offering consultative advice and providing owners with educational pamphlets, the veterinary practice can not only assist owners who are seeking medical treatment for their puppies but also serve a vital role in educating people in the community.

KITTEN HEALTH CARE

Pediatric health care usually begins when the kitten is first presented to the veterinary hospital or clinic at 8 weeks of age or older (Hoskins, 1995). The general outline of a pediatric health-care program and its implementation for kittens is presented in Table 6–2. At each office visit, a complete physical examination is done as discussed earlier for puppies.

Regularly scheduled vaccinations are a vital part of any pediatric health-care program, especially to provide for immunization of kittens against feline distemper, feline viral rhinotracheitis, feline calicivirus, feline leukemia virus, and rabies. The initial vaccination series consists of one injection of a multivalent vaccine given at 8 to 10 weeks of age and second boosters given 3 to 4 weeks later. The rabies vaccine is usually given at 12 weeks of age or older.

Although feline chlamydiosis and bordetellosis may not be as prevalent as feline viral rhinotracheitis or feline calicivirus infections, it is evident that in some young feline populations chlamydial and *Bordetella bronchiseptica*–induced infections contribute to persistent conjunctivitis and/or upper respiratory tract disease. The vaccines currently available do afford complete protection; however, clinically proven conjunctivitis and/or upper respiratory tract disease, if present, can be restricted to a short course and is mild (Hoskins et al, 1998). Intranasal feline infectious peritonitis (FIP) vaccine affords protection against FIP virus challenge. Primary vaccination with two doses should be given, with the second dose administered 3 to 4 weeks after the first, and annual revaccination with a single dose is recommended.

Owner education pamphlets on a variety of kitten-related topics can be sent home with the owner each time the kitten is seen for pediatric health care. Generally, only one or two well-written owner education pamphlets are given to the owner at the end of each office visit. By offering consultative advice and providing owners with educational pamphlets, the veterinary practice can not only assist owners who are seeking medical treatment for their kittens but also serve a vital role in educating people in the community.

INTESTINAL PARASITISM

Intestinal parasites such as hookworms, roundworms, whipworms, and tapeworms occur commonly in puppies and kittens and are treated with the same deworming products as those used for adult dogs and cats. In addition, intestinal infections with *Giardia* and *Cryptosporidium* species are extremely common in young dogs and cats. The preferred treatment for *Giardia* species infection includes metronidazole (10 to 25 mg/kg administered orally once or twice daily for 10 to 14 days), fenbendazole (50 mg/kg administered orally daily for 7 days) (Barr et al, 1994), or febantel (30 to 40 mg/kg administered orally daily for 7 days) (Barr et al, 1998). Treatment of *Cryptosporidium* species infection includes paromomycin (125 to 165 mg/kg administered orally twice daily for 5 days) or tylosin (11 mg/kg administered orally once or twice daily for 28 days) (Lappin, 1997).

Table 6-2 Outline of a Pediatric Health-Care Program for Kittens

I. First office visit for health program is usually at 8 to 10 weeks of age
  A. Perform a general physical examination, and record the body weight
  B. Check for external parasites and dermatophytes, and initiate appropriate therapy
    1. Fleas and ear mites (*Otodectes cyanotis*)
    2. Mange mites, especially *Notoedres cati*, *Demodex* species, and *Cheyletiella* species
    3. Dermatophytes, particularly *Microsporum* species and *Trichophyton mentagrophytes*
  C. Perform fecal examination, including both direct smear and flotation
  D. Administer an anthelmintic such as pyrantel pamoate for roundworms and hookworms; if tapeworms are present, administer praziquantel or epsiprantel
  E. Vaccinate with FVRC-P,*,† *Chlamydia psittaci*,‡ feline leukemia virus,§ feline infectious peritonitis,¶ *Giardia*, and *Bordetella bronchiseptica*** vaccines
  F. Advise on nutrition and routine grooming
  G. Provide the owner with client education pamphlets on topics such as
    1. Identification, treatment, and control of fleas, ticks, and ear mites
    2. Benefits of vaccination for feline leukemia virus infection
    3. Management of normal and abnormal feline behaviors
    4. "How to" on grooming and nutrition
  H. Fill in the kitten's health record for the owner

II. Second office visit for health program is usually at 12 to 14 weeks of age
  A. Perform a general physical examination, and record the body weight
  B. Check for external parasites and dermatophytes, and initiate appropriate therapy
    1. Fleas and ear mites (*Otodectes cyanotis*)
    2. Mange mites, especially *Notoedres cati*, *Demodex* species, and *Cheyletiella* species
    3. Dermatophytes, particularly *Microsporum* species and *Trichophyton mentagrophytes*
  C. Perform fecal examination, including both direct smear and flotation
  D. Administer an anthelmintic such as pyrantel pamoate for roundworms and hookworms; if tapeworms are present, administer praziquantel or epsiprantel
  E. Vaccinate with FVRC-P,* *Chlamydia psittaci*,‡ feline leukemia virus,§ rabies, feline infectious peritonitis,¶ *Giardia*, and *Bordetella bronchiseptica*** vaccines
  F. Adjust nutrition and grooming procedures
  G. Provide the owner with client education pamphlets on topics such as
    1. Identification, treatment, and control of fleas, ticks, and ear mites
    2. Benefits of vaccination for feline leukemia virus infection
    3. Dental, skin, nail, and ear care
    4. Management of normal and abnormal feline behaviors
    5. Exercise and its importance
    6. Recommendations for spaying, neutering, and declawing
  H. Fill in the kitten's health record for the owner

III. Subsequent visits for health program are usually annual visits

*This refers to the use of a vaccine to protect against FVR, feline viral rhinotracheitis; C, feline calicivirus infection; P, feline panleukopenia.

†Cats being prepared for shipment or entering a boarding kennel or veterinary hospital or clinic should be vaccinated at least 1 to 2 weeks before admission or shipment.

‡The vaccine currently available apparently produces effective protection only against *Chlamydia psittaci* infections. As is the case with other vaccines for respiratory ailments, complete protection is not afforded; however, clinically proven conjunctivitis or upper respiratory tract disease, if present, can be restricted to a short course and is mild.

§This refers to the use of a vaccine to protect against feline leukemia virus infection. These vaccines are administered subcutaneously to healthy kittens or older cats as two doses, with the second dose given 3 or 4 weeks after the first. Annual revaccination with a single dose is recommended.

¶The feline infectious peritonitis vaccine is administered intranasally to healthy cats. Primary vaccination with two doses should be given, with the second dose administered 3 to 4 weeks after the first, and single-dose annual revaccination is recommended.

**This refers to the use of vaccine to protect against feline *Bordetella bronchiseptica*–induced disease. Kittens may be vaccinated with an intranasal vaccine as young as 4 weeks of age.

EARLY SPAY-NEUTER PROCEDURES

Early spay-neuter involves the surgical removal of the gonads in sexually immature animals. Early spay-neuter of puppies and kittens as young as 8 weeks of age is now an accepted alternative to allowing sexually intact animals to leave most animal shelters or adoption agencies. Early spay-neuter allows for decreased operative time, improved visibility of intraabdominal structures, and rapid recovery from anesthesia. Puppies or kittens that undergo early spay-neuter are believed to be more people-oriented pets and are calmer, gentler, less likely to wander, and less likely to retain persistent juvenile behavior (seemingly desirable). Early spay-neuter in puppies and kittens is a safe and effective means of controlling the canine and feline population in animal control and private veterinary practice environments. The advantages of early spay-neuter far outweigh the risks.

HEREDITARY DNA TESTS

The general ideas of applying DNA testing for inherited diseases in pedigree dogs intended for breeding purposes or for specific disease recognition became a reality in the late 1990s. Information about the new DNA testing technology for the clinical practice and for dog breeders is available from the websites www.vetgen.com and www.optigen.com. The Internet may also contain other websites about similar types of genetic services.

The principles of the DNA testing technology are as follows. The gene is the basic unit of heredity. All of the genes that constitute the hereditary makeup of an organism are called the *genome*. A dog is composed of a large number of cells that are genetically identical. The canine genome is made up of 39 pairs of chromosomes (one set from each parent) that contain approximately 3 billion base pairs of DNA, or around 100,000 genes. Each gene generally occupies a particular position within a particular chromosome. Scattered throughout the chromosome are short repeated groups of these base pairs, known as *microsatellites* or *markers*, that can be used to track defective genes. Hundreds of these distinctive sequences have been isolated along the canine genome for use in mapping genes.

To find a marker that is linked to a disease, researchers often examine hundreds of markers from dogs with and without the disease before they find one that is located so close to a disease gene that it is almost always inherited along with the disease caused by that gene. The closer the marker is to the disease gene itself, the more accurate the test. Finding such a marker also narrows down where to look for the disease-causing gene, which could ultimately lead to a more specific DNA test for the gene itself.

A *mutation* is a genetic mistake that scrambles the instructions given by a gene. Mutations may be good, bad, or indifferent. In the case of inherited renal dysplasia in the Shih Tzu, Lhasa apso, and soft-coated wheaten terrier, it is believed the presence of mutations in one or perhaps two different genes causes the glomeruli of the kidney to stop developing.

What are dominant and recessive genes? A dominant gene will express itself when the puppy inherits only one copy of the gene (from sire or dam). A recessive gene will express itself only when a puppy inherits two copies of the gene (one from the sire and one from the dam). If a disease-causing gene is recessive, a dog with the gene can be bred to a dog without it and will not produce the disease, although it will produce a carrier of the gene. If the gene is dominant, both parents must be free of it to avoid producing affected puppies. Again, more than one defective gene may be needed to produce a disease.

The DNA testing procedures can be done reliably at any age, and the results are accurate. That is, the DNA test results should never change with age and should be the same whenever it is repeated. Dog breeders and veterinarians alike can separate the problem of some inherited diseases into two distinct issues: getting rid of the disease and getting rid of the defective gene. There are three possible DNA testing results obtained: Clear, Carrier, and Affected. A Clear finding indicates that the gene is not present in the tested dog. Therefore, when used for breeding purposes, Clear dogs will not pass on the disease gene. A Carrier finding indicates that one copy of the disease gene is present in the tested dog and that it is not likely to exhibit signs of the disease. Carrier dogs will probably not have medical problems as a result. Dogs with the Carrier status will not develop the medical problems and will pass on the disease gene 50% of the time. An Affected finding indicates that two copies of the disease gene are present in the tested dog, and the disease will medically affect the dog. It is always best to breed "Clear dog to Clear dog." If followed by the pedigree dog breeders, this strategy should ensure a significant reduction in the frequency of the targeted disease gene in future generations of dogs. To maintain a large enough pool of good breeding animals, however, it may be necessary for some breeders to breed Clear dogs to Carrier dogs.

At the website www.vetgen.com, the company (VetGen, 3728 Plaza Drive, Suite 1, Ann Arbor, Michigan 48108; Phone: 1-734-669-8440, Fax: 1-734-669-8441) tells about its DNA testing procedures to identify coat color predilection for the Labrador retriever, Doberman pinscher, American cocker spaniel, flat-coated retriever, poodle, and Scottish terrier. They also offer DNA tests to eliminate copper toxicosis in the Bedlington terrier and inherited renal dysplasia in the Shih Tzu, Lhasa apso, and soft-coated wheaten terrier. Other DNA tests for inherited diseases include phosphofructokinase deficiency in the English springer spaniel and American cocker spaniel, progressive retinal atrophy (PRA) in the Irish setter, and pyruvic kinase deficiency in the basenji. In addition, they perform DNA tests for von Willebrand's disease in the Doberman pinscher, Scottish terrier, Shetland sheepdog, Manchester terrier, poodle, and Pembroke Welsh corgi.

At the website www.optigen.com, the company (OptiGen, LLC, Cornell Business & Technology Park, 33 Thornwood Drive, Suite 102, Ithaca, New York 14850; Phone: 1-607-257-0301, Fax: 1-607-257-0353) tells about its

DNA testing procedures to eliminate PRA from the dog breeds Chesapeake Bay retriever, English cocker spaniel, Labrador retriever, and Portuguese water dog. They also offer DNA tests to eliminate rod-cone dysplasia and canine leukocyte adhesion deficiency in the Irish setter and congenital stationary night blindness in the briard.

References and Supplemental Reading
Preventive Health Care Programs

Barr SC, Bowman DD, Frongillo MF, et al: Efficacy of a drug combination of praziquantel, pyrantel pamoate, and febantel against giardiasis in dogs. Am J Vet Res 59:1134, 1998.

Barr SC, Bowman DD, Heller RL: Efficacy of fenbendazole against giardiasis in dogs Am J Vet Res 55:988, 1994.

Hoskins JD: Veterinary Pediatrics: Dogs and Cats from Birth to Six Months, ed 2. Philadelphia, WB Saunders, 1995.

Hoskins JD, Williams J, Roy AF, et al: Isolation and characterization of *Bordetella bronchiseptica* from cats in southern Louisiana. Vet Immunol Immunopathol 65:173, 1998.

Lappin MR: Protozoal infections. *In* Morgan RV (ed): Handbook of Small Animal Practice, ed. 3. Philadelphia, WB Saunders, 1997, p 1169.

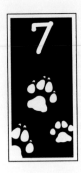

The Respiratory System

Joseph Taboada and Grant H. Turnwald

EVALUATION OF THE RESPIRATORY SYSTEM

Respiratory diseases are relatively common in puppies and kittens and can quickly result in life-threatening emergencies if not treated early. The most severe manifestation of respiratory disease is hypoxemia. Hypoxemia can result in clinical signs characterized by changes in respiratory rate, character, and effort. The respiratory rate may be increased or decreased, the depth may be impeded or exaggerated, and effort is often multiplied to the point that the puppy or kitten is weak and exhausted from the increased work effort. Mucous membrane color often ranges from cyanotic to pale. Kittens in severe respiratory distress often do not show the same degree of obvious difficulty as puppies. Tachypnea and less apparent increases in respiratory effort herald respiratory distress in kittens.

Abnormal Breathing Patterns

Care should be taken when assessing breathing patterns in puppies and kittens; their rates are more rapid and depth is shallower than those of adults. Respiratory distress and abnormal breathing patterns typically are identified in obstructive or restrictive respiratory diseases (Tables 7–1 and 7–2). Obstructive respiratory diseases are characterized by upper or lower airway obstruction in which intraluminal, mural, or extramural lesions narrow the airway lumen. An altered breathing pattern of increased depth and slower rate reduces airway resistance and is generally observed in mild obstructive disease. Severe obstructive disease generally results in increased depth and rate.

Upper airway obstruction generally produces an increase in inspiratory effort, often accompanied by stertor (snoring or snorting sounds) or stridor (high-pitched wheezing sound), whereas lower airway obstruction causes an increase in expiratory effort. Restrictive respiratory diseases are characterized by respiratory distress and restricted expansion of the lungs that may be compensated for by a rapid, shallow breathing pattern. Open-mouth breathing is usually a sign of distress in puppies and kittens. Animals with nasal obstructive disease will necessarily breath through an open mouth.

Diagnostic Approach

A thorough history and physical examination are important parts of the data used to evaluate young animals with respiratory signs. Specific evaluation of the upper or lower respiratory tract may require one or more of the following procedures—nasal cavity: rhinoscopy, nasal swab for cytology or culture, nasal lavage, aspiration biopsy, or exploratory rhinotomy; pharynx and larynx: pharyngoscopy and laryngoscopy; trachea and bronchi: tracheobronchoscopy, transtracheal wash, and/or bronchoalveolar lavage; pleural cavity: thoracocentesis for fluid analysis, cytology, culture, or ultrasonography; mediastinum: ultrasonography or fine-needle aspiration for cytology; and pulmonary parenchyma: bronchoalveolar lavage, fine-needle aspiration for cytology and culture, or open lung biopsy. These procedures performed in puppies or kittens differ little from those performed in adults, and they are described elsewhere (Hawkins, 1998; Orton and Park, 1993).

Table 7-1 Causes of Respiratory Distress

OBSTRUCTED BREATHING PATTERN		RESTRICTED BREATHING PATTERN	MISCELLANEOUS
Upper airway disorders	Lower airway disorders	The pleural cavity	Metabolic acidosis
The nasal cavity	The trachea and bronchi	Pleural effusion	Anemia
Congenital disorders	Congenital disorders	Pneumothorax	Exercise
Stenotic nares	Primary ciliary dyskinesia	The mediastinum	Heatstroke
Primary ciliary dyskinesia	Tracheal hypoplasia	Inflammation and infection	Central nervous system disease
Cleft palate	Collapsed trachea	Traumatic wounds	
Occlusive disorders	Bronchial collapse	Effusion	
Infection—bacterial, viral, fungal, and parasitic	Inflammation and infection	Pneumomediastinum	
Foreign object(s)	Infectious agents—bacterial, viral, fungal, and parasitic	Masses	
Fractures	Traumatic wounds	The diaphragm	
Hemorrhage	Compressive disorders	Congenital disorders	
Nasopharyngeal polyps	Lymphadenopathy	Pleuroperitoneal hernia	
The pharynx and larynx	Thymic lymphosarcoma	Peritoneopericardial hernia	
Congenital disorders	Other causes	Hiatal hernia	
Elongated soft palate	Osteochondral dysplasia	Acquired diaphragmatic hernia	
Laryngeal paralysis	Foreign object(s)	The thoracic wall and sternum	
Laryngeal hypoplasia	The lung parenchyma	Congenital disorders	
Subglottic stenosis	Congenital disorder	Rib abnormalities	
Inflammation and infection	Pulmonary emphysema	Pectus excavatum	
Infectious agents—bacterial, viral, and fungal	Inflammation and infection	Flat pup syndrome (swimmer puppy syndrome)	
Traumatic wounds	Infectious agents—bacterial, viral, fungal, and parasitic	Acquired disorders	
Tonsillitis	Traumatic wounds	Fractures	
Nasopharyngeal polyps	Aspiration pneumonia	Traumatic wounds	
Other causes	Pleuritis	Flail chest	
Everted laryngeal sacculi	Other causes		
Laryngeal collapse	Pulmonary edema		
Hyoid apparatus fractures	Pulmonary contusion		
Foreign object(s)	Pulmonary laceration		
Edema	Bleeding disorders		
The cervical trachea	Foreign object(s)		
Congenital disorders	Pulmonary cavitary lesions		
Primary ciliary dyskinesia	Neoplasia		
Tracheal hypoplasia	Respiratory distress syndrome		
Collapsed trachea			
Inflammation and infection			
Infectious agents—bacterial, viral, and fungal			
Traumatic wounds			
Other causes			
Osteochondral dysplasia			
Foreign object(s)			

Table 7–2	Characteristics of Abnormal Breathing Patterns	
TYPE OF BREATHING PATTERN	CAUSE	CHARACTERISTICS
Obstructed	Airway obstruction	Mild to moderate increase in respiratory rate; increase in depth of respiration
	Upper airway	Increased inspiratory effort
	Lower airway	Increased expiratory effort
Restricted	Inability to expand lungs	Rapid respiratory rate; decreased depth of respiration

THE UPPER AIRWAY: NASAL CAVITY, PARANASAL SINUS, NASOPHARYNGEAL, PHARYNGEAL, AND LARYNGEAL DISEASES

Sneezing and nasal discharge are the most common clinical signs of nasal cavity disease. Owners of puppies or kittens that are quickly cleaned by their mother or that are fastidious about licking any appearing discharge may overlook a nasal discharge. Viral disease or environmental irritants usually cause a serous or mucoid discharge; bacterial disease causes a purulent or mucopurulent discharge. Sneezing is usually prominent in acute disease but wanes with chronicity. Acute viral diseases sometimes cause enough destruction of the nasal epithelium to obliterate the sneeze reflex, despite the presence of nasal discharge and other upper respiratory signs. Less common signs of nasal disease include stertorous breathing, pawing or rubbing at the nose or mouth, facial pain, facial deformity, ocular discharge, exophthalmos, or fetid breath.

Because clinical signs related to the nose and sinuses can be manifestations of oral, pharyngeal, airway, and pulmonary disease, these areas should be carefully inspected. Evaluation of the nasal cavity should include oral and dental examination, radiographs of the nasal cavity, rhinoscopy, and visual examination of the nasopharynx and internal nares (Fig. 7–1). Pharyngeal and laryngeal disease is suggested by obstruction of airflow during inspiration, resulting in stridor, inspiratory dyspnea, loss or change of voice, exercise intolerance, or coughing. The combined signs of inspiratory dyspnea and stridor should lead the veterinarian to suspect laryngeal and/or pharyngeal disease. Diagnostic evaluation should include a thorough physical examination followed by sedation and visual inspection of the airways.

Congenital Disorders

CLEFT PALATE

Congenital incomplete closure of the primary (lip and premaxilla) and secondary (hard and soft) palate occurs in both the puppy and kitten

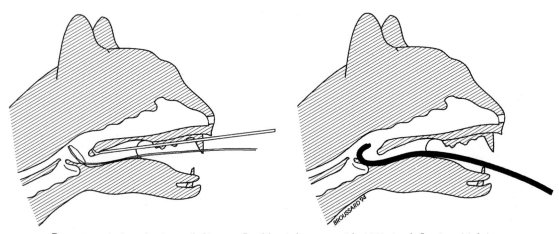

Figure 7–1. A dental mirror (left) or a flexible endoscope with 180° tip deflection (right) can be used to visually observe nasal disease such as nasopharyngeal polyps in the caudal portion of the nasal cavity.

(Nelson, 1993). Affected animals may demonstrate signs of poor growth; drainage of milk from the nares during and after nursing; and nasal discharge, sneezing, coughing, and gagging while eating. Affected animals are also predisposed to secondary bacterial rhinitis, laryngotracheitis, and aspiration pneumonia.

STENOTIC NARES

Stenotic nares occur as a congenital disorder primarily in brachycephalic breeds of dogs and cats (Nelson, 1993; Wykes, 1991). This condition is included in the characteristics of brachycephalic airway syndrome (along with elongated soft palate, eversion of laryngeal sacculi, and laryngeal collapse). The wings of affected nostrils fill most of the external nares, narrowing the transverse diameter and resulting in reduced passage of air through the nasal cavity (Fig. 7–2). Stertor, stridor, coughing, and gagging may be seen in affected animals. The primary treatment of stenotic nares is surgical resection of portions of the stenosed wings. The stenotic nares should be corrected as soon as possible, even in puppies 3 months old (Aron and Crowe, 1985).

THE BRACHYCEPHALIC AIRWAY SYNDROME

The brachycephalic airway syndrome may manifest as respiratory distress, stridor, reduced exercise and stress tolerance, and, in advanced cases, cyanosis, hyperthermia, and collapse (Wykes, 1991). Even in "normal" brachyce-

phalic animals (English bulldog, pug, Boston terrier), PaO_2 decreases significantly during sleep; sleep-disordered breathing occurs in every English bulldog older than 2 weeks (Hendricks, 1992). The syndrome occurs infrequently in brachycephalic breeds of cats. Anatomic narrowing of the upper airway results in negative intraairway pressure during inspiration and dynamic airway collapse. Prolonged increased negative pressure leads to progressive lengthening of the soft palate, redundancy/swelling of pharyngeal tissue, eversion of laryngeal sacculi, and eventually laryngeal collapse. Secondary problems that may complicate the brachycephalic airway syndrome include laryngeal and pharyngeal edema, cor pulmonale, pulmonary edema, hyperthermia, and vagally induced arrhythmias.

Diagnosis of *elongated soft palate* is made by visual examination—the soft palate should just overlap the open epiglottis. Early resection of the soft palate improves the long-term prognosis (Harvey, 1982a). *Everted laryngeal saccules* appear as small, whitish swellings or balls of tissue resting in the ventral aspect of the glottic opening. Surgical removal is usually simple and rapid (Harvey, 1982b). *Laryngeal collapse* is the most severe change associated with the brachycephalic airway syndrome—characterized by medial tipping of corniculate processes, medial flattening of the cuneiform processes of arytenoid cartilage, and narrowing of the rima glottis that appears as a slit between the collapsed arytenoids (Wykes, 1991). Because laryngeal collapse is usually associated with chronic upper airway obstruction, it is rarely seen in puppies or kittens younger than 6 months of age. Congenital malformation of the larynx may, however, result in laryngeal collapse (Burbidge et al, 1988).

AIRWAY DISEASE IN THE CHINESE SHAR-PEI

The Chinese shar-pei is a breed afflicted by a number of congenital defects. Although this is not a brachycephalic breed, a brachycephalic-like airway syndrome is seen in the young shar-pei, starting as young as 1 week. The spectrum of clinical manifestations is similar to that seen in brachycephalic dogs (CS Hedlund, personal communication, 1999). The Chinese shar-pei is also commonly afflicted with congenital hiatal hernia, and respiratory distress may occur secondary to airway disease and/or aspiration pneumonia (Johnson, 1993).

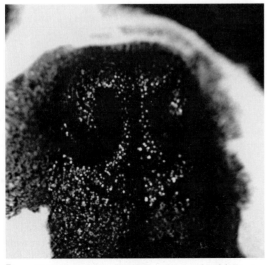

Figure 7–2. Stenotic nares in a 3-month-old Boston terrier.

LARYNGEAL PARALYSIS

Laryngeal paralysis is commonly seen as an idiopathic, naturally occurring condition of middle-aged to older large and giant breed dogs. A congenital form of the disease has been seen in Bouvier des Flandres in The Netherlands; Siberian husky, husky crosses, and Dalmatians in the United States; and bull terriers in Great Britain (Braund et al, 1992; O'Brien and Hendricks, 1986; Venker-van Haagen, 1992). In Bouviers, laryngeal paralysis is inherited as an autosomal dominant trait and results from a loss of motoneuron cells in the nucleus ambiguus (Venker-van Haagen, 1992). In bull terriers, laryngeal paralysis is associated with generalized muscular disease. Laryngeal paralysis in Dalmatians is associated with a generalized distal axonopathy and may be transmitted as an autosomal recessive trait (Braund et al, 1992). Siberian husky and husky crosses have an inherited form of laryngeal paralysis clinically similar to that described in Bouviers (O'Brien and Hendricks, 1986).

Clinical signs of congenital laryngeal paralysis are primarily due to dysfunction of laryngeal musculature and subsequent obstruction of glottic airflow during inspiration. The arytenoid cartilages are displaced ventromedially, vocal folds are passively drawn toward the midline, and a lack of normal arytenoid abduction occurs during inspiration (Greenfield, 1987). Onset of signs usually occurs at 4 and 6 months of age and includes a change in phonation, gagging, or coughing, especially during eating or drinking. Severe inspiratory dyspnea may be the first sign of laryngeal paralysis. Affected Dalmatians commonly have megaesophagus. Surgical widening of the glottic opening is the definitive treatment for congenital laryngeal paralysis. If there are concurrent motility problems in the pharynx or esophagus or both, subsequent problems with aspiration pneumonia are likely.

LARYNGEAL HYPOPLASIA

Congenital hypoplasia of the larynx is most common in brachycephalic dogs and Skye terriers (Venker-van Haagen, 1992). The laryngeal cartilages fail to adequately develop, resulting in a small, narrow, and unusually flexible larynx. The vocal folds fail to adequately abduct during inspiration, and the laryngeal ventricles evert due to the increased pharyngeal pressure. Signs, if present, vary with the degree of laryngeal narrowing. Attempts at surgical correction may result in further collapse and stenosis of the opening. In Skye terriers, the disorder is inherited as a simple autosomal recessive trait.

SUBGLOTTIC STENOSIS

Congenital subglottic stenosis has been identified in a 5-month-old dog that had signs of laryngeal stenosis (Venker-van Haagen et al, 1981). The subglottic stenosis was caudal to the glottis and cranial to the caudal margin of the cricoid cartilage. Initial signs in the dog were altered phonation and respiratory distress. Laryngeal stridor was present on both inspiration and expiration. Surgical splitting of the cricoid cartilage with or without using an internal splint will increase the glottic opening and relieve obstruction (Nelson, 1993).

Infectious/Inflammatory Disorders

NASOPHARYNGEAL POLYPS

Nasopharyngeal polyps are inflammatory lesions seen in young cats, probably arising from the tympanic cavity or auditory tube. Owners of affected cats often report signs starting before 6 months of age (Kapatkin et al, 1990). Clinical signs include inspiratory dyspnea, stertorous respiration, chronic nasal discharge, sneezing, and dysphagia. Nasopharyngeal polyp is diagnosed by direct examination of the nasopharynx under general anesthesia (Fig. 7–3); the polyp can usually be visualized after retraction of the soft palate or in the external ear canal (Boothe, 1991). Treatment is surgical excision of the polyp in combination with a ventral bulla osteotomy.

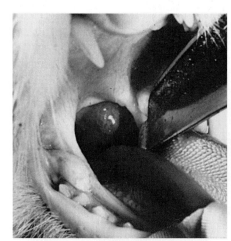

Figure 7–3. Nasopharyngeal polyp in a young cat with signs of upper respiratory disease. (Courtesy of Dr. Diana Bowen, San Jose, CA.)

INFECTIOUS UPPER RESPIRATORY DISEASE

Infectious upper respiratory disease occurs commonly in the young cat and less commonly in the young dog. Several infectious agents may be the cause of upper respiratory infections, including bacterial, viral, fungal, and parasitic agents (Ford, 1993) (Table 7–3). Viral upper respiratory infections in the cat are primarily caused by feline herpesvirus type 1 and calicivirus. Young kittens, especially those in multiple-cat households or catteries, represent the population most prone to severe, sometimes life-threatening infection. In addition, kittens persistently infected with feline calicivirus frequently develop an associated gingivitis, progressive periodontal disease, or limping kitten syndrome (Diehl and Rosychuk, 1993).

Primary bacterial upper respiratory infections occur sporadically in cats. *Bordetella* and *Chlamydia* may cause upper respiratory signs in young kittens, and mycoplasma should be considered in cases of feline upper respiratory disease that are not improving as expected.

In young dogs, canine distemper virus is the most common viral cause of upper respiratory infection, although canine adenovirus-2 and parainfluenza virus infections may also present as a rhinitis. Fungal rhinitis usually presents as a chronic condition and seldom occurs in puppies and kittens younger than 6 months old. Granulomatous rhinitis due to *Cryptococcus neoformans* infection is more likely to occur in kittens, whereas nasal infection with *Aspergillus* species is more likely in puppies (Wolf, 1992). Nasal infections with other fungal organisms

(*Penicillium* species, *Blastomyces dermatidis*, *Histoplasma capsulatum*, *Alternaria alternata*, *Exophiala spinifera*, and *Rhinosporidium seeberi*) as well as the Oomycotic organism *Pythium insidiosum* are rare.

A clinical diagnosis of upper respiratory disease in cats is based on history and clinical signs. It is seldom necessary to pursue definitive identification of the causative agent. Viral or bacterial isolation and identification and immunofluorescent studies of infected tissue can be performed during the early stage of the disease and may be of value in cattery situations. In early canine distemper infections, immunofluorescence of conjunctival scrapings can be helpful; fluorescence may be detected 5 to 21 days after infection. In cryptococcal infections, the most rapid method of diagnosis is cytologic demonstration of organisms in tissue fluid, nasal swabs, or impression smears from tissue specimens. In addition, serologic detection of capsular antigen of *Cryptococcus* organisms can be performed (Wolf, 1992). In nasal *Aspergillus* infections, organisms may be cultured, but interpretation of culture results is difficult because *Aspergillus* is a common environmental contaminant. A positive culture should be interpreted with biopsy results before making a diagnosis of nasal *Aspergillus* infection.

For kittens with mild upper respiratory infection, outpatient treatment with antimicrobial agents (Table 7–4) is indicated to decrease the severity of bacterial infection. Anorectic, dehydrated kittens may require hospitalization, fluid replacement therapy, and feeding by a nasoesophageal, esophageal, or gastrostomy tube. Other supportive measures include removal of accumulated secretions from the eyes and nose, humidification of inspired air, or saline nebulization (Povey, 1990). Intranasal administration of a pediatric phenylephrine-containing or oxymetazoline-containing decongestant once daily for a few days may help relieve upper airway obstruction. Cryptococcal rhinitis is treated with fluconazole (50 mg twice a day) (Malik et al, 1992). Canine *Aspergillus* infection can be treated with itraconazole (5 mg/kg) or fluconazole (5 mg/kg) (Sharp and Sullivan, 1986), although topical therapy with enilconazole or clotrimazole is more effective (Davidson et al, 1992; Sharp et al, 1993).

Table 7–3	Causes of Rhinitis

Bacterial Causes
  Staphylococcus intermedius, Chlamydia psittaci, and other aerobic and anaerobic bacteria
Viral Causes
  Young dogs: Canine distemper virus, canine parainfluenza virus, canine adenovirus-2, and canine herpesvirus
  Young cats: Feline rhinotracheitis (herpesvirus type I) virus, feline calicivirus, and feline reoviruses
Fungal Causes
  Cryptococcus neoformans, Blastomyces dermatitidis, Aspergillus species, and *Pythium insidiosum*
Parasitic Causes
  Cuterebra species larvae
Other Causes
  Blunt trauma, penetrating wounds, and embedded foreign object(s)

INFECTIOUS LARYNGITIS

The common causes of infectious laryngitis in puppies and kittens are the same viral and bacterial agents that cause infectious upper respira-

Table 7–4 **Therapeutic Agents Used in Respiratory Disorders**

THERAPEUTIC AGENT	DOSAGE*	COMMENTS
Analgesics		
Buprenorphine	0.005 mg/kg IV, IM q4–8h	Analgesia in dogs or cats
Butorphanol	0.1–0.4 mg/kg IV, IM, SC q2–5h	Analgesia in dogs or cats
Meperidine	3–10 mg/kg (dog) IM q2h	Analgesia in dogs or cats
	2–10 mg/kg (cat) IM q2h	
Morphine	0.2–1.0 mg/kg (dog) IM, SC q3–4h	Analgesia in dogs or cats
	0.05–0.1 mg/kg (cat) IM, SC q3–4h; given with a tranquilizer	
Oxymorphone	0.05–0.1 mg/kg (dog) IM, SC q3–4h	Analgesia in dogs or cats
	0.03–0.05 mg/kg (cat) IM, SC q3–4h; given with a tranquilizer	
Nalbuphine	0.03–0.1 mg/kg IM, SC, IV q2–4h	Analgesia in dogs or cats
Pentazocine	1–3 mg/kg IM, SC q2–4h	Analgesia in dogs or cats
Antimicrobial Agents		
Amoxicillin	22 mg/kg PO bid	Broad-spectrum antimicrobial
Amoxicillin/clavulanic acid	12.5–25 mg/kg PO bid	Broad-spectrum antimicrobial
Ampicillin	10–20 mg/kg PO tid–qid	Broad-spectrum antimicrobial
	5–10 mg/kg IV, IM, SC tid–qid	
Cefadroxil	22 mg/kg PO bid	Broad-spectrum antimicrobial
Cefaclor	4–20 mg/kg PO tid	Broad-spectrum antimicrobial
Cefazolin	10–20 mg/kg IV, IM tid	Broad-spectrum antimicrobial
Cefoxitin sodium	22 mg/kg IV, IM tid	Broad-spectrum antimicrobial
Cephalexin	20–30 mg/kg PO, SC, IV bid	Broad-spectrum antimicrobial
Cephradine	10–20 mg/kg PO tid	Broad-spectrum antimicrobial
Cefotaxime	25–50 mg/kg IV, IM, SC tid	Broad-spectrum antimicrobial
Chloramphenicol	50 mg/kg (dog) PO, IV, IM, SC tid	Broad-spectrum antimicrobial
	25–50 mg/kg (cat) PO, IV, IM, SC bid	
Clindamycin	5–10 mg/kg (anaerobic bacterial infection) PO bid	Broad-spectrum antimicrobial
	12.5 mg/kg (toxoplasmosis) PO bid	
Gentamicin	2 mg/kg IM, SC tid	Broad-spectrum antimicrobial
Metronidazole	7.5 mg/kg PO bid–tid	Antimicrobial; effective against anaerobes
Tetracycline	20 mg/kg PO tid	Broad-spectrum antimicrobial
Trimethoprim and sulfadiazine	15–30 mg (combined)/kg PO bid	Broad-spectrum antibacterial
Antitussives		
Butorphanol tartrate	0.55 mg/kg PO bid–qid	Synthetic opiate partial agonist with potent antitussive activity
	0.055–0.11 mg/kg SC bid–qid	
Codeine	1–2 mg/kg PO tid–qid	Narcotic centrally acting antitussive
Dextromethorphan	1–2 mg/kg PO tid–qid	Nonnarcotic centrally acting antitussive
Hydrocodone	0.25 mg/kg; not to exceed 0.5–1 mg/kg PO bid–qid	Narcotic centrally acting antitussive
Morphine	0.1 mg/kg SC bid–qid	Narcotic centrally acting antitussive

Table 7–4	Therapeutic Agents Used in Respiratory Disorders *(Continued)*	
THERAPEUTIC AGENT	DOSAGE*	COMMENTS
Bronchodilators		
Aminophylline	6–11 mg/kg (dog) PO tid–qid 4–6.6 mg/kg (cat) PO bid	Bronchodilation in dogs or cats
Oxtriphylline	10–15 mg/kg (dog) PO tid–qid 5–7 mg/kg (cat) PO tid–qid	Bronchodilation in dogs or cats
Terbutaline	1.25–5 mg (dog) PO bid 0.625 mg (cat) PO bid	Bronchodilation in dogs or cats
Theophylline	9 mg/kg (dog) PO qid 4 mg/kg (cat) PO bid	Bronchodilation in dogs or cats
Decongestants		
Oxymetazoline hydrochloride	0.025% 2–3 drops/nostril tid–qid	Topical decongestant
Phenylephrine hydrochloride	0.125% or 0.25% 1 drop/nostril tid–qid	Topical decongestant
Diuretics		
Ethacrynate sodium	0.2–0.4 mg/kg IV, IM bid–qid	Pulmonary edema
Furosemide	2–4 mg/kg PO, IV, SC bid–qid	Pulmonary edema
Sedatives		
Acetylpromazine	0.025–0.2 mg/kg (dog) IV, IM once 0.05–0.1 mg/kg (cat) IV, IM once	Sedation in dogs or cats
Morphine	0.1 mg/kg (dog) IM, SC bid–qid 0.1 mg/kg (cat) IM, SC bid–qid	Sedation in dogs or cats
Oxymorphone	0.05–0.1 mg/kg (dog) IM bid–qid 0.02–0.03 mg/kg (cat) IM bid–tid	Sedation in dogs or cats

*PO = Oral administration; SC = subcutaneous administration; IV = intravenous administration; IM = intramuscular administration; sid = once daily; bid = twice daily; tid = three times daily; qid = four times daily.

tory tract disease. Dogs with acute laryngitis usually demonstrate paroxysmal coughing, changes in phonation, gagging, and noisy breathing. Treatment consists of providing rest and avoiding excitement of the animal. Antitussive medications are indicated when coughing is severe enough to limit the dog's (or the owner's) ability to rest. In cats, upper respiratory viruses and *Bordetella* are the most likely causes of infectious laryngitis. Rather than cause coughing, they result in laryngeal edema and stridor.

NASAL TRAUMA AND FOREIGN BODIES

Trauma may result in facial fractures and epistaxis or blood clot formation within the nasal cavity that produces varying degrees of nasal cavity obstruction. If epistaxis is severe, owners may place ice packs over the nose before seeking veterinary care. In most cases, the bleeding will stop before hemorrhage causes significant problems. Foreign bodies occasionally lodge in the rostral portion of the nasal cavity or in the caudal portion of the nasopharynx. The presence of a foreign object in the nasal cavity may be associated with unilateral nasal discharge,

epistaxis, sneezing, and attempts to paw at the nose. Epistaxis and paroxysmal sneezing are the most likely clinical signs. Nasal and pharyngeal radiographs may be helpful. Nasal flush procedures can be used to wash foreign material out of the nasal cavity (Fig. 7–4). A flexible catheter is placed around the soft palate into the caudal nasal cavity; the head is placed down over the edge of the table, and a normal saline solution is flushed vigorously through the catheter and out the nares. Alternatively, a flush and suck technique can be used with a large catheter that is attached to a large syringe inserted through the nares into the rostral area of the nasal cavity. If nasal flush procedures are employed, the animal should be under general anesthesia, and a cuffed endotracheal tube should be in place.

LARYNGEAL TRAUMA

Laryngeal trauma is usually the result of penetrating wounds, especially bite wounds. Other causes of trauma include gunshot wounds, neck collars, and rough endotracheal intubation for inhalation anesthesia (Nelson, 1993). Bite wounds and gunshot wounds usually result in

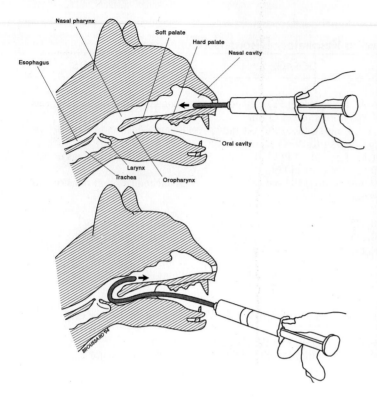

Nasal pharynx
Soft palate
Hard palate
Nasal cavity
Esophagus
Oral cavity
Larynx
Trachea
Oropharynx

BROUSSARD '94

Figure 7–4. Two techniques for nasal lavage. Sterile saline solution is flushed through a catheter into the nasal cavity either from the nares (top) or from the nasopharynx (bottom). Lavage can be useful therapeutically in young cats with severe nasal congestion or in animals suspected of having a foreign body in the nasal cavity. When the diagnosis is in question, diagnostic samples can be collected in gauze at the back of the nasopharynx (top), or the nose can be lowered and samples collected as saline solution falls from the nares. Samples of mucus, tissue, and other debris can be used for cytologic and histopathologic evaluations and for fungal culture. Nasal flushing techniques are generally not as effective diagnostically as biopsy techniques. Note that this procedure should not be performed unless a cuffed endotracheal tube is in place.

laryngeal cartilage damage, whereas neck collar trauma often results in fractures or dislocations of the hyoid apparatus. Swelling and edema resulting from the trauma may rapidly worsen and severely compromise respiration over a period of a few hours. Perforation of the upper airway may result in palpable subcutaneous emphysema around the injured site and the dorsum of the head and neck. Supportive therapy for laryngeal injury may include the use of antimicrobial agents and antiinflammatory doses of corticosteroids (see Table 7–4). Surgical intervention for debridement and alignment can be important in preventing laryngeal scarring and stenosis (laryngeal webbing) (Nelson, 1993).

NASOPHARYNGEAL STENOSIS

Nasopharyngeal stenosis is an unusual cause of nasal obstructive disease in young cats in which the normal ovoid opening of the caudal nares is reduced to a pinhole-sized orifice by the presence of a thin, tough membrane (Mitten, 1992). The signs are similar to those described previously for nasopharyngeal polyps. Diagnosis is made by visually observing the stenosed nasopharynx with a dental mirror or endoscope. Surgical enlargement of the stenotic area is the necessary treatment.

THE TRACHEA AND MAJOR BRONCHI

Cough is the most common clinical sign associated with tracheal and bronchial disease. Following a history and thorough physical examination to rule out infectious tracheobronchitis, thoracic and soft-tissue cervical radiographs may be indicated. Thoracic radiography is perhaps the single most important diagnostic test in the evaluation of the puppy or kitten that presents with cough as its primary complaint. Tracheal hypoplasia, extraluminal compressive diseases, diseases causing tracheal stenosis, intraluminal masses, and tracheal collapse may be apparent radiographically. Tracheoscopy with a small-diameter endoscope (approximately 3.5 to 5 mm in diameter or a rigid arthroscope) is useful in evaluating the trachea when obstructive or mucosal disease is suspected. It is especially useful in the diagnosis of tracheal collapse, tracheal foreign body, tracheal stenosis, parasitic tracheobronchitis, and tracheal osteochondroma.

Congenital Disorders
PRIMARY CILIARY DYSKINESIA

Primary ciliary dyskinesia is a congenital respiratory disorder that is characterized by absent or deficient mucociliary clearance (Edwards et al, 1992). The ciliary dysfunction reduces mucociliary transport, which frequently leads to persistent or recurrent rhinitis, sinusitis, bronchitis, and bronchopneumonia. Chronic cough, nasal discharge, and recurrent bronchopneumonia are the most common complaints. Affected dogs may experience signs from birth. Breeds affected include the bichon frise, Border collie, Chihuahua, Chinese shar-pei, chow chow, English springer spaniel, English pointer, English setter, Dalmatian, Doberman pinscher, golden retriever, miniature poodle, Old English sheepdog, and Rottweiler. The condition is likely inherited as an autosomal recessive trait (Edwards et al, 1992). Definitive diagnosis depends on demonstration of decreased mucociliary clearance and abnormal structural appearance of the cilia by electron microscopy. Decreased mucociliary clearance can be detected by using nuclear imaging to monitor the clearance of a small drop of ^{99m}Tc-labeled macroaggregated albumin from the nasal cavity or distal region of the trachea. Treatment of primary ciliary dyskinesia requires the periodic or continuous use of antimicrobial agents and supportive care (see Table 7–4).

HYPOPLASIA OF THE TRACHEA

Hypoplasia of the trachea is a congenital defect in which there is apposition or overlap of the free ends of each of the tracheal rings, resulting in narrowing of the cross-sectional tracheal diameter (Coyne and Fingland, 1992). The disease is seen most commonly in English bulldogs, Boston terriers, and boxers, but both brachycephalic and nonbrachycephalic breeds can be affected. The disorder has also been diagnosed in the cat (Suter, 1984a). Although most affected animals will show clinical signs early in life, not all animals with hypoplasia of the trachea will be symptomatic. When present, signs of hypoplasia of the trachea are usually evident within the first 5 months of life and may include coughing, gagging, respiratory distress, stridor, decreased exercise tolerance, and syncope. Crackles or wheezes may be heard on thoracic auscultation. Other associated congenital anomalies include elongated soft palate, stenotic nares, megaesophagus, cardiac defects, and cleft palate. Radiographic diagnosis can be made with the aid of a lateral thoracic radiograph by dividing the tracheal diameter at the thoracic inlet (TD) by the diameter of the thoracic inlet (TI) (Fig. 7–5). The TD/TI should be less than 0.16 in brachycephalic dogs with tracheal hypoplasia and less than 0.2 in affected nonbrachycephalic dogs. Dyspnea does not appear to be related to the degree of narrowing of the tracheal lumen. In most cases, dogs with dyspnea have concurrent anomalies that can account for the respiratory distress (Coyle and Fingland, 1992). Treatment of dogs showing signs of hypoplasia of the trachea is directed toward treatment of underlying respiratory tract infection if present and correction of concurrent anomalies if possible.

CONGENITAL TRACHEAL COLLAPSE

Congenital tracheal collapse is uncommon but was reported in a dog that demonstrated respiratory distress and an obstructed breathing pattern. The cause of the tracheal collapse was an absence of cartilage in the tracheal rings (Davies and Mason, 1968).

CONGENITAL BRONCHIAL COLLAPSE

Congenital bronchial collapse is also uncommon, having been reported in a 6-week-old Pekingese that suffered severe respiratory distress (Sartin and Dubielzig, 1984). At necropsy, pneumothorax and pulmonary emphysema were identified and believed to be the result of the bronchial collapse.

Infectious Tracheobronchitis

CANINE INFECTIOUS TRACHEOBRONCHITIS

Canine infectious tracheobronchitis, commonly referred to as "kennel cough," usually occurs where dogs are housed together (i.e., animal shelters, pet shops, boarding kennels, and veterinary hospitals). *Bordetella bronchiseptica*, canine parainfluenza virus, and *Mycoplasma* species are the most frequent causative agents (Ford and Vaden, 1990). Other agents that may be involved include canine distemper virus, canine adenovirus-2, canine adenovirus-1, canine reovirus-1, canine reovirus-2, canine reovirus-3, and canine herpesvirus. Affected dogs usually have had recent exposure to other dogs and experienced sudden onset of a paroxysmal cough. Other signs may include oculonasal discharge, conjunctivitis, depression, and fever. Coughing is usually self-limiting, resolving within 2 weeks. A more serious form of the disease, characterized by chronic bronchopneumonia, is seen in young puppies and young adult dogs with congenital airway abnormalities.

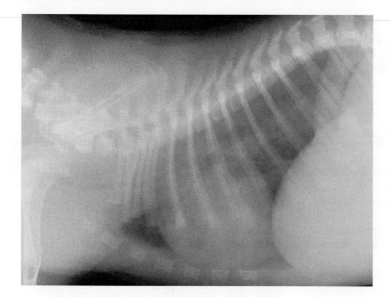

Figure 7–5. A lateral thoracic radiograph of a Boston terrier puppy with a hypoplastic trachea.

Diagnosis is primarily based on clinical signs and a history of exposure to other dogs. Thoracic radiographs are usually not necessary but if taken are normal unless secondary bronchopneumonia is present. Culture of tracheobronchial lavage solutions should be performed in dogs that have systemic illness, have radiographic evidence of bronchopneumonia, or fail to improve after symptomatic therapy to treat the signs.

Affected dogs should be isolated from other dogs and maintained in a warm, stress-free environment. Antimicrobial therapy, although not always needed, is indicated for puppies and young adults because of the likely involvement of *Bordetella bronchiseptica* or *Mycoplasma* species and the potential severity of bronchopneumonia as a sequela (see Table 7–4). Ideally, antimicrobial therapy should be based on bacterial culture and sensitivity testing. Chloramphenicol or amoxicillin/clavulanate combinations are initial choices for antimicrobial therapy because they are usually effective treatment for both *Bordetella bronchiseptica* and *Mycoplasma* species (Bemis, 1992). Antitussives can be used to suppress excessive nonproductive coughing in animals without evidence of bronchopneumonia (see Table 7–4). Prevention is based on vaccination programs and avoidance of potentially infected dogs. Sodium hypochlorite bleach (diluted 1 to 32 with water and a freshly prepared solution) may be used for disinfection of the infected premises.

FELINE INFECTIOUS TRACHEOBRONCHITIS

Infectious tracheobronchitis is uncommon in adult cats, but in cats younger than 1 year of age it can be especially common and associated with *Bordetella bronchiseptica* infection and the same viral agents that cause infectious upper respiratory infections (Wallace et al, 1992). Cats housed together in confined quarters frequently contain inapparent, chronic carrier cats that shed feline herpesvirus intermittently and/or feline calicivirus continuously. Active upper respiratory disease in these carrier cats is often triggered by stressful situations such as weaning, overcrowding, and poor husbandry.

In dogs, *Bordetella bronchiseptica* causes paroxysms of a dry, hacking cough. Although coughing may occur in cats, it is usually mild. More typical signs include fever, sneezing, oculonasal discharge, submandibular lymphadenopathy, and increased lung sounds. Most illness is usually self-limiting, with spontaneous resolution occurring after about 10 to 14 days. Severe bronchopneumonia associated with *Bordetella bronchiseptica* may occur, especially in kittens younger than 12 weeks of age (Willoughby et al, 1991).

Specific diagnosis of feline bordetellosis is difficult because the signs associated with it mimic those seen with the viral respiratory disease agents. Oropharyngeal and tracheobronchial cultures may be used to identify active *Bordetella bronchiseptica* infection. Isolation of the organism from active cases is relatively easy; however, chronic carrier cats often shed few organisms and require repeated oropharyngeal cultures.

Infected cats can be treated with tetracycline or amoxicillin/clavulanate combinations for 10 to 14 days (Speakman et al, 1997). Antimicrobial therapy does not eliminate the carrier state but does reduce the severity of the disease.

Proper husbandry can minimize the impact of *Bordetella bronchiseptica* infection in a group. Good nutrition, sanitation, ventilation, parasite control, and control of other respiratory agents minimize the occurrence of clinical disease in these environments.

Although feline bordetellosis is not as prevalent as feline herpesvirus or feline calicivirus infections, it is evident that in some young feline populations *Bordetella bronchiseptica* infections significantly contribute to persistent acute respiratory tract disease. The intranasal vaccine currently available affords complete protection; however, upper respiratory disease, if it does occur, can be restricted to short courses and is mild (Jacobs et al, 1993). Kittens may be vaccinated with the intranasal *Bordetella bronchiseptica* vaccine as young as 4 weeks of age.

PARASITIC TRACHEOBRONCHITIS

Capillaria aerophila of dogs and cats and *Oslerus (Filaroides) osleri* of dogs are occasionally found in the trachea and bronchi of young animals. The clinical sign is usually a nonproductive cough. Nodules containing masses of mature and immature *Oslerus (Filaroides) osleri* may be detected near the tracheal bifurcation during endoscopy. Eggs or larvae of the parasites may be identified by fecal examination using a modified Baermann technique or cytologic examination of lavage solution obtained by transtracheal aspiration or tracheobronchial lavage. Successful treatment is usually possible with fenbendazole (50 mg/kg daily given orally for 10 to 21 days) or ivermectin (300 µg/kg given orally or subcutaneously once). One month after therapy, eggs and larvae should have disappeared from the animal's feces.

TRACHEAL AND BRONCHIAL TRAUMA

Tracheal and bronchial trauma are seen with penetrating wounds or blunt trauma to the cervical region or thorax. Overinflation of the cuff of an endotracheal tube during anesthesia can also result in trauma to the tracheal mucosa. Coughing, dyspnea, and persistent peritracheal, subcutaneous, or mediastinal emphysema after cervical or thoracic trauma indicate thorough evaluation of the airways. Small wounds are often self-limiting, but extensive tissue damage, which may accompany penetrating bites or gunshot wounds, may require immediate care. Immediate treatment of tracheal or bronchial trauma should center on maintaining a patent airway, providing oxygen, and treating shock and/or hemorrhage. Antiinflammatory doses of glucocorticoids may decrease edema and inflammation that is contributing to airway obstruction. Wounds may require surgical debridement and apposition after the animal is stable.

TRACHEAL AND BRONCHIAL FOREIGN BODY

Foreign objects that lodge in the trachea or bronchi are more commonly seen in puppies than in kittens, having been inhaled during normal play activities or while eating. Varying degrees of tracheal obstruction result in an obstructed breathing pattern and coughing. Subcutaneous emphysema may also be evident in the cervical area if tracheal integrity has been breached. Diagnosis of tracheal foreign objects is made by radiographic examination or, if necessary, endoscopy. Tracheal foreign objects that are free in the tracheal or bronchial lumen can occasionally be removed by holding the animal with the head down and rapidly compressing its thorax or by inducing a cough by tracheal palpation while the head is held in a lowered position. Otherwise, tracheal or bronchial foreign objects can be removed with a retrieving instrument passed through or along the side of a small endoscope (Dimski, 1991). Failing endoscopic removal, surgical intervention will be necessary.

Neoplasia

Tracheal neoplasia of dogs and cats is uncommon. Tracheal osteochondroma (also referred to as tracheal osteochondral dysplasia), however, occurs in dogs younger than 6 months (Carlisle et al, 1991). These growths are benign and are not aggressive locally. Affected dogs usually demonstrate coughing, exercise intolerance, and an obstructed breathing pattern. The growths are readily seen radiographically as solitary distinct intratracheal masses that may, on occasion, be ossified. Surgical removal is the treatment of choice.

THE LOWER AIRWAY: SMALL BRONCHI AND LUNGS
Abnormal Lung Sounds

Lung sounds in puppies and kittens older than 6 weeks of age may be characterized as normal breath sounds (those sounds that accompany air movement in the normal tracheobronchial tree) and adventitious sounds (abnormal sounds that are superimposed on breath sounds) (Table 7–5) (Kotlikoff and Gillespie, 1983, 1984). Breath sounds are evenly distributed over all of the lung fields and are usually loudest on inspiration. Intensity of breath sounds may be characterized as normal or abnormally loud or soft. The sound intensity is generally much louder in the young animal than the adult because of less attenuation of sounds by a thinner thoracic wall. Changes in intensity of breath sounds can be attributed to either changes in airflow velocity or altered transmission of sound to the thoracic wall. Pleural effusion and pneumothorax diminish the transmission of these lung sounds. A consolidated lung lobe, despite reduced ventilation, will transmit sound more effectively than a well-ventilated lung. Increased respiratory efforts, which might be seen with exercise, anemia, hyperthermia, hypoxemia, and acidemia, will result in increased intensity of breath sounds as well.

Adventitious sounds are never heard in healthy animals (Kotlikoff and Gillespie, 1984). Adventitious sounds are produced by pathologic processes and are either crackles (rales) or wheezes (rhonchi) (see Table 7–5). Crackles are short, nonmusical, sharp, or explosive sounds that are produced by equalization of pressure following reopening of a collapsed airway. Crackles are best heard in cases of restrictive lung disease characterized by reduced compliance and associated decrease in lung volume, which leads to airway closure. Crackles may also be heard when there is disruption of liquid films or bubbles in the airways as may occur in pulmonary edema. Crackles should be characterized as to where in the respiratory cycle they are most evident. Fine crackles associated with interstitial pulmonary edema or interstitial pneumonia are usually heard late in inspiration, whereas coarse crackles associated with excessive airway secretions are heard throughout the respiratory cycle. Wheezes are continuous musical sounds. They are produced by vibration of airway walls that are in close contact. Wheezes may be of a single tone (monophonic) or multiple tones (polyphonic) and may occur in either the inspiratory or expiratory phase of the respiratory cycle. They are generally associated with airway obstruction and subsequent airway narrowing; inspiratory wheezes generally signify upper airway obstruction, and expiratory wheezes are more likely to represent obstruction of the lower respiratory tract.

Congenital Disorders

Most congenital diseases of the lung are uncommon in puppies and kittens. Agenesis or hypoplasia of the lungs causes death shortly after birth. If only one lung lobe is hypoplastic, signs are not present and the condition is only diagnosed as an incidental finding if radiographs are taken or necropsy is performed. Congenital tracheoesophageal or bronchoesophageal fistulas are uncommon.

CONGENITAL PULMONARY EMPHYSEMA

Pulmonary emphysema is an increase beyond normal size of the airspaces distal to the terminal bronchi that results from the destruction of alveolar walls. Congenital pulmonary emphysema in young puppies may be associated with an absence of cartilaginous plates or cartilaginous tissue around the bronchi (Hoover et al, 1992). Affected animals may show signs of progressively worsening respiratory distress com-

Table 7–5	Characteristics of Lung Sounds	
TYPE OF SOUNDS	**CAUSE**	**ASSOCIATION**
Normal breath sounds	Turbulent flow of air	Normal breathing activity
Adventitious sounds		
Crackles	Rapid opening of small airways and/or fluid in the airways	Bronchopneumonia Space-occupying pleural disorders Pulmonary edema Chronic interstitial disease
Wheezes	Vibration of airway walls in close contact	Inspiratory: extrathoracic airway obstruction, laryngeal paralysis, neoplasia, foreign object(s), collapsed trachea Expiratory: intrathoracic airway obstruction, bronchial disease, collapsed trachea

mencing as early as 6 weeks of age. An expiratory obstructed breathing pattern, as well as crackles and wheezes, may be evident. Radiographically, the emphysematous areas are generally hyperlucent (Suter, 1984c). Cats can also be affected with a similar problem (LaRue et al, 1990).

PULMONARY CAVITARY LESIONS

Pulmonary cavitary lesions, seen infrequently in puppies and kittens, include cysts, bullae, blebs, abscesses, cystic bronchiectasis, and pneumatoceles (Anderson, 1987; Nelson, 1993). These lesions may be either congenital or acquired and typically are air or fluid filled. Bronchogenic cysts are lined by respiratory epithelium and are poorly developed terminal bronchioles (Suter, 1984b). Blebs are subpleural airspaces within the pulmonary parenchyma that arise from breakdown of alveolar septa (Anderson, 1987; Suter, 1984c). Pneumatoceles are large cavitary lesions that form in the lung parenchyma when necrotic tissue is replaced by air (Anderson, 1987). The cavitary lesions are often incidental findings on thoracic radiographs but may rupture and lead to pneumothorax. If the cavitary lesions are incidental radiographic findings, treatment is usually not necessary. If pneumothorax is present, continuous or repeated pleural space drainage should be tried for 2 to 3 days. If pneumothorax cannot be controlled, thoracotomy is indicated to find and remove the leaking cystic lesion (Nelson, 1993).

Infectious/Inflammatory Disorders

INFECTIOUS PNEUMONIA

Pneumonia of an infectious source generally represents a primary lung disorder, extension of an existing tracheobronchial disease, opportunistic invasion, or the spread of a systemic disease to the lungs. Bacterial pneumonia (i.e., *Bordetella bronchiseptica*, *Streptococcus zooepidemicus*, and other gram-negative bacteria) is more common in puppies than in kittens (Roudebush, 1990). In kittens, *Bordetella bronchiseptica* and *Pasteurella* species are the most likely organisms to cause a primary bacterial pneumonia. Bacterial pneumonias are, however, often secondary, following viral infection; or, in animals with preexisting upper airway anomalies, immunocompromise; or in association with gastrointestinal disease that results in dysphagia, regurgitation, or vomiting. *Toxoplasma gondii* and, rarely, *Pneumocystis carinii* infections can cause pneumonia in puppies and kittens (Taboada and Merchant, 1995). Infections with *Aelurostrongylus abstrusus* in cats, *Paragonimus kellicotti* in dogs and cats, and *Filaroides hirthi* in dogs are the most common pulmonary parasitic causes of pneumonia, although they are uncommon in animals younger than 6 months (Barsanti and Prestwood, 1983). In addition, pulmonary migration of larval stages of *Toxocara canis* may infrequently produce a verminous pneumonia (Barsanti and Prestwood, 1983). Fungal pneumonia rarely occurs in dogs or cats younger than 6 months (Hodgin et al, 1987).

Typically, puppies or kittens with primary or secondary bacterial pneumonia will show tachypnea, respiratory distress, fever, and a productive cough. Lung sounds are often normal, but there may be an increased intensity of normal lung sounds, crackles, or, less frequently, wheezes (Thayer and Robinson, 1984). Radiographs may demonstrate an interstitial and alveolar lung pattern with a cranioventral distribution, typical of bacterial pneumonia; a diffuse interstitial lung pattern, typical of viral pneumonia; or a mixed lung pattern, that is, a combination of alveolar, interstitial, and peribronchial lung patterns, such as that seen in pulmonary toxoplasmosis, *Aelurostrongylus* pneumonia, or secondary bacterial pneumonia (Table 7–6).

Antimicrobial agents are an important component of the medical therapy for bacterial pneumonia. The choice of an antimicrobial agent should be based on bacterial culture and sensitivity test results. Therapy should, however, be commenced before the culture results are available. The antimicrobial agents generally preferred for the initial treatment of an uncomplicated bacterial pneumonia are amoxicillin/clavulanate or trimethoprim/sulfonamide combinations for dogs or a first-generation cephalosporin for cats (see Table 7–4). Chloramphenicol or amoxicillin/clavulanate combinations should be used for dogs or cats with suspected *Bordetella* infections. In severe cases, gentamicin or amikacin and a first-generation cephalosporin are usually effective when used in combination. Antimicrobial therapy should be modified based on culture results and continued for at least 4 weeks. Alternatively, antimicrobial therapy should be continued for at least 10 days beyond radiographic resolution (Stone and Pook, 1992).

The animal's hydration should be adequate to ensure mucociliary clearance in the lower airways. Crystalloid solutions should be given intravenously or subcutaneously to prevent dehydration. Additionally, airway hydration can be

Table 7-6 Radiographic Changes of Selected Pulmonary Diseases

DISEASE	DISTRIBUTION	LUNG PATTERN	BLOOD VESSELS	AIRWAY PATTERN	ASSOCIATED RADIOGRAPHIC LESIONS
Broncho-pneumonia	Asymmetric: cranioventral, or no preference	Alveolar or mixed	Normal	May be increased bronchial pattern	None
Aspiration pneumonia	Asymmetric: affecting ventral, middle, and accessory lobes	Mixed	Normal	May be increased bronchial pattern	May be megaesophagus
Viral pneumonia (canine distemper)	Generalized	Interstitial or mixed	Normal	May be increased bronchial pattern	Pulmonary edema
Cardiogenic	Perihilar to generalized	Alveolar or mixed	Increased diameter of veins	May be increased bronchial pattern	Cardiomegaly, left atrial enlargement, elevation of left mainstem bronchus
Caused by electrical cord bites	Generalized: often most prominent in caudal lung lobes	Mixed	Normal	May be increased bronchial pattern	
Neoplasia (lympho-sarcoma)	Symmetric	Fine nodular interstitial	Normal	Normal	Enlarged thymus and mediastinal lymphadenopathy ± pleural effusion

Adapted from Suter PF: Lower airway and pulmonary parenchymal disease. *In* Suter PF (ed): Thoracic Radiography: A Text Atlas of Thoracic Diseases of the Dog and Cat. Wettswil, Switzerland, Peter F. Suter, 1984, p 554.

maximized by nebulization with normal saline solution. Oxygen and bronchodilator therapy may be needed for hypoxemic animals. Cough suppressants should not be given to animals with pneumonia. *Aelurostrongylus* and *Paragonimus* infections can be treated successfully with fenbendazole at 50 mg/kg orally once a day for 10 to 14 days. Fenbendazole therapy is terminated when larvae or eggs are not found in the feces or when anorexia develops. Another therapy for *Aelurostrongylus* infection is ivermectin (400 μg/kg subcutaneously once) (Stone and Pook, 1992). *Paragonimus* infection can also be treated with praziquantel (25 mg/kg orally 3 times a day for 3 days) (Stone and Pook, 1992). Toxoplasmosis can be effectively treated with clindamycin at a total daily dosage of 25 mg/kg divided twice a day for 4 weeks (Lappin, 1994).

ASPIRATION PNEUMONIA

Aspiration pneumonia occurs more frequently in puppies than in kittens; most often it is asso-ciated with congenital megaesophagus or im-proper feeding of milk-replacement formula. Aspiration may also result from esophageal or pharyngeal dysfunction, chronic vomiting, or a depressed state of consciousness. Anesthesia is always a risk factor for aspiration pneumonia because an animal may regurgitate gastric con-tents into the pharynx during general anesthesia or vomit during recovery. Typically, once a sig-nificant quantity of material is aspirated, rapid onset of clinical signs occurs. The signs are similar to those observed with a bacterial pneu-monia; the severity depends on the amount and content of the aspirated material. Aspiration of acidic gastric contents will cause the most se-vere damage.

Radiographic abnormalities may not be ap-parent until 12 to 24 hours after aspiration and include consolidation and alveolar and intersti-tial infiltration of dependent lung lobes (Fig. 7–6). The right cranial and middle lung lobes are most commonly affected in animals that aspirate while in a sternal position, whereas

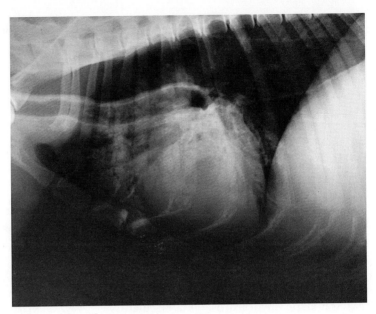

Figure 7–6. A lateral thoracic radiograph of a young dog with megaesophagus secondary to myasthenia gravis. Alveolar consolidation in the right cranial and middle lung lobes is due to aspiration pneumonia. Note the air-filled esophagus indicative of megaesophagus and the consolidation with air bronchograms indicative of alveolar disease in the ventral portions of the cranial and middle lung lobes.

other lung lobes are likely affected in animals that are in prone positions. Aspiration pneumonia should be treated similarly to other types of pneumonia. Immediately on aspiration, if possible, mechanical suction of the airways should be attempted.

Pulmonary Edema

Pulmonary edema is uncommon in puppies and even less common in kittens. When seen, it is usually secondary to congenital or acquired heart disease, head trauma or seizures, severe upper airway obstruction, or electric shock (Taboada et al, 1992). Parvoviral myocarditis can cause pulmonary edema in young puppies (Jezyk et al, 1979). In addition, pulmonary edema is seen in cases of aspiration and inhalation pneumonia and acute respiratory distress syndrome (ARDS). Regardless of the cause of pulmonary edema, clinical signs are the same—productive cough, dyspnea, cyanosis, orthopnea, apprehension, and, in severe cases, hemorrhagic froth from the nose and mouth. Thoracic auscultation may reveal increased intensity of normal lung sounds, end-inspiratory crackles, and/or expiratory wheezes. With suspected pulmonary edema, the lips, gingiva, tongue, and palate should be examined closely for burns associated with biting into an electric cord (Kolata and Burrows, 1981). Thoracic radiographs are extremely helpful in the diagnosis of pulmonary edema (see Table 7–6) but should be taken when the animal is stable.

Successful treatment of pulmonary edema requires attention to the cause and rigorous treatment of the signs. The principal objectives of therapy are to (1) decrease oxygen demands (cage rest); (2) improve alveolar oxygen delivery (oxygen therapy, bronchodilators); (3) decrease excessive pulmonary fluid (diuretics); (4) support and maintain pulmonary circulation (myocardial support); and (5) treat the underlying disorder (Taboada et al, 1992). The consequences of overzealous treatment are minimal compared with the consequences of inadequate therapy. Oxygen can be administered via mask, cage, nasal catheter, or endotracheal tube. Furosemide should be given to reduce intravascular volume by diuresis and to increase systemic venous capacitance. Treatment of noncardiogenic edema is similar but generally less effective. Corticosteroids may be useful in cases of electric shock or ARDS.

ACUTE RESPIRATORY DISTRESS SYNDROME

ARDS is a condition in which there is life-threatening respiratory failure due to noncardiogenic pulmonary edema associated with severe illness. In puppies and kittens, ARDS may be seen with septicemia, trauma, and other shock states (Orsher and Kolata, 1982). Clinically, ARDS is characterized by sudden onset of respiratory distress in a critically ill animal. No characteristic hematologic or serum chemistry profile abnormalities occur, but thrombocytopenia and leukopenia are inconsistent findings. Thoracic radiographs confirm pulmonary edema. Hypoxemia is present, and the PaO_2 level fails to significantly increase with the administration of oxygen—a finding indicative of ventilation-perfusion mismatch and right-to-left pulmonary shunting. ARDS has been reported in newborn and young puppies (Manktelow and Baskerville, 1972). Affected puppies may be found dead or develop respiratory distress and die within a few hours. Most likely, a similar respiratory distress syndrome occurs in young kittens. The ARDS may be part of the "fading puppy and kitten syndromes."

Pulmonary Contusions and Lacerations

Contusions usually result from being hit by a car or from bite wounds inflicted by another animal. Associated conditions include rib fractures, pleural hemorrhage, diaphragmatic hernia, traumatic myocarditis, and circulatory shock. On examination of the animal, varying degrees of respiratory distress are usually evident, and crackles and wheezes may be heard on auscultation. Radiographic evidence of pulmonary contusion includes alveolar and/or interstitial lung densities and atelectasis (Fig. 7–7). These changes may not be evident until 12 hours after trauma and are expected to regress within 24 to 72 hours and resolve within 3 to 10 days (Gibbons, 1992; Suter, 1984f). Signs of pulmonary lacerations are similar to those of pulmonary contusions, but they tend to be more severe because of coexisting hemothorax, pneumothorax, and hemoptysis. Specific treatment for pulmonary contusions is usually supportive care.

Pulmonary Neoplasia

Pulmonary neoplasia rarely occurs in dogs and cats younger than 6 months. Lymphosarcoma can, on occasion, involve the pulmonary parenchyma and be manifested radiographically as diffuse, indistinct nodules (see Table 7–6). These lesions are usually associated with enlargement of surrounding thoracic lymph nodes (Suter, 1984c). Metastatic neoplasia is uncommon in animals younger than 6 months.

THE PLEURAL CAVITY

Pneumothorax

Trauma is the most common cause of pneumothorax in the young dog or cat. Penetrating thoracic wall injuries from animal bites or projectiles, laceration of the tracheobronchial airway, blunt trauma to the thorax, rib fractures, alveolar rupture due to overzealous assisted positive pressure ventilation, and/or ruptured cystic lesions can all cause pneumothorax. Signs of pneumothorax may vary from mild polypnea to severe respiratory distress and cyanosis. Radiographically, retraction of lung lobes toward the hilum is noted; in the lateral view, the heart is separated from the sternum (Fig. 7–8) (Suter, 1984c). Pneumothorax in the puppy or kitten is managed in a similar way as in the adult.

Pleural Effusion

Pleural effusions are generally characterized as being transudate, modified transudate, exudate, or hemorrhage (Duncan and Prasse, 1986).

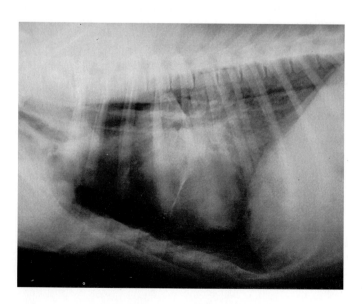

Figure 7–7. A lateral thoracic radiograph of a young dog hit by a car. Note the pneumomediastinum and pulmonary contusions. Air within the mediastinum allows visual observation of the outer wall of the trachea. (Courtesy of Dr. Beth Partington, School of Veterinary Medicine, Louisiana State University.)

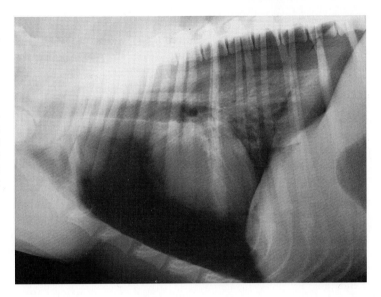

Figure 7–8. A lateral thoracic radiograph of a pneumothorax in a young dog hit by a car. The cardiac silhouette is pulled away from the sternum, and the dorsal lung lobes are sharply outlined due to the air in the pleural space.

Characteristics of the various types of pleural effusions are presented in Table 7–7. The most common causes of pleural effusion in puppies and kittens are pyothorax, cardiomyopathy, and the effusive form of feline infectious peritonitis. Thoracocentesis of pleural effusion is always required to characterize the fluid. Cytologic findings of the different types of pleural effusions are presented in Table 7–7. Specimens of pleural fluid that have the cytologic characteristics of an exudate should be cultured for aerobic and anaerobic bacteria and tested for antimicrobial sensitivity. Management of pleural effusion in puppies and kittens is similar to that in adults.

THE DIAPHRAGM
Congenital Diaphragmatic Hernia

Two types of congenital diaphragmatic hernias are seen in young dogs and cats—peritoneopericardial and pleuroperitoneal diaphragmatic hernias (Johnson, 1993; Wallace et al, 1992).

Congenital Peritoneopericardial Hernia

Congenital peritoneopericardial hernias are much more common in the dog and cat than are congenital pleuroperitoneal hernias (Johnson, 1993). A ventral diaphragmatic defect allows abdominal viscera into the pericardial sac. The defect is developmental but does not appear to be inherited. The defect has been reported in the collie and cocker spaniel to affect multiple animals from a single litter (Bellah et al, 1989). Other congenital defects, including sternal defects, cranial midline abdomi-

nal wall hernia, umbilical hernia, abnormal swirling hair along the ventrum, cardiac defects, congenital portosystemic vascular shunt, and pulmonary vascular disease may be seen in conjunction with peritoneopericardial hernia. Signs depend somewhat on the organ(s) that protrude through the diaphragmatic defect and the amount of displaced tissue contained in the hernia. Gastrointestinal, cardiovascular, or respiratory signs may be noted (Johnson, 1993; Wallace et al, 1992). Liver incarceration or a concurrent congenital portosystemic vascular shunt may cause encephalopathic signs. In addition, there may be a displacement of the apex beat of the heart, and intestinal sounds may be auscultated in the thorax. Gastrointestinal signs of vomiting, anorexia, and/or diarrhea are seen most commonly (Wallace et al, 1992). Diagnosis of peritoneopericardial hernia can usually be made radiographically or ultrasonographically (Fig. 7–9). The cardiac silhouette is usually enlarged and appears round or ovoid. The density of the cardiac silhouette may be nonhomogeneous owing to the presence of soft tissue, fat, and/or gas densities. Pericardial ultrasonography is useful in differentiating a peritoneopericardial hernia from pericardial effusion or cardiomegaly when it is not obvious from the radiographs (Johnson, 1993). Treatment for congenital peritoneopericardial diaphragmatic hernia is surgical, especially if the animal is showing signs of the hernia (Johnson, 1993).

Congenital Pleuroperitoneal Hernia

Congenital defects in the diaphragm resulting in pleuroperitoneal hernia are uncommon in

Table 7–7	Causes and Characteristics of Pleural Effusion

Transudate
  Causes: Hypoalbuminemia, right heart failure
  Characteristics: Colorless, clear. Protein content
    <2.5 g/dl. Nucleated cells <500 cells/μl

Modified Transudate
  Causes: Persistent transudation with added cells
    and protein content, lymphatic obstruction,
    chylous and pseudochylous effusions
  Characteristics: Appearance variable according to
    the cause. Protein content generally >2.5 g/dl.
    Nucleated cells generally >500 cells/μl. In
    chylous effusions, lymphocytes and/or
    neutrophils are the predominant cell types; the
    triglyceride content of the effusion is greater
    than that of serum

Exudate
  Causes: Increased vascular permeability and
    inflammation
  Characteristics: Turbid. Protein content generally
    >3 g/dl. Nucleated cells >3000 cells/μl and
    predominantly neutrophils. Neutrophils may be
    nondegenerate in nonseptic inflammatory
    processes or degenerate in septic processes

Hemorrhage
  Causes: Usually trauma, bleeding disorders
  Characteristics: Recent hemorrhage: bright red.
    Protein content and nucleated cell numbers are
    less than those of peripheral blood.
    Cytologically, intact red blood cells and white
    blood cells are in morphologic condition and
    distribution to those of peripheral blood. Long-
    standing hemorrhage: buff red. Protein content
    and nucleated cell numbers are less than those
    of peripheral blood. Cytologically, red blood
    cells and white blood cells are distorted, and
    hypersegmented neutrophils and phagocytized
    red blood cells are seen

dogs and cats. When present, the defect is usually in the dorsolateral part of the diaphragm and may result in stillbirth or death shortly after birth, especially if the defect is on the left side. This form of hernia is likely to be inherited as an autosomal recessive trait (Valentine et al, 1988).

THE THORACIC WALL

Congenital Disorders

RIB DEFORMITIES

Deformities in the number, position, and shape of the ribs do occur but usually are of little if any significance to health (Orton, 1993). If the deformity does cause a restriction in ventilation, surgical correction may be indicated. Surgery is also occasionally performed for cosmetic reasons.

PECTUS EXCAVATUM

Pectus excavatum results from intrusion of the sternum into the thorax. This disorder has been identified in both puppies and kittens (Orton, 1993). Other signs that may be present in addition to the sternal malformations are uncommon; they include poor growth rate, respiratory distress, and exercise intolerance. Radiographically, the ventral ends of the ribs are turned medially to join the dorsally displaced sternebrae (Fig. 7–10) (Suter, 1984b). Mild cases require no treatment. The reader is referred elsewhere for treatment of more severe cases (Shires et al, 1988).

Trauma

Rib and sternebra fractures are usually the result of blunt trauma. The flexibility of the thoracic wall in young animals is highly protective against such fractures; nevertheless, these fractures, with or without intrathoracic injuries, do occasionally occur. Accompanying injuries may include pulmonary contusion, intercostal artery laceration, pulmonary parenchymal and diaphragm laceration, and possibly concurrent laceration of abdominal structures (Fig. 7–11). Intrathoracic injuries may also occur in the absence of rib or sternebra fractures. Signs vary depending on the degree of respiratory distress, severity of the fracture(s), and accompanying intrathoracic lesions. Rib and sternebra fractures can usually be identified by thorough palpation and confirmed radiographically. Rib and sternebra fractures that do not interfere with the overall integrity of the thoracic wall are usually left to heal undisturbed. If shock and/or intrathoracic injuries are present, appropriate medical and surgical treatment is indicated. A grossly unstable thoracic wall that is causing severe respiratory compromise is best managed surgically (Orton, 1993).

THE MEDIASTINUM

Mediastinitis

Mediastinitis can result from a tracheal or esophageal rupture or from extension of an infection from an adjacent area (Suter, 1984d). If a mediastinal infection is present, it may extend

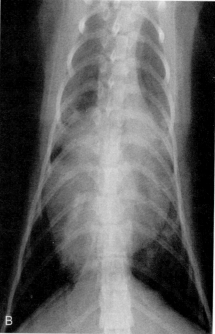

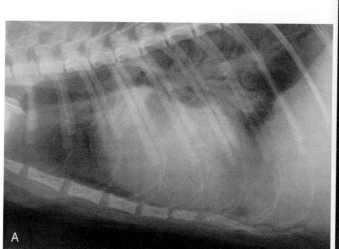

Figure 7–9. A, Lateral thoracic radiograph of a young Himalayan cat with a peritoneopericardial diaphragmatic hernia and a congenital portosystemic vascular anomaly. Note the markedly enlarged cardiac silhouette. **B,** Ventrodorsal projection of the same cat.

into the fascial planes of the neck. Fever, thoracic pain, restricted breathing pattern, and, less commonly, regurgitation and/or coughing may be present, depending somewhat on the origin of the mediastinitis. Radiographically, mediastinitis is usually identified by a diffuse widening of the mediastinum (Suter, 1984d). Pneumomediastinum and/or pneumothorax may also be evident. Treatment of mediastinitis is directed toward correction of the underlying cause and supportive care.

Mediastinal Masses

Mediastinal masses are characterized by their location in the mediastinum, that is, involving the cranial, middle, or caudal portion of the mediastinum. Craniodorsal mediastinal masses tend to depress the trachea ventrally and include esophageal dilations such as those caused by megaesophagus, vascular ring anomalies, and esophageal foreign bodies. Thymic lymphosarcoma is the most common mediastinal mass in

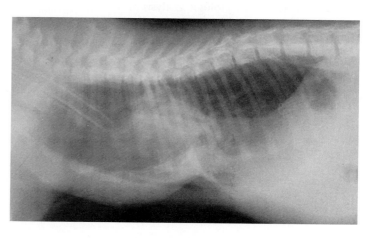

Figure 7–10. A lateral thoracic radiograph of a puppy with pectus excavatum.

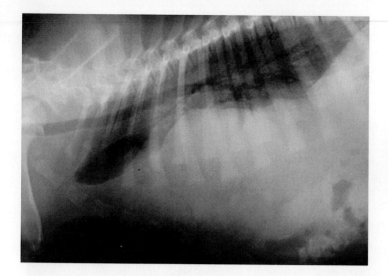

Figure 7–11. A lateral thoracic radiograph of a 2-month-old puppy with a traumatic diaphragmatic hernia after being hit by a car. Note the loss of the diaphragmatic border, pleural effusion, and dorsal displacement of the cardiac silhouette.

the young cat and tends to elevate the trachea. Signs associated with mediastinal masses depend on the region of the mediastinum involved and tissue of origin. Signs may include coughing, respiratory distress, restricted or obstructed breathing pattern, exercise intolerance, regurgitation, neck and forelimb edema, Horner's syndrome, changes in phonation, and fever (Suter, 1984d). Inability to compress the thoracic wall cranial to the heart in a young cat is suggestive of thymic lymphosarcoma. Granulomatous masses of the cranial mediastinum in cats younger than 6 months have also been reported (Jang et al, 1975).

Survey thoracic radiographs usually reveal the presence of mediastinal masses and their location (Suter, 1984d). To identify the cellular or tissue origin of a mediastinal mass, a transthoracic aspiration for cytology or ultrasound-guided percutaneous biopsy is required. If pleural fluid is present, removal of the fluid may be required before thoracic radiographs can identify a mediastinal mass. Cytologic analysis of the fluid may yield a definitive diagnosis, particularly if the mass is caused by lymphosarcoma. Treatment of mediastinal masses is directed at the underlying cause and supportive care.

References and Supplemental Reading

Anderson GI: Pulmonary cavitary lesions in the dog: A review of seven cases. J Am Anim Hosp Assoc 23:89, 1987.

Aron DN, Crowe DT: Upper airway obstruction: General principles and selected conditions in the dog and cat. Vet Clin North Am Small Anim Pract 15:891, 1985.

Barsanti JA, Prestwood AK: Parasitic diseases of the respiratory tract. In Kirk RW (ed): Current Veterinary Therapy VIII. Philadelphia, WB Saunders, 1983, p 241.

Bellah JR, Spencer CP, Brown DJ, et al: Congenital cranioventral abdominal wall, caudal sternal, diaphragmatic, pericardial, and intracardiac defects in cocker spaniel littermates. J Am Vet Med Assoc 194:1741, 1989.

Bemis DA: Bordetella and mycoplasma respiratory infections in dogs and cats. Vet Clin North Am Small Anim Pract 22:1173, 1992.

Boothe HW: Surgery of the tympanic bulla (otitis media and nasopharyngeal polyps). Prob Vet Med 3:254, 1991.

Braund KG, Shores A, Di Pinto N, et al: Laryngeal paralysis in Dalmatians. J Vet Intern Med 3:117, 1992 (Abstract).

Burbidge HM, Goulden BE, Dickson GB: Surgical relief of severe laryngeal malformation in an English bulldog. N Z Vet J 36:29, 1988.

Carlisle CH, Biery DN, Thrall DE: Tracheal and laryngeal tumors in the dog and cat: Literature review and 13 additional patients. Vet Radiol 32:229, 1991.

Coyne BE, Fingland RB: Hypoplasia of the trachea in dogs: 103 cases (1974–1990). J Am Vet Med Assoc 201:768, 1992.

Davidson A, Komtebedde J, Pappagianis D, et al: Treatment of nasal aspergillosis with topical clotrimazole. Proc Am Coll Vet Intern Med 10:807, 1992.

Davies RC, Mason RS: Abnormalities of the trachea in a dog. Vet Rec 82:191, 1968.

Diehl K, Rosychuk AW: Feline gingivitis-stomatitis-pharyngitis. Vet Clin North Am Small Anim Pract 23:139, 1993.

Dimski DS: Tracheal obstruction caused by tree needles in a cat. J Am Vet Med Assoc 199:477, 1991.

Duncan JR, Prasse KW: Cytology. In Duncan JR, Prasse KW (eds): Veterinary Laboratory Medicine, 2nd ed. Ames, Iowa State University Press, 1986, p 201.

Edwards DF, Patton CS, Kennedy JR: Primary ciliary dyskinesia in the dog. Prob Vet Med 4:291, 1992.

Ford RB: Role of infectious agents in respiratory disease. Vet Clin North Am Small Anim Pract 23:17, 1993.

Ford RB, Vaden SL: Canine infectious tracheobronchitis. In Greene CE (ed): Infectious Diseases of the Dog and Cat. Philadelphia, WB Saunders, 1990, p 259.

Gibbons G: Respiratory emergencies. In Murtaugh RJ, Kaplan PM (eds): Veterinary Emergency and Critical Care Medicine. St. Louis, Mosby Year Book, 1992, p 399.

Greenfield CL: Canine laryngeal paralysis. Compend Contin Educ Pract Vet 9:1011, 1987.

Harvey CE: Upper airway obstruction surgery: Part II. Soft palate resection in brachycephalic dogs. J Am Anim Hosp Assoc 18:538, 1982a.

Harvey CE: Upper airway obstruction surgery: Part III. Everted laryngeal saccule surgery in brachycephalic dogs. J Am Anim Hosp Assoc 18:545, 1982b.

Hawkins EC: Respiratory disorders. In Nelson RW, Couto CG (eds): Small Animal Internal Medicine. St. Louis, Mosby, 1998, p 214.

Hendricks JC: Brachycephalic airway syndrome. Vet Clin North Am Small Anim Pract 22:1145, 1992.

Hodgin EC, Corstvet RE, Blakewood BW: Cryptococcosis in a pup. J Am Vet Med Assoc 191:697, 1987.

Hoover JP, Henry GA, Panciera RJ: Bronchial cartilage dysplasia with multifocal lobar bullous emphysema and lung torsions in a pup. J Am Vet Med Assoc 201:599, 1992.

Jacobs AAC, Chalmers WSK, Pasman FV, et al: Feline bordetellosis: Challenge and vaccine studies. Vet Rec 133:260, 1993.

Jang SS, Lock A, Biberstein EL: A cat with Corynebacterium equi lymphadenitis clinically simulating lymphosarcoma. Cornell Vet 65:232, 1975.

Jezyk PF, Haskins ME, Jones CL: Myocarditis of probable viral origin in pups of weaning age. J Am Vet Med Assoc 174:1204, 1979.

Johnson KA: Diaphragmatic, pericardial, and hiatal hernia. In Slatter D (ed): Textbook of Small Animal Surgery, vol 1, 2nd ed. Philadelphia, WB Saunders, 1993, p 455.

Kapatkin AS, Matthiesen DT, Noone KE, et al: Results of surgery and long-term follow-up in 31 cats with nasopharyngeal polyps. J Am Anim Hosp Assoc 26:387, 1990.

Kotlikoff MI, Gillespie JR: Lung sounds in veterinary medicine. Part 1. Terminology and mechanisms of sound production. Compend Contin Educ Pract Vet 5:634, 1983.

Kotlikoff MI, Gillespie JR: Lung sounds in veterinary medicine. Part II. Deriving clinical information from lung sounds. Compend Contin Educ Pract Vet 6:462, 1984.

Lappin MR: Diagnosis of toxoplasmosis. In August JR (ed): Consultations in Feline Internal Medicine 2. Philadelphia, WB Saunders, 1994, p 41.

LaRue MJ, Garlick DS, Lamb CR, et al: Bronchial dysgenesis and lobar emphysema in an adult cat. J Am Vet Med Assoc 197:886, 1990.

Malik R, Wigney DI, Gregory DJ, et al: Cryptococcosis in cats: Clinical and mycological assessment of 29 cases and evaluation of treatment using orally administered fluconazole. J Med Vet Mycol 30:133, 1992.

Manktelow BW, Baskerville A: Respiratory distress syndrome in newborn puppies. J Small Anim Pract 13:329, 1972.

Mitten RW: Acquired nasopharyngeal stenosis in cats. In Kirk RW, Bonagura JD (eds): Current Veterinary Therapy XI. Philadelphia, WB Saunders, 1992, p 801.

Nelson AW: Upper respiratory system. In Slatter D (ed): Textbook of Small Animal Surgery, vol 1, 2nd ed. Philadelphia, WB Saunders, 1993, p 777.

O'Brien JA, Hendricks J: Inherited laryngeal paralysis. Analysis in the husky cross. Vet Q 8:301, 1986.

Orsher AN, Kolata RJ: Acute respiratory distress syndrome: Case report and literature review. J Am Anim Hosp Assoc 18(1):41, 1982.

Orton EC: Thoracic wall. In Slatter D (ed): Textbook of Small Animal Surgery, vol 1, 2nd ed. Philadelphia, WB Saunders, 1993, p 370.

Orton EC, Park RD: Evaluation of the surgical respiratory patient. In Slatter D (ed): Textbook of Small Animal Surgery, vol 1, 2nd ed. Philadelphia, WB Saunders, 1993, p 724.

Povey RC: Feline respiratory diseases. In Greene CE (ed): Infectious Diseases of the Dog and Cat. Philadelphia, WB Saunders, 1990, p 346.

Roudebush P: Bacterial infections of the respiratory system. In Greene CE (ed): Infectious Diseases of the Dog and Cat. Philadelphia, WB Saunders, 1990, p 114.

Sartin EA, Dubielzig RR: Congenital abnormalities in the respiratory tree of a dog. J Am Anim Hosp Assoc 20:775, 1984.

Sharp NJH, Sullivan M: Treatment of canine nasal aspergillosis with systemic ketoconazole and enilconazole. Vet Rec 118:560, 1986.

Sharp NJH, Sullivan M, Harvey CE, et al: Treatment of canine nasal aspergillosis with enilconazole. J Vet Intern Med 7:40, 1993.

Shires PK, Waldron DR, Payne J: Pectus excavatum in three kittens. J Am Anim Hosp Assoc 24:203, 1988.

Speakman AJ, Binns SH, Dawson S, et al: Antimicrobial susceptibility of Bordetella bronchiseptica isolates from cats and a comparison of the agar dilution and E-test methods. Vet Microbiol 54:63, 1997.

Stone MS, Pook H: Lung infections and infestations: Therapeutic considerations. Prob Vet Med 4:279, 1992.

Suter PF: Diseases of the nasal cavity, larynx and trachea. In Suter PF (ed): Thoracic Radiography: A Text Atlas of Thoracic Diseases of the Dog and Cat. Wettswil, Switzerland, Peter F. Suter, 1984a, p 205.

Suter PF: Lesions of the thoracic wall, extra pleural diseases. *In* Suter PF (ed): Thoracic Radiography: A Text Atlas of Thoracic Diseases of the Dog and Cat. Wettswil, Switzerland, Peter F. Suter, 1984b, p 161.

Suter PF: Lower airway and pulmonary parenchymal disease. *In* Suter PF (ed): Thoracic Radiography: A Text Atlas of Thoracic Diseases of the Dog and Cat. Wettswil, Switzerland, Peter F. Suter, 1984c, p 517.

Suter PF: Mediastinal abnormalities. *In* Suter PF (ed): Thoracic Radiography: A Text Atlas of Thoracic Diseases of the Dog and Cat. Wettswil, Switzerland, Peter F. Suter, 1984d, p 253.

Suter PF: Pleural abnormalities. *In* Suter PF (ed): Thoracic Radiography: A Text Atlas of Thoracic Diseases of the Dog and Cat. Wettswil, Switzerland, Peter F. Suter, 1984e, p 683.

Suter PF: Trauma to the thorax and the cervical airways. *In* Suter PF (ed): Thoracic Radiography: A Text Atlas of Thoracic Diseases of the Dog and Cat. Wettswil, Switzerland, Peter F. Suter, 1984f, p 127.

Taboada J, Hoskins JD, Morgan RV: Respiratory emergencies. *In* Emergency Medicine and Critical Care in Practice. Trenton, NJ, Veterinary Learning Systems, 1992, p 50.

Taboada J, Merchant SR: Protozoal and miscellaneous infections. *In* Ettinger SJ, Feldman EC (eds): Textbook of Veterinary Internal Medicine, 4th ed. Philadelphia, WB Saunders, 1995, p 384.

Thayer GW, Robinson SK: Bacterial bronchopneumonia in the dog: A review of 42 cases. J Am Anim Hosp Assoc 20:731, 1984.

Valentine BA, Cooper BJ, Dietze AE, et al: Canine congenital diaphragmatic hernia. J Vet Intern Med 2:109, 1988.

Venker-van Haagen AJ: Diseases of the larynx. Vet Clin North Am Small Anim Pract 22:1155, 1992.

Venker-van Haagen AJ, Engelse EJJ, van den Ingh ThSGAM: Congenital subglottic stenosis in a dog. J Am Anim Hosp Assoc 17:223, 1981.

Wallace J, Mullen HS, Lesser MB: A technique for surgical correction of peritoneal pericardial diaphragmatic hernia in dogs and cats. J Am Anim Hosp Assoc 28:503, 1992.

Willoughby K, Dawson S, Jones RC, et al: Isolation of *B. bronchiseptica* from kittens with pneumonia in a breeding cattery. Vet Rec 129:407, 1991.

Wolf AM: Fungal diseases of the nasal cavity of the dog and cat. Vet Clin North Am Small Anim Pract 22:1119, 1992.

Wykes PM: Brachycephalic airway obstructive syndrome. Prob Vet Med 3:188, 1991.

The Cardiovascular System

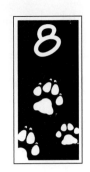

Janice McIntosh Bright

DEVELOPMENT OF THE CARDIOVASCULAR SYSTEM

The circulatory physiology of newborn and young animals is different from that of adults. Therefore, evaluation of the cardiovascular system requires awareness of the structural and functional changes occurring in dogs and cats from birth to 6 months of age.

Although the stroke work of the ventricles is nearly equal in utero, stroke work of the right ventricle decreases relative to that of the left ventricle after birth. Consequently, the relative masses of the right and left ventricles progressively change from a 1:1 ratio in the newborn to 1:2 to 1:3 ratio in the adult (Kirk et al, 1975; Lee et al, 1975). In dogs, the left ventricular geometry also changes with age, the chamber becoming less elliptical and more globular during maturation (Lee et al, 1975). These anatomic differences may affect the appearance of the electrocardiogram, echocardiogram, and thoracic radiographs.

Compared with the adult, the puppy or kitten has a lower blood pressure, stroke volume, and peripheral vascular resistance. The young animal, however, has a greater heart rate, cardiac output, plasma volume, and central venous pressure (Table 8–1). In puppies, these parameters will simultaneously and progressively change to adult values during the first 7 months of life (Adelman and Wright, 1985; Magrini, 1978). During infancy, the cardiovascular system appears to operate as a high-blood-flow, low-arteriolar-resistance, and possibly a low-venous-capacitance system, providing high tissue perfusion to meet the metabolic needs of growing tissues.

Table 8–1	Body Weight and Hemodynamic Findings in Five Conscious Dogs at Different Ages*	
	1 MONTH OF AGE	9 MONTHS OF AGE
Body weight (kg)	2.12 ± 0.15	17.57 ± 0.62
Heart rate (beats/min)	173 ± 6	71 ± 4
Cardiac index (L/min/kg)	0.22 ± 0.025	0.12 ± 0.018
Stroke volume (ml/kg)	1.23 ± 0.9	1.69 ± 0.6
Mean arterial pressure (mmHg)	49 ± 5	94 ± 2
Total peripheral resistance (mmHg • min/L)	188 ± 23	765 ± 30
Central venous pressure (mmHg)	8 ± 2	2 ± 1
Plasma volume (L/kg)	0.068 ± 0.006	0.049 ± 0.005

*Values are expressed as mean ± standard error.
Adapted with permission from Magrini F: Haemodynamic determinants of the arterial blood pressure rise during growth in conscious puppies. Cardiovasc Res 12:422, 1978.

Autonomic innervation of the heart and vasculature is incomplete in newborn puppies and kittens, providing them with little baroreflex control of circulation (Hageman et al, 1986; Hutchinson et al, 1962; Mace and Levy, 1983a,b; Tynan et al, 1977; Vatner and Mand-

103

ers, 1979). In addition, myocardial contractility is decreased compared with that in the adult (Davies et al, 1975; Horton and Coln, 1985; Suga et al, 1986). Young animals, therefore, have a limited ability to compensate for circulatory stresses in situations such as hyperthermia, acid-base shifts, and hemorrhage (Horton and Coln, 1985).

EVALUATION OF THE CARDIOVASCULAR SYSTEM

History

A thorough history can be extremely useful in establishing the diagnosis and prognosis of a suspected cardiovascular abnormality. Identifying the presence or absence of illness in the dam, sire, littermates, and kennel mates may be helpful for identifying certain infectious diseases or heritable defects. Determining the nature and progression of clinical signs, if present, is also important. Signs of illness often associated with cardiovascular disease in young animals include lethargy, stunted growth, exercise intolerance, cough, ascites, edema, syncope, cyanosis, dyspnea, and sudden death.

Examination

Procedurally, examination of the cardiovascular system of a kitten or puppy is similar to the examination of an adult (Gompf, 1988). The smaller size and more rapid heart rate of the young animal may, however, limit one's ability to localize heart sounds and to evaluate pulses.

Particularly important when examining a young animal is inspection of the oral, conjunctival, and genital mucous membranes for pallor or cyanosis. Pallor due to anemia is common in heavily parasitized puppies and kittens. The anemia, if severe, may produce an audible murmur and a hyperdynamic circulatory state, which should not be confused with primary cardiac disease. Cyanosis, the presence of blue-tinged mucosa, is an important finding in young animals because it indicates severe hypoxemia. Cyanosis may result from hypoventilation, primary pulmonary disease, heart failure with pulmonary edema, or cardiovascular malformations with shunting of unoxygenated blood. Because cyanosis is apparent only when there is more than 5 g/dl of unoxygenated hemoglobin in the peripheral circulation, anemic animals may have severe hypoxemia without detectable cyanosis. Preputial or vaginal membranes should be examined to identify differential cyanosis that may occur in an animal with reverse patent ductus arteriosus (PDA). Differential cyanosis refers to the presence of normal mucous membranes of the head with cyanosis of the genital mucous membranes and is typical of a right-to-left shunting PDA.

Healthy, unanesthetized, full-term puppies and kittens during the first 4 weeks of life have average heart rates of 209 ± 16 and 240 ± 20, respectively (Adelman and Wright, 1985; Finley and Kelly, 1986; Haddad et al, 1984). The chronotropic responses to either parasympathetic or sympathetic stimuli are greatly attenuated during the first 2 months of life owing to functional immaturity of the autonomic nervous system (Hageman et al, 1986; Mace and Levy, 1983a,b).

Auscultation

Auscultation of the heart is one of the most useful and sensitive means of detecting the presence of heart disease in a young dog or cat. It is important to recognize, however, that significant cardiac disease may occur in the absence of a murmur. Furthermore, functional murmurs, which are murmurs unrelated to an anatomic defect, are common in young animals. The small size of most young dogs and cats makes definition of the exact anatomic location of the heart sounds difficult. Generally, heart sounds can be localized to the left side of the thorax at the cardiac apex (left fifth to sixth intercostal space, ventral third of thorax), the left side of the thorax at the cardiac base (left third to fourth intercostal space above the costochondral junction), or the right side of the thorax at the cardiac apex (right fourth to fifth intercostal space opposite the mitral valve area). A stethoscope with a pediatric-sized chest piece (2 cm bell; 3 cm diaphragm) is helpful for auscultation of young animals.

A heart murmur is the most common type of abnormal sound heard in young dogs or cats. Functional murmurs and those associated with congenital disease are particularly common. The location, timing, and quality of the murmur are helpful in determining cause and significance. Functional murmurs are usually soft, early systolic murmurs heard best at the left base. Functional murmurs in kittens and puppies generally result from increased blood velocity, such as during fever, sepsis, or high sympathetic tone, or from decreased blood viscosity that occurs during anemia or hypoproteinemia. Innocent murmurs that are not associated with pathology are common, especially in large and giant breed dogs. Such innocent murmurs are usually enhanced with excitement or exercise and often disappear by 4 to 5 months of age. If a murmur is associated with a precordial thrill, an abnormal arterial or venous pulse, polycythemia, or cardiomegaly or if the murmur persists beyond 4 months of age, the animal should be evaluated thoroughly by a cardiologist.

Electrocardiography

The electrocardiogram (ECG) is used to diagnose arrhythmias and conduction disturbances in the young dog and cat. It may also be used together with other diagnostic techniques to detect cardiac chamber enlargement or hypertrophy. The clinician must, however, recognize the age-related variations of the normal ECG. When possible, a standard 10-lead ECG should be recorded with the animal in right lateral recumbency and the forelimbs positioned perpendicular to the spine (Hill, 1968; Trautvetter et al, 1981b). Any ECG lead with easily recognizable P waves and QRS complexes can be used to identify arrhythmias.

In newborn puppies the mean QRS vector is directed cranially, ventrally, and to the right. By 12 weeks of age, however, the vector is oriented leftward and caudally, with progressive changes occurring in the first, second, and third weeks of life (Trautvetter et al, 1981b). This shift in mean electrical axis is presumed to result from the increase in left ventricular mass that develops during maturation. In contrast, puppies born with severe pulmonic stenosis have abnormally deep negative deflections in leads I, II, III, and aVF that may be recognized immediately after birth if compared with those of age-matched normal puppies (Trautvetter et al,

1981a). These abnormal puppies fail to develop the left ventricular dominant ECG pattern of normal puppies.

Echocardiography

Diagnostic ultrasound is a useful, noninvasive method of evaluating young animals with cardiac disease. Lesions readily identified with M-mode or two-dimensional echocardiography include pericardial effusion, valvular vegetations, chamber dilation, myocardial hypertrophy, and abnormal cardiac motion. Although specific cardiac lesions cannot always be directly imaged, the echocardiogram usually demonstrates the secondary effects of a lesion on the heart (i.e., dilation, hypertrophy, and hyperkinesis). Contrast echocardiography may be helpful in confirming a right-to-left shunting lesion (Bonagura and Pipers, 1983). Doppler ultrasonography has become widely available as a noninvasive means of assessing and quantitating the direction and velocity of blood flow within the heart and blood vessels (Darke, 1992; Darke et al, 1996; Moise, 1989). Doppler imaging of high-velocity, retrograde, or turbulent flow through valves or intracardiac communications provides useful diagnostic and prognostic information in young animals with congenital lesions (Fig. 8–1).

Interpretation of an echocardiogram from an immature animal requires an awareness of the growth pattern and developmental anatomy of the heart during the first year of life. After birth there is a decrease in right ventricular mass relative to the left ventricle and to body weight, a decrease that occurs by the third week of life in dogs (Bishop, 1988). Sequential M-mode

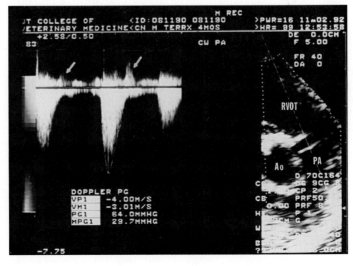

Figure 8–1. Continuous wave Doppler spectral velocity recording and simultaneous two-dimensional echocardiographic image of pulmonic stenosis and insufficiency from a puppy. Flow away from the transducer (below the zero line) reaches 4.0 m/s in systole, predicting a 64-mmHg instantaneous systolic pressure gradient. The brief, abnormal diastolic flow toward the transducer (arrows) represents pulmonic insufficiency. RVOT = right ventricular outflow tract; Ao = aorta; PA = pulmonary artery.

Table 8–2	Relationships of M-Mode Echocardiographic Measurements to Body Weight in Growing Dogs

COEFFICIENTS FOR EQUATION $y = ax^{b*}$

ECHOCARDIOGRAPHIC VARIABLE	A	B
RVIDd (mm)	3.723	0.454
LVIDd (mm)	11.63	0.409
LIVDs (mm)	6.764	0.445
LVWd (mm)	2.471	0.348
IVSd (mm)	2.357	0.367
LA (mm)	7.218	0.380
Ao (mm)	7.283	0.401
FS (%)	41.14	− 0.053
LA/Ao	0.991	− 0.021

*y = Echocardiographic measurement (variable) in units as listed; x = body weight in kilograms.

RVIDd = right ventricular internal dimension at end diastole; LVIDd = left ventricular internal dimension at end diastole; LVIDs = left ventricular internal dimension during systole; LVWd = left ventricular wall thickness at end diastole; IVSd = interventricular septal thickness at end diastole; LA = left atrial dimension; Ao = aortic dimension; FS = fractional shortening.

Adapted with permission from Sisson D, Schaeffer D: Changes in linear dimensions of the heart, relative to body weight, as measured by M-mode echocardiography in growing dogs. Am J Vet Res 52:1591, 1991.

echocardiographic measurements obtained during maturation have been reported for healthy English pointers (Sisson and Schaeffer, 1991). These measurements reveal that, at least in this breed, the linear dimensions of the growing canine heart can be expressed as exponential functions of body weight (Table 8–2). To the author's knowledge, echocardiographic mea-

surements of healthy, growing kittens have not been reported.

CARDIAC RHYTHM

The normal rhythm of the heart in puppies and kittens is a regular sinus rhythm. In young animals there is little to no variation in rhythm associated with breathing (Egbert and Katona, 1980; Haddad et al, 1984). The absence of a respiratory arrhythmia is consistent with the fact that vagal reflexes responsible for cardiac inhibition during expiration are immature at birth and develop shortly after 8 weeks of age in the dog (Mace and Levy, 1983b). Normal puppies older than 8 weeks may, however, have sinus arrhythmia, a wandering pacemaker, or incomplete atrioventricular block due to parasympathetic predominance (Fig. 8–2) (Branch et al, 1975; Haddad et al, 1984). These vagally mediated rhythm changes are unusual and usually pathologic in young cats (Tilley, 1985).

As in the adult animal, arrhythmias can occur in puppies and kittens from a variety of both cardiac and extracardiac abnormalities. Because the effective refractory period of the atria is relatively shorter in younger animals than in adults, newborns are particularly susceptible to the initiation and perpetuation of atrial tachycardias (Dunnigan and Benson, 1983; Pickoff et al, 1985b). Also common are ventricular extrasystoles and tachycardias secondary to inflammation, stretching, or hypoxia of the myocardium in animals with myocarditis or congenital heart disease. Because neural innervation of the heart is immature in the puppy and kitten younger than 8 weeks of age, the usual autonomic responses to conditions such as fever, pain, fear, hypovolemia, hypoxemia, and toxe-

CN 040115

50mm/s 1mV/cm

A

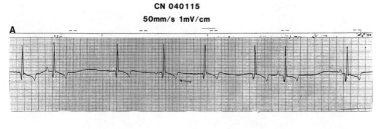

LII

B

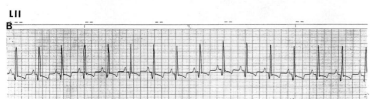

Figure 8–2. **A,** Marked sinus arrhythmia and a wandering pacemaker in a healthy 4-month-old Tibetan terrier. **B,** Rhythm strip from the same dog after atropine (0.02 mg/kg IM) administration.

mia may be attenuated or absent during this time.

The treatment of arrhythmias in young dogs and cats is similar to treatment in adults, and arrhythmia management is discussed elsewhere (Bonagura, 1985a; Sisson, 1988). It is important to note, however, the difference in responsiveness of the immature myocardium to many antiarrhythmic agents. Both increased and decreased sensitivities to antiarrhythmic agents have been demonstrated in the hearts of young animals, depending on the agent used and the specific physiologic parameter studied (Ezrin et al, 1980; Gaum et al, 1983; Mary-Rabine and Rosen, 1977; Pickoff et al, 1983, 1985a; Woods et al, 1978). Puppies younger than 39 days of age have a paradoxical negative chronotropic response to atropine and a marked sensitivity to the depressant effects of propranolol on the sinus node (Woods et al, 1978). Whereas verapamil has a more profound effect on sinus automaticity and atrial refractoriness in puppies than in adults, suppression of atrioventricular conduction is comparable at all ages (Pickoff et al, 1985a). Common antiarrhythmic agents with suggested dosages for young dogs and cats are listed in Table 8–3. It should be mentioned that the pharmacokinetic and toxicologic data that

Table 8–3	Antiarrhythmic Agents—Suggested Dosages and Indications in Young Animals		
DRUG	**DOSAGE***	**INDICATIONS**	**COMMENTS**
Atropine	Dog and cat: 0.01–0.02 mg/kg IV, IM 0.02–0.04 mg/kg SC	Vagally induced bradyarrhythmias and atrioventricular block	Do not give to animals younger than 8 weeks old
Isoproterenol	Dog and cat: 0.4 mg in 250 ml isotonic dextrose, drip slowly to effect IV	Sinus bradycardia; sinoatrial arrest; atrioventricular block; cardiac arrest with asystole	May induce tachycardia; ventricular extrasystoles
Digoxin	Dog: 0.01 mg/kg PO divided bid; 0.005 mg/kg IV; repeat with ½ this dose in 30–60 min if necessary Cat: 0.007 mg/kg PO qod	Supraventricular tachycardia; atrial fibrillation	
Propranolol	Dog and cat: 0.02–0.06 mg/kg IV 0.2–1.0 mg/kg PO q48h	Supraventricular tachycardia; atrial fibrillation; premature ventricular contractions	Do not give to animals younger than 40 days old
Lidocaine	Dog: 2–4 mg/kg IV followed by 25–75 µg/kg/min Cat: 0.25 mg/kg slowly IV	Premature ventricular contractions; ventricular tachycardia	May cause seizures, emesis
Procainamide	Dog: 3–6 mg/kg slowly IV 10 mg/kg IM 4–6 h 10 mg/kg PO qid–tid	Premature ventricular contractions; ventricular tachycardia	May cause hypotension, gastrointestinal upset; prolonged QRS duration and prolonged QT interval
Quinidine	Dog: 10 mg/kg IM or PO qid	Premature ventricular contractions; ventricular tachycardia; supraventricular tachycardias	
Verapamil	Dog and cat: 0.05–0.15 mg/kg slowly IV	Supraventricular tachycardias	May cause bradycardia, hypotension, and AV block

*IV = intravenous administration; IM = intramuscular administration; SC = subcutaneous administration; PO = oral administration; bid = twice a day; tid = three times a day; qid = four times a day; qod = every other day.

are needed to optimally administer antiarrhythmic agents to puppies and kittens are not available. The listed dosages in Table 8–3 have, therefore, been extrapolated from pharmacodynamic studies and from experience with these agents in older animals.

CONGENITAL HEART DISEASE

The prevalence of congenital heart defects in dogs has been estimated to be 0.67 to 0.85% (Buchanan, 1992). Because many animals dying of congenital cardiac anomalies are not evaluated by necropsy, this estimate may be low. Congenital heart disease appears to occur less frequently in cats than in dogs, with an overall prevalence in cats of approximately 0.2% (Harpster and Zook, 1987). It is estimated that 15% of cardiac diseases in cats are congenital (Bolton and Liu, 1977).

Although cardiac anomalies usually occur singly in puppies, variation in the severity of a defect and combinations of defects can be found. In a group of 290 dogs with congenital heart defects, 17 different malformations were found (Patterson, 1968). Of these heart defects, 72% were PDA, pulmonic stenosis, aortic stenosis, vascular ring anomaly, ventricular septal defect, or tetralogy of Fallot. There does not seem to be an overall sex predilection for congenital heart defects, except for an increased incidence of PDA in female dogs (Patterson, 1968; Buchanan, 1992). Purebred puppies have a higher incidence of congenital heart defects than mixed-breed puppies (Patterson, 1968; Patterson et al, 1974; Pyle et al, 1976), and certain cardiac anomalies occur more frequently in specific dog breeds (Table 8–4).

Congenital heart disease appears to be less prevalent in cats than in dogs (Liu, 1974; Harpster and Zook, 1987). Kittens, however, have a greater frequency of serious cardiovascular anomalies that are less amenable to surgical correction (Harpster, 1977; Liu, 1974, 1977). Cats also have a higher incidence of multiple cardiovascular anomalies than dogs (Harpster, 1977). For most congenital heart defects in cats, no breed predisposition has been found (Bolton and Liu, 1977). Endocardial fibroelastosis, however, occurs most frequently in the Siamese (Harpster, 1977) and Burmese (Zook and Paasch, 1982) breeds. Hypertrophic cardiomyopathy has been recognized as a heritable disorder in Maine coon (Kittleson et al, 1996), Persian (Martin et al, 1994), and some American short-haired cats (Meurs et al, 1997). Cats inheriting hypertrophic cardiomyopathy often de-

Table 8–4	Breeds of Dogs Predisposed to the Common Congenital Heart Defects
DEFECT	**BREEDS**
Patent ductus arteriosus	Poodle,* Pomeranian, collie, German shepherd, Shetland sheepdog, Maltese, keeshond, English springer spaniel, Welsh corgi (Ackerman et al, 1978; Buchanan, 1992; Mulvihill and Priester, 1973; Patterson, 1968; Orton, 1995)
Subaortic stenosis	Newfoundland,* boxer, German shepherd, golden retriever, German short-haired pointer, Rottweiler, English bull terriers (Bonagura, 1987; Buchanan, 1992; Mulvihill and Priester, 1973; Patterson, 1968, 1971; Darke et al, 1996)
Pulmonic stenosis	Beagle,* English bulldog, Chihuahua, fox terrier, Samoyed, miniature schnauzer (Mulvihill and Priester, 1973; Patterson, 1968)
Vascular ring anomaly	German shepherd,* Irish setter, Great Dane (Buchanan, 1992; Mulvihill and Priester, 1973; Patterson, 1968, 1971)
Ventricular septal defect	English bulldog (Buchanan, 1992; Mulvihill and Priester, 1973)
Tetralogy of Fallot	Keeshond* (Patterson, 1968, 1971)
Mitral/tricuspid valve dysplasia	Labrador retriever, Great Dane, Weimaraner, English bulldog, Chihuahua (Buchanan, 1992; Mulvihill and Priester, 1973; Patterson, 1968)

*Hereditary transmission confirmed by breeding trials.

velop severe left ventricular hypertrophy at a young age, often as early as 3 months old (Fig. 8–3). Common congenital anomalies in the cat include mitral and tricuspid valve malformations, persistent common atrioventricular canal (endocardial cushion defect), ventricular septal defect, endocardial fibroelastosis, aortic stenosis, PDA, and tetralogy of Fallot (Buchanan, 1992; Harpster, 1977; Liu, 1974). A male predominance has been reported for most of these anomalies (Buchanan, 1992).

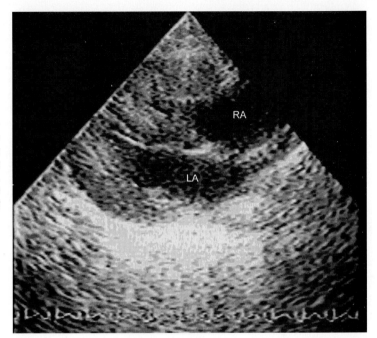

Figure 8–3. Still-frame two-dimensional echocardiographic image obtained from a 12-week-old Persian kitten with inherited hypertrophic cardiomyopathy (long axis view). The right and left ventricular walls exceed 7 mm in thickness during diastole. RA = right atrium; LA = left atrium.

Litters of kittens and puppies have been identified in which multiple siblings have similar single or multiple defects (Eyster et al, 1977c; Malik et al, 1991; Ogburn et al, 1981; Paasch and Zook, 1980; Pyle and Patterson, 1972). The defects in these animals may reflect hereditary lesions but could also result from environmental stress on the dam, infection, or drug-induced toxicity (Khera, 1964). Although any of the common defects can occur as isolated events, the heritability of many cardiac anomalies has been proved. It is recommended that animals with congenital heart defects not be used as breeding animals (Patterson, 1986). A congenital heart disease registry has recently been established for the purposes of gathering data regarding congenital heart disease in dogs and identifying dogs that are phenotypically normal before use in a breeding program.*

Patent Ductus Arteriosus

The most common congenital heart defect in dogs is PDA (Buchanan, 1992; Hunt et al, 1990; Patterson, 1968). This defect is occasionally seen in cats. The PDA is inherited as a polygenetic threshold trait, with a high degree of inheritability in poodles (Patterson, 1971). It frequently occurs in Pomeranians, collies, Shetland sheepdogs, Maltese, Welsh corgis, and English

*OFA Congenital Heart Disease Registry, Orthopedic Foundation for Animals, Columbia, MO.

springer spaniels but may be found in any breed. Trial breedings of normal dogs and dogs with PDA have shown an increased occurrence in females (Patterson, 1968). Additional matings in which both animals were affected, however, demonstrated an equal incidence of PDA in either sex (Ackerman et al, 1978). Patent ductus arteriosus may have a graded expression, ranging from a large patent ductus to a blind-ended diverticulum (Patterson et al, 1971). Animals with either PDA or ductus diverticulum, however, have a similar capability of transmitting the defective ductal closure to their young.

A PDA occurs when the normal fetal vessel (ductus arteriosus) that shunts blood past the nonfunctional fetal lungs into the aorta fails to close within the first 2 to 3 days of life. Because the systolic and diastolic pressures are generally greater in the aorta than in the pulmonary artery, PDA most commonly results in a continuous shunting of blood from the aorta to the pulmonary artery (classic left-to-right shunting PDA). The characteristic "machinery" murmur of a classic PDA is loudest high in the left axillary region over the left cardiac base. Commonly, this continuous murmur can be heard only in a very localized area, whereas the systolic component of the murmur may radiate over a larger area of the thoracic wall. Although some affected animals present with lethargy, poor growth, or left heart failure, most will present with only a murmur found during routine physical examination. Animals with PDA frequently have hyperdynamic or bounding femoral arterial pulses and a palpable thrill over the left hemithorax.

In most animals with PDA there is a left-to-right shunt that causes a volume overload of the pulmonary circulation and the left side of the heart. The left atrium and left ventricle dilate to accommodate the augmented pulmonary blood flow (Weirich et al, 1978). The ECG often shows wide P waves suggestive of left atrial enlargement and abnormally tall R waves in the cranial-caudal and left precordial leads consistent with left ventricular enlargement (Fig. 8–4). Atrial fibrillation is a common finding in dogs with severe left atrial dilation.

Thoracic radiographs of animals with classic PDA usually show cardiomegaly with enlargement of the left atrium and left ventricle. Pulmonary overcirculation is apparent (Fig. 8–5). There is usually an aortic aneurysmal dilation that appears on the dorsoventral projection as a leftward bulge of the descending aorta (ductus bump). There may also be a dilated pulmonary

artery segment due to turbulent blood flow (Suter and Lord, 1984) (Fig. 8–6).

Standard echocardiography is of limited value in the diagnosis of PDA because the ductus can rarely be directly imaged. Echocardiography may, however, be used to confirm the increase in size of the left atrium and left ventricle (Bonagura, 1983). Doppler echocardiography may be used to confirm the presence of left-to-right flow through a patent ductus by demonstrating continuous retrograde flow from the aorta into the pulmonary artery (O'Grady and Allen, 1987; Pearlman, 1985).

Cardiac catheterization is generally unnecessary in puppies with clinical findings typical of PDA because most dogs do not have associated cardiac anomalies. In cats, however, multiple anomalies with PDA appear to be particularly common.

Surgical correction of a PDA in an asymptomatic animal should be done at a young age to minimize secondary damage to the myocardium and pulmonary vasculature (Eyster et al, 1976d).

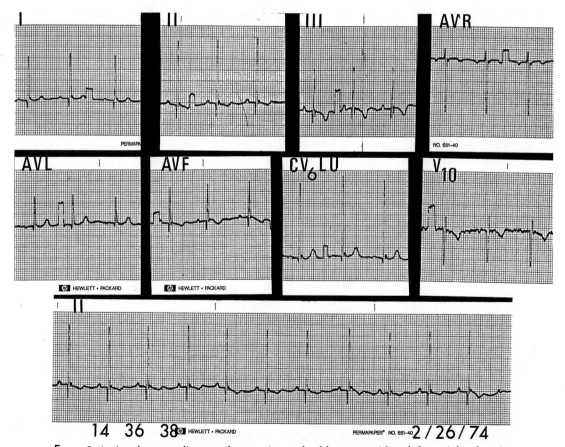

Figure 8–4. An electrocardiogram from a 4-month-old puppy with a left-to-right shunting patent ductus arteriosus. There are abnormally tall R waves in leads I, II, aVF, and CV_6LU, consistent with left ventricular enlargement. (Paper speed = 50 mm/s.)

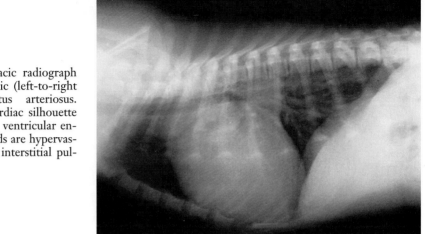

Figure 8–5. Lateral thoracic radiograph from a puppy with classic (left-to-right shunting) patent ductus arteriosus. There is an enlarged cardiac silhouette due to left atrial and left ventricular enlargement. The lung fields are hypervascular, and there is early interstitial pulmonary edema.

Surgery is usually performed before the puppy or kitten is 5 months old. Closure of the shunt is accomplished through a left fourth intercostal incision (sixth intercostal space in kittens) and involves simple ligation in most cases (Bolton

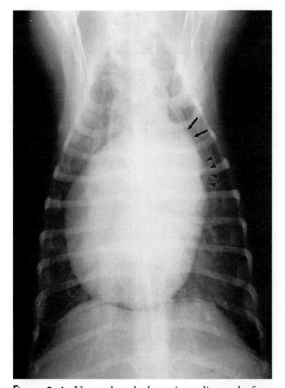

Figure 8–6. Ventrodorsal thoracic radiograph from the same puppy as in Figure 8–5. In addition to left-sided heart enlargement, this view illustrates dilatation of the descending aorta at the level of the ductus (arrowheads) and an enlarged pulmonary artery segment (arrows).

and Liu, 1977; Cohen et al, 1975; Jackson and Henderson, 1979) (Fig. 8–7). Postoperatively, a systolic murmur of mitral insufficiency or relative aortic stenosis may be heard over the left thorax (Weirich et al, 1978). This turbulence is the result of increased blood volume secondary to the shunt and usually disappears within a few days to several weeks after the surgery.

Transcatheter closure of left-to-right shunting PDAs in puppies has been described as an alternative to surgical ligation (Miller et al, 1999; Fox et al, 1998). Using a snare or biopsy forceps to position an occluding spring coil appears to work well and is less invasive and less costly than surgical ligation (Miller et al, 1999; Fox et al, 1998).

The prognosis for an animal with a corrected left-to-right shunting PDA is excellent. Older animals undergoing surgery for PDA have a much higher incidence of postoperative complications than those corrected early (Eyster et al, 1976d). Dogs with untreated PDA may develop left heart failure, and untreated cats usually die before they are 1 year of age (Bolton and Liu, 1977; Patterson et al, 1971).

Right-to-left shunting PDA may occur in young animals as a result of persistent pulmonary hypertension (failure to adapt to extrauterine life), or the right-to-left shunt may develop in older animals with PDA as a late complication of chronically increased pulmonary blood flow (Pyle et al, 1981). Augmented pulmonary flow stimulates fibromuscular proliferation of the tunica media and intima of the pulmonary arterioles, which then results in increased pulmonary vascular resistance and reversal of blood flow through the shunt (blood flows from the pulmonary artery into the aorta through the

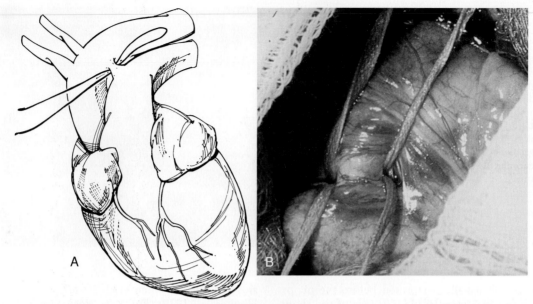

Figure 8–7. A, A schematic drawing of the heart and great vessels illustrating ligation of a classic patent ductus arteriosus. (Drawing by Ms. Carol Haynes, University of Tennessee, Knoxville, TN.) **B,** An intraoperative photograph showing ligatures placed around the patent ductus before closure. The descending aorta is seen at the top, with the pulmonary artery visible below. (Courtesy of Dr. Walter Weirich, Purdue University, West Lafayette, IN.)

ductus) (Fig. 8–8). Trial breedings of dogs with PDA have resulted in 15% of their young having either right-to-left or bidirectional shunts (Patterson, 1971; Pyle et al, 1981). Animals with reverse PDA commonly present with lethargy, hindlimb weakness, elevated hematocrit, and differential cyanosis (Pyle et al, 1981). These

animals do not have the characteristic continuous murmur associated with PDA. Instead, most have a soft systolic murmur at the left heart base and increased intensity of the second heart sound (Pyle et al, 1981). Dogs with right-to-left shunting PDA have a very poor prognosis. They are not candidates for surgical correction if pul-

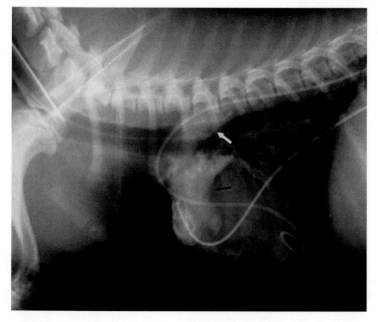

Figure 8–8. Radiopaque contrast material has been injected into the main pulmonary artery of a young Maltese terrier with a right-to-left shunting patent ductus arteriosus. Note that the contrast material is apparent in the descending aorta (white arrow) and the pulmonary trunk (black arrow) as a result of flow through the ductus. The contrast material is not seen in the ascending aorta, brachiocephalic artery, or left subclavian artery, indicating that the unoxygenated, shunted blood is directed caudally.

monary artery pressures exceed systemic pressures because ductal ligation will precipitate immediate right heart failure and death. Periodic phlebotomy may be helpful if seizures occur secondary to the polycythemia (Legendre et al, 1974; Pyle et al, 1981).

Aortic Stenosis

The second most common congenital heart defect in dogs is aortic stenosis (AS) (Buchanan, 1992; Patterson, 1968). Aortic stenosis is inherited as a polygenetic trait in Newfoundland dogs (Pyle et al, 1976). It occurs commonly in golden retrievers, German shepherds, Rottweilers, English bull terriers, and boxers as well (Buchanan, 1992; Darke et al, 1996). Although AS is heritable in most of these breeds, the exact mode of transmission is unclear. The obstruction can be supravalvular, valvular, or subvalvular, but the subvalvular form is most common in dogs. Subvalvular AS results from a ridge of fibrocartilaginous tissue located below the aortic valve. The severity of this lesion has been graded 1 to 3. With grade 3 the stenosis is severe, and the ridge extends completely around the outflow tract to include the ventral leaflet of the mitral valve (Pyle et al, 1976). Phenotypic expression of the lesion develops during the postnatal period and may not be fully apparent until 2.5 years of age (Nakayama et al, 1996).

Aortic stenosis is recognized less frequently in cats than in dogs. As in dogs, the lesion in cats is usually a fibrous subaortic band (Fig. 8–9) (Stepien and Bonagura, 1991). This lesion can be difficult to distinguish from asymmetric septal hypertrophy found in some cats with primary hypertrophic cardiomyopathy.

Aortic stenosis causes a systolic murmur that is loudest over the left fourth intercostal space near the costochondral junction. The murmur may also be heard on the right hemithorax, at the thoracic inlet, and radiating up the carotid arteries. Occasionally, the murmur radiates along the vertebral arteries to the occipital protuberance of the skull. In many affected animals

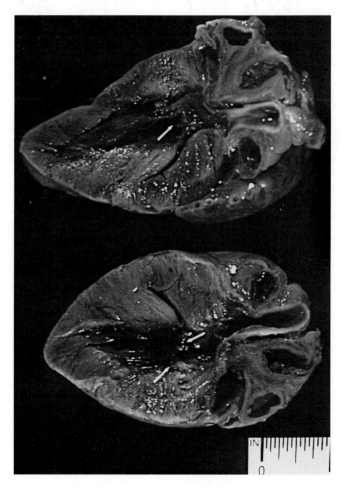

Figure 8–9. Necropsy specimen obtained from a cat with congenital subaortic stenosis. In addition to concentric left ventricular hypertrophy and left atrial enlargement, the lesion is visible as a subaortic band encircling the left ventricular outflow tract (arrows).

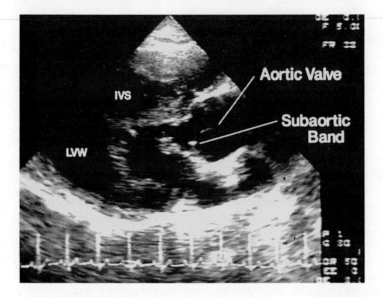

Figure 8–10. Still-frame two-dimensional image obtained from an 11-week-old Rottweiler puppy with congenital subaortic stenosis. IVS = interventricular septum; LVW = left ventricular wall.

the arterial pulses are weak, and there may be a palpable thrill over the left hemithorax.

ECGs obtained from puppies with aortic stenosis are usually normal. In some affected animals, however, the ECG may show a left axis deviation (less than 40°) and tall R waves. Depression of the ST segment and cardiac arrhythmias, especially premature ventricular contractions, are common ECG abnormalities and probably reflect compromised coronary blood flow (Pyle et al, 1976; Tilley and Owens, 1985).

In some cases of AS the cardiac silhouette is normal on thoracic radiographs. The lateral view, however, usually shows tracheal elevation and left ventricular enlargement (Ettinger and Suter, 1970). Dilatation of the ascending aortic arch is common and may cause a loss of the cranial cardiac waist. Left atrial enlargement and congestion of the pulmonary veins occur in severe cases. Echocardiographic features of AS may include significant enlargement of the ascending aorta during systole and diastole, narrowing of the left ventricular outflow tract, and concentric myocardial hypertrophy (Bonagura, 1983; Wingfield et al, 1983). Two-dimensional echocardiography often reveals the subvalvular fibrous obstruction (Fig. 8–10). These abnormalities are also seen angiocardiographically (Fig. 8–11). Doppler echocardiography is useful for assessing the severity of the obstruction and may demonstrate secondary aortic regurgitation in some animals.

Catheter or continuous wave Doppler measurement of the systolic pressure gradient across

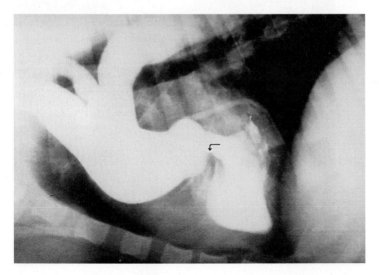

Figure 8–11. A left ventricular angiogram obtained from a puppy with subaortic stenosis. Narrowing of the outflow tract is visible, and there is a filling defect due to the presence of a subvalvular obstruction (arrow). There is tremendous enlargement of the ascending aorta, common brachiocephalic trunk, and left subclavian artery.

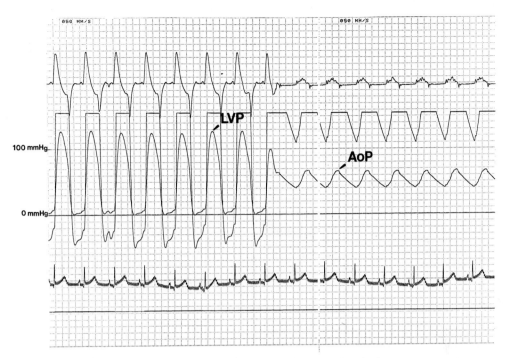

Figure 8–12. A pressure tracing recorded from a young cat with valvular aortic stenosis as a catheter is pulled from the left ventricle into the aorta across the obstruction. Note that the peak systolic pressure decreases from 126 mmHg in the left ventricle (LVP) to 66 mmHg in the aortic root (AoP), indicating a moderately severe aortic stenosis.

the stenotic lesion is useful for determining severity of the obstruction and thereby providing prognostic information (Fig. 8–12). Gradients of less than 50 mmHg, measured in an awake, unsedated animal, are considered hemodynamically insignificant, whereas those over 100 mmHg are likely to result in the development of clinical signs and a shortened lifespan (Eyster and Probst, 1985; Orton, 1995). The significance of pressure gradients between 50 and 100 mmHg is unclear. Young animals with small gradients should be re-evaluated at maturity and at 2½ to 3 years of age to determine the degree of progression of the lesion. A palliative procedure (surgical or balloon catheter dilation) should be considered for animals developing clinical signs such as decreased exercise tolerance, coughing, dyspnea, or syncope. Unfortunately, one of the common signs of AS is sudden death without previous evidence of illness, and neither surgical nor catheter correction appears to improve survival despite reduction in gradient and clinical signs (DeLellis et al, 1993; Orton et al, 2000).

Administration of β-adrenergic antagonists or calcium channel blocking agents to animals with AS decreases the myocardial oxygen requirement. The effect of these agents on survival has not, however, been critically evaluated. Dilatation of the stenotic lesion can be performed surgically or by cardiac catheterization with a balloon catheter (DeLellis et al, 1993; Orton et al, 1993), but dilation by either method may not provide sustained benefit. Surgery may also be done with cardiopulmonary bypass, hypothermic cardioplegia, and direct resection of the stenosis (Eyster et al, 1975; Orton et al, 1995). Even with direct surgical excision the long-term prognosis for animals with AS is guarded because of myocardial damage that often occurs before surgery. Dogs with subaortic stenosis are predisposed to secondary bacterial endocarditis of the aortic valve, and antibiotics should be administered prophylactically before elective surgery or dental procedures.

Pulmonic Stenosis

The third most common congenital heart defect in dogs is pulmonic stenosis (PS) (Buchanan, 1992). PS is, however, rare as an isolated defect in cats (Hawe, 1981). Pulmonic stenosis occurs frequently in beagles, Chihuahuas, English bulldogs, fox terriers, Samoyeds, and miniature schnauzers and is most likely heritable in these breeds. In beagles pulmonary valve dysplasia is inherited as a polygenetic trait (Patterson et al, 1981). Although stenosis may occur in the supravalvular, valvular, or subvalvular area, pulmonic stenosis due to valvular dysplasia is most common in dogs. Characteristics of a dysplastic pulmonary valve include thickening and hypoplasia of the cusps, fusion of the valve commissures, and hypoplasia of the annulus (Fingland et al, 1986; Patterson et al, 1981). Obstruction of right ventricular outflow results in hypertrophy of the right ventricular musculature, which may ultimately contribute to the obstruction. In English bulldogs, anomalous coronary arteries often coexist with PS. Specifically, bulldogs may have a single coronary artery with an anomalous left coronary artery (Fig. 8–13). In some cases the anomalous left coronary artery may pass cranial to the pulmonary artery, resulting in compression of the pulmonary orifice and significant limitation of the available treatment options.

Most dogs with PS are asymptomatic at the time of diagnosis, but, when present, the most common signs of illness are those of right heart failure or syncope (Fingland et al, 1986). The murmur of pulmonic stenosis is a systolic murmur heard loudest over the left heart base. There may be a second systolic murmur heard over the right hemithorax due to tricuspid insufficiency.

The ECG is typically normal in animals with mild PS but usually shows deviation of the mean electrical axis to the right (greater than 100°) in moderately to severely affected dogs. The ECG may suggest right atrial enlargement (tall P waves) or right ventricular enlargement (deep S waves in leads I, II, III, and aVF) (Tilley, 1985) (Fig. 8–14). Radiographs generally reveal right ventricular enlargement and a poststenotic dilatation of the main pulmonary artery (Fingland et al, 1986; Suter and Lord, 1984). The peripheral pulmonary vasculature may be normal or decreased in size (Fingland et al, 1986). Two-dimensional echocardiography demonstrates the stenotic lesion and the secondary right ventricular hypertrophy. Valve motion, valve orifice size, and the poststenotic dilation may also be evaluated. Doppler echocardiography or cardiac catheterization is used to confirm the presence of PS and to quantitate severity (see Fig. 8–1). Doppler is also used to determine whether patent foramen ovale or secondary tricuspid regurgitation is present.

The severity of PS should be assessed by Doppler echocardiographic or catheter measurement of the systolic pressure gradient to determine whether surgical correction is needed (i.e., the difference in the systolic pressure across the PS). Peak systolic pressure gradients have been classified as mild (less than 50 mmHg), moderate (50 to 100 mmHg), and severe (greater than 100 mmHg) (Fingland et al,

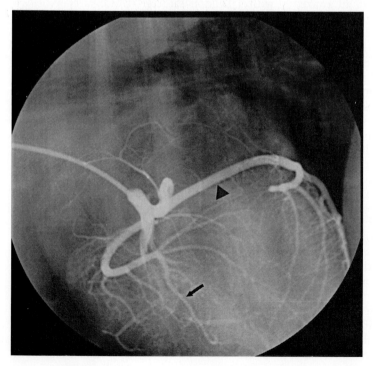

Figure 8–13. A coronary angiogram obtained from an English bulldog puppy with pulmonic stenosis and an anomalous single coronary artery. The contrast has been injected into the sole coronary artery from which the right coronary as well as the intraventricular paraconal (arrow) and the left circumflex (arrowhead) arteries arise. (Courtesy of Dr. Greg Daniel, University of Tennessee, Knoxville, TN.)

CN # 35045

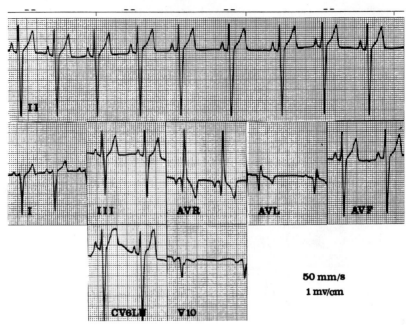

50 mm/s
1 mv/cm

Figure 8–14. An electrocardiogram recorded from a puppy with severe pulmonic stenosis. Note the abnormally deep S waves in leads I, II, III, aVF, and CV₆LU, which suggest right ventricular enlargement. There is also a right axis deviation in the frontal plane (mean electrical axis is 220°).

1986). Animals appear to be able to tolerate a mild pressure gradient without developing signs of illness. Severe stenosis is, however, associated with a strain on the myocardium and leads to fibrosis and infarction (Weirich et al, 1971). Arrhythmias, congestive heart failure, and sudden death are possible sequelae of this myocardial degeneration.

Although Doppler echocardiography will, in most cases, define the anatomy and physiologic significance of the lesion, right ventricular angiography may also be used to demonstrate PS and secondary changes (Fig. 8–15). Poststenotic dilatation of the pulmonary artery cannot be used to quantitate the severity of the PS, but enlargement of the vessel in excess of its size at the level of the pulmonary sinus is useful in diagnosis of the condition angiocardiographically (Fingland et al, 1986).

Correction of PS is recommended for animals with severe obstruction because severe, uncorrected PS is associated with high mortality (Fingland et al, 1986). Valvular lesions may be corrected surgically by open or closed valvulotomy. Supravalvular obstructions can be corrected by outflow tract reconstruction using the placement of a pericardial or synthetic patch graft (Breznock and Wood, 1976). The patch graft technique has also been advocated for correction in animals with severe valvular hypoplasia, marked infundibular hypertrophy, or both (Breznock and Wood, 1976; Orton and Monnet, 1994). Percutaneous balloon valvuloplasty, frequently used to correct PS in humans (Walls et al, 1984), has been used successfully in dogs as well (Bright et al, 1987; Brownlie et al, 1991; Martin et al, 1992). This procedure is most suitable for patients lacking annular hypoplasia or severe infundibular stenosis (Lau and Hung, 1993). There are some data suggesting that balloon valvuloplasty provides greater immediate and greater long-term survival rates than surgical corrective procedures (Ewey et al, 1992).

Vascular Ring Anomalies

Vascular ring anomalies (VRAs) are the fourth most common congenital heart defect in dogs (Buchanan, 1992; Patterson, 1968). German shepherds and Great Danes are predisposed to VRA, and a hereditary basis has been demonstrated in German shepherds. Cats are less frequently affected than dogs (Ellison, 1980; McCandlish et al, 1984; Wheaton et al, 1984). The VRAs constitute a group of defects that result from abnormal maturation of the embry-

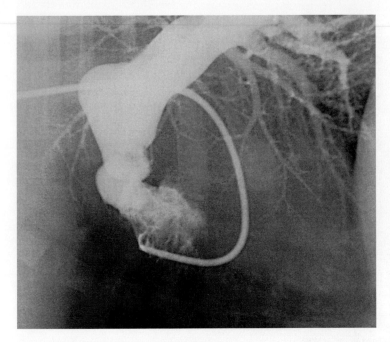

Figure 8–15. A right ventricular angiocardiogram obtained from the same puppy as in Figure 8–13. This puppy has congenital pulmonic stenosis and an anomalous single coronary artery. There is hypertrophy of the right ventricular wall and christasupraventricularis with distortion of the conus arteriosus. The pulmonary sinuses are asymmetric, and the main pulmonary artery is dilated. (Courtesy of Dr. Greg Daniel, University of Tennessee, Knoxville, TN.)

onic aortic arches (Moore, 1973). Persistent right aortic arch with a left ductus arteriosus is the most common form of VRA (Ellison, 1980; Shires and Liu, 1981).

Animals are usually asymptomatic until weaning, when regurgitation of solid food becomes apparent. Retarded growth of the animal and regurgitation of undigested food within minutes or hours of eating are typical clinical signs (Ellison, 1980). Most cases of VRA are diagnosed before the animal reaches maturity. Physical examination is often unremarkable except for generalized emaciation. Abnormal lung sounds, such as crackles and increased large airway sounds, may be auscultated if a secondary aspiration pneumonia is present. A food bolus may occasionally be palpated in the dilated cervical esophagus.

The hemogram and serum chemistry panel of an animal with VRA are usually normal unless pneumonia or hypoproteinemia is present. Similarly, ECG findings are unremarkable. Thoracic radiographs are generally diagnostic for VRA. Radiographic signs include ventral tracheal displacement, widening of the cranial mediastinum, and dilatation of the esophagus anterior to the base of the heart (Ellison, 1980). Feeding a mixture of radiopaque contrast medium in a food slurry will aid in making the diagnosis. Occasionally, the esophagus caudal to the heart is also dilated. The incidence, cause, and significance of this caudal esophageal dilation are uncertain, but the dilation may be asso-

ciated with a poor postoperative prognosis. The secondary loss of myenteric ganglion cells from the dilated esophagus has been documented (Clifford et al, 1971). Whether a poor prognosis is related to this loss of neural tissue is not known.

Treatment of VRA is directed at "opening" the ring anomaly. In most cases, correction involves double ligation and transection of the left ligamentum arteriosus (Ellison, 1980; Shires and Liu, 1981). Similar correction of an aberrant subclavian artery may result in temporary weakness of the forelimb, but collateral circulation usually obviates long-term problems. Resection or ligation of the esophagus is not needed. Although the survival rate of the surgical procedure is high, continuing problems related to the dilated esophagus are common (Shires and Liu, 1981). Early surgical correction and controlled postoperative feeding of a gruel with elevation of the dog's front quarters often minimize these problems.

Ventricular Septal Defect

A ventricular septal defect (VSD) is a common congenital heart defect in cats, often occurring in conjunction with other cardiac anomalies (Liu, 1977). Ventricular septal defect is also common in dogs. No breed predilection for VSDs has been clearly established. The defect possibly occurs with an increased frequency in English bulldogs (Buchanan, 1992).

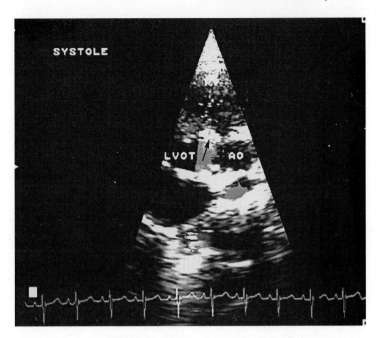

Figure 8–16. Still-frame color Doppler image obtained from a 6-month-old kitten with a membranous ventricular septal defect. The arrow on the image is over a turbulent jet flowing from left to right immediately below the aortic valve during systole. LVOT = left ventricular outflow tract; AO = aorta.

A VSD is usually a single defect located high in the septum, just below the tricuspid and aortic valves (Fig. 8–16) (Eyster and DeYoung, 1985). Abnormalities involving the endocardial cushion, namely the lower atrial septum, upper ventricular septum, and septal leaflets of the atrioventricular valves, may also be present and are frequently seen in cats (Liu, 1977).

The clinical and hemodynamic features associated with a VSD are variable and are determined primarily by the size of the defect, the relative pulmonary and systemic vascular resistances, and the presence of other cardiac defects. Most commonly there is left-to-right shunting of blood at the level of the outflow tracts during systole, which produces a volume overload to the pulmonary circulation, left atrium, and left ventricle. With very large VSDs there is, essentially, a common ventricle, and significant right ventricular dilation and hypertrophy occur. In this case, bidirectional shunting of blood across the defect is common. If there is increased resistance to right ventricular outflow due to pulmonic stenosis or pulmonary hypertension, there is usually bidirectional or right-to-left shunting. Animals with a small, uncomplicated VSD may be asymptomatic. If the animal develops clinical signs, these usually occur by 1 year of age and include cough, exercise intolerance, and poor growth (Eyster and DeYoung, 1985; Weirich and Blevins, 1978). Animals with right-to-left shunting of blood often present with generalized cyanosis, exercise in-

tolerance, and polycythemia (elevated hematocrit).

In most animals with an uncomplicated VSD, blood is shunted from the left to the right ventricular outflow tract during systole, producing a harsh holosystolic murmur that is best heard along the right cranial sternal border. There may also be a murmur over the left cardiac base resulting from increased right ventricular outflow. Less commonly, there is a soft, early diastolic murmur caused by aortic regurgitation due to prolapse of an aortic valve leaflet into a subpulmonic VSD.

The secondary manifestations of a VSD on chest radiographs, ECG, echocardiogram, and Doppler echocardiogram depend on the direction and quantity of shunted blood. Generally, the chest radiographs reveal pulmonary overperfusion, left atrial enlargement, and varying degrees of left ventricular and right ventricular enlargement (Weirich and Blevins, 1978). The ECG is often normal but may suggest either left or right ventricular enlargement. Conduction abnormalities associated with the defect may also be recognized. Echocardiography and Doppler flow studies are useful for demonstrating the defect and blood flow across the defect (Fig. 8–16). Cardiac catheterization and angiography are also used to demonstrate the defect as well as the degree and direction of shunting. Small ventricular septal defects impose a minimal hemodynamic burden, and most animals with small defects remain normal. Some VSDs in dogs have been known to close spontaneously (Breznock, 1973). Animals with pulmonary to systemic blood flow ratios of approximately 2:1 or greater are likely, however, to develop clinical signs and may benefit from surgical correction (Eyster and DeYoung, 1985; Weirich and Blevins, 1978).

Definitive correction of a VSD requires cardiopulmonary bypass with suturing or patching of the defect (Weirich and Blevins, 1978). Palliative surgery with pulmonary artery banding increases the right ventricular pressure, thereby decreasing the degree of left-to-right shunting. This, it is hoped, protects the pulmonary vasculature and left heart from the deleterious effects of augmented flow (Eyster et al, 1977d; Mann et al, 1971). Congestive heart failure or cardiac arrhythmias associated with VSD should be medically managed. As with a reversed-shunting patent ductus arteriosus, surgical correction of animals with a right-to-left shunting VSD is contraindicated if pulmonary artery pressures exceed those of the systemic circulation.

Tetralogy of Fallot

Tetralogy of Fallot (TF) includes a VSD, right ventricular outflow tract obstruction, hypertrophy of the right ventricle, and a dextropositioned aorta that accepts blood from both ventricles. TF occurs when the conotruncal septum between the aorta and pulmonary artery fails to develop and fuse normally with the interventricular septum (Bolton et al, 1972; Patterson et al, 1974).

The right ventricular hypertrophy described by Fallot is not actually an anomaly but, rather, a manifestation of the increased right ventricular afterload. Typically, the PS is severe enough to offer more resistance to flow through the pulmonary arterial system than that offered to systemic flow through the systemic vessels. Unoxygenated blood is, therefore, shunted across the septal defect into the aorta. The mixture of arterialized and venous blood in the aorta accounts for the arterial hypoxemia and cyanosis observed clinically. The severity of hypoxemia and, hence, the severity of clinical signs depend on the relative resistance to blood flow through the pulmonary and systemic vasculature (Bolton et al, 1972). Tetralogy of Fallot is common in cats (Harpster, 1977; Liu, 1974) and has been shown to be a polygenetic threshold trait in keeshonds (Patterson et al, 1974).

Animals with TF rarely develop congestive heart failure but instead have tachypnea, exercise intolerance, depression, and/or syncope. Cerebral or myocardial embolism may cause sudden death. Secondary polycythemia is common and often produces hyperviscosity with central nervous system signs (e.g., seizures, stroke). Cyanosis may develop quickly if the animal is stressed. Tetralogy of Fallot may occur without cyanosis if the PS is not severe enough to produce severe arterial desaturation (Bolton et al, 1972).

Most animals with TF have a systolic ejection murmur characteristic of PS unless there is pulmonary artery hypoplasia or marked polycythemia. There may be a holosystolic murmur associated with the septal defect (Bolton and Liu, 1977). Some animals with TF have no audible murmur.

A right ventricular enlargement pattern characterized by right axis deviation and deep S waves in leads I, II, III, and aVF is commonly seen on the ECG of animals with TF. Some cats may have a left axis deviation on the ECG, most likely a result of intraventricular conduction abnormalities (Bonagura, 1987). Typical radiographic features of TF include a normal to slightly enlarged cardiac silhouette with rounding of the right ventricular border, a hyperlucent lung field with attenuated pulmonary vasculature, a normal to small pulmonary artery trunk, and an enlarged aortic arch (Suter and Lord, 1984) (Fig. 8–17). Doppler echocardiography, contrast echocardiography, or angiocardiography can be used to demonstrate the VSD, right ventricular hypertrophy, dextropositioned aorta, right-to-left shunting, right ventricular outflow tract obstruction, and small left atrium and left ventricle. Cardiac catheterization and angiocardiography are useful for assessing the degree of pulmonary vascular and bronchial collateral blood flow. This assessment is important when considering palliative surgical procedures (Bonagura, 1987).

Definitive correction of TF can be done but requires cardiopulmonary bypass. More commonly palliative surgical procedures are done to create a left-to-right pulmonary shunt in order to increase pulmonary perfusion and reduce arterial hypoxemia. Pulmonary balloon valvuloplasty has been used safely and effectively as a nonsurgical palliative procedure in children with tetralogy of Fallot and should be considered as a therapeutic option for puppies as well (Boucek et al, 1988). Medical palliation with β-adrenergic blockade (propranolol) may provide symptomatic relief in some animals. The mechanism responsible for the beneficial effects of

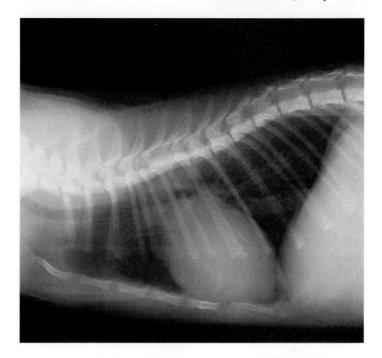

Figure 8–17. Lateral thoracic radiograph from a 3-month-old kitten with tetralogy of Fallot. There is slight enlargement of the cardiac silhouette due to right ventricular enlargement and hyperlucency of the lung fields.

β-adrenergic blocking agents is complex and includes increased peripheral resistance, decreased myocardial contractility, prevention of tachycardia, and a favorable shift in the hemoglobin-oxygen dissociation curve (Garson et al, 1981). β-Adrenergic blockade may be used as the only treatment or may be used to improve an animal's condition before surgery. Phlebotomy may be needed to relieve the hyperviscosity caused by polycythemia.

Without some form of palliative therapy, most animals with TF develop severe polycythemia or are incapacitated by hypoxemia. Many die suddenly. Surgical palliation may control clinical signs for 4 years or more (Bonagura, 1987).

Tricuspid Valve Dysplasia

Dysplasia of the tricuspid (right atrioventricular) valve (TD) has been reported in cats and large breed dogs, with Labrador retrievers being overrepresented (Liu and Tilley, 1976; Weirich et al, 1974; Kornreich and Moise, 1997). The term *dysplasia* refers to a spectrum of abnormalities including focal or diffuse thickening or fenestration of the valve leaflets; shortening, absence, or fusion of the chordae tendineae and papillary muscles; abnormal numbers of papillary muscles; incomplete separation of the valve leaflets from the ventricular wall; and agenesis

of valvular tissue (Becker et al, 1971; Liu and Tilley, 1976). Enlargement of the right atrium and ventricle occurs secondary to valvular incompetence.

Clinical signs of TD are usually recognized before maturity and typically include lethargy, weight loss, and right heart failure. Most affected animals have a systolic regurgitant murmur over the tricuspid valve area. Some have atrial fibrillation.

Right axis deviation and increased amplitude of the P waves are common ECG findings (Liu and Tilley, 1976). Splintering of the QRS complexes is also a common ECG abnormality in affected animals (Fig. 8–18) (Kornreich and Moise, 1997). Marked enlargement and rounding of the cardiac silhouette (due mainly to dilatation of the right atrium) are seen on thoracic radiographs of animals with TD (Liu and Tilley, 1976; Weirich et al, 1974) (Fig. 8–19). Echocardiography and angiocardiography confirm the dilatation of the right atrium and may show thickened valve leaflets. Contrast studies or Doppler studies will document valve incompetence. Animals with TD often have additional anomalies such as septal defects or pulmonic stenosis. Therapy consists of medical management of congestive heart failure and arrhythmias. Surgical correction using ring annuloplasty or valvular prosthesis should be considered before the development of end-stage heart

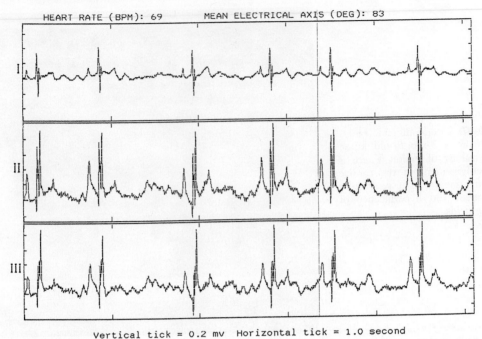

HEART RATE (BPM): 69   MEAN ELECTRICAL AXIS (DEG): 83

Vertical tick = 0.2 mv   Horizontal tick = 1.0 second

Figure 8–18. An electrocardiogram recorded from a young Labrador retriever with tricuspid valve dysplasia illustrating the splintering of QRS complexes often noted in dogs and cats with this anomaly.

failure in dogs with severe dysplasia (Orton, 1995). The prognosis without surgical repair is poor in severe cases.

Ebstein's anomaly is a variant of TD that has been reported in the dog (Eyster et al, 1977a). This defect differs from TD by a downward displacement of the tricuspid valve and a hypoplastic right ventricle. Antemortem diagnosis of Ebstein's anomaly and its differentiation from TD require ultrasonography or the ability to monitor an intracardiac ECG simultaneous with recording pressure within the cardiac chambers.

Mitral Valve Malformation

Malformation of the mitral valve (MVM) has been reported to be the most common isolated congenital heart defect found at necropsy in cats (Liu, 1977). Great Danes, German shepherds, mastiffs, English bull terriers, and various retrievers may also have MVM (Hamlin and Harris, 1969; Liu and Tilley, 1975; Darke et al, 1996). Abnormalities found with MVM include dilatation of the mitral annulus, short thickened valve leaflets, clefts in the leaflets, long thin chordae tendineae allowing valve prolapse, short thick chordae tendineae limiting valve movement, malalignment of the papillary muscles causing abnormal pull on the valves, and

diffuse thickening of the endocardium (Liu and Tilley, 1975). These anomalies invariably result in chronic regurgitation, but some animals have concurrent mitral stenosis as well (Fox et al, 1992; Stamoulis and Fox, 1993; Lehmkuhl et al, 1994).

Presenting signs of MVM range from left heart failure with coughing and lethargy to sudden death. Physical examination reveals a systolic murmur of mitral regurgitation, auscultated low on the fifth left intercostal space. The ECG and radiographic abnormalities are consistent with left atrial and ventricular enlargement. Pulmonary venous congestion is also common, and atrial fibrillation may occur secondary to the atrial dilation. The structural abnormalities of the mitral valve apparatus are usually easily appreciated with two-dimensional echocardiographic imaging (Fig. 8–20). Echocardiography reveals normal myocardial systolic function in most animals with MVM, although contractility may be decreased in chronic cases (Lord et al, 1975). Angiography or Doppler echocardiography can be used to document the regurgitant flow.

Animals with symptomatic mitral regurgitation may be managed with diuretics and arteriolar vasodilators. Antiarrhythmic therapy may also be needed. Some dogs become asympto-

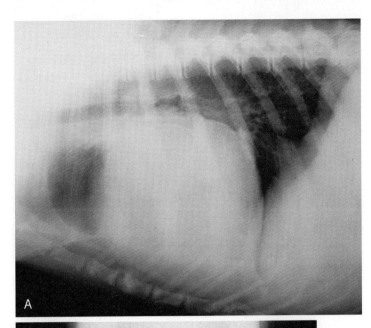

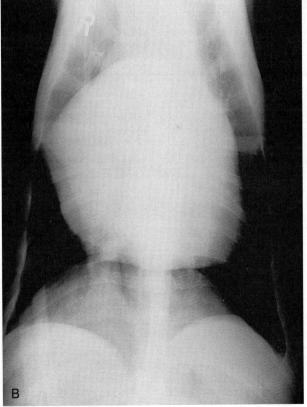

Figure 8–19. Survey lateral **(A)** and ventrodorsal **(B)** thoracic radiographs from a young Newfoundland dog with congenital tricuspid regurgitation due to valvular dysplasia. There is tremendous right-sided cardiomegaly as a result of right atrial and right ventricular dilatation.

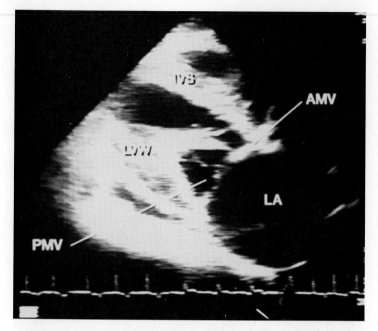

Figure 8–20. A single-frame echocardiographic image from a young German shepherd with congenital mitral valve dysplasia. Note the presence of a single giant papillary muscle. The chordae tendineae are abnormally short and thick, and some attach aberrantly to the interventricular septum (IVS). The anterior mitral valve leaflet (AMV) is abnormally short and thickened as well. The left atrium (LA) is enlarged as a result of chronic mitral regurgitation. LVW = left ventricular wall; PMV = posterior mitral valve leaflet.

matic with medical management (Hamlin and Harris, 1969). Surgical repair of MVM by annuloplasty and leaflet reconstruction can be successful in some affected dogs (Orton EC, unpublished data).

Atrial Anomalies

Atrial septal defects (ASDs) are seldom recognized as individual anomalies and are usually identified with other cardiac defects at the time of necropsy (Patterson, 1968). Atrial septal defect has been reported as one of a group of cardiac anomalies in a family of boxer dogs, but no trial breedings were performed (Pyle and Patterson, 1972).

ASDs are classified according to their location in the septum, with ostium secundum defects the most prevalent type in dogs. Ostium primum defects occur in the ventral atrial septum close to the atrioventricular valves, and defects in this location are common in cats. Ostium primum ASDs are nearly always associated with other abnormalities affecting the interventricular septum, mitral valve, and tricuspid valve constituting a complex lesion called *complete atrioventricular septal defect* or *endocardial cushion defect* (Fig. 8–21).

The hemodynamic and clinical sequelae of an atrial septal defect depend on the size of the defect, the diastolic compliance of the right and left ventricles, and the ratio of pulmonary to systemic vascular resistance (Hamilton et al, 1987). Most ASDs cause shunting of blood primarily in a left-to-right direction, with resulting right ventricular and right atrial volume overload. Many animals are asymptomatic, but large defects may induce decreased exercise tolerance and right-sided congestive heart failure. Secondary pulmonary hypertension, tricuspid or pulmonary valve regurgitation, and supraventricular tachyarrhythmias may develop (Eyster et al, 1976b). Surgical repair is recommended for large ASDs, particularly in those animals with clinical signs or Doppler evidence of bidirectional shunting (Orton, 1995; Monnet et al, 1997).

Another atrial defect recognized in dogs and cats is cor triatriatum, a rare congenital cardiac anomaly in which a membrane separates the atrium into two chambers. This abnormal septation may occur in either the left atrium (cor triatriatum sinister) or the right atrium (cor triatriatum dexter). Cor triatriatum sinister has been reported in kittens (Gordon et al, 1982; Wander et al, 1998). Cor triatriatum dexter has been described in dogs (Stern et al, 1986; Miller et al, 1989: Otto et al, 1990; Tobias et al, 1993), with an increased prevalence in chow chows (Miller and Fossum, 1994).

Cor triatriatum dexter results from persistence of the embryonic eustachian valves within the right atrium. The persistent embryonic valves effectively segment the atrium and obstruct venous return from the caudal vena cava and coronary sinus. Presenting signs are those of right heart failure with severe ascites. Abnormal septation of the atrium may be dem-

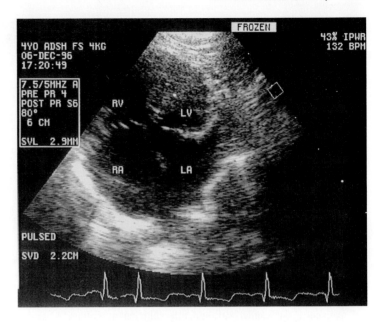

Figure 8–21. Still-frame two-dimensional echocardiographic image obtained from a young cat. This apical view image shows an ostium primum atrial septal defect (ASD) that is contiguous with a high membranous ventricular septal defect. The lesion is a complete atrioventricular septal defect (endocardial cushion defect). RA = right atrium; RV = right ventricle; LA = left atrium; LV = left ventricle.

onstrated with two-dimensional echocardiography or venography. Venography also demonstrates the obstructed flow (Stern et al, 1986; Tobias et al, 1993). A pressure gradient is present across the restrictive membrane. Surgical correction or balloon dilation of this anomaly eliminates obstruction to venous flow.

Endocardial Fibroelastosis

Endocardial fibroelastosis (EF) is a rare congenital disorder characterized by proliferation of elastic and collagenous fibers within the endocardium. Grossly, the endocardium is abnormally thickened and has a smooth, milky white or "porcelain" appearance. The left atrium and left ventricle are usually exclusively involved. There is marked cardiac dilation. Microscopically, the subendocardium is thickened by proliferation of collagen and elastic fibers.

Endocardial fibroelastosis occurs commonly in young cats in the absence of other cardiac anomalies (Harpster, 1977; Liu, 1974). The defect is hereditary in Burmese (Paasch and Zook, 1980; Zook and Paasch, 1982) and Siamese (Harpster, 1977; Patterson, 1986) cats but may occur in other breeds as well. Results of one study suggest that male kittens are more commonly affected than females (Harpster, 1977). The onset of clinical signs usually occurs at 12 to 16 weeks of age (Harpster, 1977; Liu, 1974). The most common presenting complaint is sudden onset of dyspnea. Other clinical features include tachycardia, signs of congestive heart failure, cardiomegaly, and often terminal cyano-

sis. There may be a gallop rhythm or systolic murmur in some kittens. The electrocardiographic and radiographic changes reflect atrial and ventricular enlargement and heart failure with a high incidence of pleural and abdominal effusion (Harpster, 1977). Echocardiography of kittens with EF demonstrates a markedly dilated left ventricle, a thin free wall, and greatly diminished contractility (Fig. 8–22). Some human infants with EF respond to treatment with L-carnitine, but it is not yet known whether myocardial carnitine deficiency plays a role in EF in kittens.

Endocardial fibroelastosis is less common in puppies than in kittens. In puppies, the disorder is often associated with other congenital heart anomalies (Lombard and Buergelt, 1984; Wegelius and von Essen, 1969).

CONGENITAL RHYTHM DISORDERS

Several disorders of impulse formation and conduction have been recognized in young dogs and cats. Ventricular preexcitation occurs as an isolated abnormality and also in association with anatomic congenital lesions (Hill and Tilley, 1985). The ECG features of this abnormality depend on the location of the accessory atrioventricular conduction pathway. Typically, there is a decrease in the PR interval ($\leq$0.05 second). There may also be a wide QRS complex that is slurred at its onset, a delta wave. Animals with ventricular preexcitation may be asymptomatic,

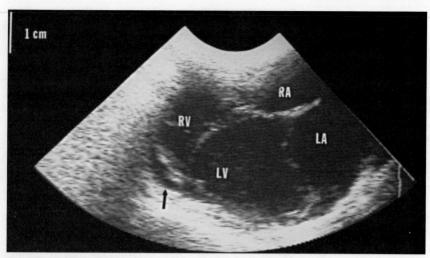

Figure 8–22. A single-frame, two-dimensional echocardiographic image obtained from a 14-week-old domestic short-haired kitten with endocardial fibroelastosis (right, long-axis view). The image demonstrates dilatation of all four cardiac chambers, with a thinning of the left ventricular caudal wall and interventricular septum. A small amount of pleural fluid is also visible (arrow). The kitten had severe, diffuse myocardial hypokinesis with less than a 10% decrease in the measured left ventricular minor axis during systole. LV = left ventricle; LA = left atrium; RV = right ventricle; RA = right atrium.

or they may present with weakness or syncope resulting from paroxysmal reentry tachycardias.

Fatal ventricular arrhythmias are heritable in some bloodlines of purebred German shepherds (Moise et al, 1997). Affected puppies die suddenly, usually during sleep, and have no identifiable gross or microscopic lesions of the heart. Death commonly occurs between the ages of 4 and 18 months. Electrocardiographic studies of puppies from affected bloodlines have revealed variations in the severity of ventricular ectopia, ranging from isolated (single) ventricular premature contractions to episodes of nonsustained ventricular tachycardia (Fig. 8–23). Whereas puppies with six or more consecutive premature complexes appear to have the highest risk of experiencing sudden death, those without ventricular tachycardia on ambulatory ECG recordings (Holter monitoring) do not have fatal events. Although it is not known which, if any, antiarrhythmic medications can be given to prevent sudden death, ambulatory ECG monitoring may be used to identify puppies likely to have a fatal arrhythmia.

Persistent atrial standstill has been reported in young dogs, usually in English springer spaniels. In some cases, the disorder is associated with features of scapulohumeral-type muscular dystrophy (Tilley and Liu, 1979). Other cases have been associated with atrial myocarditis of uncertain cause (Robinson et al, 1981). The ECG diagnosis of this disorder is made by noting the absence of P waves and the presence of a junctional or ventricular escape rhythm in an animal with normal serum potassium concentrations (Fig. 8–24) (Bonagura and O'Grady, 1983). The bradycardia of persistent atrial standstill does not respond to atropine, and symptomatic dogs must be treated by permanent pacemaker implantation.

Hereditary stenosis of the atrioventricular bundle associated with sinus arrest has been described in pugs (James et al, 1975). Dogs with this condition may have syncopal attacks that begin during the first several months of life. Sinoatrial block and sinoatrial arrest have also been reported in association with congenital deafness in patched Dalmatian coach hounds (James, 1967). Pacemaker implantation is required for treatment of these congenital bradyarrhythmias. Congenital bradycardias are extremely rare in young cats.

ACQUIRED HEART DISEASE

Although it is less common than congenital disease, acquired heart disease, especially of an infectious nature, may affect young animals. Many of the acquired cardiac abnormalities in puppies and kittens are associated with disease of other organ systems, and extracardiac signs are frequently more obvious and more life-threatening than circulatory dysfunction.

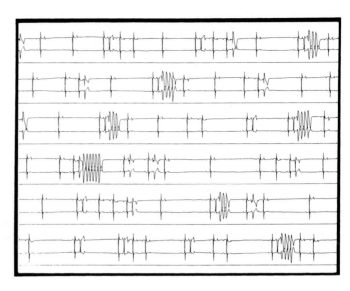

Figure 8–23. Selected electrocardiographic rhythm strips obtained from a German shepherd puppy by 24-hour ambulatory monitoring of the cardiac rhythm. The puppy is related to shepherds known to have died suddenly. The rhythm strips shown, which were obtained during sleep, reveal multiple episodes of paroxysmal ventricular tachycardia. (Courtesy of Dr. N. Sydney Moise, New York State College of Veterinary Medicine, Ithaca, NY.)

Primary Myocardial Diseases

Primary myocardial diseases constitute a heterogeneous group of cardiac muscle disorders, including the dilated, hypertrophic, and restrictive forms of cardiomyopathy as well as boxer cardiomyopathy, Doberman cardiomyopathy, and excessive left ventricular moderator bands. Of these, feline dilated cardiomyopathy (Fox, 1983), feline hypertrophic cardiomyopathy (Kittleson et al, 1996; Meurs et al, 1997), and canine hypertrophic cardiomyopathy (Swindle et al, 1984; Thomas et al, 1984) have been recognized in animals less than 6 months old. Puppies and kittens with hypertrophic cardiomyopathy are usually asymptomatic except for the presence of an apical systolic murmur. It is not, however, unusual for cats with inherited hypertrophic cardiomyopathy to develop heart failure when they reach maturity.

Secondary Myocardial Diseases

Secondary cardiomyopathy results from myocardial injury of known cause. Often the underlying disease process causes ionic changes, altered membrane permeability, and inflammation or necrosis with subsequent arrhythmogenesis. The contractile function of the heart may also be affected, however, producing symptoms similar to those of primary myocardial disease. Even histopathologically the distinction between primary and secondary myocardial disease may be unclear because chronic processes or sublethal injuries may produce degeneration and fibrosis resembling idiopathic cardiomyopathy. In young animals an underlying cause of secondary myocardial disease should always be sought. When possible, specific treatment is then administered along with supportive therapy for the heart. Of the many recognized causes of

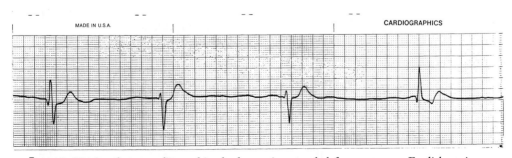

Figure 8–24. An electrocardiographic rhythm strip recorded from a young English springer spaniel with atrial myocarditis and left heart failure. There are a lack of atrial activity and a ventricular escape rhythm. (Paper speed = 50 mm/s.)

secondary myocardial disease, several are more common in puppies and kittens and are discussed.

INFECTIOUS MYOCARDITIS

Inflammation of the myocardium may occur with a variety of systemic diseases, usually of an infectious nature. The inflammatory process may be acute or chronic, and both functional and structural damage may persist after the initial myocardial inflammation resolves (Lenghaus and Studdert, 1984). Clinical manifestations usually include arrhythmias, conduction disturbances, and congestive heart failure. There may also be systemic evidence of inflammation such as fever or leukocytosis and evidence of dysfunction in other organs.

Canine parvovirus causes myocarditis in young puppies. Although puppies can be infected with this agent in utero (Lenghaus et al, 1980; Lenghaus and Studdert, 1984), there are ample experimental and epidemiologic data to suggest that puppies stricken with myocarditis are probably born of seronegative dams and exposed to canine parvovirus shortly after birth (Meunier et al, 1981, 1984). Usually, parvoviral myocarditis causes sudden death or pulmonary edema in 4- to 10-week old puppies (Hezel et al, 1979; Mulvey et al, 1980). Some dogs may, however, survive the early inflammation and develop congestive heart failure as older puppies or young adults (Atwell and Kelly, 1980). The diagnosis of parvoviral myocarditis can be confirmed histopathologically by identifying the characteristic myocardial lesions and basophilic intranuclear inclusion bodies (Gagnon et al, 1980; Robinson et al, 1980). Canine distemper virus may also cause myocarditis in puppies less than 10 days old (Higgins et al, 1981). Histopathologic lesions in the myocardium caused by canine distemper virus can usually be easily distinguished from those of parvoviral myocarditis (Higgens et al, 1981).

Parvoviral myocarditis similar to that in puppies has also been seen in kittens with generalized parvovirus infection (feline panleukopenia) (Bestetti and Wahlen, 1985). Feline infectious peritonitis virus has been implicated as a cause of left heart failure and sudden death in kittens (Scott et al, 1979). However, conclusive evidence relating this virus to dilated cardiomyopathy and death in kittens is lacking.

Bacterial myocarditis or endomyocarditis may occur in kittens and puppies, usually developing secondary to hematogenous spread from a septic focus elsewhere or from a generalized septicemia. Although kittens may be infected with *Toxoplasma gondii*, toxoplasma-induced myocarditis is rare and injection is more likely to produce symptoms related to encephalitis, pneumonitis, or enteritis (Dubey, 1986). Fungal myocarditis and other types of parasitic myocarditis are rare in dogs and cats younger than 6 months of age.

INBORN ERRORS OF METABOLISM

There are several hereditary defects in metabolism that can affect the electrophysiologic and mechanical functions of the myocardium. Specifically, mucopolysaccharidosis I, a deficiency of the lysosomal enzyme α-L-iduronidase, has been recognized in cats (Haskins et al, 1979) and in young Plott hounds (Shull et al, 1982, 1984). Affected animals may have radiographic, electrocardiographic, pathologic, and echocardiographic evidence of ventricular dilation and thickening of the atrioventricular valve leaflets. α-Glucosidase deficiency involving the heart, skeletal muscle, and liver has been identified in Lapland dogs (Walvoort et al, 1984). Cardiac abnormalities described in these puppies include generalized cardiomegaly, atrial fibrillation, increased QRS complex voltage, and prolonged QRS complex duration. With either of these storage diseases, cardiac manifestations are usually less obvious and less life-threatening than the coexisting neurologic, muscular, and hepatic alterations.

TRAUMATIC INSULT

Penetrating or blunt trauma of the thorax may cause contusion, laceration, or infarction of the myocardium, producing cardiac arrhythmias or failure. Occasionally, supportive therapy or antiarrhythmic agents are warranted, and anesthesia should be avoided until the cardiac abnormalities have resolved.

Electrical shock occurs more commonly in puppies and kittens than in adults. The shock may cause sudden death from ventricular fibrillation. Animals surviving immediate electrocution may subsequently develop acute left ventricular failure. The pathogenesis of this heart failure is not well understood. In addition to oxygen, diuretics, and vasodilators for the pulmonary edema, prednisolone sodium succinate is recommended (Wood, 1983). For a more complete description of electrical shock injuries, the reader is referred to Chapter 23 on environmental injuries.

DISEASES OF THE PULMONARY AND PERIPHERAL VASCULATURE

Vascular abnormalities in young dogs and cats are usually congenital, arising most often from anomalous development of the systemic veins (persistent left cranial vena cava) or the aortic arches (vascular ring anomalies). Anomalous pulmonary venous return is less common but has been reported in association with an ASD and right heart failure in a 5-month-old puppy (Hilwig and Bishop, 1975). Extracardiac arterial-venous (A-V) fistulas can be either congenital or acquired and have been reported in both kittens and puppies (Bolton et al, 1976; Easley and Carpenter, 1975; Jones et al, 1981). The A-V fistulas may affect any part of the vascular system but usually affect the great vessels, internal organs, or distal extremities. Signs associated with an A-V fistula depend on its location and the size of the A-V shunt. Often there is a continuous murmur or bruit in the area of the shunt. Temporary occlusion of the A-V shunt, when possible, may result in bradycardia or in external collapse of an affected lesion. Large shunts may produce high-output cardiac failure.

Vascular hamartomas are congenital or developmental anomalies similar to A-V fistulas. When present in the pulmonary vasculature, hamartomas produce signs similar to those of other types of right-to-left shunts such as hypoxemia and polycythemia.

Pulmonary hypertension usually occurs in adult dogs and cats as an acquired abnormality, but occasionally it occurs in the young dog or cat. Pulmonary hypertension may be associated with hypertrophy of the media of the pulmonary arteries, which is reversible. With time, however, plexiform arteriopathy characterized by intimal proliferation, thickening, and plexiform lesions; atherosclerosis; thrombosis; necrotizing arteritis; and occlusion occur that make the vascular disease irreversible (Geer et al, 1965). Necrotizing pulmonary arteritis with right heart failure has occurred in puppies with peritoneopericardial diaphragmatic hernia, PDA, and Eisenmenger's syndrome (Nimmo-Wilkie and Feldman, 1981; Turk et al, 1981, 1984). Canine heartworm disease (due to *Dirofilaria immitis*), the most common cause of pulmonary hypertension and pulmonary arteritis in adult dogs, does not occur in dogs younger than 6 months of age. *Dirofilaria immitis* microfilaremia may, however, occur in puppies subsequent to placental transfer (Atwell, 1981). Medial hypertrophy, intimal proliferation, and pulmonary hypertension have been described in

kittens with *Toxocara cati* infection (Weatherly and Hamilton, 1984).

Peripheral vascular diseases are uncommon in kittens and puppies. Arterial thromboembolism is unusual in this age group but may occasionally occur secondary to myocardial disease, protein-losing nephropathy, endocarditis, or traumatic injury. Immune-mediated vasculitis resembling polyarteritis nodosa and experimental serum sickness has been described in young beagle dogs (Harcourt, 1978). These puppies had severe pain and neurologic dysfunction due to involvement of the meningeal arteries.

Vasculitis may also be seen in young dogs with infectious canine hepatitis (ICH) (Greene, 1990). This disease, caused by canine adenovirus-1 (CAV-1), affects unvaccinated puppies and puppies who lack sufficient protective maternal antibody. The CAV-1 produces severe, generalized endothelial damage with subsequent widespread tissue damage. Disseminated intravascular coagulation frequently results. The treatment of dogs with ICH is symptomatic and supportive (Greene, 1990). Infectious vasculitis in young dogs may also develop after infection with *Ehrlichia canis* or *Rickettsia rickettsii*, the causative agents of canine ehrlichiosis and Rocky Mountain spotted fever, respectively (Troy and Forrester, 1990; Greene and Breitschwerdt, 1990). These rickettsial diseases are similar and are characterized by fever, anorexia, depression, lymphadenopathy, and oculonasal discharge. The rickettsia-induced endothelial damage occurring with either agent commonly produces petechial and ecchymotic hemorrhages. Puppies with canine ehrlichiosis or Rocky Mountain spotted fever should receive tetracycline or chloramphenicol therapy in addition to general supportive care.

References and Supplemental Reading

Ackerman N, Burk R, Hahn AW, et al: Patent ductus arteriosus in the dog: A retrospective study of radiographic, epidemiologic, and clinical findings. Am J Vet Res 39:1805, 1978.

Adelman RD, Wright J: Systolic blood pressure and heart rate in the growing beagle puppy. Dev Pharmacol Ther 8:396, 1985.

Atwell RB: Prevalence of *Dirofilaria immitis* microfilaraemia in 6- to 8-week-old pups. Aust Vet J 57:479, 1981.

Atwell RB, Kelly WR: Canine parvovirus: A cause of chronic myocardial fibrosis and adolescent congestive heart failure. J Small Anim Pract 21:609, 1980.

Becker AE, Becker MJ, Edwards JE: Pathologic spectrum of dysplasia of the tricuspid valve. Arch Pathol 91:167, 1971.

Bestetti G, Wahlen R: Generalized parvovirus infection with inclusion-body myocarditis in two kittens. J Comp Pathol 95:393, 1985.

Bishop SP: Developmental anatomy of the heart and great vessels. In Fox PR (ed): Canine and Feline Cardiology. New York, Churchill Livingstone, 1988, p 3.

Blackstone EH, Kirklin JW, Bradley EL, et al: Optimal age and results in repair of large ventricular septal defects. J Thorac Cardiovasc Surg 72:661, 1976.

Bolton GR, Edwards NJ, Hoffer RE: Arteriovenous fistula of the aorta and caudal vena cava causing congestive heart failure in a cat. J Am Anim Hosp Assoc 12:463, 1976.

Bolton GR, Ettinger SJ, Liu SK: Tetralogy of Fallot in three cats. J Am Vet Med Assoc 160:1622, 1972.

Bolton GR, Liu SK: Congenital heart diseases of the cat. Vet Clin North Am 7:341, 1977.

Bonagura JD: M-mode echocardiography. Vet Clin North Am 13:299, 1983.

Bonagura JD: Antiarrhythmic therapy. In Tilley LP (ed): Essentials of Canine and Feline Electrocardiography, 2nd ed. Philadelphia, Lea & Febiger, 1985a, p 281.

Bonagura JD: Congenital heart diseases. Proc 9th Kal Kan Symp 1985b, p 96.

Bonagura JD: Congenital heart disease. In Bonagura JD (ed): Cardiology. Contemporary Issues in Small Animal Practice, vol 7. New York, Churchill Livingstone, 1987, p 1.

Bonagura JD, O'Grady M: ECG of the month. J Am Vet Med Assoc 183:658, 1983.

Bonagura JD, Pipers FS: Diagnosis of cardiac lesions by contrast echocardiography. J Am Vet Med Assoc 182:396, 1983.

Boucek MM, Webster HE, Orsmond GS, et al: Balloon pulmonary valvulotomy: Palliation for cyanotic heart disease. Am Heart J 115:318, 1988.

Branch CE, Robertson BT, Williams JC: Frequency of atrioventricular block in dogs. Am J Vet Res 36:925, 1975.

Breznock EM: Spontaneous closure of ventricular septal defects in the dog. J Am Vet Med Assoc 162:399, 1973.

Breznock EM, Whiting P, Pendray D, et al: Valved apicoaortic conduit for relief of left ventricular hypertension caused by discrete subaortic stenosis in dogs. J Am Vet Med Assoc 182:51, 1983.

Breznock EM, Wood GL: A patch-graft technique for correction of pulmonic stenosis in dogs. J Am Vet Med Assoc 169:1090, 1976.

Bright JM, Jennings J, Toal R, et al: Percutaneous balloon valvuloplasty for treatment of pulmonic stenosis in a dog. J Am Vet Med Assoc 191:995, 1987.

Brownlie SE, Cobb MA, Chambers J, et al: Percutaneous balloon valvuloplasty in four dogs with pulmonic stenosis. J Small Anim Pract 32:165, 1991.

Buchanan JW: Radiographic aspects of patent ductus arteriosus in dogs before and after surgery. Acta Radiol (Suppl) 319:271, 1972.

Buchanan JW: Pulmonic stenosis caused by single coronary artery in dogs: Four cases (1965–1984). J Am Vet Med Assoc 196:115, 1990.

Buchanan JW: Causes and prevalence of cardiovascular disease. In Kirk RW, Bonagura JD (eds): Current Veterinary Therapy XI. Small Animal Practice. Philadelphia, WB Saunders, 1992, p 647.

Clifford DH, Ross JN, Waddell ED, et al: Effect of persistent aortic arch on the ganglial cells of the canine esophagus. J Am Vet Med Assoc 158:1401, 1971.

Cohen JS, Tilly LP, Liu SK, et al: Patent ductus arteriosus in five cats. J Am Anim Hosp Assoc 11:95, 1975.

Darke PGG: Doppler echocardiography. J Small Anim Pract 33:104, 1992.

Darke PGG, Bonagura JD, Kelly DF: Color Atlas of Veterinary Cardiology. London, Mosby-Wolfe, 1996, pp 47–91.

Davies PJ, Dewar J, Tynan M, et al: Postnatal developmental changes in the length-tension relationship of cat papillary muscles. J Physiol (Lond) 253:95, 1975.

DeLellis LA, Thomas WP, Pion PD: Balloon dilation of congenital subaortic stenosis in the dog. J Vet Intern Med 7:153, 1993.

Dubey JP: Toxoplasmosis in cats. Feline Pract 16:12, 1986.

Dunnigan A, Benson DW Jr: Atrial flutter in infancy: Clinical features and modes of termination. Pediatr Cardiol 4:308, 1983.

Easley JC, Carpenter JL: Hepatic arteriovenous fistula in two Saint Bernard pups. J Am Vet Med Assoc 166:167, 1975.

Egbert JR, Katona PG: Development of autonomic heart rate control in the kitten during sleep. Am J Physiol 238:H829, 1980.

Ellison GW: Vascular ring anomalies in the dog and cat. Compend Contin Educ Pract Vet 11:693, 1980.

Ettinger SJ, Suter PF: Congenital heart disease. In Ettinger SJ (ed): Canine Cardiology. Philadelphia, WB Saunders, 1970, p 528.

Ewey DM, Pion PD, Hird DW: Survival in treated and untreated dogs with congenital pulmonic stenosis. Proc ACVIM 10:797, 1992.

Eyster GE: Pulmonic stenosis. In Bojrab MJ (ed): Current Techniques in Small Animal Surgery, 2nd ed. Philadelphia, Lea & Febiger, 1983, p 462.

Eyster GE, Anderson LK, Cords GB: Aortic regurgitation in the dog. J Am Vet Med Assoc 168:138, 1976a.

Eyster GE, Anderson L, Evans AT, et al: Ebstein's anomaly: A report of 3 cases in the dog. J Am Vet Med Assoc 170:709, 1977a.

Eyster GE, Anderson LK, Krehbeil JD, et al: Surgical repair of atrial septal defect in a dog. J Am Vet Med Assoc 169:1081, 1976b.

Eyster GE, Anderson LK, Sawyer DC, et al: Beta adrenergic blockade for management of tetralogy of Fallot in a dog. J Am Vet Med Assoc 169:637, 1976c.

Eyster GE, Braden TD, Appleford M, et al: Surgical

management of tetralogy of Fallot. J Small Anim Pract 18:387, 1977b.

Eyster GE, DeYoung B: Cardiac disorders. *In* Slatter DH (ed): Textbook of Small Animal Surgery, vol 1. Philadelphia, WB Saunders, 1985, p 1076.

Eyster GE, Evans AT, Blanchard GL, et al: Congenital pericardial diaphragmatic hernia and multiple cardiac defects in a litter of collies. J Am Vet Med Assoc 170:516, 1977c.

Eyster GE, Eyster JT, Cords GB, et al: Patent ductus arteriosus in the dog: Characteristics of occurrence and results of surgery in one hundred consecutive cases. J Am Vet Med Assoc 168:435, 1976d.

Eyster GE, Hough JD, Evans AT, et al: Surgical repair of patent ductus arteriosus, aortic stenosis, and aortic regurgitation in a dog. J Am Vet Med Assoc 167:942, 1975.

Eyster GE, Probst M: Basic cardiac procedures. *In* Slatter DH (ed): Textbook of Small Animal Surgery, vol 1. Philadelphia, WB Saunders, 1985, p 1128.

Eyster GE, Weber W, Chi S, et al: Mitral valve prosthesis for correction of mitral regurgitation in a dog. J Am Vet Med Assoc 168:1115, 1976e.

Eyster GE, Whipple RD, Anderson LK, et al: Pulmonary artery banding for ventricular septal defect in dogs and cats. J Am Vet Med Assoc 170:434, 1977d.

Ezrin AM, Epstein K, Bassett AL, et al: Effects of procainamide on cellular physiology of neonatal and adult dog myocardium. Dev Pharmacol Ther 1:352, 1980.

Feldman EC, Nimmo-Wilkie JS, Pharr JW: Eisenmenger's syndrome in the dog: Case reports. J Am Anim Hosp Assoc 17:477, 1981.

Fingland RB, Bonagura JD, Myer CW: Pulmonic stenosis in the dog: 29 cases (1975–1984). J Am Vet Med Assoc 189:218, 1986.

Finley JP, Kelly C: Heart rate and respiratory patterns in mild hypoxia in unanaesthetized newborn mammals. Can J Pharmacol 64:122, 1986.

Fox PR: Feline myocardial disease. *In* Kirk RW (ed): Current Veterinary Therapy VIII. Philadelphia, WB Saunders, 1983, p 337.

Fox PR, Bond BR, Sommer RJ: Nonsurgical transcatheter coil occlusion of patent ductus arteriosus in two dogs using a preformed nitrol snare delivery technique. J Vet Intern Med 12:182, 1998.

Fox PR, Miller MW, Liu S-K: Clinical, echocardiographic, and Doppler imaging characteristics of mitral valve stenosis in two dogs. J Am Vet Med Assoc 201:1575, 1992.

Gagnon AN, Crowe SP, Allen DG, et al: Myocarditis in puppies: Clinical, pathologic, and virological findings. Can Vet J 21:195, 1980.

Garson A, Gilette PC, McNamara DG: Propranolol: The preferred palliation for tetralogy of Fallot. Am J Cardiol 47:1099, 1981.

Gaum WE, Lathrop DA, Kaplan S: Age-related changes in electrophysiological properties of canine Purkinje fibers: Effect of ouabain. Dev Pharmacol Ther 6:145, 1983.

Geer JC, Glass BA, Albert HM: The morphogenesis and reversibility of experimental hyperkinetic pulmonary vascular lesions in the dog. Exp Mol Pathol 4:399, 1965.

Gompf RE: The clinical approach to heart disease: History and physical examination. *In* Fox PR (ed): Canine and Feline Cardiology. New York, Churchill Livingstone, 1988, p 29.

Gordon B, Trautvetter E, Patterson DF: Pulmonary congestion associated with cor triatriatum in a cat. J Am Vet Med Assoc 180:75, 1982.

Greene CE: Infectious canine hepatitis and canine acidophil cell hepatitis. *In* Greene CE (ed): Infectious Diseases of the Dog and Cat. Philadelphia, WB Saunders, 1990, p 242.

Greene CE, Breitschwerdt EB: Rocky Mountain spotted fever and Q fever. *In* Greene CE (ed): Infectious Diseases of the Dog and Cat. Philadelphia, WB Saunders, 1990, p 419.

Haddad GG, Jeng HJ, Lee SH, et al: Rhythmic variations in R-R interval during sleep and wakefulness in puppies and dogs. Am J Physiol 247:H67, 1984.

Hageman GR, Neely BH, Urthaler F: Cardiac autonomic efferent activity during baroreflex in puppies and adult dogs. Am J Physiol 251:H443, 1986.

Hamilton WT, Haffajee CI, Dalen JE, et al: Atrial septal defect secundum: Clinical profile with physiologic correlates. *In* Roberts WC (ed): Adult Congenital Heart Disease. Philadelphia, FA Davis, 1987, p 395.

Hamlin RL, Harris SG: Mitral incompetence in Great Dane pups. J Am Vet Med Assoc 154:790, 1969.

Harcourt RA: Polyarteritis in a colony of beagles. Vet Rec 102:519, 1978.

Harpster NK: Cardiovascular diseases of the domestic cat. Adv Vet Sci Comp Med 21:39, 1977.

Harpster NK, Zook BC: The cardiovascular system. *In* Holzworth J (ed): Diseases of the Cat: Medicine and Surgery. Philadelphia, WB Saunders, 1987, p 820.

Haskins ME, Jezyk PF, Desnick RJ, et al: Alpha-L-iduronidase deficiency in a cat: A model of mucopolysaccharidosis I. Pediatr Res 13:1294, 1979.

Hawe RS: Pulmonic stenosis in a cat. J Am Anim Hosp Assoc 17:777, 1981.

Herrtage ME, Hall LW, English TAH: Surgical correction of the tetralogy of Fallot in a dog. J Small Anim Pract 24:51, 1983.

Hezel B, Thornburg LP, Kintner LD: Inclusion body myocarditis: Cause of acute death in puppies. Vet Med Small Anim Clinician 74:1627, 1979.

Higgins RJ, Krakowka S, Metzler AE, et al: Canine distemper virus–associated cardiac necrosis in the dog. Vet Pathol 18:472, 1981.

Hill BL, Tilley LP: Ventricular preexcitation in seven dogs and nine cats. J Am Vet Med Assoc 187:1026, 1985.

Hill JD: The electrocardiogram in dogs with standardized body and limb positions. J Electrocardiol 1:175, 1968.

Hilwig RW, Bishop SP: Anomalous pulmonary venous return in a Great Dane. J Am Vet Med Assoc 36:229, 1975.

Horton JW, Coln D: Cardiovascular function and fluid compartments in newborn canine hemorrhagic shock. Am J Physiol 248:R724, 1985.

Hunt GB, Church DB, Malik R, et al: A retrospective analysis of congenital cardiac anomalies (1977–1989). Aust Vet Pract 20:70, 1990.

Hutchinson RA, Percival CJ, Young IM: Development of cardiovascular responses in the kitten. J Exp Physiol 47:201, 1962.

Jackson WF, Henderson RA: Ligature placement in closure of patent ductus arteriosus. J Am Anim Hosp Assoc 15:55, 1979.

James TN: Congenital deafness and cardiac arrhythmias. Am J Cardiol 19:627, 1967.

James TN, Robertson BT, Waldo AL, et al: De subitaneis mortibus XV. Hereditary stenosis of the His bundle in pug dogs. Circulation 52:1152, 1975.

Jones DGC, Allen WE, Webbon PM: Arteriovenous fistula in the metatarsal pad of a dog: A case report. J Small Anim Pract 22:635, 1981.

Kelly WR: Fatal diffuse subacute myocarditis in pups. Mod Vet Pract 60:719, 1979.

Khera KS: Fetal cardiovascular and other defects induced by thalidomide in cats. Anat Rec 149:299, 1964.

Kirk GR, Smith DM, Hutcheson DP, et al: Postnatal growth of the dog heart. II. J Anat 119:461, 1975.

Kittleson MD: Drugs used in the management of heart failure. In Kirk RW (ed): Current Veterinary Therapy VIII. Philadelphia, WB Saunders, 1983, p 285.

Kittleson MD, Kittleson JA, Mekhamer Y: Development and progression of inherited hypertrophic cardiomyopathy in Maine coon cats. Proc Am Coll Vet Intern Med 14:747, 1996.

Kornreich BG, Moise NS: Right atrioventricular valve malformation in dogs and cats: An electrocardiographic survey with emphasis on splintered QRS complexes. J Vet Intern Med 11:226, 1997.

Lau KW, Hung JS: Controversies in percutaneous balloon pulmonary valvuloplasty: Timing, patient selection, and technique. J Heart Valve Dis 2:321, 1993.

Lee JC, Taylor JFN, Downing SE: A comparison of ventricular weights and geometry in newborn, young, and adult mammals. J Appl Physiol 38:147, 1975.

Legendre AM, Appleford MD, Eyster GE, et al: Secondary polycythemia and seizures due to right to left shunting patent ductus arteriosus in a dog. J Am Vet Med Assoc 164:1198, 1974.

Lehmkuhl LB, Ware WA, Bonagura JD: Mitral stenosis in 15 dogs. J Vet Intern Med 8:2, 1994.

Lenghaus C, Studdert MJ: Animal model of human disease: Acute and chronic viral myocarditis. Am J Pathol 115:316, 1984.

Lenghaus C, Studdert MJ, Finnie JW: Acute and chronic canine parvovirus myocarditis following intrauterine inoculation. Aust Vet J 56:465, 1980.

Liu SK: Pathology of feline heart disease. In Kirk RW (ed): Current Veterinary Therapy V. Philadelphia, WB Saunders, 1974, p 341.

Liu SK: Pathology of feline heart diseases. Vet Clin North Am 7:323, 1977.

Liu SK, Tilley LP: Malformation of the canine mitral valve complex. J Am Vet Med Assoc 167:465, 1975.

Liu SK, Tilley LP: Dysplasia of the tricuspid valve in the dog and cat. J Am Vet Med Assoc 169:623, 1976.

Lombard CW, Buergelt CD: Endocardial fibroelastosis in four dogs. J Am Anim Hosp Assoc 20:271, 1984.

Lord PF, Wood A, Liu SK, et al: Left ventricular angiocardiography in congenital mitral valve insufficiency of the dog. J Am Vet Med Assoc 166:1069, 1975.

Mace SE, Levy MN: Autonomic nervous control of heart rate: Sympathetic-parasympathetic interactions and age related differences. Cardiovasc Res 17:547, 1983a.

Mace SE, Levy MN: Neural control of heart rate: A comparison between puppies and adult animals. Pediatr Res 17:491, 1983b.

Magrini F: Haemodynamic determinants of the arterial blood pressure rise during growth in conscious puppies. Cardiovasc Res 12:422, 1978.

Malik R, Turnbull GR, Black AP: Patent ductus arteriosus in five related female border collies. Aust Vet Pract 21:2, 1991.

Mann PGH, Stock JE, Sheridan JP: Pulmonary artery banding in the cat: A case report. J Small Anim Pract 12:45, 1971.

Martin L, VandeWoude S, Boon J, et al: Left ventricular hypertrophy in a closed colony of Persian cats. Proc Am Coll Vet Intern Med 12:974, 1994.

Martin MWS, Godman M, Luis Fuentes V, et al: Assessment of balloon pulmonary valvuloplasty in six dogs. J Small Anim Proc 33:443, 1992.

Mary-Rabine L, Rosen MR: Lidocaine effects on action potentials of Purkinje fibers from neonatal and adult dogs. J Pharmacol Exp Ther 205:204, 1977.

McCandlish IAP, Nash AS, Peggram A: Unusual vascular ring in a cat: Left aortic arch with right ligamentum arteriosum. Vet Rec 114:338, 1984.

Meunier PC, Cooper BJ, Appel MJG, et al: Experimental viral myocarditis: Parvoviral infection of neonatal pups. Vet Pathol 21:509, 1984.

Meunier PC, Glickman LT, Appel MJG, et al: Canine parvovirus in a commercial kennel. Epidemiologic and pathologic findings. Cornell Vet 71:96, 1981.

Meurs K, Kittleson MD, Towbin J, et al: Familial systolic anterior motion of the mitral valve and/or hypertrophic cardiomyopathy is apparently inherited as an autosomal dominant trait in a family of American shorthair cats. Proc Am Coll Vet Intern Med 15:685, 1997.

Miller CW, Holmberg DL, Bowen V, et al: Microsurgical management of tetralogy of Fallot in a cat. J Am Vet Med Assoc 186:708, 1985.

Miller MW, Bonagura JD, DiBartola SP, et al: Budd-Chiari-like syndrome in two dogs. J Am Anim Hosp Assoc 25:277, 1989.

Miller MW, Meurs KM, Gordon SG, et al: Transarterial ductal occlusion using Gianturco vascular occlusion coils: 43 cases (1994–1998). Proc Am Coll Vet Intern Med 17:247, 1999.

Moise NS: Doppler echocardiographic evaluation of congenital heart disease: An introduction. J Vet Intern Med 3:195, 1989.

Moise NS, Gilmour RF, Riccio ML, et al: Diagnosis of inherited ventricular tachycardia in German shepherd dogs. J Am Vet Med Assoc 210:403, 1997.

Monnet E, Orton EC, Gaynor J, et al: Diagnosis and surgical repair of partial atrioventricular septal defects in two dogs. J Am Vet Med Assoc 211:569, 1997.

Moore KL: The Developing Human. Philadelphia, WB Saunders, 1973, p 273.

Mulvey JJ, Bech-Nielsen S, Haskins ME, et al: Myocarditis induced by parvoviral infection in weanling pups in the United States. J Am Vet Med Assoc 177:695, 1980.

Mulvihill JJ, Priester WA: Congenital heart disease in dogs: Epidemiologic similarities to man. Teratology 7:73, 1973.

Nakayama T, Wakao Y, Ishikawa R, et al: Progression of subaortic stenosis detected by continuous wave Doppler echocardiography in a dog. J Vet Intern Med 10:97, 1996.

Nimmo-Wilkie JS, Feldman EC: Pulmonary vascular lesions associated with congenital heart defects in three dogs. J Am Anim Hosp Assoc 17:485, 1981.

Ogburn PN, Peterson M, Jeraj K: Multiple cardiac anomalies in a family of Saluki dogs. J Am Vet Med Assoc 179:57, 1981.

O'Grady MR, Allen DG: Doppler echocardiographic findings in the dog and cat with patent ductus arteriosus. Proc Am Coll Vet Intern Med 5:939, 1987.

Orton EC: Small Animal Thoracic Surgery. Baltimore, Williams & Wilkins, 1995, p 177.

Orton EC, Boon J, Wagner A, et al: Open resection of discrete subvalvular aortic stenosis: Early results. Proc ACVIM 11:929, 1993.

Orton EC, Monnet E: Pulmonic stenosis and subvalvular aortic stenosis: Surgical options. Semin Vet Med Surg Small Anim 9:221, 1994.

Orton EC, Herndon GD, Boon JA, et al: Influence of open surgical correction on intermediate-term outcome in dogs with subvalvular aortic stenosis: 44 cases (1991–1998). J Am Vet Med Assoc 216:364, 2000.

Otto CM, Mahaffey M, Jacobs C, et al: Cor triatriatum dexter with Budd-Chiari syndrome and a review of ascites in young dogs. J Sm Anim Pract 31:385, 1990.

Paasch LH, Zook BC: The pathogenesis of endocardial fibroelastosis in Burmese cats. Lab Invest 42:197, 1980.

Patterson DF: Epidemiologic and genetic studies of congenital heart disease in the dog. Circ Res 23:171, 1968.

Patterson DF: Canine congenital heart disease: Epidemiology and etiologic hypotheses. J Small Anim Pract 12:263, 1971.

Patterson DF: Hereditary defects of the cardiovascular system in the dog and cat. Proc Am Coll Vet Intern Med 4:7, 1986.

Patterson DF, Haskins ME, Schnarr WR: Hereditary dysplasia of the pulmonary valve in beagle dogs. Pediatr Cardiol 47:631, 1981.

Patterson DF, Pyle RL, Buchanan JW, et al: Hereditary patent ductus arteriosus and its sequelae in the dog. Circ Res 29:1, 1971.

Patterson DF, Pyle RL, Van Mierop L, et al: Hereditary defects of the conotruncal septum in keeshond dogs: Pathologic and genetic studies. Am J Cardiol 34:187, 1974.

Pearlman AS: The use of Doppler in the evaluation of cardiac disorders and function. In Hurst JW (ed): The Heart, 6th ed. New York, McGraw-Hill, 1985, p 1978.

Pickoff AS, Flinn CJ, Singh S, et al: The effects of verapamil on the electrophysiology of the intact immature mammalian heart. J Cardiovasc Pharmacol 7:125, 1985a.

Pickoff AS, Singh S, Flinn CJ, et al: Dose-dependent electrophysiologic effects of amiodarone in the immature canine heart. Am J Cardiol 52:621, 1983.

Pickoff AS, Singh S, Flinn CJ, et al: Atrial vulnerability of the immature canine heart. Am J Cardiol 55:1402, 1985b.

Pyle RL, Park RD, Alexander AF, et al: Patent ductus arteriosus with pulmonary hypertension in the dog. J Am Vet Med Assoc 178:565, 1981.

Pyle RL, Patterson DF: Multiple cardiovascular malformations in a family of boxer dogs. J Am Vet Med Assoc 160:965, 1972.

Pyle RL, Patterson DF, Chacko S: The genetics and pathology of discrete subaortic stenosis in the Newfoundland dog. Am Heart J 92:324, 1976.

Robinson WF, Huxtable CR, Pass DA: Canine parvoviral myocarditis: A morphologic description of the natural disease. Vet Pathol 17:282, 1980.

Robinson WF, Thompson RR, Clark WT: Sinoatrial arrest associated with primary atrial myocarditis in a dog. J Small Anim Pract 22:99, 1981.

Scott FW, Weiss RC, Post JE, et al: Kitten mortality complex (neonatal FIP?). Feline Pract 9:44, 1979.

Shires PK, Liu W: Persistent right aortic arch in dogs: A long term follow-up after surgical correction. J Am Anim Hosp Assoc 17:773, 1981.

Shull RM, Helman RG, Spellacy E, et al: Morphologic and biochemical studies of canine mucopolysaccharidosis. I. Am J Pathol 114:487, 1984.

Shull RM, Munger RJ, Spellacy E, et al: Canine alpha-L-iduronidase deficiency: A model of mucopolysaccharidosis I. Am J Pathol 109:244, 1982.

Sisson D: The clinical management of cardiac arrhythmias in the dog and cat. In Fox PR (ed): Canine and Feline Cardiology. New York, Churchill Livingstone, 1988, p 289.

Sisson D, Schaeffer D: Changes in linear dimensions of the heart, relative to body weight, as measured by M-mode echocardiography in growing dogs. Am J Vet Res 52:1591, 1991.

Sisson D, Thomas WP: Endocarditis of the aortic valve in the dog. J Am Vet Med Assoc 184:570, 1984.

Stamoulis ME, Fox PR: Mitral valve stenosis in three cats. J Small Anim Pract 34:9, 1993.

Stepien RL, Bonagura JD: Aortic stenosis: Clinical findings in six cats. J Small Anim Pract 32:341, 1991.

Stern A, Fallon RK, Aronson E, et al: Cor triatriatum dexter in a dog. Compend Contin Educ Pract Vet 8:401, 1986.

Suga H, Yamada O, Goto Y, et al: Peak isovolumic pressure-volume relation of puppy left ventricle. Am J Physiol 250:H167, 1986.

Suter PF, Lord PF: Thoracic Radiography. A Text Atlas of Thoracic Diseases of the Dog and Cat. Davis, CA, Stonegate Publishing, 1984, p 498.

Swindle MM, Huber AC, Kan JS, et al: Mitral valve prolapse and hypertrophic cardiomyopathy in a pup. J Am Vet Med Assoc 184:1515, 1984.

Thomas WP, Mathewson JW, Suter PF, et al: Hypertrophic obstructive cardiomyopathy in a dog: Clinical, hemodynamic, angiographic, and pathologic studies. J Am Anim Hosp Assoc 20:253, 1984.

Tilley LP: Essentials of Canine and Feline Electrocardiology, 2nd ed. Philadelphia, Lea & Febiger, 1985, pp 64, 207.

Tilley LP, Liu SK: Persistent atrial standstill in the dog with muscular dystrophy. Proc Am Coll Vet Intern Med, 1979, p 111.

Tilley LP, Owens LM: Congenital heart disease. In Manual of Small Animal Cardiology. New York, Churchill Livingstone, 1985, p 252.

Tobias AH, Thomas WP, Kittleson MD, et al: Cor triatriatum dexter in two dogs. J Am Vet Med Assoc 202:285, 1993.

Trautvetter E, Detweiler DK, Bohn FK, et al: Evolution of the electrocardiogram in young dogs with congenital heart disease leading to right ventricular hypertrophy. J Electrocardiol 14:275, 1981a.

Trautvetter E, Detweiler DK, Patterson DF: Evolution of the electrocardiogram in young dogs during the first 12 weeks of life. J Electrocardiol 14:267, 1981b.

Troy GC, Forrester SD: Canine ehrlichiosis. In Greene CE (ed): Infectious Diseases of the Dog and Cat. Philadelphia, WB Saunders, 1990, p 404.

Turk JR, Miller LM, Miller JB, et al: Necrotizing pulmonary arteritis in a dog with patent ductus arteriosus. J Small Anim Pract 22:603, 1981.

Turk MAM, Turk JR, Rantanen NW, et al: Necrotizing pulmonary arteritis in a dog with peritoneo-pericardial diaphragmatic hernia. J Small Anim Pract 25:25, 1984.

Tynan M, Davies P, Sheridan D: Postnatal maturation of noradrenaline uptake and release in cat papillary muscles. Cardiovasc Res 11:206, 1977.

Vatner SF, Manders WT: Depressed responsiveness of the carotid sinus reflex in conscious newborn animals. Am J Physiol 237:H40, 1979.

Walls JT, Lababidi Z, Curtis JJ, et al: Assessment of percutaneous balloon pulmonary and aortic valvuloplasty. J Thorac Cardiovasc Surg 88:352, 1984.

Walvoort HC, van Nes JJ, Stokhof AA, et al: Canine glycogen storage disease type II: A clinical study of four affected Lapland dogs. J Am Anim Hosp Assoc 20:279, 1984.

Wander KW, Monnet E, Orton EC: Surgical correction of cor triatriatum sinister in a kitten. J Am Anim Hosp Assoc 34:383, 1998.

Weatherly AJ, Hamilton JM: Possible role of histamine in the genesis of pulmonary arterial disease in cats infected with Toxocara cati. Vet Rec 114:347, 1984.

Wegelius O, von Essen R: Endocardial fibroelastosis in dogs. Acta Pathol Microbiol Scand 77:66, 1969.

Weirich WE, Bisgard GE, Will JA, et al: Myocardial infarction and pulmonic stenosis in a dog. J Am Vet Med Assoc 159:315, 1971.

Weirich WE, Blevins WE: Ventricular septal defect repair. Vet Surg 7:2, 1978.

Weirich WE, Blevins WE, Conrad CR, et al: Congenital tricuspid insufficiency in a dog. J Am Vet Med Assoc 164:1025, 1974.

Weirich WE, Blevins WE, Rebar AH: Late consequences of patent ductus arteriosus in the dog: A report of six cases. J Am Anim Hosp Assoc 14:40, 1978.

Wheaton LG, Blevins WE, Weirich WE: Persistent right aortic arch associated with other vascular anomalies in two cats. J Am Vet Med Assoc 184:848, 1984.

Whiting PG, Breznock EM, Pendray DL, et al: Double-outlet right ventricle for relief of pulmonic stenosis in dogs, an experimental study. Vet Surg 13:64, 1984.

Wingfield WE, Boon JA, Miller CW: Echocardiographic assessment of congenital aortic stenosis in dogs. J Am Vet Med Assoc 183:673, 1983.

Wood GL: Canine myocardial diseases. In Kirk RW (ed): Current Veterinary Therapy VIII. Philadelphia, WB Saunders, 1983, p 329.

Woods WT, Urthaler F, James TN: Progressive postnatal changes in sinus node response to atropine and propranolol. Am J Physiol 234:H412, 1978.

Yasui H, Yoshitoshi M, Miyamoto AT, et al: Ventricular septal defect: Selection of patients and timing for surgery. Am Heart J 93:40, 1977.

Zook BC, Paasch LH: Endocardial fibroelastosis in Burmese cats. Am J Pathol 106:435, 1982.

Dental Disease and Care

B. Jean Hawkins

An oral examination should be performed each time a puppy or kitten is presented. Many pathologic or potentially pathologic conditions can be detected at an early age and corrective measures taken. Introducing the pet owner to the concept of oral home care and regular professional dental prophylaxis are the two most important responsibilities of the veterinarian with regard to dental disease care and prevention.

TOOTH MORPHOLOGY

There are three types of teeth in the deciduous dentition of puppies and kittens: incisor (I), canine (C), and premolar (P); a fourth type, molar (M), is found in the permanent dentition. Each type is designed to be self-cleaning in the noncrowded scissors occlusion, when the animal eats a natural diet, that is, catches its prey.

Each tooth type serves a specific function. Incisor teeth are for grooming and nibbling, canine teeth are for grasping and tearing, premolars are for shearing, and molars are for grinding. The cat, a true carnivore, has no occlusal surface on the mandibular molar. The maxillary molar is small and vestigial in the cat (Hawkins, 1992). Each tooth is covered with enamel, the hardest body substance. The bulk of the tooth is dentin, a living tissue that continues to be deposited by the odontoblasts lining the pulp chamber in viable teeth. Cementum, modified bone, covers the tooth root.

Many factors may affect the normal development of the permanent tooth bud. Interference can produce dens-in-dente, fusion, gemination, and various other abnormalities (Wiggs and Lobprise, 1997).

TOOTH ERUPTION

Deciduous Dentition

Deciduous dentition begins to erupt at 2 to 3 weeks of age in puppies and kittens. All deciduous teeth should be in place by 12 weeks in puppies and 6 weeks in kittens (Wiggs and Lobprise, 1997). The deciduous teeth are much smaller and have relatively longer roots than the permanent teeth (Fig. 9–1) (Ellenport, 1975).

The deciduous dentition for puppies is 2 (I 3/3 C 1/1 P 3/3) = 28. If a deciduous tooth is missing developmentally, there will be no permanent tooth because both develop from the same embryonic tissues (Wiggs and Lobprise, 1997). The last maxillary premolar has three roots; the other two premolars have two roots each. Each mandibular deciduous premolar has two roots. There are no deciduous precursors

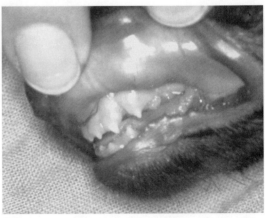

Figure 9–1. Normal dentition in a 3-week-old puppy.

for permanent premolar 1 or the molar teeth in dogs (Hawkins, 1992).

The deciduous dentition for kittens is 2 (I 3/3 C 1/1 P 3/2) = 26. The last maxillary premolar has three roots. Deciduous teeth are normally shed as the permanent counterparts erupt. There are no deciduous premolars for the permanent molar teeth in cats.

Permanent Dentition

The permanent dentition in the older puppy is 2 (I 3/3 C 1/1 P 4/4 M 2/3) = 42. The permanent dentition in the older kitten is 2 (I 3/3 C 1/1 P 3/2 M 1/1) = 30. The older kitten is missing maxillary premolar 1 and mandibular premolars 1 and 2 (Orsini and Hennet, 1992). The permanent toothbuds lie lingual to deciduous teeth. The maxillary canine tooth moves to a mesial location before eruption (Emily and Penman, 1990). The crowns of the permanent teeth are formed by 11 weeks (Fig. 9–2) (Emily and Penman, 1990). In the puppy, the presence or absence of a permanent tooth crown is visible radiographically at 8 to 12 weeks (Lobprise, 1993).

THE PERIODONTIUM

The periodontium consists of the tissue surrounding the tooth. It is composed of the gingiva, cementum (a bone-like tissue that covers the roots), periodontal ligaments that insert into the cementum, the alveolus, periodontal tissues, and the alveolar bone that houses the teeth.

The gingival tissues are tough and nonelastic around the teeth. The gingiva protects the underlying bone and tooth structure from the trauma of chewing and gnawing. Inflammation of the gingiva occurs with the eruption of the deciduous and the permanent dentition. The gingiva probably causes an itchy sensation that causes puppies and kittens to chew excessively during the time period of tooth growth and eruption.

The attachment of the gingiva to the tooth, that is, the epithelial attachment, creates a moat around each tooth called the *gingival sulcus*. Immunoglobulin A is secreted within the gingival sulcus where neutrophils, lymphocytes, and plasma cells reside. The gingival sulcus is the active zone of protection against inflammation around the teeth (Hawkins, 1992). The mucogingival junction or mucogingival line marks the area where the alveolar mucosa joins the gingiva. Alveolar mucosa is mobile and forms the lining of the cheeks and sublingual tissues.

SALIVA AND ITS FUNCTION

Saliva is released from salivary gland duct openings that are located primarily in the buccal pouch area, adjacent to the maxillary cheek teeth (P4 and M1) and sublingually. Saliva helps lubricate food for easier swallowing and keeps the oral tissues moist. Mucopolysaccharides within saliva help form the base for developing dental plaque. Dental plaque is the soft sticky material that coats the teeth if they are not brushed. It is about 80% bacteria and unless removed daily leads to halitosis and the beginning of gingivitis even in young puppies and kittens. Gingivitis is a reversible form of periodontal disease, that is, no tissue attachment is lost.

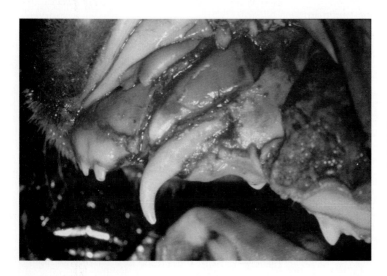

Figure 9–2. Permanent maxillary canine tooth bud (nonerupted) located mesial to deciduous maxillary canine tooth in a 9-week-old puppy.

NORMAL DENTAL OCCLUSION

The normal dental occlusion in the dog and cat is the "scissors" occlusion (Harvey and Emily, 1993). The maxillary incisors slightly overlap the mandibular incisors, and the mandibular canine tooth lies equidistant between the maxillary third incisor and maxillary canine tooth. In the dog, the mandibular first premolar is the most rostral (mesial) cheek tooth, with the cusps of the other cheek teeth interdigitating in a pinking shear effect (DeBowes, 1995). In the cat, the maxillary second premolar is the most rostral (mesial) cheek tooth. Cats have little, if any, curvature to the maxillary and mandibular incisor arches. Often cats have a level occlusion (DeBowes, 1995) with no detectable changes in the incisor and canine tooth relationship.

ABNORMAL DENTAL OCCLUSIONS

Abnormal dental occlusions can be part of the expected breed standard in both adult dogs and cats. Examples are the brachycephalic breeds such as the Pekingese dog and the Persian cat. Owners may be distressed to learn that the abnormal anatomy of their dog or cat is causing significant oral pathology even though it is the perfect breed standard.

Anterior Crossbite

Anterior crossbite, also referred to as *class 1 malocclusion*, involves the incisor teeth. One or more of the maxillary incisors lies caudal to the mandibular incisors, but there is still equidistance between the maxillary third incisor and maxillary canine tooth with the mandibular canine tooth. Also the cusp of mandibular premolar 4 interdigitates perfectly between maxillary premolars 3 and 4. Anterior crossbite could develop into a mandibular prognathism (or maxillary brachygnathism) in the mature adult (Fig. 9–3) (Emily and Penman, 1990).

Posterior Crossbite

Posterior crossbite occurs when the mandible is wider than the maxilla (Emily and Penman, 1990). The mandibular molars and/or some premolars may be buccal to the maxillary cheek teeth. The abnormal anatomy causes dental calculus to accumulate on the maxillary and mandibular cheek teeth rapidly and predisposes them to periodontal disease. Home care and

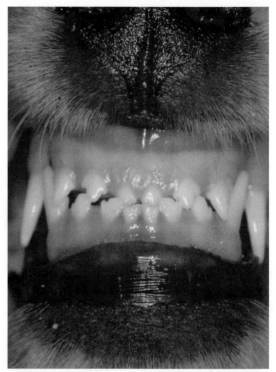

Figure 9–3. Anterior crossbite of maxillary central incisors in a 3-month-old puppy.

frequent dental prophylaxis is the treatment of choice for preventing periodontal disease.

Maxillary Brachygnathism

Maxillary brachynathism is often referred to as *mandibular prognathism* or *class 3 malocclusion*. In maxillary brachynathism, the mandibular arch is longer than the maxillary arch (Emily and Penman, 1990). This is the standard in the brachycephalic canine and feline breeds. There may be hard or soft tissue trauma and overcrowding of the maxillary cheek teeth that predisposes the adult to early periodontal disease. Extraction or reshaping of the overcrowded occlusion is recommended. Also seen with increasing frequency are dogs that should have a scissors occlusion but are "going undershot." In the deciduous dentition, extraction of the teeth in the maxilla (the short arch) is generally recommended. Extraction of the teeth does not alter the genetic potential of the animal; it simply removes mechanical interference that may be restraining the maxillary growth (Wiggs and Lobprise, 1997). As a result, there may be three postextraction scenarios: (1) the occlusion may remain the same, (2) the maxilla may lengthen, or (3) the mandible may grow longer faster. The pet owner should understand these possibilities before any deciduous interceptive orthodontia (extraction) is performed. Each case should be judged individually; the dental interlock may prevent the development of even more severe mandibular prognathism (Wiggs and Lobprise, 1997).

Mandibular Brachygnathism

Mandibular brachygnathism is often referred to as *maxillary prognathism* or *class 2 malocclusion*. This occlusion is not accepted breed standard for any breed, yet it is seen with increasing frequency. It seems to occur most often in those breeds with dolichocephalic heads (Fig. 9–4). Mandibular brachygnathism has been seen in breeds as diverse as German shepherd and Chihuahua (Fig. 9–5) dogs and Siamese cats. The

shortened mandible is usually more narrow and predisposes the affected dog to base-narrow mandibular canine teeth that can traumatize hard and soft tissue. Orthodontia by means of a palatally positioned incline plane appliance or mandibular expansion device is the preferred corrective procedure to crown height reduction and a pulp cap procedure. Tipping the mandibular canine teeth into an atraumatic occlusion maintains the integrity of the tooth and preserves more aesthetic function of the teeth than does crown height reduction.

Wry Mouth

Wry mouth is most commonly present when just one of the jaw quadrants grows to an inappropriate length—either too short or too long. The net result is deviation of either the mandi-

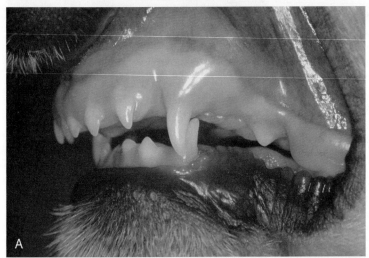

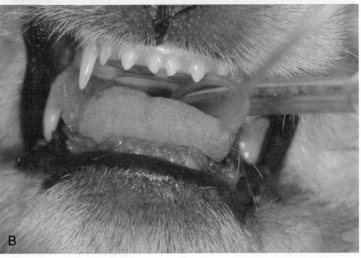

Figure 9–4. **A,** Mandibular brachygnathism with maxillary mechanical interlock in an 8-week-old keeshond puppy. **B,** Interceptive orthodontics performed by extraction of mandibular deciduous canine and incisor teeth.

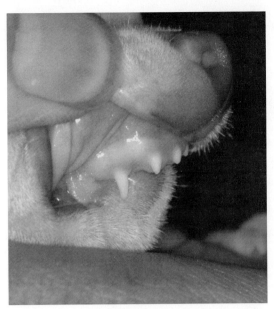

Figure 9–5. Severe mandibular brachygnathism (class 2 malocclusions) in an 8-week-old Chihuahua puppy.

ble or the maxilla to one side or the other. Therefore, head symmetry should be evaluated in each puppy or kitten examined. Mild to severe malocclusion can develop (Emily and Penman, 1990). Adjustment by interceptive orthodontia or active orthodontia is appropriate to relieve trauma.

ABNORMAL NUMBERS OF TEETH

Oligodontia

Oligodontia, or *hypodontia*, refers to too few teeth (Harvey and Emily, 1993). Anodontia, the total absence of teeth, is rare in dogs and cats (Harvey and Emily, 1993). Missing teeth occur most commonly in small breed and in certain large-breed dogs (Harvey and Emily, 1993). Large breeds such as the Doberman pinscher, Rottweiler, and German shepherd are often affected. These large breeds must have a full dentition, that is, 42 teeth, to be exhibited (American Kennel Club, 1973). There is a familial tendency in Tibetan and wheaten terriers for delayed eruption (Aller, 1990). Dental radiographs can determine the presence or absence of nonerupted permanent teeth at 8 to 12 weeks of age (Wiggs and Lobprise, 1997). Operculectomy (removal of the gingiva covering the tooth) may be necessary for complete eruption to occur (Wiggs and Lobprise, 1997).

Polyodontia

Polyodontia (extra teeth) occurs occasionally in young dogs and cats (Harvey and Emily, 1993). Extra teeth may not need to be extracted unless oral trauma or overcrowding results. Extraction of teeth in the overcrowded area helps deter the development of early periodontal disease. The extra teeth are usually in the incisor or premolar area (Fig. 9–6), although an occasional extra canine tooth is found (Hawkins, 1992).

RETAINED DECIDUOUS TEETH

Retained deciduous teeth usually remain in place with the corresponding permanent teeth positioned lingually. The exception to this rule is the maxillary permanent canine tooth that is mesial (rostral) to the retained deciduous canine

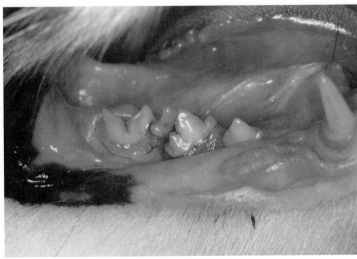

Figure 9–6. Extra mandibular premolar 4 in a cat. Extraction of extra mandibular premolar 4 is recommended.

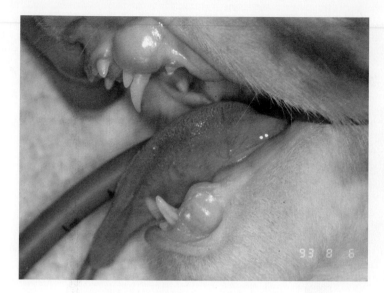

Figure 9-7. Retained deciduous maxillary canine tooth in a 6-month-old kitten with an overbite occlusion.

tooth (Fig. 9–7) (Hawkins, 1992). A retained deciduous tooth may remain in the dentition for several years when there is no permanent tooth to replace it (Wiggs and Lobprise, 1997). Retained deciduous teeth occur most commonly in small dog breeds but are seen occasionally in large-breed dogs and cats. Occasionally, a permanent maxillary fourth premolar erupts buccal to a retained deciduous maxillary premolar in small breeds such as the Pomeranian.

Extraction of retained deciduous teeth is best accomplished using a very small root tip elevator (Fig. 9–8) such as the Henry Schein H1, H2, or H3. The long, slender deciduous roots fracture easily. If the retained deciduous tooth is preventing a permanent tooth from moving into normal position, the root, if it fractures, should be carefully removed. The crown of an extracted retained deciduous tooth can be trimmed to a wedge shape and forced into the alveolar space on the lingual aspect of its respective permanent tooth. This temporary wedge will help lever the permanent tooth into the space vacated by the retained deciduous tooth. The wedge will fall out in 2 to 3 days (Fig. 9–9).

ABNORMAL TOOTH POSITIONS
Undescended Maxillary Canine Teeth

Nondescended maxillary canine teeth that are rostrally deviated are seen in small dogs such as

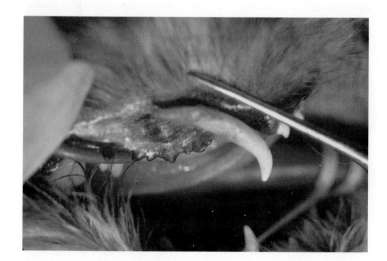

Figure 9-8. Extraction of a deciduous canine tooth, with the root intact, using an H1 root tip elevator. The tooth and root tip elevator are overlaid.

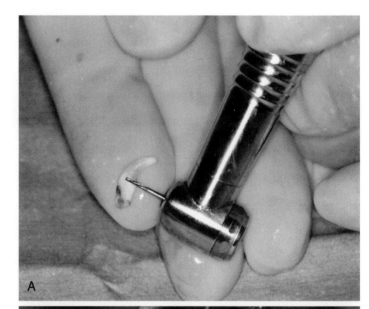

Figure 9–9. **A,** Crown of extracted deciduous canine tooth shaped into a dental wedge. **B,** Two deciduous crown tooth wedges are positioned distal to slightly mesially to displace the maxillary central incisor tooth. The dental wedges will fall out in 2 to 3 days.

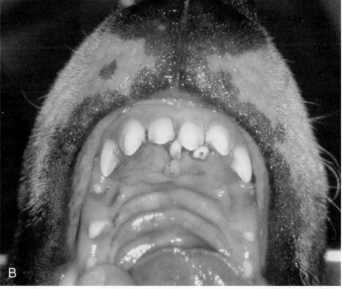

Shetland sheepdogs and less frequently in cats (Harvey and Emily, 1993). These teeth usually respond well to orthodontic movement once the roots have developed. Changing the anchor tooth from maxillary premolar 4 to mandibular molar 1 every 3 to 5 days decreases the possibility of movement of the anchor tooth. Orthodontic treatment is not instituted until the roots of the anchor tooth develop at 9 to 10 months of age.

Narrow-Base Mandibular Canine Teeth

Narrow-base mandibular canine teeth refer to the lingually displaced mandibular canine teeth (Fig. 9–10). The positioning of the mandibular canine teeth lingually usually occurs in conjunction with retained deciduous teeth or with mandibular brachygnathism (Oakes, 1993; Harvey and Emily, 1993). The condition can occur when there is insufficient space between the maxillary third incisor and the maxillary canine tooth for the mandibular canine tooth to interdigitate. Significant oral trauma such as oronasal fistula and attrition of opposing teeth may occur (Fig. 9–11).

Orthodontic treatment with an acrylic incline plane appliance or mandibular expansion device can be used to reposition the mandibular canine teeth. Extraction of the maxillary third incisor and alveoloplasty is satisfactory when the cause is insufficient interdental space. An acrylic

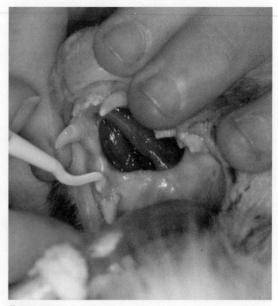

Figure 9–11. Severe, large hard palate defect (oronasal fistula) that probably originated secondary to an electrical cord burn.

bite opener is usually positioned around the maxillary incisor teeth until the soft tissue heals. Crown height reduction is a last choice because it decreases the functionality of the canine tooth. A pulp cap is not always 100% successful, that is, the tooth may need endodontic treatment or extraction secondary to abscessation from a failed pulp cap procedure. If the mandibular canine teeth are only slightly base-narrow and there is sufficient space for the mandibular canine tooth in the maxilla, a gingivoplasty of the interdental space between maxillary canine tooth and maxillary third incisor may be the only treatment needed to correct the problem.

TUMORS OF DENTAL ORIGIN

Fibromatous epulis has been reported in a 4-month-old German shepherd puppy (Hernandez and Negro, 1996). Other tumors of dental origin occur with abnormal tooth development. For instance, if the tooth germ becomes cystic before enamel and dentin formation, a *primordial cyst* develops; a cystic enamel organ forms a *dentigerous cyst*, which usually surrounds the nonerupted crown; and teeth that form in an irregular mass constitute an *odontoma* (Wiggs and Lobprise, 1997). When a permanent tooth does not erupt, especially if a swelling develops in the area, dental radiographs can help identify the problem. Tumors of dental origin should be removed surgically.

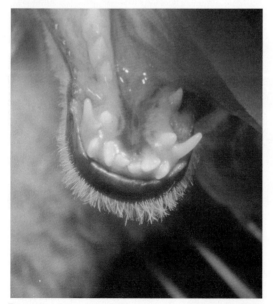

Figure 9–10. Narrow-base mandibular canine teeth in a 5-month-old puppy with retained deciduous mandibular canine teeth.

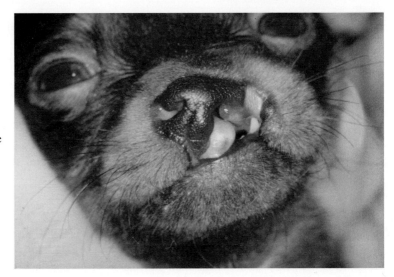

Figure 9–12. Primary cleft palate in a 3- to 4-week-old puppy.

CRANIOMANDIBULAR OSTEOPATHY

Craniomandibular osteopathy is likely to be a genetic condition in West Highland white, Scottish, cairn, and bull terriers and affects young dogs. The jaw may appear swollen due to the bilateral mandibular enlargement from periosteal proliferation of the horizontal ramus, with extension into the temporomandibular joint region at times. Oral discomfort and reluctance to eat may affect some individuals, and symptomatic treatment may make them more comfortable. The condition typically regresses by around 11 to 13 months of age as bone maturation and ossification are completed (Harvey and Emily, 1993).

TIGHT LIP SYNDROME

Chinese shar-pei dogs are predisposed to the condition of tight lip syndrome, which is caused by a band of collagenous fibers in the mandibular lip that extends between the mandibular frenula. This fibrous band prevents forward growth of the mandible, and soft tissue trauma occurs when the lip rolls over the mandibular incisor and canine teeth. Surgical intervention to transect the fibrous band at multiple sites releases the pressure and eliminates the soft tissue trauma. Evaluation of the occlusion is necessary after complete surgical healing has occurred. In very young puppies, surgical intervention is usually successful.

CLEFT PALATE

Primary cleft palate occurs early embryonically (Wiggs and Lobprise, 1997) and involves the incisive bone and/or the lip (Fig. 9–12 and Fig. 9–13). Secondary cleft palate occurs later in development and involves the hard palate and/or soft palate (Wiggs and Lobprise, 1997). Surgical treatment is possible, but most affected puppies and kittens die from aspiration pneumonia or are euthanized.

ORONASAL FISTULAS

Damage secondary to chewing on electric cords is considered hard palate or arch defects. The tissue necrosis can affect soft tissue, bone, and developing tooth structures. Mild to severe oronasal fistulas as well as scar tissue in the tongue and lips can result (see Fig. 9–11).

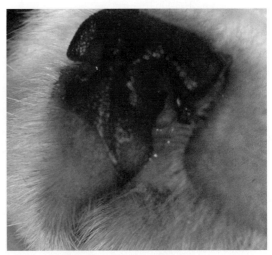

Figure 9–13. Primary cleft palate in a 6-month-old Japanese Chin puppy with no surgery performed.

MISCELLANEOUS DENTAL PROBLEMS

Enamel Hypocalcification

Canine distemper teeth was the term used for years to describe the discolored chalky irregular crown surface that was observed in the permanent dentition of dogs surviving canine distemper. Ameloblasts, which form tooth enamel, require perfect physiologic conditions for effective enamel formation. Because of this, enamel may not be laid down evenly in young dogs and cats during abnormal health periods, such as high fever, heavy parasitism, extreme nutritional deficiency, or even multiple surgeries in young puppies or kittens. The result is a weakened tooth with less organized matrix than normal (Wiggs and Lobprise, 1997). Management of these teeth may include smoothing of the tooth surface, application of dentinal sealer, weekly stannous fluoride applications, or placement of composite restorations for cosmetic purposes.

Enamel Hypoplasia

Enamel hypoplasia is thinning of enamel over all or part of the tooth crown. It often occurs in conjunction with enamel hypocalcification (Wiggs and Lobprise, 1997).

Malformed Permanent Teeth

Malformed erupted or nonerupted permanent teeth can be the result of trauma to the face or

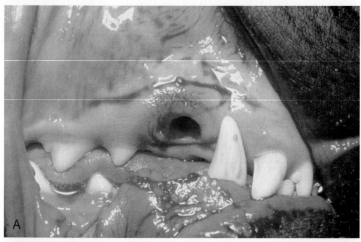

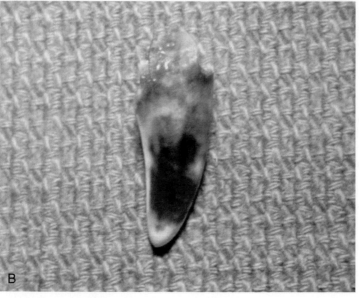

Figure 9–14. A, Site of permanent maxillary canine tooth in a 7-month-old Chesapeake Bay retriever. The deciduous tooth had been fractured but not extracted at the time. **B,** The crown of the tooth in **A.** No root developed presumably because of infection of the permanent tooth bud through the fractured deciduous tooth site.

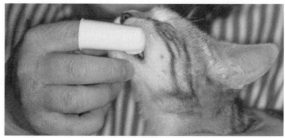

Figure 9–15. Brushing a young cat's teeth with a fingerbrush.

iatrogenic damage secondary to the extraction of a deciduous tooth. In the early stage of crown development, the calcified crown tip can be moved slightly off the developing permanent tooth bud. The result can be a tooth with a short, angulated crown that has a self-induced trauma related pulp cap on the remaining root and crown.

Tetracycline Discoloration

Tetracycline discoloration occurs in deciduous teeth (or other calcium-forming tissues) if the mother is given tetracycline or its derivatives during the formation of the deciduous teeth in utero. If puppies or kittens are given tetracycline or its derivative during formation of the permanent tooth buds, tetracycline can be incorporated into the enamel and dentin, resulting in yellow discoloration. Enamel hypoplasia has been reported in these dogs (Bennett and Law, 1965). Discoloration may, however, be the only adverse effect in tetracycline-treated teeth (Wiggs and Lobprise, 1997).

Fractured Teeth

Deciduous teeth that are fractured should be extracted (Hawkins, 1996). The open endodontic system can shuttle bacteria to the area of the developing permanent tooth bud. Infection of the permanent tooth bud may then result in malformation and/or destruction of the remaining crown or root (Fig. 9–14). Fractured immature permanent teeth should be treated endodontically with calcium hydroxide to encourage the closure of the apex if patent and to thicken the dental walls (Wiggs and Lobprise, 1997). Conventional root canal therapy should follow when further development of the dentinal walls has ended (Wiggs and Lobprise, 1997).

Avulsed Teeth

Avulsed teeth should be gently lavaged with sterile saline solution before reimplantation. The tooth (or teeth) is stabilized with a figure-of-eight wire that can then be overlaid with orthodontic acrylic powder and liquid (cooled with water during the exothermic polymerization). Root canal therapy is necessary after healing occurs (Hawkins, 1996).

Periodontal Disease and Home Care

Periodontal disease is caused by the accumulation of plaque on the teeth (Hawkins, 1992). Periodontal disease is the most common disease found in young dogs and cats (Harvey and Emily, 1993). The daily removal of plaque by brushing from the teeth of puppies and kittens begins a life-long prevention of periodontal disease (Fig. 9–15). There are many good home care products available for dogs and cats. Some contain enzymatic compounds, and others have calculus complexing ingredients or are antiseptic. A dry toothbrush will, however, work well in removing accumulation of plaque. The most important aspect of home care is that it be performed on a daily basis.

Annual dental prophylaxis usually begins at 2 years of age for most dogs and cats. The first dental prophylaxis may need to be performed at about 9 to 12 months of age. A brief dental prophylaxis, that is, brushing the teeth with chlorhexidine, charting the teeth, polishing the teeth, and giving a fluoride treatment, can be performed in the healthy puppy or kitten at the time of the standard neutering procedure. This early exposure to proper dental prophylaxis gives owners an indication of the importance of dental care for their pets.

References and Supplemental Reading

Aller S: Retained deciduous teeth and delayed development of dentition of Tibetan terriers. Vet Dent Forum '90, p 75, 1990.

American Kennel Club: The Complete Dog Book: An Official Publication of the American Kennel Club. New York, Howell Book House, 1973, pp 252, 256, 304.

Bennett IC, Law DB: Incorporation of tetracycline in developing dog enamel and dentin. J Dent Res 44:788, 1965.

DeBowes LJ: Dental disease and care. *In* Hoskins JD (ed): Veterinary Pediatrics: Dogs and Cats From Birth to Six Months, 2nd ed. Philadelphia, WB Saunders, 1995, p 125.

Ellenport CR: Carnivore digestive system. *In* Sisson S, Grossman JD (eds): Anatomy of the Domestic Animals, vol 2, 5th ed. Philadelphia, WB Saunders, 1975, p 1543.

Emily P, Penman S: Handbook of Small Animal Dentistry. Oxford, Pergamon Press, 1990, p 6.

Harvey CE, Emily PP: Periodontal disease. *In* Harvey CE, Emily PP (eds): Small Animal Dentistry. St. Louis, Mosby-Year Book, 1993, pp 3, 89.

Hawkins BJ: Applied Dentistry for Veterinary Hospital Staff. Waltham Video Series, Trenton, New Jersey, 1992, p 3.

Hawkins BJ: Broken face and other dental traumas. Vet Dent Forum '96, p 70, 1996.

Hernandez S, Negro V: Fibromatous epulis in a puppy. Vet Dental Forum '96, p 188, 1996.

Lobprise HB: Pedodontics. *In* Harvey CE, Emily PP (eds): Small Animal Dentistry. St. Louis, CV Mosby-Year Book, 1993, p 25.

Oakes AB: Lingually displaced mandibular canine teeth in dogs. Compend Contin Educ Pract Vet 15:961, 1993.

Orsini P, Hennet P: Anatomy of the mouth and teeth of the cat. Vet Clin North Am Small Anim Pract 22:1265, 1992.

Wiggs RB, Lobprise HB: Pedodontics. *In* Wiggs RB, Lobprise HB (eds): Veterinary Dentistry: Principles and Practice. Philadelphia, Lippincott-Raven, 1997, p 167.

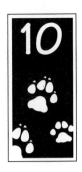

The Digestive System

Johnny D. Hoskins

THE ORAL CAVITY

The oral cavity of the young dog and cat is easily examined; its examination should be consistent and systematic and include inspection and palpation of the gingiva, teeth, tongue, lingual frenulum, floor of the mouth, buccal surface, and hard and soft palates. In a young puppy or kitten, the right hand can be easily replaced by a moistened cotton-tipped applicator to accommodate the animal's smaller oral cavity. The healthy oral cavity is generally pink with a scattering of pigment, appears smooth and glistening, and has limited accumulation of secretions. The surface tissue is pliable and easily blanched with light touch. Gentle opening and palpation of the oral cavity should not be painful or cause prompt withdrawal of the head. Consequently, a painful reaction or inability to fully open the mouth should be obvious. The breath of a growing, healthy dog or cat is not unpleasant; the breath of nursing puppies or kittens generally has a characteristic milky smell. Alterations in the odor of the breath usually indicate a disease state, food the animal has eaten, or medication it has received. Offensive, foul-smelling breath may be caused by oral lesions, necrotic respiratory disease, or alimentary tract disease associated with belching. Periodontal disease is not as likely in the young dog or cat to cause bad breath. Teeth should always be inspected and the number of teeth and their arrangement within the dental arcade evaluated at each examination. The occlusal pattern of the jaws and teeth should also be examined regardless of the animal's age.

The ingestive and masticatory functions of the oral cavity depend largely on the ability of the oral cavity to form a closed, hollow compartment, requiring labial and palatal competence. Most anatomic or functional disturbances of the oral cavity may to varying degrees disrupt fluid or food ingestion and/or interfere with the mastication of food. Cleft palate, cleft lip, or other causes of altered competence of the oral cavity should be identified during the oral examination. In addition, observation of eating, drinking, licking, and yawning helps to identify such disturbances.

Stomatitis

Any infectious, physical, or chemical agent or traumatic insult that significantly alters the replication, maturation, or exfoliation of the healthy mucosa favors the occurrence of stomatitis (Table 10–1).

Viral Stomatitis. Feline rhinotracheitis virus (FRV) and feline calicivirus (FCV) cause most of the oral lesions seen in young cats (Scott, 1986). Buccal, lingual, and nasal ulcers frequently accompany these viral respiratory infections, although ulcers are generally more severe in FCV than in FRV infections. Feline leukemia virus and feline immunodeficiency virus may also be associated with oral lesions as a persistent glossitis, periodontitis, palatitis, and/or gingivitis, presumably because of virus-induced immunosuppression (Pedersen et al, 1987). Canine distemper virus, canine parvovirus type 2, and feline parvovirus (feline panleukopenia virus) may cause stomatitis also, although these viruses typically produce more severe symptoms referable to other organ systems. Because oral lesions from most viral infec-

Table 10–1	Causes of Stomatitis

Infectious Agents
Viral diseases: Feline viral rhinotracheitis, feline calicivirus infection, feline leukemia virus infection, feline immunodeficiency virus infection, feline panleukopenia, canine distemper, canine parvovirus-2 infection, and canine oral papillomatosis
Bacterial diseases: Actinomycosis, mycobacteriosis, leptospirosis, and other aerobic or anaerobic bacterial-induced oral lesions
Fungal disease: Pythiosis and systemic fungal diseases (i.e., blastomycosis, cryptococcosis, histoplasmosis, coccidioidomycosis, and sporotrichosis)

Physical Agents
Foreign objects: Needles, wood splinters, fishhooks, dried weeds, grass awns, porcupine quills, plastic toys, and bones
External trauma: Fight wounds and automobile accidents
Electrical cord burns
Insect bites/stings: Bees, spiders, scorpions, and ants

Chemical Agents
Strong alkalis and acids: Lye
Petroleum distillates
Heavy metals: Thallium
Pesticides
Fertilizers
Irritant plants and insect bites/stings

Other Disorders
Immune-mediated diseases: Pemphigus diseases, bullous pemphigoid, lupus erythematosus, drug eruptions, and ulcerative gingivitis-stomatitis of Maltese terriers
Feline lymphoplasmacytic stomatitis
Metabolic diseases: Diabetes mellitus and renal failure
Vitamin and mineral deficiencies
Coagulation abnormalities: Rodenticide poisoning, disseminated intravascular coagulation, thrombocytopenia, and congenital clotting factor deficiencies
Adverse drug reactions
Cyclic hematopoiesis of silver-gray collies
Eosinophilic granulomata of Siberian huskies
Feline eosinophilic granuloma complex
Ulcerative eosinophilic stomatitis of Cavalier King Charles spaniels

tions are only part of the disease, their treatment is usually supportive.

Physical Agent-Induced Stomatitis. Foreign objects frequently cause traumatic insult to the oral mucosa of young dogs and cats, probably owing to the animals' curious natures and normal developmental chewing habits. The animal generally presents in varying phases of recovery, with secondary bacterial infection and scar tissue often camouflaging the foreign object(s). Removal of the foreign object(s) usually effects a cure. Intermittent problems from migrating grass awns or porcupine quills may be eliminated only by thorough dissection of irritated tissue. Traumatic injury to the tongue, palate, or lips is common, and the original wound is often aggravated by secondary bacterial infections. Oral burns from electrical cords are especially common in young dogs and cats that chew through the insulation of the cords. Pulmonary edema, seizures, and cardiac arrhythmias frequently accompany these electrical shock injuries.

Chemical Agent–Induced Stomatitis. Oral lesions from ingestion of caustic or corrosive substances are uncommon. When they occur, immediate, liberal flushing of the mouth with copious amounts of water should be done. Generally, chemical neutralization with homemade antidotes is ineffective because of the delay from time of exposure to presentation of the animal to the veterinarian. Continual exposure to chemicals, especially pesticides, fertilizers, and irritant plants, in the environment may cause severe oral lesions, which is more common in rural settings. Supportive care includes cleansing and occasional debridement of the oral lesions, treatment of secondary bacterial infection, and frequent feeding of a nutritionally complete, soft, palatable diet to ensure adequate caloric intake.

Immune-Mediated Stomatitis. In the immune-mediated diseases (i.e., pemphigus diseases, bullous pemphigoid, and lupus erythematosus), it is unusual in either the dog or cat for oral lesions to occur without skin involvement, especially at other mucocutaneous junctions, such as eyelids, nostrils, anus, vagina, and prepuce (Scott et al, 1987a, b). In pemphigus vulgaris, the presence of autoantibodies to intercellular epidermal antigens causes acantholysis and intraepidermal vesicobullous ulceration of the skin and oral cavity. Pemphigus foliaceus, the most common of the pemphigus diseases, rarely affects the oral cavity. In bullous pemphigoid, the presence of autoantibodies against antigens at the basement membrane zone causes subepidermal vesicobullous ulceration of the skin and oral cavity. In systemic lupus erythematosus, oral ulceration may occur in conjunction with its other multisystemic manifestations. Any of these immune-mediated diseases may first appear in the dog or cat at 4 to 6 months of age and typically follow the same lesion(s) development and patterns as seen in the adult. Their treatment follows the same regimens as used for the adult.

Feline Lymphoplasmacytic Stomatitis. Lymphoplasmacytic stomatitis commonly affects young to middle-aged cats, but a cat as young as 4 months of age may be affected. Calicivirus has been isolated from some affected cats. The definitive cause of the oral lesions is unknown, but an immunologic basis has been suspected. Abyssinian and Somali are commonly affected cat breeds. Lymphoplasmacytic stomatitis typically follows the same lesion(s) development (i.e., small erythemic papules to severe mucosal proliferation of gingiva and/or palatal arches) as seen in the adult cat. Cytologic examination of biopsy material or deep scrapings will show mucosal hyperplasia with large numbers of lymphocytes and plasma cells and variable numbers of neutrophils and macrophages. Oral lesion(s) treatment follows the same regimens as used for the adult.

Other Causes. Mineral and vitamin deficiencies, heavy-metal poisoning, and coagulation abnormalities may also cause oral lesions. Black tongue, caused by niacin deficiency in dogs, is no longer seen as a clinical entity (Dillon, 1980). Although rarely seen, deficiencies in many of the B-complex vitamins and possibly in zinc may contribute to the appearance of oral lesions in growing, malnourished dogs or cats (Lewis et al, 1987; Lyon, 1988). Thallium is generally the heavy-metal cause of oral lesions. Petechiation of the oral mucosa or gingival bleeding may occur with coagulation abnormalities, that is, rodenticide poisoning, thrombocytopenia, clotting factor deficiencies, and disseminated intravascular coagulation. Silver-gray collies affected with cyclic hematopoiesis often develop a recurrent stomatitis that coincides with absolute neutropenia (Cheville, 1968). Proliferative eosinophilic granulomas have been seen in the oral cavity of Siberian huskies and in many breeds of young cats (i.e., in kittens as young as 8 weeks of age) (Madewell et al, 1980; Potter et al, 1980).

General Therapy. The definitive cause of a stomatitis cannot always be determined by history, physical examination, cytologic examination, bacterial and fungal culture, or tissue biopsy. In many cases, bacterial cultures reveal the normal mixed flora of the oral cavity (Table 10–2); therefore, antimicrobial sensitivities are

Table 10–2	Bacteria Commonly Isolated from the Oral Cavity

Corynebacterium
Enterobacter
Streptococcus
Staphylococcus
Acinetobacter
Actinomyces
Escherichia coli
Proteus
Pasteurella
Pseudomonas
Capnocytophaga canimorsus (DF-2)
Unclassified rod (EF-4)
Caryophanon
Mycoplasma
Actinobacter
Moraxella
Neisseria
Bacillus
Bacteroides
Fusobacterium
Propionibacterium
Peptostreptococcus
Clostridium
Veillonella
Simonsiella

often unreliable. In these cases, therapy to treat the symptoms is often efficacious. A gauze sponge can be used for mechanical cleaning of the mucosal surface. Daily flushing of the mouth with chlorhexidine (diluted to 0.1% to 0.2% solution in tepid water) followed by rinsing the mouth with copious amounts of fresh water will help cleanse the affected areas. Soft, palatable food may need to be provided for several days during the initial healing phase. Ampicillin, amoxicillin, or cephalosporins may be administered daily in an oral liquid form for both a local antimicrobial effect and subsequent systemic effect after absorption. Antimicrobial therapy may be indicated for up to 3 weeks.

Cleft Palate–Cleft Lip Complex

A high degree of variability exists in the cleft palate–cleft lip complex. The cleft lip usually occurs as a unilateral defect in the lip or in the floor of the nostril (Figs. 10–1 and 10–2) and is occasionally seen in conjunction with cleft palate. Thorough examination of the nostril is required to identify an extension of the defect into the nasal passage. Cleft palate may be identified as offset palatal rugae on the roof of the

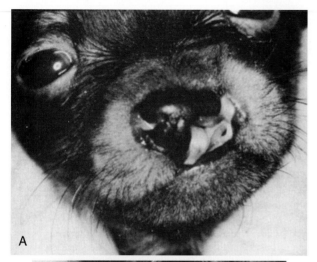

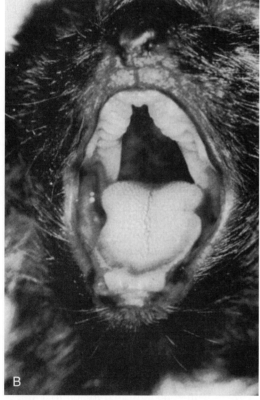

Figure 10–1. A, Cleft lip that extends along the floor of the nostril in a puppy. (From Dillon AR: The oral cavity. *In* Jones BD, Liska WD [eds]: Canine and Feline Gastroenterology. Philadelphia, WB Saunders, 1986, p 35.) **B,** A cleft palate in a young cat.

oral cavity, incomplete fusion of the soft palate, or an oronasal fistula through a cleft palate. The incidence of cleft palate–cleft lip complex is higher in brachycephalic dog breeds (e.g., Boston terrier and Pekingese), although other breeds (e.g., schnauzer, Labrador retriever, cocker spaniel, dachshund, and German shepherd) have a high incidence (Jurkiewicz and Bryant, 1968). Cleft palate may also be seen in young cats, especially the Siamese, Abyssinian, and Manx breeds (Saperstein et al, 1976; Wardrip, 1982).

The cause of the cleft palate–cleft lip complex may be congenital or inherited. Administration of corticosteroids, metronidazole, or griseofulvin and metabolic disturbances during pregnancy are incriminated as the primary causes of congenital cleft palate–cleft lip com-

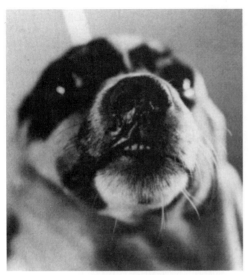

Figure 10–2. Incomplete cleft lip in a young dog.

plex (Dillon, 1980). The inheritance pattern of the complex is a simple recessive or irregular dominant trait. Signs associated with cleft palate vary with the extent of the defect and may include poor growth; drainage of milk from the nostrils during and after nursing; coughing, gagging, and sneezing while eating; and recurrent respiratory tract infections. Aspiration pneumonia is a common sequela in most severely affected animals. Tube-feeding is an effective method of providing adequate nutrition to the most severely affected animals until repair of palatal defects is possible.

Surgical repair of the complex should not be attempted until the puppy or kitten is 7 to 9 weeks of age. A temporary prosthesis made of acrylic resins can be used to cover the defect until surgical repair is possible (Dillon, 1986). During this delay in surgical closure, the cleft in the hard palate often decreases in width, making more tissue available for reconstruction. The tissue also has more time to mature and gain better holding strength, and there is more operative room in the small oral cavity. Surgical techniques for repair of cleft palate–cleft lip complex are described elsewhere (Pope and Constantinescu, 1998). Multiple surgical procedures may be necessary for complete restoration of palatal defects. Although minor mucosal or soft palate defects are compatible with life, the affected animals should not be used for breeding purposes.

Tumors of the Oral Cavity

Papillomas. Oral papillomas are caused by papillomavirus, commonly occur in dogs younger than 1 year of age, and may spread through a kennel in 2 to 4 weeks. The cauliflower-like growths begin as smooth, cream-colored elevations, which later become rough and gray (Fig. 10–3). Histologically, a thick squamous epithelium covers branching cords of dermal papillae. The oral mucosa and commissures of the lips are most commonly affected (Bredal et al, 1996). The number and size of lesions are variable. Although usually not necessary, a biopsy may be required with early atypical lesions or hyperpigmented, contracted lesions that form during regression (Dillon, 1986). In most cases, therapy is usually unnecessary because the lesions regress spontaneously in 6 to 12 weeks. Surgical excision may be a means of stimulating regression and eliminating confluent pedunculated masses, which may impair the prehension and mastication of food. Lifetime immunity generally follows recovery.

Epulides. Epulides are the most common benign oral tumors of dogs. They arise from the periodontal membrane, an origin that differentiates epulides from odontogenic tumors (Dubielzig et al, 1979). The cause of epulides is unknown, but persistent inflammation and irritation are considered the primary inciting factors. Affected dogs are generally over 6 years old; however, an epulis may first appear at 4 to 6 months of age. The diagnosis and treatment in the younger dog generally follow the same approaches as those described for the adult (Richardson et al, 1983). Epulides recur if not successfully managed.

Odontogenic Tumors. Odontogenic tumors in young dogs and cats are rare (Figueiredo et al, 1974; Geake, 1982; Nold et al, 1984; Valentine et al, 1985). They generally originate from the dental laminar epithelium and contain enamel inclusions, dental pulp stroma, or organized dental structures (Fig. 10–4). Of various odontogenic tumors, ameloblastoma is the most common (Richardson et al, 1983). Radical surgical excision usually effects a cure.

THE TONSILS

The tonsils serve as regional lymph nodes of the pharynx and should be closely examined if disease is suspected. With the tongue pulled forward, the tonsils in the young dog and cat normally appear as pink, elongated structures that prolapse from their crypts when pressure is applied to the base of the tongue. Depending on the animal's age and breed, the tonsils differ

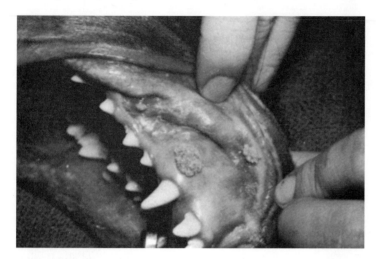

Figure 10–3. Papillomatosis appearing as a small cauliflower-like growth on the gingiva.

greatly in size, shape, and amount of tonsil tissue within the crypt. The physical size and shape of the tonsils generally have no correlation with disease. Observation of the tonsils protruding from their crypts or of phlegm in the pharynx is not sufficient evidence to support a diagnosis of tonsillitis (Table 10–3). Color is considered the best criterion for diagnosing tonsillitis. Unilateral involvement prompts close inspection for tonsillar cysts, lodged foreign object(s), or localized pharyngeal abscesses.

Primary Tonsillitis

Small-breed young dogs are most commonly affected with primary tonsillitis. Anorexia, lethargy, dysphagia, coughing, gagging, and fever

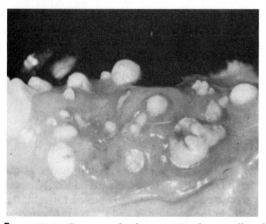

Figure 10–4. Compound odontoma in the maxilla of a dog producing many tooth-like structures. (From Norris AM, Withrow SJ, Dubielzig RR: Oropharyngeal neoplasms. *In* Harvey CE [ed]: Veterinary Dentistry. Philadelphia, WB Saunders, 1985, p 133.)

are the usual complaints. The absence of tonsillar swelling does not necessarily preclude the diagnosis of tonsillitis, especially in cats. Improvement of the animal, observed with antimicrobial therapy, generally precedes resolution of the inflammation, although tonsillar swelling may continue to be present. Recurrence is com-

Table 10–3	Characteristics of Tonsillitis	
ITEM	**REMARKS**
Size of tonsils	Uniform enlargement; may be two to three times normal size for the age and breed; usually bilateral involvement
Color of tonsils	Reddened; may be petechial hemorrhages noted on tonsillar surfaces; may be minute foci of necrosis or suppuration
Consistency of tonsils	Often soft and friable and bleed easily when manipulated
Surrounding tissue	Normal or inflamed
Regional lymph nodes (mandibular and retropharyngeal)	Slight uniform enlargement; may be hot and painful; usually bilateral involvement
Superficial body lymph nodes	Not affected
Signs	Fever, gagging, cough, lethargy, and anorexia
Hematologic findings	May be leukopenia or leukocytosis, depending on stage and cause of tonsillar involvement

mon, with exacerbations lasting several days. Tonsillectomy is rarely required in recurrent tonsillitis unless the tonsillar enlargement obstructs the pharynx. Most dogs can be effectively treated medically and appear to "outgrow" the problem. Medical treatment of tonsillitis includes using broad-spectrum antimicrobial agents and supportive care as discussed for stomatitis. Bacterial culture of inflamed tonsillar tissue usually produces β-hemolytic streptococci, coliforms, or other bacteria of the normal oral flora (see Table 10–2); therefore, antimicrobial sensitivities may be unreliable.

Secondary Tonsillitis

Secondary tonsillitis may be associated with systemic disease or local predisposing anatomic or pathologic factors. The presence of tonsillitis does not indicate the site of primary disease. Any persistent irritation or inflammatory process of the oral cavity or pharynx (e.g., abscesses, gingivitis, lodged foreign object(s), or persistent vomiting or regurgitation) may induce a secondary tonsillitis. The gagging, regurgitation, and vomiting of foam in cases of tonsillitis necessitate differentiation from megaesophagus, pyloric disorders, cricopharyngeal achalasia, productive cough, retropharyngeal abscesses, and lodged foreign object(s) in the pharynx, larynx, or esophagus (Dillon, 1986). Treatment should be directed toward eliminating the underlying secondary cause of the tonsillitis.

PERIODONTAL DISEASE

Periodontal disease starts soon after birth and continues until death. For this reason, examining for the presence of periodontal disease should be part of each examination of the oral cavity. The owner should be informed of the degree of periodontal disease present and the treatment recommended. For the young dog or cat, regular home treatments of the teeth are important for the prevention of periodontal disease. Starting early in the animal's life, the owner can effectively brush the animal's teeth with a soft child-sized toothbrush. Human dentifrices should not be used because the animal will typically swallow enough of the detergent-based dentifrice to cause gastric upset. Use of a nondetergent toothpaste or commercial dog/cat dentifrice is recommended. If the animal will not tolerate the brushing procedure, simply rubbing the tooth surface with a soft cloth dipped in one of the previously mentioned sub-

stances will assist in controlling early stages or mild cases of periodontal disease. These home treatments should be done at least two or three times a week. The use of treat biscuits, chew toys, and dry crunchy food, which exercise the teeth and gingiva, has been advocated to aid in reducing periodontal disease. A dog or cat is never too young to start on a dental hygiene program at home.

THE JAW
Prognathism

Prognathism, or "undershot jaw," describes the jaw occlusion pattern in which the mandibular incisors contact or are rostral to the maxillary incisors. The brachycephalic breeds, such as the Boston terrier, English bulldog, and pug, show this typical pattern as a normal breed characteristic (Weigel and Dorn, 1985). In these breeds, the prognathic deformity results from the inherited defect in development of the bones in the base of the skull. The length of the mandible is determined primarily by genetic factors that are different from those affecting skull development.

Positioning of the teeth and the resulting dental interlock guide the longitudinal growth of the maxilla and mandible toward their genetically predetermined lengths, which are evident when the growing animals are 3 to 9 months of age (Ross, 1975a). The normal bite of the dog and cat exists when the maxillary incisors overlap the mandibular incisors, the mandibular canine teeth articulate rostral to the maxillary canine teeth, and the mandibular premolars close the interproximal space rostral to their maxillary counterparts—all of which constitutes the dental interlock (Fig. 10–5) (Ross, 1975a). The loss of the dental interlock, or the presence of abnormal interlock, results in an inappropriate positioning of the teeth, which affects the development of the dental arcade and causes the loss of forces required to maintain correct jaw length.

Prognathism occurs very early in life and may be evident before the permanent dentition appears. Extraction of the deciduous canine and incisor teeth that seem to be inhibiting the forward growth of an obviously shorter mandible is done at 8 to 12 weeks of age (Ross, 1975b). The reasoning is that the caudal position of these teeth in relation to the position of the corresponding upper teeth blocks the normal rostral growth of the mandible. If an animal's occlusion corrects itself after extraction of the deciduous teeth, one can be reasonably assured

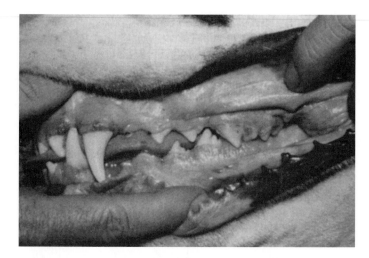

Figure 10–5. The normal relationship between the canine teeth and the premolar teeth combined with normal occlusion of incisors is characteristic of a normal dental interlock.

that the prognathism was not inherited. If no improvement occurs, however, breeding of the affected animal is not recommended.

Brachygnathism

Brachygnathism, or "overshot jaw," occurs when the upper jaw is longer than the lower jaw (Fig. 10–6). It can occur in most breeds of dogs and cats and to different degrees of severity (Weigel and Dorn, 1985). It is an inherited defect, and animals showing brachygnathism should not be used for breeding.

THE SALIVARY GLANDS

The occurrence of disorders of the salivary glands in young dogs and cats is rare (Bedford,

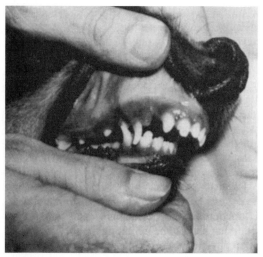

Figure 10–6. Extreme brachygnathism in this dog involves malocclusion of all teeth in the arcade.

1980; Harvey, 1981; Moraes Barros et al, 1985; Wallace, 1972). Of these salivary gland disorders, sialadenitis, inflammation of a salivary gland, is likely to occur most often. Sialadenitis may be caused by bite wounds, lacerations, blunt trauma, or extension from cellulitis and abscesses of the head and neck. Sudden swelling in the region of a salivary gland, fever, inappetence, and pain on opening the mouth are usually evident on physical examination. Diagnosis of sialadenitis is usually obvious, but cytologic examination confirms salivary tissue involvement. Treatment should be aimed at the underlying cause. Ways of providing symptomatic relief include the administration of antimicrobial agents, application of warm compresses, replacement fluid therapy, drainage if abscess is present, and frequent feeding of small amounts of a nutritionally complete, soft, palatable food.

A sialocele is a collection of saliva in tissue. Any age, sex, and breed of dog or cat can be affected. Sialocele formation most commonly involves the sublingual and mandibular salivary glands, where blockage of a duct or rupture of the gland causes extravasation of saliva into the surrounding connective tissue. The saliva may gravitate to the sublingual area (often referred to as a *ranula*), intermandibular space, mediastinum, or pharyngeal area (Fig. 10–7). Swelling may develop suddenly but is more likely to be in the form of a slowly developing, fluctuant sac. Diagnosis of sialocele is based on physical appearance of the cervical swelling and on cytologic evaluation. Needle aspiration of the swelling yields a viscous, mucoid fluid that is usually clear or brown. Hemorrhage and exudate, which will cytologically show clumps of polymorphonuclear leukocytes and red blood cells

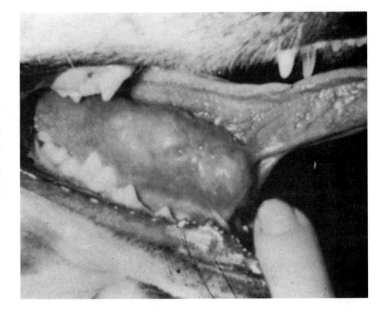

Figure 10–7. Mouth of a dog with a ranula (sialocele of the sublingual tissue). (From Harvey CE, O'Brien JA, Rossman LE, et al: Oral, dental, pharyngeal and salivary gland disorders. *In* Ettinger SJ [ed]: Textbook of Veterinary Internal Medicine, vol 2, 2nd ed. Philadelphia, WB Saunders, 1983, p 1184.)

with saliva, may develop after excessive manipulation of the sialocele or with infection (Fig. 10–8). The injection of water-soluble contrast medium through the ducts may help to identify the affected gland, but in the young dog or cat the openings of the ducts are extremely small and usually impossible to find. Therefore, a thorough physical examination and cytologic examination of aspirated fluid are more reliable. Total excision of the affected gland, which is usually the sublingual or mandibular gland, and drainage of the sialocele provide the only long-term therapy for sialoceles. Removal of an elliptic portion of the wall of a ranula allows direct drainage of saliva into the oral cavity. The surgical techniques for the management of salivary gland disorders are described elsewhere (Harvey, 1989).

Congenital enlargement of the parotid salivary glands has been reported in dogs (Bedford, 1980; Harvey, 1981). The dogs typically present with hypersalivation (drooling) and are treated effectively with parotid duct ligation. Neoplasia of a salivary gland in the young dog or cat is extremely rare and is diagnosed and treated as for an adult animal.

THE OROPHARYNX
Dysphagia

The events of swallowing can be divided into oral, pharyngeal, and cricopharyngeal stages

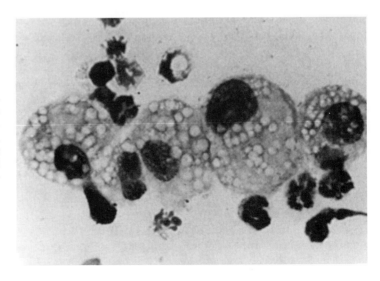

Figure 10–8. Cytologic examination of swelling from sialocele reveals polymorphonuclear leukocytes and red blood cells with saliva. (From Dillon AR: The oral cavity. *In* Jones BD, Liska WB [eds]: Canine and Feline Gastroenterology. Philadelphia, WB Saunders, 1986, p 49.)

(Watrous and Suter, 1979). The oral stage includes prehension of food and delivery of the food bolus to the base of the tongue. The pharyngeal stage occurs when the food bolus is propelled from the base of the tongue to the cricopharyngeal passage. The cricopharyngeal stage involves relaxation of the cricopharyngeal sphincter, passage of the food bolus into the esophagus, closure of the cricopharyngeal sphincter, and relaxation of the pharyngeal muscles (Suter and Watrous, 1980). Difficulty in swallowing during any one of these stages is defined as dysphagia (Shelton, 1982). Dysphagia is uncommon in dogs and rare in cats. Dysphagia is usually recognized in puppies and kittens shortly after weaning.

Oral Dysphagias. Oral dysphagias may result from disturbances to various motor and sensory tracts and peripheral nerves. Branches of cranial nerves V, IX, and X provide sensory innervation for swallowing, and cranial nerves V, VII, IX, X, XI, and XII deliver motor innervation via the nucleus ambiguus and the respiratory centers (Strombeck and Guilford, 1990). Signs of oral dysphagia may include difficulty in prehension of food and lapping water, excessive chewing or chomping, hypersalivation, and diminished or absent gag reflex (Fig. 10–9). Evidence of denervation of the tongue may exist, and food may drop from the animal's mouth or be retained in the buccal cavity (Shelton, 1982). The cineradiographic features of oral dysphagia are reduction in tongue movements, diminished or absent plunger action of the tongue, decreased bolus accumulation, and retention of bolus or contrast medium in the oropharynx.

Pharyngeal Dysphagias. Pharyngeal dysphagias are less consistent, and related signs are more difficult to localize. The most common signs are coughing with repeated unsuccessful attempts at swallowing and laryngotracheal aspiration of swallowed material. Often, the puppy or kitten will regurgitate masticated food several hours after ingestion, or food or liquid material will be misdirected into the nasopharynx, leading to nasal discharge (Shelton, 1982). Cineradiographic features are generally more diagnostic than the presenting signs. These features include residual air and contrast medium in the pharynx with normal cricopharyngeal sphincter function; slow initiation and progress of pharyngeal peristaltic contractions; retention of contrast medium in the oropharynx, pharynx, and piriform recesses; and passage of contrast medium into the larynx (Suter and Watrous, 1980).

Cricopharyngeal Dysphagias. Cricopharyngeal dysphagias typically manifest as problems of asynchrony (i.e., incoordination of pharyngeal contraction and cricopharyngeal sphincter relaxation) or as achalasia (i.e., failure of cricopharyngeal sphincter relaxation) (Shelton, 1982). In asynchrony, the cricopharyngeal muscle may contract too early or too late in relation to contraction of the pharyngeal muscles. Cricopharyngeal achalasia results from the failure of the cricopharyngeus muscle and part of the thyropharyngeus muscle to relax and thus permit a food bolus to move from the pharynx into the cranial esophagus (Rosin and Hanlon, 1972; Sokolovsky, 1967). Signs of cricopharyngeal dysphagias can vary, depending on whether there is an achalasia or asynchrony. Because presenting signs of cricopharyngeal dysphagias are similar to those seen with pharyngeal dysphagias, cricopharyngeal and pharyngeal dysphagias can be differentiated only by means of cineradiographic studies. If there is incomplete relaxation of the cricopharyngeal sphincter, cricopharyngeal dysphagias usually show a dorsal indentation of the food bolus as it passes through the sphincter. If there is incoordination of sphincter and pharynx, the food bolus will be misdirected into the nasopharynx (Fig. 10–10) (Shelton, 1982; Suter and Watrous, 1980).

Treatment of Dysphagia

Differentiation of oral, pharyngeal, and cricopharyngeal dysphagias is important. Myotomy of the muscles of the cricopharyngeal sphincter gives dramatic improvement in cricopharyngeal achalasia (Gourley and Leighton, 1972; Sokolovsky, 1967). Oral and pharyngeal dysphagias are generally, however, made worse by the myotomy procedures (Suter and Watrous, 1980). Oral and pharyngeal dysphagias are best managed by treating any underlying medical illness, changing the consistency of the animal's usual diet, and feeding the animal in an elevated position (Hoffer, 1986). Other valuable techniques for short-term therapy are feeding by means of a nasogastric, esophagostomy, or gastrostomy tube. If conservative therapy is not helpful and the owner does not wish to continue feeding by one of the enteral methods, cricopharyngeal myotomy may be considered. In this situation, the owner should be aware that cricopharyngeal myotomy may make the animal's condition worse.

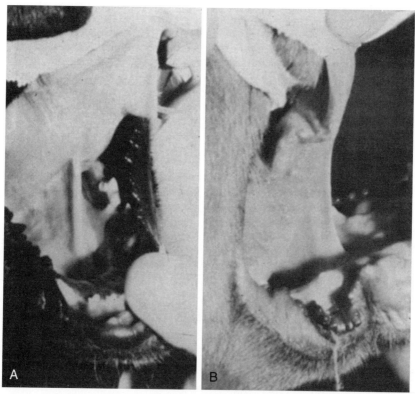

Figure 10–9. A, Frenulum linguae of a 12-week-old Great Dane puppy with a "tongue-tied" anomaly. **B,** Normal frenulum of a puppy of similar age. (From Watrous BJ: Clinical presentation and diagnosis of dysphagia. Vet Clin North Am 13:440, 1983.)

Figure 10–10. Cricopharyngeal achalasia. Note the contrast material filling the nasopharynx and adhering to the wall of the trachea. (From Aronson E, Carrig CB, Lattimer JC: Radiology of the gastrointestinal system. *In* Jones BD, Liska WD [eds]: Canine and Feline Gastroenterology. Philadelphia, WB Saunders, 1986, p 395.)

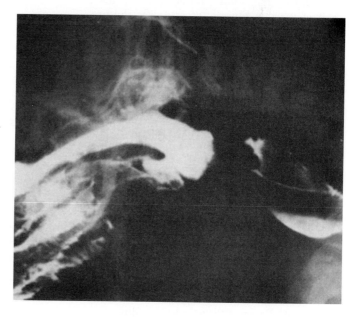

THE ESOPHAGUS

Congenital Vascular Ring Anomalies

Causes. Vascular ring anomalies are congenital malformations of the great vessel system that interfere with esophageal function. These anomalies produce an extramural obstruction of the esophagus at the base of the heart and rarely affect the trachea or cardiovascular system. The most frequently encountered vascular ring anomaly in the young dog or cat is persistent right aortic arch (Watrous, 1983). Other vascular ring anomalies that occur infrequently are a double aortic arch due to persistence of both right and left fourth arches, anomalous origin of the subclavian or intercostal arteries, and an aberrant patent ductus arteriosus associated with the left or right aortic arches. The incidence of vascular ring anomalies is higher in young dogs than in young cats. Irish setters, Boston terriers, and German shepherds are the most commonly affected dog breeds (Leipold, 1977; Patterson, 1968). Cats of all breeds are equally susceptible to persistent right aortic arch and the other vascular ring anomalies (Harpster, 1987).

Diagnosis. Signs caused by the vascular ring anomalies result from esophageal entrapment and obstruction, with subsequent precordial megaesophagus. When weaning to solid food, puppies and kittens will repeatedly regurgitate. Although regurgitation is usually associated with eating when solid food is first fed, it will occur at variable times after eating as the precordial megaesophagus worsens. Occasionally, signs in the puppy or kitten are associated with ingestion of maternal milk. The food-distended megaesophagus may be palpated at the thoracic inlet. Affected animals are obviously malnourished and underweight. Auscultation of the thorax may reveal coarse lung sounds due to laryngotracheal aspiration of ingested food and water, although heart sounds are usually normal. The diagnosis of a vascular ring anomaly–induced megaesophagus can usually be confirmed by a positive contrast esophagogram (Fig. 10–11).

Treatment. Treatment is early surgical correction by ligation and transection of the stricturing ligament or vessel and complete mobilization of the esophagus from the connective tissue in the area of entrapment. The surgical technique has been described elsewhere (Ellison, 1998). Prognosis is guarded pending complete postoperative recovery because of frequent complicating factors (e.g., existing malnourishment, weakened state of the animal, aspiration pneumonia, and persistent megaesophagus despite surgical correction). Most animals show substantial improvement if they survive the immediate postoperative period. Persistent megaesophagus occurs if the esophagus develops sacculations, an extensive dilation that fills the anterior region of the mediastinum, or dilatation of the esophagus caudal to the vascular ring anomaly. These sacculations probably represent neuromuscular disease of the esophagus in conjunction with the vascular ring anomaly.

Vascular compression of the esophagus by the left subclavian artery and brachiocephalic artery has also been described in English bulldogs (Woods et al, 1978). Presenting signs of these dogs included recurrent regurgitation and aspiration pneumonia. Their esophagograms have shown an abrupt ventral deviation (compression) of the esophagus at the level of the first or second rib. Transection and anastomosis of the left subclavian artery relieve the regurgitation (Woods et al, 1978). This type of vascular compression of the esophagus should be considered in any young brachycephalic dog presenting with recurrent regurgitation.

Esophagitis

Esophagitis is unusual in the young dog and cat and usually occurs because of traumatic insult, ingestion of a chemical or thermal irritant, or gastric acid reflux. Thermal injuries may occur when eager eaters bolt hot food or when puppies or kittens are fed hot gruel. Gastric acid reflux is uncommon as a primary event, but can occur any time the lower esophageal sphincter pressure is compromised, such as during anesthesia or severe blunt trauma directly to the thorax or abdomen. Esophagitis can be limited to mucosal damage or may extend into the submucosa and musculature. If only the mucosa is involved, the esophagitis is usually mild and self-limiting. Esophagitis with submucosal and musculature involvement, however, often leads to severe ulceration with subsequent perforation, fibrotic stricture formation, persistence of inflammation, and/or disturbed motor activity (acquired megaesophagus). The possibility of gastric acid reflux–induced esophagitis should be minimized during surgical procedures by fasting surgical patients for 6 to 12 hours before surgery and avoiding surgical positions that promote gastric acid reflux (e.g., positioning the head lower than the body).

Signs of esophagitis are regurgitation and dysphagia. The diagnosis of esophagitis can be

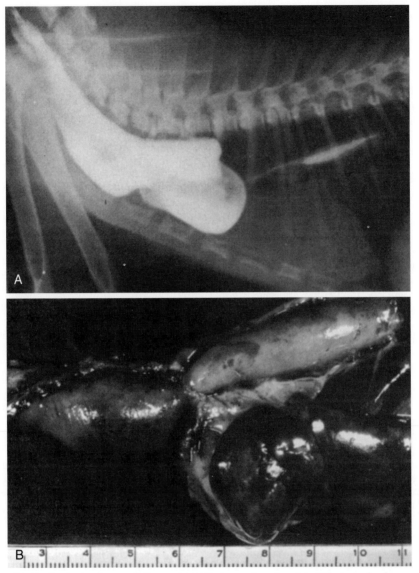

Figure 10–11. **A,** A persistent right aortic arch constricts the esophagus at the base of the heart, permitting small amounts of contrast material to pass. The esophagus cranial to the stricturing ligament or vessel is dilated. **B,** In the same 3-month-old cat as in **A,** the ligamentum arteriosum was excised at surgery, but a thin band of fascia persisted, producing a moderate constriction over the dorsal aspect of the esophagus. The dilated portion of the esophagus measured about 3 cm in diameter. The kitten failed to recover from anesthesia. (From Harpster NK: The cardiovascular system. *In* Holzworth J [ed]: Diseases of the Cat: Medicine and Surgery, vol 1. Philadelphia, WB Saunders, 1987, p 881.)

difficult because the esophagogram may appear normal, especially when only the surface mucosa is involved. Esophagoscopy may then be required to make a definitive diagnosis by visualization of mucosal changes; questionable cases may be confirmed by histopathology. Treatment of esophagitis is aimed at eliminating the underlying cause and symptomatic management of

the esophagus and the systemic effects that the esophagitis created. Means of providing symptomatic relief include esophageal rest by feeding through a gastrostomy tube or by frequent small feedings of nutritionally complete, soft, bland food and administration of antimicrobial agents, H_2-receptor antagonists, metoclopramide, and sucralfate slurry (crush 1 g sucralfate and mix with 10 ml water; give 5 ml of slurry four to six times daily).

Esophageal Foreign Objects

Causes. Foreign objects frequently lodge in the esophagus despite its normal distensibility. Indiscriminant eating habits and inadequate mastication of food contribute to the occurrence of lodged foreign objects in young dogs, whereas cats are usually more fastidious eaters and ingest foreign objects because of their hunting or playing behavior. Common types of foreign objects that partially or completely obstruct the esophagus are bones, wood, string, fishhooks, needles, and other metallic or plastic objects. The normal esophagus has several narrow areas where swallowed objects tend to lodge. These areas include the cricopharyngeal sphincter region (Fig. 10–12); the thoracic inlet, where adjacent soft tissue impedes esophageal distensibility (Fig. 10–13); the heart base area, where the aorta deflects the esophagus to the right; and the gastroesophageal junction at the level of the diaphragm.

Diagnosis. Diagnosis of a lodged foreign object in the esophagus is generally based on a history of ingestion. Signs are attributed to the partial or complete obstruction of the esophagus and/or the size and shape of the lodged foreign object and length of time since its becoming lodged. Early signs may include regurgitation of all ingested solids and possibly liquids, painful dysphagia, hypersalivation, repeated gulping, and anorexia. Later the signs may include profound depression, anorexia, weight loss, and other signs that relate to associated complications. These complications may include perforated esophagus, pleuritis, mediastinitis, pyothorax, mucosal lacerations, esophageal stricture, diverticula, and severe esophagitis (Houlton et al, 1985). Confirmation of the presence of a lodged foreign object requires a physical examination (which includes a thorough oral examination), cervical and thoracic radiographs, and esophagoscopy (Fig. 10–14).

Treatment. A foreign object lodged in the esophagus must be considered an emergency situation because the frequency of complications increases with the duration of the problem. In most cases of a suspected foreign object lodged in the esophagus, the use of esophagoscopy is advisable. Flexible endoscopes allow easy passage into an anesthetized young dog's or cat's esophagus to visualize a foreign object and to inspect for extent of esophageal damage. If the foreign object is small, it can often be removed by passing a flexible four-prong grasping forceps through the endoscope, grasping the foreign object, and pulling it retrogradely through the mouth. If the foreign object is too large for the flexible grasping forceps, rigid grasping forceps may be passed in conjunction with a flexible endoscope (Figs. 10–15 and 10–16). Once the object is grasped, it and the endoscope can then be pulled retrogradely through the mouth. Frequently, the object becomes dislodged from the grasper as it is passing through the cricopharyngeal sphincter region. The object can then be easily retrieved by grasping it with long alligator forceps through the sphincter and thus removing it. If the object cannot be removed in a

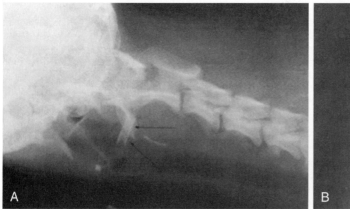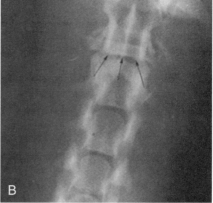

Figure 10–12. Lateral **(A)** and ventrodorsal **(B)** radiographs of pheasant bone (*arrows*) caught in the cricopharyngeal sphincter region of the esophagus. (From Aronson E, Carrig CB, Lattimer JC: Radiology of the gastrointestinal system. *In* Jones BD, Liska WD [eds]: Canine and Feline Gastroenterology. Philadelphia, WB Saunders, 1986, p 392.)

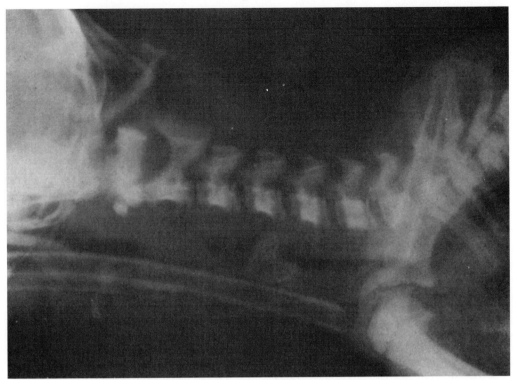

Figure 10–13. A lateral radiograph of a puppy that had been observed eating chicken 2 days before presentation. Large or sharp foreign objects frequently lodge in the cervical esophagus at the thoracic inlet. (From Watrous B: Esophageal disease. *In* Ettinger SJ [ed]: Textbook of Veterinary Internal Medicine, vol 2, 2nd ed. Philadelphia, WB Saunders, 1983, p 1202.)

retrograde manner, one may attempt to push it directly into the stomach. Careful manipulation is necessary when pushing the object into the stomach because the caudal portion of the esophagus deviates slightly at the gastroesophageal junction.

When the foreign object is being removed by endoscopy, by retrograde retrieval, or by pushing it into the stomach, the esophagus needs to be distended with insufflated air so that the object is freed from the esophageal wall. Once in the stomach, the foreign object may be digested and passed in the feces within 7 to 10 days or removed by gastrotomy. For passage of foreign objects, serial abdominal radiographs should be taken to confirm that the object(s) have indeed left the stomach and passed aborally through the intestinal tract without causing a subsequent obstruction.

After the foreign object has been successfully removed via endoscopy, the extent of esophageal damage should be assessed. The esophageal mucosa is examined visually by passing the endoscope through the length of the esophagus. Usually, the degree of mucosal damage is directly proportional to the length of time that the foreign object was in the esophagus. Erythema and mild ulceration at the site of entrapment are common. Special attention should be given to any evidence of tears or perforations of the esophageal wall. Thoracic radiographs should also be taken after the removal of all esophageal foreign objects because pneumothorax or pneumomediastinum may have occurred if the esophagus was indeed perforated.

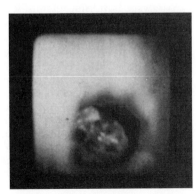

Figure 10–14. Esophagoscopy. Note the presence of a foreign object lodged in the esophagus.

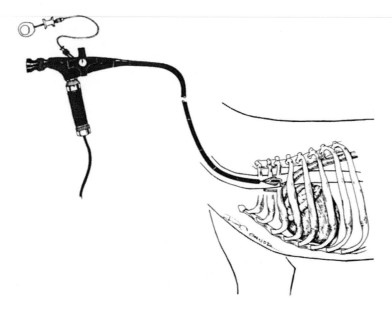

Figure 10–15. The use of a flexible endoscope with a four-prong grasping forceps being passed through the operating channel. The forceps is grasping the foreign object (bone). Small foreign object(s) can then be removed by pulling the endoscope and grasping forceps retrogradely through the mouth. (From Roudebush P, Jones BD, Vaughan RW: Medical aspects of esophageal disease. *In* Jones BD, Liska WD [eds]: Canine and Feline Gastroenterology. Philadelphia, WB Saunders, 1986, p 69.)

Idiopathic Megaesophagus

Idiopathic megaesophagus is characterized by motor disturbances of the esophagus that result in abnormal or unsuccessful transport of ingesta between the pharynx and stomach. Although a complete understanding of the pathophysiology of idiopathic megaesophagus is still lacking, it is believed by most investigators that idiopathic megaesophagus results from a dysfunction of the primary motor system of the esophagus with or without secondary dysfunction of the gastroesophageal sphincter (Hoffer, 1986; Rogers et al, 1979; Strombeck, 1978; Strombeck and Guilford, 1990; Strombeck and Troya, 1976).

Causes. Both congenital and acquired forms of idiopathic megaesophagus occur in young dogs and cats. There is evidence that congenital idiopathic megaesophagus is inherited in both the dog (e.g., wire-haired fox terrier and miniature schnauzer) and cat (Clifford et al, 1971;

Cox et al, 1980; Osborne et al, 1967; Strating and Clifford, 1966). The incidence is highest in Great Danes, German shepherds, Irish setters, Labrador retrievers, and Chinese shar-peis. Esophageal dysfunction in Chinese shar-peis may result from segmental hypomotility and esophageal redundancy (Stickle et al, 1992). In the cat, Siamese and Siamese-related breeds have the highest incidence (Watrous, 1983).

Acquired idiopathic megaesophagus may occur spontaneously in any young dog or cat. In most instances, the underlying cause is undetermined; however, megaesophagus may occur in several systemic diseases that affect the nervous system or skeletal muscles. These diseases include myasthenia gravis, polymyositis, toxoplasmosis, canine distemper, hypothyroidism, hypoadrenocorticism, and myotonia with myopathy. Other potential diseases that could contribute to megaesophagus are systemic lupus erythematosus, tick paralysis, botulism, tetanus, lead poi-

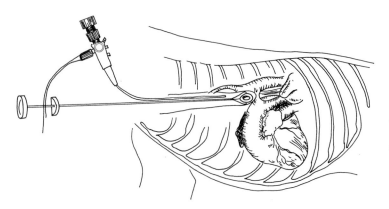

Figure 10–16. The grasping forceps and flexible endoscope in place. These two instruments are then both pulled retrogradely to extract the foreign object from the esophagus. (From Roudebush P, Jones BD, Vaughan RW: Medical aspects of esophageal disease. *In* Jones BD, Liska WD [eds]: Canine and Feline Gastroenterology. Philadelphia, WB Saunders, 1986, p 70.)

soning, ganglioradiculitis, dysautonomia, anti-cholinesterase compounds, and polyneuritis (Shelton, 1982; Watrous, 1983). Megaesophagus has also been associated in cats with pyloric dysfunction (Pearson et al, 1974) and feline dysautonomia, often referred to as the Key-Gaskell syndrome (Sharp et al, 1984). Canine or feline dysautonomia, the main features of which are dilated pupils, dry mucous membranes, megaesophagus, constipation, and dysuria and urinary incontinence with urinary bladder distention, is a dysfunction of the autonomic nervous system. The cause of dysautonomia is currently unknown.

Diagnosis. The onset of signs associated with congenital idiopathic megaesophagus usually begins around the time of weaning (Boudrieau and Rogers, 1985; Harvey et al, 1974). Signs may include effortless regurgitation of esophageal contents, weight loss, polyphagia, weakness, dehydration, impaired skeletal mineralization, ballooning of the cervical esophagus that is synchronized with respiration, and recurrent laryngotracheal aspiration that often leads to recurrent pneumonia. Oral fetor may be present owing to stagnation of fermenting ingesta retained in the dilated esophagus. Regurgitation may be seen immediately upon feeding or up to 12 or more hours later. The time interval between eating and regurgitation can be related to the degree of dilation or to the general activity of the animal. Usually both liquids and solids are poorly tolerated.

Survey thoracic radiographs consistently reveal a dilated esophagus (Watrous, 1983). The esophageal lumen typically contains sufficient air and ingesta to allow visual observation on the lateral projection a pair of soft tissue stripes that arise in the midthorax and converge toward the gastroesophageal junction. Cranially, the dorsal wall of the esophagus may merge with the longus coli muscle to outline a sharp margin. Ventrally, the ventral wall of the esophagus will create a silhouette with the dorsal wall of the air-filled trachea, creating a wide soft tissue band called the "tracheal stripe" (Fig. 10–17). When the cervical esophageal segment is dilated, a saber-shaped radiolucent shadow is seen dorsal to the trachea and tapering toward the thoracic inlet. A partially fluid-filled esophagus will present as a homogeneous gray shadow with a similar relationship to that described. With marked esophageal dilation, ventral displacement of the trachea and heart occurs. In the dorsoventral or ventrodorsal projection, the caudal thoracic esophagus is seen as a V-shaped pair of lines to either side of the midline with

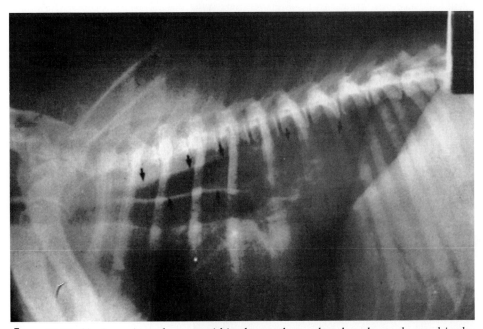

Figure 10–17. Air *(arrows)* can be seen within the esophagus dorsal to the trachea and in the caudal thorax. The two lower arrows, dorsal to the heart, indicate a tracheal stripe sign. Air in the esophagus, except in very small quantities, is unusual and is often indicative of abnormality. This was a megaesophagus. (From Kealy JK: Diagnostic Radiology of the Dog and Cat, 2nd ed. Philadelphia, WB Saunders, 1987, p 45.)

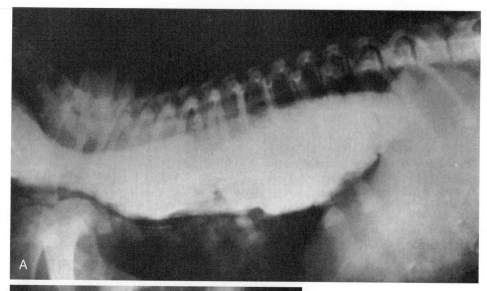

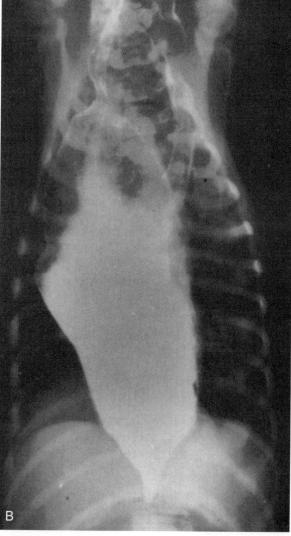

Figure 10–18. A, Megaesophagus. The trachea is depressed by a markedly dilated esophagus. A contrast study shows the extent of the dilation. **B,** In megaesophagus, the esophagus narrows sharply at the gastroesophageal junction. (From Kealy JK: Diagnostic Radiology of the Dog and Cat, 2nd ed. Philadelphia, WB Saunders, 1987, pp 46, 49.)

the convergence at the gastroesophageal junction. Evidence of aspiration pneumonia is frequently present and consistent with the signs of dysphagia and regurgitation.

When the esophagus is not observed visually on survey radiographs, a contrast esophagogram is required (Watrous, 1983). A barium contrast study better defines the degree of esophageal dilation, lack of function, and extent of involvement (Fig. 10–18). The study helps rule out congenital vascular ring anomalies or other causes of localized obstruction that might contribute to megaesophagus and outlines the funnel shape of the caudal region of the esophagus to rule out invasive processes that may cause irregular or asymmetric narrowing. If no contrast medium enters the stomach, as noted on initial contrast radiographs, the animal's forequarters should be elevated for several minutes to allow for gravitational flow of the contrast medium into the stomach, and follow-up radiographs should be obtained.

Treatment. In the treatment of congenital idiopathic megaesophagus, proper dietary management in terms of frequent, elevated feedings (Fig. 10–19) with foods of appropriate consistency for the particular animal (some handle bulky foods well; others tolerate gruels better) generally results in spontaneous improvement in a number of animals (Watrous, 1983). This had led investigators to believe that congenital idiopathic megaesophagus may be due to delayed neurologic development of esophageal innervation (Diamant et al, 1974; Kipnis, 1978). With the elevated feedings, minimal stress and

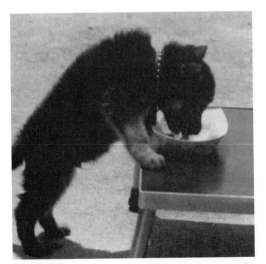

Figure 10–19. Megaesophagus. Feeding a puppy from an elevated stand.

distention of the esophagus occur until such time as normal esophageal motor function develops. If stasis of esophageal contents is allowed, however, gradual overdistention and atony result, contributing to persistent megaesophagus. The earlier the dysfunction is recognized and the dietary management instituted, the better the prognosis. Puppies and kittens diagnosed at the time of weaning and managed appropriately have a better prognosis than those whose condition is recognized later, at around 4 to 6 months of age. Once severe megaesophagus occurs, complete recovery is unlikely. Aspiration pneumonia and malnourishment limit the longevity of these animals.

If the underlying cause of acquired idiopathic megaesophagus can be identified and successfully treated, the signs of megaesophagus may subside (Watrous, 1983). The development of megaesophagus secondary to systemic disease is, however, correlated with an extremely poor response to therapy. Death results from aspiration pneumonia, gastroesophageal intussusception, malnutrition, and other related organ dysfunctions.

Esophageal Diverticula

Congenital esophageal diverticula are extremely rare in young dogs and cats. The areas of the esophagus typically involved are the area just cranial to the thoracic inlet (Fig. 10–20) and the area just cranial to the diaphragm. Congenital diverticula have been attributed to abnormal separation of tracheal and esophageal embryonic buds, development of eccentric vacuoles in the formation of the esophageal lumen, and inherent weakness of the esophageal wall (Lantz et al, 1976). Periodic diverticularization of the esophagus at the thoracic inlet is considered to be a normal finding for most young English bulldogs (Woods et al, 1978). Periodic diverticularization or a redundancy of the esophagus at the thoracic inlet may be detected as a coincidental finding during evaluation of vomiting or regurgitation problems or may, in a few cases, cause transient regurgitation (Fig. 10–21).

Signs of esophageal diverticula are quite varied and are related to the size of the diverticula (Fukata, 1984; Pearson et al, 1978). Signs may include distress or gagging soon after eating, postprandial regurgitation, intermittent anorexia and lethargy, reluctance to move, and incoordination or ataxia after eating. Diagnosis requires the differentiation of diverticula from other esophagus-related causes of regurgitation. To identify esophageal diverticula, contrast eso-

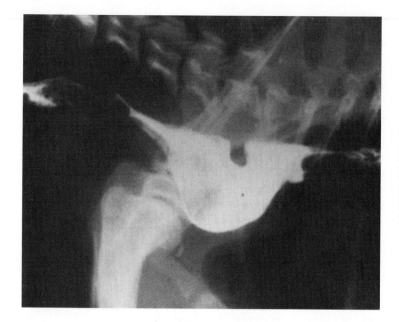

Figure 10–20. Lateral esophagogram demonstrating a large diverticulum at the thoracic inlet. (From Aronson E, Carrig CB, Lattimer JC: Radiology of the gastrointestinal system. *In* Jones BD, Liska WD [eds]: Canine and Feline Gastroenterology. Philadelphia, WB Saunders, 1986, p 402.)

phagography, fluoroscopic observation, and esophagoscopy are used. Esophagoscopy, in particular, may confirm the hernia-like outpouching from the esophageal lumen, determine the presence of associated esophagitis, and facilitate the removal of entrapped material in the diverticulum.

Small diverticula with no other associated esophageal lesions may be treated conservatively by feeding a nutritionally complete, soft, bland diet, feeding the animal in an elevated position, and administering ample liquids after feedings (Lantz et al, 1976). Symptomatic diverticula usually require surgical excision and reconstruction of the esophageal wall for adequate control of the signs.

Disorders of the Gastroesophageal Junction

Disorders affecting the function of the gastroesophageal junction are uncommon. The disorders more commonly associated with its altered function are hiatal hernia with reflux esophagitis (Alexander et al, 1975; Gaskell et al, 1974; Robotham, 1977) and gastroesophageal intussusception (Leib and Blass, 1984; Morris and Turnwald, 1980; Singer, 1975). *Hiatal hernia* is the result of a congenital or acquired defect of the phrenoesophageal ligament that allows displacement of the gastroesophageal junction forward into the thoracic cavity (Fig. 10–22). Hiatal hernia may also be associated with an upper respiratory obstruction, especially common in young Chinese shar-peis. Gastric contents reflux

through the incompetent junction into the caudal region of the esophagus, where they produce varying degrees of irritation to the esophageal mucosa. Signs may include regurgitation with possible hematemesis, dysphagia, altered breathing pattern, and weight loss. Diagnosis requires a high index of suspicion followed by a barium contrast study performed under fluoroscopic observation. The hiatal hernia may be a sliding type hernia (Gaskell et al, 1974), which moves in and out of its normal position, or a fixed hernia (Alexander et al, 1975), which remains out of position. The amount of stomach that protrudes through the esophageal hiatus determines the radiographic appearance of the hernia. Usually, external abdominal pressure is necessary to demonstrate a sliding hiatal hernia (Hoffer, 1986). The hiatal hernia may be repaired surgically. If excessive gastric reflux occurs, the gastroesophageal junction may be surgically strengthened by a gastric fundoplication (Nissen's operation) procedure (Hoffer, 1986).

Gastroesophageal intussusception or invagination involves the telescoping of all or part of the stomach into the esophageal lumen (Fig. 10–23). Occasionally, the spleen and pancreas are also included (Singer, 1975). The cause of this condition is not understood, but an incompetent gastroesophageal junction must be suspected. Gastroesophageal intussusception generally occurs in puppies of large breeds and in kittens, particularly those with congenital megaesophagus. A puppy or kitten will be presented to the veterinarian with sudden onset of difficulty in breathing, impending shock, and a

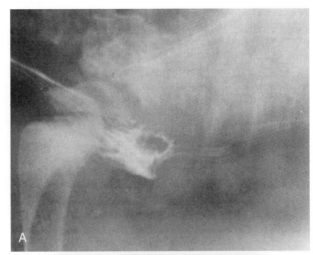

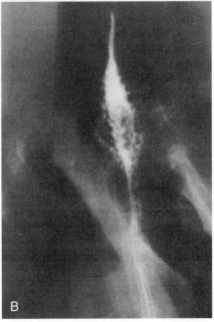

Figure 10–21. Lateral **(A)** and ventrodorsal **(B)** esophagograms. Note the irregular mucosal pattern at the thoracic inlet, often seen in young dogs presenting with transient regurgitation. (From Aronson E, Carrig CB, Lattimer JC: Radiology of the gastrointestinal system. *In* Jones BD, Liska WD [eds]: Canine and Feline Gastroenterology. Philadelphia, WB Saunders, 1986, p 402.)

history of vomiting. Radiographically, a mass that has a surface contour of rugal folds is seen just cranial to the diaphragm filling the caudal region of the esophagus. When the intussusception includes the spleen, its shadow will be absent on survey abdominal radiographs. The sudden onset of signs and radiographic appearance of the mass are the keys to the diagnosis. Treatment is surgical reduction of the intussusception and a gastropexy (Hoffer, 1986).

THE STOMACH

Gastritis

Gastritis frequently occurs in dogs and cats from the time of weaning through adulthood.

By definition, gastritis is inflammation and mucosal damage that has occurred in response to an insult to the gastric mucosa. Vomiting is typically the primary sign of gastric disorders. Vomiting as an event first appears in puppies and kittens with a full stomach at 3 days and 10 days of age, respectively (Brizzee and Vitale, 1959; Smith et al, 1974). The veterinarian can identify gastric disorders by observation of vomiting, which differs from regurgitation associated with esophageal disorders or from coughing and expulsion of phlegm associated with respiratory or cardiovascular disorders. Vomiting is usually preceded by a short period of nausea with licking, hypersalivation, or multiple attempts at swallowing. This period is fol-

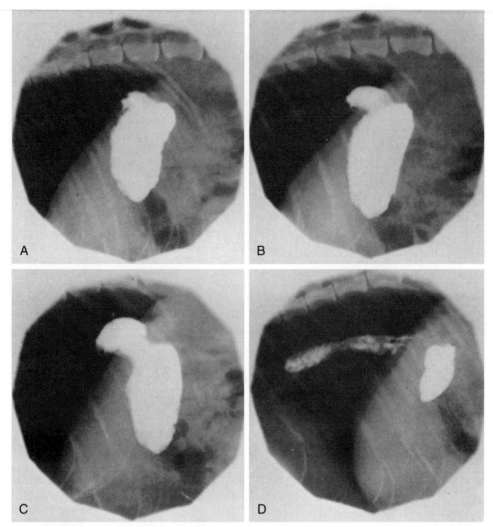

Figure 10–22. A cat with a history of persistent vomiting that had been increasing in frequency for 4 to 6 weeks. Fluoroscopic study shows the progression **(A–D)** of the stomach as it enters the esophagus and returns to its normal position. Diagnosis: recurring hiatal hernia. (From Dehoff WD: Surgery of the stomach. *In* Jones BD, Liska WD [eds]: Canine and Feline Gastroenterology. Philadelphia, WB Saunders, 1986, p 158.)

lowed by retching or several forceful, simultaneous diaphragmatic and abdominal contractions and, with the head lowered, expulsion of gastric contents (Wingfield and Twedt, 1986).

Observation of the amount, color, and consistency of vomitus is useful for obtaining insight into the origin of a gastric disorder and the degree of mucosal damage. If the vomitus consists of food, the degree of digestion indicates the length of time food has remained in the stomach. Vomitus can contain varying amounts of mucus and fluid from gastric and swallowed salivary secretions. Yellow- or green-stained vomitus indicates intestinal reflux of bile into the stomach. Vomitus containing feces usually indicates intestinal stasis or possibly intestinal obstruction. Fresh blood from gastric bleeding may be present as small red flecks or as large blood clots. Blood that has been retained in the stomach soon becomes partially digested and has a brown "coffee grounds" appearance. The presence of blood in vomitus usually signifies a more serious gastric disorder. Other signs associated with gastric disorders may include nausea, belching, inappetence, polydipsia, and pica. Melena, or black tarry stools, is seen with upper gastrointestinal bleeding and may imply gastric mucosal damage (Wingfield and Twedt, 1986).

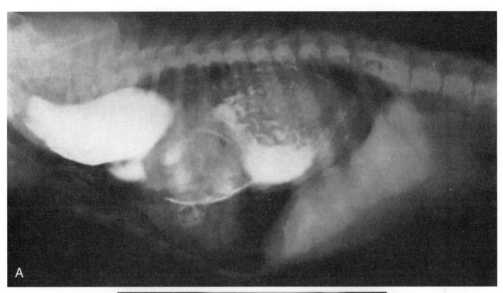

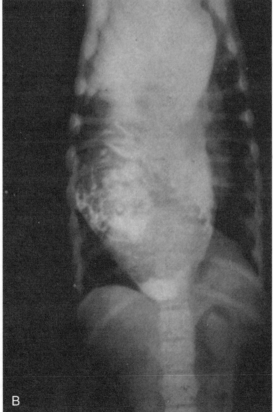

Figure 10–23. Gastroesophageal intussusception. A 9-week-old German shepherd with a history of vomiting and respiratory distress for 2 days. There is an associated megaesophagus. Gastric rugal folds can be seen within the thorax. The typical stomach shadow is not seen in the abdomen. (From Kealy JK: Diagnostic Radiology of the Dog and Cat, 2nd ed. Philadelphia, WB Saunders, 1987, p 57.)

Causes. Gastritis can be associated with a multitude of factors but more commonly results from dietary indiscretions, infectious diseases, and possibly endoparasites. It is often associated with ingestion of rancid or contaminated foodstuffs that leads to food intoxication. The contaminated foodstuffs generally contain products of fermentation or putrefaction, various bacterial enterotoxins, and possibly mycotoxins (Harris, 1975). Ingestion of foreign material such as bones, pins, needles, plastic objects, food wrappings, rocks, and small toys mechanically irritates the gastric mucosa and thereby causes gastritis. The incidence of ingested foreign material is much higher in young dogs and cats, possibly owing to their developmental chewing habits and curious natures. Trichobezoars (hairballs) are frequently seen in the vomitus of long-haired cats and some dogs. Many drugs (e.g., antimicrobial agents, nonsteroidal antiinflammatory drugs, anthelmintics, and corticosteroids) and chemicals (e.g., heavy metals, cleaning agents, fertilizers, and herbicides) may also contribute to gastritis in the young animal (Atkins and Johnson, 1975; Harris, 1975).

Many types of ingested plants and plant toxins may cause gastritis. The ingestion of grass and plants by seemingly healthy animals is not uncommon, possibly owing to their natural, instinctual behaviors. Many young dogs and cats with gastric disorders, for some unknown reason, frequently ingest and then vomit grass or plant material. The incidence of bacterial-induced gastritis is extremely low because the acidic gastric lumen does not favor the growth and colonization of bacteria (Strombeck and Guilford, 1990). A gastric chlamydial infection has been identified in young cats (Gaillard et al, 1984). Viruses such as canine distemper virus, canine herpesvirus, canine adenovirus-1, coronaviruses, and parvoviruses may cause gastric lesions and vomiting as a part of a more extensive disease condition. Mycotic infections of the stomach are extremely rare and generally not an important cause of gastritis in dogs and cats younger than 6 months (Ader, 1979; Foil et al, 1984). Endoparasites seldom produce gastric lesions or signs. *Physaloptera* species, *Ollulanus tricuspis* (cats), ascarids, and, occasionally, tapeworms are endoparasites that may be associated with gastric irritation and vomiting. Other conditions, including renal failure, liver disease, neurologic disease, shock, sepsis, and possibly altered behavior, may also play a role in the cause of gastritis in the young dog and cat.

Diagnosis and Treatment. Gastritis is generally diagnosed and treated on the basis of the animal's history, signs, and physical findings. Symptomatic treatment of most cases of gastritis and vomiting is begun without extensive diagnostic procedures. Most animals show improvement within 12 to 24 hours after little or no therapy and usually are treated on an outpatient basis. Those animals with persistent vomiting, evidence of dehydration, abdominal pain, organomegaly or palpable abdominal mass, or failure to respond to previous symptomatic treatment require further medical and laboratory evaluation. The general principles of the treatment of gastric disorders include removing the inciting cause; providing proper conditions to promote mucosal repair; correcting fluid, electrolyte, and acid-base abnormalities; and alleviating secondary complications of gastritis, such as abdominal pain and diarrhea (Wingfield and Twedt, 1986).

Dietary restriction is the initial management for gastritis. An animal with gastritis should be withheld food for 24 to 48 hours and water for 12 to 24 hours. If no vomiting occurs during this period of management, over the next 2 to 5 days the animal is gradually returned to full feed and water. Water is offered initially in small, frequent amounts or provided in ice cubes, enough to keep the mouth moist and to supply a modest fluid replacement. Until vomiting is well controlled, small amounts (three to six times daily) of a highly digestible, low-fiber diet are fed frequently, including cooked rice or cooked cereals supplemented in a 50:50 ratio with low-fat cottage cheese, boiled chicken, lean boiled ground beef, or commercial baby foods. Commercial diets formulated for gastrointestinal disease may also be prescribed. One can expect most cases of vomiting in young dogs and cats to respond to just dietary and water intake management.

Administration of parenteral fluids is initiated when electrolyte or acid-base imbalances or dehydration occurs. The quantity of fluids given should be enough to supply daily maintenance needs (approximately 40 to 60 ml/kg per day), to correct existing dehydration, and to replace fluid losses caused by continued vomiting. Vomiting in gastritis generally results in volume depletion and losses of sodium, chloride, and potassium with a metabolic acidosis. An isotonic, balanced electrolyte solution such as lactated Ringer's solution is usually given (Twedt and Grauer, 1982).

Antiemetic drugs may be given to control refractory vomiting in dogs and cats older than

3 months (Table 10–4) and when the presence of a pyloric dysfunction or a gastric foreign object has been ruled out. These drugs inhibit vomiting but do little for primary treatment of gastritis. Antiemetic drugs act centrally by suppressing either the chemoreceptor trigger zone (CRTZ), the emetic center, or the vestibular apparatus. The phenothiazine tranquilizers (chlorpromazine) have a broad-spectrum pharmacologic effect in blocking the emetic center and the CRTZ and some anticholinergic action (Davis, 1980; DeNovo, 1986). These drugs are effective in blocking viscerally stimulated vomiting caused by gastritis and can be given to animals with protracted vomiting. The phenothiazines should not be given to a dehydrated or a hypotensive animal or when a hepatopathy is suspected (DeNovo, 1986).

Anticholinergic drugs reduce gastric motility and smooth muscle spasms. In addition to blocking the parasympathetic stimulation of smooth muscles, these drugs block the cephalic and gastric phases of gastric acid secretion, but they do not block histamine or gastrin-stimulated acid secretion. These drugs have the adverse effect of slowing gastric emptying, which results in gastric distention and further gastric acid secretion. Overuse of the anticholinergic drugs can cause gastric atony and a pharmacologic gastric outflow obstruction, resulting in further vomiting. Anticholinergic drugs used in the therapy of gastric disorders include atropine and propantheline (DeNovo, 1986). These drugs often are combined with an antiemetic for veterinary use.

Oral protectants, such as kaolin and pectin, and antimicrobial agents are usually not indicated for the treatment of gastritis in the young dog or cat. Protectants may bind certain bacteria or toxins, but they do not coat or protect the irritated gastric mucosa. Any potential benefit is frequently outweighed by difficulty in owner administration and vomiting that occurs because of gastric distention. Sucralfate in tablet form or given as a slurry (crush 1 g sucralfate and mix with 10 ml water; give 5 ml of slurry four to six times daily) may, however, be protective when the gastric mucosa is irritated or ulcerated. Antimicrobial agents are not required unless a bacterial infection is suspected.

Secretory blockers (H_2-receptor antagonists), such as cimetidine, ranitidine, and famotidine, are effective in reducing gastric acid production by blocking the H_2 receptors of the parietal cells (see Table 10–4). Use of these drugs has been recommended in the symptomatic treatment of gastric and duodenal ulcers and in syndromes resulting in gastric acid hypersecretion (Wingfield and Twedt, 1986). They may be useful as adjunctive therapy in some types of gastritis; however, they probably should not be administered to dogs or cats younger than 2 months of age. Cimetidine inhibits hepatic blood flow and microsomal enzymes and should not be given to puppies and kittens with liver disease or those receiving other hepatically metabolized drugs. Severe gastric hemorrhage should be treated as an emergency. Whole blood and parenteral fluids should be given to replace blood and fluid loss. Attempts at controlling bleeding are generally made with the use of gastric lavages with ice water or surgical gastrectomy.

Gastric Foreign Objects

With ingestion of small objects such as needles or pins with no evidence of vomiting, one may elect to allow for natural passage of the object(s). A high-fiber diet is given, and the animal is kept under strict observation. Failure to pass the object(s) in 48 hours or lack of movement of the object(s), as determined by serial abdominal radiographs, requires surgical removal of the object(s). Emetic drugs to initiate vomiting should be used with extreme caution. They should be attempted only when the foreign object(s) are small and have smooth surfaces that will not cause gastric or esophageal laceration, perforation, or obstruction. Vaseline or other petroleum-based products may be used to promote passage of small hairballs aborally through the gastrointestinal tract. Owners should not be advised to administer oily-liquid products such as mineral oil orally, as it may cause laryngotracheal aspiration and a subsequent pneumonia.

Endoscopy can be used because many gastric foreign objects can be removed successfully with grasping forceps or snares under endoscopic visual observation. The methods used to retrieve foreign objects from the stomach via endoscopy are quite similar to those used to remove lodged foreign objects from the esophagus. Surgical removal of gastric foreign objects offers the advantage of examining the other sections of the gastrointestinal tract for foreign objects or other abnormalities.

Gastric Retention Disorders

Causes. Gastric retention and paresis are most often associated with pyloric dysfunction, motility disturbances of the stomach, or both (Strombeck and Guilford, 1990). Pyloric dys-

Table 10–4 Summary of Therapeutic Products Available for Management of Gastrointestinal Disorders

THERAPEUTIC AGENT	DOSAGE AND ROUTE*	COMMENTS
Antidiarrheal Agents		
Chlordiazepoxide and clidinium	1–2 tablets bid–tid PO (dogs)	Combination CNS depressant and anticholinergic effects; contraindicated in infectious enteritis and gastrointestinal obstructions; not recommended for dogs weighing less than 10 kg
Dicyclomine	0.15 mg/kg tid PO (pediatric dosage)	Anticholinergic effects; no well-established dosage for dogs or cats
Diphenoxylate	0.05–0.1 mg/kg tid–qid PO (dogs) 0.063 mg/kg tid PO (cats)	Narcotic analgesic effects
Loperamide	0.08 mg/kg tid–qid PO (dogs) 0.04 mg/kg sid–bid PO (cats; use with caution)	Available in tablet and liquid formulations; narcotic analgesic effects
Paregoric	0.05–0.06 mg/kg bid–tid PO (dogs)	Useful when treating dogs weighing less than 10 kg; narcotic analgesic effects
Propantheline	0.25 mg/kg bid–tid PO	Anticholinergic effects; contraindicated in infectious enteritis and gastrointestinal obstructions
Antiemetic Agents		
Chlorpromazine	0.25–0.5 mg/kg sid–qid IM, SC (dogs and cats) 1.0 mg/kg tid–qid PO, rectal (dogs) 0.05 mg/kg tid–qid IV (dogs) 0.01–0.025 mg/kg IV (cats)	Effective phenothiazine antiemetic
Dimenhydrinate	4 mg/kg sid–tid PO (dogs) 2 mg/kg sid–tid PO (cats)	Effective antihistamine antiemetic; good for motion sickness if given before travel
Diphenhydramine	2–4 mg/kg PO (dogs) 2 mg/kg bid–tid IM, IV slowly	Effective antihistamine antiemetic; good for motion sickness if given before travel
Metoclopramide	0.2–0.4 mg/kg tid–qid PO, SC 1–2 mg/kg/24 hours as a slow IV infusion can be used for severe vomiting (dogs) 0.1–0.2 mg/kg tid PO, SC 0.05–1 mg/kg/24 hours as a slow IV infusion can be used for severe vomiting (cats)	For gastric motility disorders, reflux esophagitis, and dysautonomia, give 30 min before meals and at bedtime; quickly eliminated by IV route; adverse effects seen at dosage greater than 1 mg/kg
Prochlorperazine	0.1 mg/kg tid–qid IM (dogs)	Effective phenothiazine antiemetic
Trimethobenzamine	3 mg/kg bid–tid IM (dogs)	Effective antihistamine antiemetic; no experience with use in cats
Antimicrobial Agents		
Amoxicillin	22 mg/kg bid PO	Possible alternative to ampicillin
Ampicillin	10–20 mg/kg tid–qid PO 5–10 mg/kg tid–qid IV, IM, SC	Combine with aminoglycoside for systemic infections
Cefadroxil	22 mg/kg bid PO	Combine with aminoglycoside for systemic infections
Cefoxitin sodium	22 mg/kg tid IV, IM	Combine with aminoglycoside for systemic infections
Cephalexin	20 mg/kg tid PO, SC, IV	Combine with aminoglycoside for systemic infections
Cephradine	10–20 mg/kg tid PO	Combine with aminoglycoside for systemic infections
Chloramphenicol	50 mg/kg IV, IM, SC, PO tid for dogs, bid for cats	*Salmonella, Campylobacter, Yersinia* usually sensitive
Clindamycin	3–5 mg/kg bid PO, IV, IM	*Campylobacter* and *Toxoplasma* usually sensitive
Erythromycin	10 mg/kg tid PO	May cause anorexia and vomiting
Gentamicin	2 mg/kg tid IM, SC	Maintain adequate hydration; evaluate renal function often; *Shigella* and *Yersinia* usually sensitive; combine with cephalosporin for systemic salmonellosis
Metronidazole	7.5 mg/kg bid–tid PO	Combine with penicillins and cephalosporins for systemic infections
Spectinomycin	5–12 mg/kg bid IM, 20 mg/kg bid PO	Possible alternative to aminoglycoside
Sulfasalazine	10–25 mg/kg tid–qid PO	Safe dosage for cats not established; adverse effects are uncommon—vomiting, hemolytic anemia, leukopenia, icterus, keratoconjunctivitis sicca

Table continued on opposite page

Table 10–4 **Summary of Therapeutic Products Available for Management of Gastrointestinal Disorders** *Continued*

THERAPEUTIC AGENT	DOSAGE AND ROUTE*	COMMENTS
Antimicrobial Agents		
Trimethoprim-sulfadiazine	15 mg/kg bid SC, IM, PO	Long-term (40- to 60-day) therapy may eliminate carrier state of salmonellosis; *Yersinia* usually sensitive
Tylosin (powdered)	20–40 mg/kg bid PO (dogs) 5–10 mg/kg bid PO (cats)	One tsp supplies approximately 400 mg tylosin; mix thoroughly with food to camouflage bitter taste; *Cryptosporidium* usually sensitive
Gastric Protectants		
Cimetidine—H₂-receptor blockers	5 mg/kg bid–tid IM, IV, PO	Indicated for esophageal and gastric disease; impedes hepatic biotransformation enzymes; probably should not be used in dogs and cats younger than 2 mo
Famotidine—H₂-receptor blockers	0.5–1.0 mg/kg sid–bid PO, SC	Indicated for esophageal and gastric disease; probably should not be used in dogs and cats younger than 2 mo
Misoprostol	2–5 µg/kg tid–qid PO (dogs)	Indicated for gastric disease; may cause diarrhea
Omeprazole	1–2 mg/kg sid PO (dogs)	Indicated for esophageal and gastric disease; prolonged administration not recommended
Ranitidine—H₂-receptor blockers	2–4 mg/kg bid–tid PO, SC, IV	Indicated for esophageal and gastric disease; similar precautions as for cimetidine; does not affect hepatic biotransformation enzymes; probably should not be used in dogs and cats younger than 2 mo
Sucralfate	100–1000 mg (dogs) 100–200 mg (cats)	Requires acidic pH for activation; administer 30–40 minutes before H₂-receptor blockers; higher doses are for dogs or cats older than 4 mo of age; constipation often occurs with daily use; is not absorbed systemically
Laxative Agents		
Bisacodyl	5 mg sid PO	Available in 5-mg tablet and 5-mg suppository; takes 6–12 hours for tablets to take effect; animal should be well hydrated and feces softened before its use
Bran	1–2 tbsp mixed in 400 g of canned food and given sid or bid	Available in powder form; takes 12–24 hours to take effect
Dioctyl sodium sulfosuccinate	1–4 capsules (50 mg) sid PO (dogs) 1 capsule (50 mg) sid PO (cats)	Available in 50- and 100-mg capsules, 1% liquid, 4 mg/ml syrup; takes 12–72 hours to take effect; animal should be well hydrated before its use
Dioctyl calcium sulfosuccinate	2–3 tablets (50 mg) sid PO (dogs) 1–2 tablets (50 mg) sid PO (cats)	Available in 50- and 240-mg tablets; similar activity and precautions as for dioctyl sodium sulfosuccinate
Lactulose	1 ml/4.5 kg tid PO for dogs to start; then adjust dosage to stool consistency and 2–3 soft bowel movements per day 0.25–1 ml for cats sid–bid PO to start; then adjust dosage to stool consistency and 2–3 soft bowel movements per day Retention enema procedure: 5–10 ml of lactulose diluted 1:3 in water tid—qid (this procedure is only used for management of hepatoencephalopathy)	Overdosage may cause diarrhea, flatulence, intestinal cramping (colic), dehydration, and acidosis
Psyllium (natural)	1–3 tsp mixed with food and given sid or bid	Available in powder form; takes 12–24 hours to take effect
White petrolatum	1–5 ml sid PO initially; then 2–3 days/week	Available in paste form; should be given only between meals; takes 12–24 hours to take effect
Motility Smooth Muscle Stimulator		
Cisapride	0.1–0.5 mg/kg bid–tid PO (dogs) 2.5–5 mg per cat bid–tid PO	Administer 30 min before feeding; may cause increased heart rate

*PO = oral administration; SC = subcutaneous administration; IV = intravenous administration; IM = intramuscular administration; sid = once daily; bid = twice daily; tid = three times daily; qid = four times daily.

function in the young dog or cat usually results from congenital pyloric stenosis or from an intraluminal foreign object obstructing the gastric outflow area. Traumatic injury and inflammatory disease can reduce motility throughout the gastrointestinal tract, resulting in the retention of gastric contents. Drugs, hypokalemia, recurring gastric dilation, and long-term obstruction of the pylorus may also contribute to altered gastric motility and gastric retention.

Congenital pyloric stenosis is recognized most often in the boxer and Boston terrier dog breeds. It rarely occurs in the young cat, although Siamese cats have the highest reported incidence (Boehringer, 1973; Pearson et al, 1974). Congenital pyloric stenosis probably is caused by excessive secretion of gastrointestinal hormones (Wingfield and Twedt, 1986). Gastrin, produced by the G cells in the stomach wall, has a potent trophic effect on pyloric circular smooth muscle as well as on the mucosa. With altered gastric motility and antral distention, the G cells are stimulated to release gastrin, ultimately leading to an increase in gastric acid production and pyloric stenosis from hypertrophy of the circular smooth muscle.

Diagnosis. Gastric retention either is present at birth or develops with advancing age. Vomiting at variable intervals after ingestion of solid food, with accompanying gastric distention, is the primary sign of gastric retention (Wingfield and Twedt, 1986). The vomitus is usually undigested food and is rarely bile stained. Animals with gastric retention may exhibit projectile vomiting; the vomiting occurs abruptly and without the warning of hypersalivation and retching. In most instances, the vomitus is propelled a considerable distance and readily empties the stomach. After vomiting, the animal will usually resume feeding, only to vomit again at variable intervals.

On survey abdominal radiographs, the presence of gastric distention with food or air, long after the ingesta should be in the intestine (within 6 to 8 hours after eating), is suggestive of gastric retention. In the cat with a gastric retention problem, although the fundus and body become elongated craniocaudally because of an increase in gastric volume, the fundus and body remain on the left side of the midline (Pearson et al, 1974). Contrast medium studies are useful for assessing the rate of gastric emptying of liquids in those animals suspected of having an abnormal gastric retention problem. Less than 30 minutes is generally considered to

be a normal gastric emptying time for a quiet, well-behaved animal. The presence of contrast medium or food in the stomach for longer than 12 to 24 hours is definitely abnormal and should be considered evidence of gastric retention. Chemical or manual restraint of the young animal will slow gastric emptying for a variable length of time (Zontine, 1973). Fluoroscopic studies with contrast medium are required for assessing altered gastric motility as a cause of a gastric retention problem. In gastric retention caused by altered motility, the motor activity is usually of normal rate and intensity but results only in a dilation of the antrum, with little contrast medium passing aborally through the pyloric canal (Wingfield and Twedt, 1986).

Endoscopy in dogs and cats younger than 6 months with hypertrophy of the pyloric musculature is not well documented. One should remember that the pyloric orifice of the mature dog is usually partially open, and passage of the flexible endoscope through the pylorus may be possible in a nonobstructed pyloric canal. In dogs younger than 6 months and in cats, however, the animal's pyloric canal may not be large enough to accommodate the standard endoscope. Failure of passage of a flexible endoscope through the pyloric canal of the mature dog is suggestive of pyloric stenosis, and biopsy specimens should be obtained to determine diagnosis and prognosis. This may not necessarily be true for the young dog or cat.

Treatment. Congenital pyloric stenosis is generally managed surgically with pyloroplasty (DeHoff, 1986; Walter et al, 1985). Medical therapy has been generally directed toward the control of signs, mainly through the use of dietary management and antiemetic drugs. Gastric stimulation with metoclopramide is helpful in animals with functional, but not anatomical, gastric retention (see Table 10–4). Metoclopramide increases gastric antral contractions, promotes relaxation of the pylorus, and increases smooth muscle contraction in the proximal small intestine. This enhances coordination of the antral and duodenal contractions, with subsequent acceleration of gastric emptying and small intestinal transit. Metoclopramide is contraindicated whenever increased gastrointestinal motility might be harmful. It should not be administered to animals with central nervous system disease, given in conjunction with phenothiazines or narcotic analgesics, or administered to animals younger than 2 months of age.

Gastric Dilation-Volvulus

Gastric dilation-volvulus syndrome is most frequently seen in dogs between the ages of 2 and 10 years and seldom in cats or dogs younger than 6 months (Key, 1977). Overeating or signs of altered gastric motility may begin immediately after weaning to solid food, leading to gastric dilation-volvulus later in life.

Diagnosis. Gastric dilation usually precedes the volvulus (Figs. 10–24 and 10–25). Young dogs presenting with gastric dilation rarely have tympany on percussion of the abdomen (Wingfield and Twedt, 1986). The animals are often lethargic and reluctant to move and make grunting sounds with each respiratory effort. Attempts to palpate the abdomen encounter abdominal splinting and increased grunting sounds. In most instances, the animals make no attempt to retch or vomit. If the animal exhibits sudden onset of gastric tympany, there will be cranial abdominal distention and the abdomen will be tensed upon palpation. Increased respiratory efforts, hyperpnea, and open-mouthed panting are frequently noted. Abdominal palpation may also reveal splenomegaly, with the spleen oriented cranially to caudally along the ventral midline of the abdomen. Retching with an inability to vomit may be observed. The retching may become quite violent without pro-

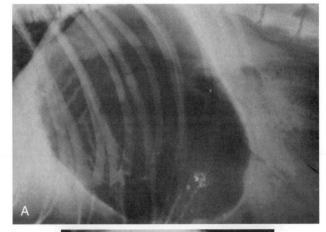

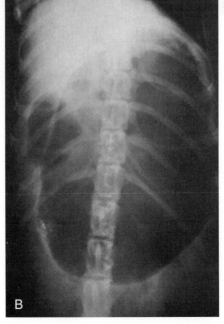

Figure 10–24. Lateral **(A)** and ventrodorsal **(B)** radiographs of a young Labrador retriever with gastric dilation. Note that, although the stomach is greatly distended with gas, the relationship of the stomach within the abdomen remains normal. (From Aronson E, Carrig CB, Lattimer JC: Radiology of the gastrointestinal system. *In* Jones BD, Liska WD [eds]: Canine and Feline Gastroenterology. Philadelphia, WB Saunders, 1986, p 428.)

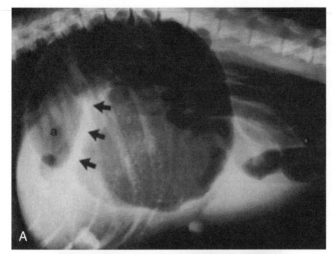

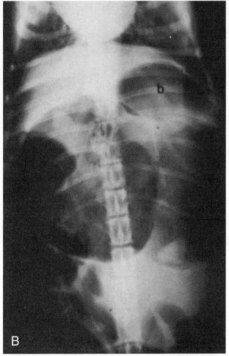

Figure 10–25. Lateral (A) and ventrodorsal (B) radiographs of a dog with gastric volvulus. There is marked distention of the stomach with gas and fluid. Note on the lateral view that the pyloric antrum (a) is displaced dorsally, and a soft tissue dense band *(arrows)* suggests compartmentalization of the stomach. In the ventrodorsal view, the pyloric antrum (b) is present in the left cranial abdomen. In both radiographs, the small intestines are enlarged and gas filled. (From Aronson E, Carrig CB, Lattimer JC: Radiology of the gastrointestinal system. *In* Jones BD, Liska WD [eds]: Canine and Feline Gastroenterology. Philadelphia, WB Saunders, 1986, p 428.)

ducing vomitus. With increasing efforts to retch, the abdomen further distends from swallowed air.

As gastric distention progresses, signs of shock become evident. A weak femoral pulse, tachycardia, and prolonged capillary refill time of the mucous membranes are commonly noted. Increased venous pressures can be observed by placing the dog in lateral recumbency and observing the saphenous vein (Wingfield and Twedt, 1986). As the leg of a healthy dog is slowly raised to the level of the right atrium,

this vein disappears. In the dog with gastric dilation-volvulus, the leg may be raised well above the level of the right atrium before the vein collapses, suggesting increased venous pressure.

Passage of an orogastric tube does not eliminate the possibility of gastric volvulus; the definitive diagnosis is confirmed by abdominal radiographs. Radiographs are obtained after the initial therapy for circulatory shock and gastric decompression because positioning for radiographs increases stress and risk to the animal

(Wingfield and Twedt, 1986). Barium contrast medium will assist in identifying the position of the pylorus, which is most important in determining the presence of a gastric volvulus. Because the stomach may partially derotate after decompression, position of the pylorus in other than the far right cranial abdominal quadrant must be considered evidence that gastric dilation-volvulus existed before decompression.

Treatment. Baseline laboratory samples should be collected before large-volume fluid replacement and gastric decompression. A packed cell volume and a total plasma solids value (total plasma protein) provide information useful in assessing the need for fluid replacement. Determining a complete blood count and blood glucose level is useful in assessing the presence of endotoxic shock. Leukopenia (<3000 leukocytes/μl), a prominent left shift, and hypoglycemia (<60 mg glucose/dl) suggest septicemia (Wingfield and Twedt, 1986).

Gastric decompression is immediately accomplished by passing a large-bore, firm, flexible, well-lubricated orogastric tube or by gastrocentesis (trocarization). When the orogastric tube cannot be passed, the stomach may be decompressed with a 12- to 16-gauge needle. Partial relief of gastric air often allows subsequent passage of the orogastric tube. Cardiovascular function generally improves following gastric decompression and is further improved by rapid volume replacement using intravenous, balanced electrolyte solution supplemented with potassium chloride. A transient hyperkalemia results from gastric decompression (Wingfield et al, 1975); however, a deficit in total body potassium levels is usually present owing to gastrointestinal loss and reduced intake of potassium. Corticosteroids are routinely used in the management of shock (Rawlings et al, 1976). Fluid replacement therapy should always precede corticosteroid therapy. Additionally, broad-spectrum antimicrobial agents are used to control preoperative and postvolvulus bacterial numbers and to lessen the severity of endotoxemia (Wingfield and Twedt, 1986).

Surgical procedures to correct gastric dilation-volvulus have been described elsewhere (Lantz, 1998). After either surgical correction or radiographic evidence that the stomach has returned naturally to its proper position, small amounts of water are gradually provided in a bowl or in the form of ice cubes. Food is withheld until the dog has not vomited for at least 24 hours; then one third of the daily requirement of a highly digestible diet, divided into three to six small meals, is fed. Over the next 3 to 7 days, the amount of food fed is gradually increased up to the animal's maintenance caloric needs.

Prevention. Several surgical techniques have been described to prevent recurrence of gastric dilation-volvulus. These include gastropexy, gastrocolopexy, permanent gastropexy, tube gastrostomy, circumcostal gastropexy, belt loop gastropexy, and ventral midline gastropexy. Of these techniques, the circumcostal gastropexy, belt loop gastropexy, and ventral midline gastropexy appear to be the most successful procedures for preventing recurrence and provide a greater adhesion strength than the permanent or tube gastrostomy techniques. Application of feeding techniques that promote gastric emptying is also useful in preventing gastric dilation-volvulus. During the animal's growth period it is important to provide a high-quality, low-fiber, highly digestible, and nutritionally balanced diet. All dogs should be fed throughout their lives at least twice daily or "free choice." Dogs previously affected with gastric dilation-volvulus syndrome should be fed a highly digestible diet at least three times a day, and their physical activity and excitement should be minimized before, during, and for 1 hour after feeding. Feeding the dog by itself and in a quiet location may also be helpful.

THE INTESTINE
Congenital Disorders

Congenital disorders of the intestinal tract are rarely encountered in puppies and kittens, probably because most such affected animals die at birth or become fading puppies or kittens. The congenital disorders that have been reported include atresia of intestinal segment (Ladds and Anderson, 1971; Martin, 1977; Mullen, 1982; Smart et al, 1978; van der Gaag and Tibboel, 1980) and duplication of intestinal segment (Jakowski, 1977). These disorders in the newborn puppy or kitten are usually incompatible with life unless corrected surgically.

Enterocolitis

Enterocolitis frequently occurs in dogs and cats from the time of weaning through adulthood. Enterocolitis is inflammation and mucosal damage that has occurred in response to an insult to the small and large intestine. Diarrhea is the primary sign of enterocolitis and often occurs secondary to many nonintestinal diseases. Diarrhea of young dogs and cats typically is of abrupt onset and has a short course that ranges from transient and self-limiting to fulminating and explosive. With the aid of history, physical examination, and stool characteristics (i.e., frequency, volume, consistency, color, odor, and composition), diarrhea can be localized to the small intestine, large intestine, or both (Table 10–5), and a search for the cause and treatment can be undertaken.

Causes. Enterocolitis is associated with many factors but more commonly results from dietary indiscretions, infectious diseases, and endoparasitism. Dietary causes may include intestinal overload from overeating; ingestion of rancid or spoiled foodstuffs from scavenging of decomposing garbage or carrion; ingestion of indigestible and abrasive foreign material, such as bones, rocks, plants, wood, cloth, thread and sewing needles (Felts et al, 1984), and plastic objects; intolerance of lactose ingested as milk; and intolerance of miscellaneous types of food, such as fatty or spicy food. The incidence of ingesting foreign objects is much higher for young dogs and cats, probably because of their developmental chewing habits and curious natures. Trichobezoars (hairballs) are frequently encountered in the diarrheic stools of long-haired cats and some dogs. Many drugs (e.g., corticosteroids, nonsteroidal antiinflammatory drugs, antimicrobial agents, and anthelmintics) and chemicals (e.g., heavy metals, cleaning agents, fertilizers, and herbicides) may cause enterocolitis (Atkins and Johnson, 1975; Harris, 1975). Many ingested plants and plant toxins may cause diarrhea and an associated enterocolitis.

Many infectious agents are generally associated with varying degrees of enterocolitis. Bacteria (e.g., *Salmonella* species, *Escherichia coli*, *Campylobacter* species, *Yersinia enterocolitica*, *Bacillus piliformis*, and *Clostridium perfringens*) reside in, and may contribute to severe mucosal damage in, the small and/or large intestine. Viruses (e.g., canine distemper virus, parvovirus-2, coronavirus, and rotavirus) are important causes of enterocolitis in young dogs. Other viruses that have been identified in unformed stools of dogs are a minute parvovirus (canine parvovirus-1), adenovirus, caliciviruses (Evermann et al, 1985), paramyxovirus-like virus, astrovirus, picornavirus, and human echovirus and coxsackievirus (Greene, 1990). Feline parvovirus-1 (feline panleukopenia virus) and coronaviruses are the most prominent viruses in young cats; other viruses have been identified,

Table 10–5	Differentiation of Small Intestinal Diarrhea from Large Intestinal Diarrhea	
SIGNS	**SMALL INTESTINE**	**LARGE INTESTINE**
Feces		
Volume	Always increased	Normal or increased (small quantities)
Mucus	Absent	Invariably present
Blood	Dark black (digested)	Red (fresh)
Fat droplets	Present with maldigestive or malabsorptive disease	Absent
Undigested food	May be present with maldigestion	Absent
Color	Color variations occur; lighter colored (e.g., creamy brown), orange, green, or gray	May appear bloody
Defecation		
Frequency	Normal or slightly increased	Very frequent
Urgency	Absent	Usually present
Tenesmus	Absent	Usually present
Associated Signs		
Vomiting	May be present	Uncommon
Generalized malaise	May be present	Uncommon
Flatulence and borborygmus	May be present	Absent
Belching	May be present	Uncommon
Altered breath odor in the absence of stomatitis	May be present	Absent
Weight loss or failure to gain weight	May be present	Uncommon

including rotavirus, astrovirus, calicivirus, reovirus type 3, and nonculturable enteric Picornaviridae-like virus (Greene, 1990). In refractory diarrheal problems, feline leukemia virus, feline immunodeficiency virus, and feline infectious peritonitis virus should be considered in the diagnosis. The primary fungi infecting the intestinal tract are *Histoplasma capsulatum*, *Aspergillus* species, and *Pythium* species; however, they are uncommon in dogs and cats younger than 6 months.

Endoparasites generally do not produce intestinal lesions but contribute importantly to generalized unthriftiness, diarrhea, and weight loss or failure to gain adequate body weight. The younger the animal, the more frequent are endoparasites present and the more severe the consequences of endoparasitism. Endoparasitism often complicates other existing intestinal disorders such as virus- or bacterial-induced enterocolitis. The more common endoparasites that are identified in the intestinal tract of young dogs and cats are listed in Table 10–6. Other disorders, including renal failure, liver disease, neurologic disease, shock, sepsis, hypoadrenocorticism, stress, and even altered behavior, may play a prominent role in the cause of enterocolitis (Strombeck and Guilford, 1990).

Diagnosis. The diagnosis of acute enterocolitis is usually made on the basis of an animal's history, signs, and physical findings, often without detailed diagnostic procedures. A review of the animal's vaccination status, diet, current medications, and possible exposure to chemicals or infectious diseases is warranted. Endoparasites, ingestion of questionable food or foreign material, and/or infectious diseases should always be considered the primary cause of enterocolitis in the young dog or cat until proved otherwise. Animals that experience severe illness or fail to respond to symptomatic therapy usually require a more detailed medical and laboratory evaluation. Diagnostic efforts should then be aimed at detection of an underlying nonintestinal disease as the contributing cause of the diarrhea. Diagnostic evaluations considered for short-term diarrhea are fecal identification of endoparasites, virologic tests, fecal cultures for bacteria, and survey abdominal radiographs for detection of intestinal foreign material or an obstruction.

Treatment. Enterocolitis is generally treated on the basis of the animal's history, signs, and physical findings. Symptomatic treatment is given initially for most cases of enterocolitis and diarrhea without extensive diagnostic procedures. Most animals with enterocolitis show improvement within 24 to 48 hours with little or no therapy and usually are treated on an outpatient basis. The basic principles in the treatment of enterocolitis include removing the inciting cause; providing proper conditions to promote mucosal repair; correcting fluid, electrolyte, and acid-base abnormalities; and alleviating secondary complications of enterocolitis, such as vomiting, abdominal pain, and infection.

Dietary restriction is the initial step in the management of enterocolitis. Animals with severe intestinal disturbances should be deprived of food for 24 to 48 hours or longer. Water may be offered in small amounts during the first 24 hours. If the animal is vomiting, however, water should be restricted. Restriction of food and possibly water allows for restoration of mucosal integrity and a more rapid return of gastrointestinal function. In most cases, fasting reduces or eliminates diarrhea by removing the osmotic or irritating effects of undigested or unabsorbed nutrients. If no diarrhea has occurred during the 24- to 48-hour fast, small amounts of a highly digestible, low-fiber, moderately low-fat diet are fed three to six times daily, such as cooked rice or cooked cereals supplemented in a 4:1 ratio with low-fat cottage cheese, lean boiled ground beef or chicken, or commercial baby foods. Commercial diets formulated for gastrointestinal disease may also be prescribed. With the commercial diets, the animal is first fed one third the amount needed

Table 10–6	Common Endoparasites Associated with Enterocolitis

Helminths

Ascarids: *Toxocara canis*, *Toxocara cati*, and *Toxascaris leonina*

Hookworms: *Ancylostoma caninum*, *Ancylostoma tubaeforme*, *Ancylostoma braziliense*, and *Uncinaria stenocephala*

Whipworms: *Trichuris vulpis* (puppies older than 4 mo of age)

Tapeworms (cestodes): *Dipylidium caninum* and *Taenia* species

Strongyloides: *Strongyloides stercoralis* (*S. canis*, *S. felis*) and *Strongyloides tumefaciens*

Flukes: *Nanophyetus salmincola* and *Alaria* species

Protozoa

Coccidia: *Cystoisospora* (*Isospora*) species, *Toxoplasma gondii*, and *Cryptosporidium* species

Giardia species

Pentatrichomonas (*Trichomonas*) species

to meet normal maintenance caloric needs. Over the next several days, the amount of food is gradually increased to meet the animal's needs in order to maintain body weight.

Parenteral fluids are initiated when electrolyte or acid-base imbalances or dehydration occurs. The quantity of fluids given should be enough to supply daily maintenance needs (approximately 40 to 60 ml/kg per day), to correct existing dehydration, and to replace fluid losses that may occur with continued diarrhea and vomiting. Diarrhea in enterocolitis generally results in volume depletion and losses of sodium, chloride, bicarbonate, and potassium with metabolic acidosis. An isotonic, balanced electrolyte solution such as lactated Ringer's solution is usually recommended (Twedt and Grauer, 1982). Potassium levels are often depleted, particularly if inappetence has accompanied profuse diarrhea, and additional potassium chloride should be added to the fluids. The amount of potassium chloride added is based on the existing serum potassium levels.

Protectants are used frequently in the general treatment of diarrhea, although they are probably not beneficial in animals (DeNovo, 1986). There is, however, some evidence that pectin plus salicylates can absorb and inactivate enterotoxins, such as those produced by *Escherichia coli*. Of the salicylates, bismuth subsalicylate appears to be more effective as an oral antidiarrheal compound. The dose is about 0.25 ml/kg body weight divided into four to six equal daily doses. Bismuth subsalicylate probably should be administered with caution in cats because of their increased sensitivity to aspirin and should not be administered to cats younger than 3 months of age. Its taste is unpleasant, but some of the resistance to administration may be overcome by keeping the product in the refrigerator and administering it cold.

The use of narcotic analgesics as antimotility drugs is warranted in the treatment of some diarrheas (see Table 10–4). The rationale behind their use is based on their direct action on the smooth muscle of the small intestine and colon, causing increasing tone and segmentation (DeNovo, 1986). This produces increased resistance to luminal transit of ingesta. These drugs effectively relieve abdominal pain and tenesmus and reduce the frequency of stools. Anticholinergic and related antispasmodic drugs have an uncertain role in the management of diarrhea. Anticholinergic drugs block the effect of acetylcholine, the major neurotransmitter of the gastrointestinal smooth muscle, resulting in both decreased peristalsis and decreased segmenta-

tion. With their use, motility of the small intestine and colon can be stopped, which allows the occurrence of bacterial overgrowth, thus compounding the hypomotility and possibly the diarrhea problem. Therefore, the narcotic analgesics, such as diphenoxylate hydrochloride and loperamide hydrochloride, are the preferred motility modifiers to be used in the symptomatic treatment of diarrhea. If the diarrhea is caused by an infectious agent such as *Salmonella*, the narcotic analgesics may be detrimental because they may trap organisms and their toxins within the intestine, and the infection may persist longer.

Because of the frequent occurrence of endoparasites as the primary or secondary cause of enterocolitis in the young dog or cat, routine administration of an appropriate antiparasitic drug is recommended. Currently available antiparasitic drugs for dogs and cats are listed in Table 10–7. The use of antimicrobial agents in the treatment of diarrhea is controversial. If antimicrobial agents only succeed in inhibiting the normal intestinal flora, they are detrimental. In diarrhea, antimicrobial therapy is warranted only when there is evidence of inflammation in the gastrointestinal tract (numerous inflammatory cells in the feces), damaged intestinal mucosa (blood in the stool), a systemic inflammatory reaction (fever and leukocytosis), and/or abnormal fecal culture results (Strombeck and Guilford, 1990).

Protein-Losing Enteropathy

Causes. Protein-losing enteropathies are characterized by the loss of protein into the intestinal lumen. Causes of protein-losing enteropathies in young dogs and cats include congenital lymphangiectasia, congestive heart failure, and infectious inflammatory and ulcerative enteric diseases. Congenital lymphangiectasia results from malformation of the lymphatic system; it rarely occurs in puppies and kittens. Two breeds of dogs are reported to be predisposed to a form of lymphangiectasia and protein-losing enteropathy, that is, the Norwegian lundehund (Flesja and Torstein, 1977) and the basenji (Breitschwerdt et al, 1984). In the Norwegian lundehund, the disorder appears to have a hereditary basis and is characterized by intermittent diarrhea, vomiting, weight loss, anorexia, hypoalbuminemia, ascites, and edema.

In the basenji, the lymphangiectasia occurs secondary to a unique intestinal disease that has been referred to as *immunoproliferative enteropathy of basenjis* (Breitschwerdt et al, 1984). This

Table 10-7	Antiparasitic Drugs for Dogs and Cats		
GENERIC NAME	**INDICATIONS**	**DOSAGE***	**COMMENTS**
Albendazole	*Giardia*	25 mg/kg PO twice a day for four doses	Cessation of diarrhea within 72 h of initiation of treatment; not routinely recommended in dogs because of possible bone marrow toxicosis
Amprolium	Coccidia	Capsule or feed: 6-wk-old puppies of small breeds, one 100-mg capsule containing 20% amprolium soluble powder daily for 7–10 d; 200 mg for puppies of large breeds; capsule contents can be added to food Drinking water: 7.8 ml of 9.6% amprolium solution is mixed in 1 liter drinking water for 7–10 d; no other source of water is provided	Either regimen can be used for treatment or prevention (especially before stress when shipping kenneled puppies); amprolium is a thiamine inhibitor; side effects (neural disturbances, anorexia, diarrhea) are rare
Butamisole hydrochloride	Hookworms, whipworms	2.4 mg/kg SC	Approved for dogs; do not use in heartworm-positive or debilitated dogs or in puppies less than 8 wk of age
Dichlorvos	Hookworms, ascarids, whipworms	Dogs: 27–33 mg/kg Puppies and cats: 11 mg/kg	Contraindicated in heartworm disease, liver or kidney damage, and severe diarrhea accompanied by anemia and lethargy in puppies with hookworms; do not use in conjunction with other cholinesterase inhibitors; split-dosage schedule should be used for heavily parasitized, anemic, or debilitated animals; do not use in animals weighing less than 0.9 kg (2 lb) or under 10 d of age
Diethylcarbamazine	Heartworm prevention, ascarids	6.6 mg/kg PO as a heartworm-preventive drug	Adult ascarid burden is diminished when it is given as a heartworm-preventive drug; contraindicated if microfilaremia is present
Epsiprantel	Tapeworms	Dogs: 5 mg/kg PO Cats: 2.5 mg/kg PO	Minimally absorbed after oral administration; do not use in kittens and puppies less than 7 wk of age

Table continued on following page

Table 10–7	Antiparasitic Drugs for Dogs and Cats *Continued*		
GENERIC NAME	**INDICATIONS**	**DOSAGE***	**COMMENTS**
Febantel	Ascarids, hookworms, whipworms, *Taenia* tapeworms, *Giardia*	Mature dogs and cats: 10 mg/kg Puppies and kittens: 15 mg/kg given once daily for 3 consecutive days	Not labeled for use in dogs and cats; administer to adults by mouth or in food without regard to feeding schedule; administer only by mouth on full stomach to puppies and kittens less than 6 mo of age
Febantel and praziquantel	Ascarids, hookworms, whipworms, tapeworms, *Giardia*	Mature dogs and cats: 10 mg/kg febantel and 1 mg/kg praziquantel given once daily for 3 consecutive days Puppies and kittens: 15 mg/kg febantel and 1.5 mg/kg praziquantel given once daily for 3 consecutive days	Administer to adults by mouth or in food without regard to feeding schedule; administer only by mouth on full stomach to puppies and kittens less than 6 mo of age
Fenbendazole	Hookworms, ascarids, whipworms, *Taenia* tapeworms, *Giardia*	50 mg/kg/day for 3–7 consecutive days	No known contraindications in either dogs or cats
Ivermectin	Hookworms, ascarids, whipworms; heartworm prevention	200 µg/kg PO	Not approved for use in dogs and cats as intestinal dewormer; not effective for tapeworms, flukes, or protozoa; may be contraindicated in collies; monthly dose for heartworm prevention is 6.0 µg/kg PO for dogs and 24 µg/kg PO for cats
Mebendazole	Hookworms, ascarids, whipworms, *Taenia* tapeworms	22 mg/kg in food once daily for 3 consecutive days	Occasionally in dogs, hepatic dysfunction, sometimes fatal, especially following retreatment
Metronidazole	*Giardia, Balantidium, Entamoeba, Trichomonas*	30 mg/kg PO once daily for 10–14 consecutive days	Cessation of diarrhea within 72 h of initiation of treatment; may split the daily dosage into two doses, especially for puppies and kittens
Milbemycin oxime	Heartworm prevention; aids in control of hookworms, whipworms, and ascarids	0.5 mg/kg PO	Dosed on a monthly basis; contraindicated if microfilaremia is present
Moxidectin	Heartworm prevention	3 µg/kg	Used as a monthly heartworm preventive drug; can be used in puppies 8 wk and older

Table continued on opposite page

Table 10–7	Antiparasitic Drugs for Dogs and Cats *Continued*		
GENERIC NAME	**INDICATIONS**	**DOSAGE***	**COMMENTS**
Oxibendazole and diethylcarbamazine citrate	Hookworms, whipworms, ascarids; heartworm prevention	5 mg oxibendazole/kg and 6.6 mg diethylcarbamazine/kg PO daily	Used as a heartworm preventive drug; aids in control of hookworms, whipworms, and ascarids; contraindicated if microfilaremia is present; occasionally in dogs, hepatic dysfunction, sometimes fatal; can be used in puppies 8 wk and older
Piperazine salts	Ascarids	45–65 mg base/kg PO; maximum of 150 mg for puppies under 2.5 kg and for cats and kittens	No contraindications except long-standing renal or liver disease
Praziquantel	Tapeworms	Dogs: 5 mg/kg, single PO, SC, or IM dose Cats: 11 mg total (1–3 lb), 22 mg total (3–11 lb), or 33 mg total (>11 lb)	Effective against tapeworm larvae in many intermediate hosts; 10 mg/kg required for *Echinococcus* juveniles; not intended for use in puppies less than 4 wk of age or kittens less than 6 wk of age
Pyrantel pamoate	Hookworms, ascarids	15 mg/kg in tablet or suspension	Used in dogs and cats of all ages, including nursing young; no known contraindications for either dogs or cats
Quinacrine hydrochloride	*Giardia, Trichomonas*	6.6 mg/kg PO twice a day for 5 d	Not approved for use in dogs or cats; cholinesterase inhibitor; may cause anorexia, fever, and lethargy
Selamectin	Heartworm prevention; aids in control of hookworms and ascarids	6 mg/kg applied topically at the base of the neck	Dosed on a monthly basis; contraindicated if microfilaremia is present; recommended for use in dogs and cats 6 wk of age and older
Sulfadiazine and trimethoprim	Coccidia	30 mg/kg daily for 7–10 days (may be divided into two doses for administration)	Folic acid inhibitor; generally no contraindications for treatment of coccidia in the well-hydrated dog or cat; efficacy of treatment for coccidia is questionable
Sulfadimethoxine	Coccidia	55 mg/kg daily the first day; 25 mg/kg once daily for 14–20 d thereafter (may be divided into two doses for administration)	Folic acid inhibitor; generally no contraindications for treatment of coccidia in the well-hydrated dog or cat; efficacy of treatment for coccidia is questionable

Table continued on following page

Table 10-7	Antiparasitic Drugs for Dogs and Cats *Continued*		
GENERIC NAME	**INDICATIONS**	**DOSAGE***	**COMMENTS**
Thenium closylate	Hookworms	1 tablet (500 mg) for dogs over 5 kg (10 lb) regardless of weight; 1/4 tablet (125 mg) for 2.5–5 kg (5–10 lb)	Recently weaned puppies respond better to split-dose administration (twice daily); cannot give to nursing puppies or those less than 2.3 kg (5 lb); do not feed milk or other fatty foods during treatment; occasionally deaths (Airedales); some vomiting and hypersalivation
Thenium closylate and piperazine phosphate	Hookworms, ascarids	2 doses, 8 h apart; each dose: 0.9–2.3 kg (2–5 lb), 1/2 tablet; 2.3–4.5 kg (5–10 lb), 1 tablet; 4.5 kg (10 lb), 2 tablets. First dose AM before feeding; feed between first and second doses; no milk or fatty foods	Cannot use in puppies less than 5 wk of age or those less than 0.9 kg (2 lb); some vomiting and hypersalivation
Thiabendazole	*Strongyloides*	50–100 mg/kg once daily PO for 3–5 d	To check results of treatment, examine stools passed on 2–3 consecutive days because larvae are discharged sporadically; no known contraindication in either dogs or cats
Tinidazole	*Giardia, Trichomonas*	44 mg/kg PO once a day for 3 d	Very effective for *Trichomonas* and somewhat effective for *Giardia*; no known contraindication in either dogs or cats

*PO = oral administration; SC = subcutaneous administration; IM = intramuscular administration.

Retreatment is advisable to kill mature worms that were immature larvae during earlier treatments. Retreatment schedule: *Hookworms*—for litter from a bitch that previously lost puppies from hookworm anemia or heavily parasitized puppies, treat weekly for 5–6 treatments, beginning at 2 wk of age; others, retreat in 2–3 wk. *Ascarids*—for puppies and kittens with heavy ascarid infection, treat every week for 3–4 treatments, beginning at 2 wk of age; for older animals retreatment is done in 3–4 wk. *Whipworms*—for severe infections, retreat in 2–4 wk; recheck at 3-mo intervals. *Tapeworms*—retreatment is in 3–4 wk, and for *Dipylidium caninum* infection, flea eradication program is enforced. *Strongyloides*—repeat treatment monthly if needed.

disorder appears to have a hereditary basis and is characterized by bouts of intermittent diarrhea, weight loss, hypoalbuminemia, hyperglobulinemia (an unusual finding in protein-losing enteropathy), and widespread lymphocytic-plasmacytic infiltration of the gastrointestinal tract. In puppies, swelling of buccal lymph nodes, adverse effects from routine vaccinations, and transient neurologic signs are additional features of the disorder. Neurologic signs may include incoordination, paresis, seizures, and contracture of the facial musculature.

Diagnosis. The diagnosis of protein-losing enteropathy and lymphangiectasia is established by the animal's history, signs, physical findings, and histologic confirmation of the characteristic lesions in intestinal biopsy specimens (Sherding, 1986). Biopsy specimens may be obtained via laparotomy or less invasively by endoscopy or peroral suction biopsy capsule. Surgery in dogs with severe hypoalbuminemia or emaciation is not without risk. Full-thickness surgical biopsy tissue from the intestine often leads to dehiscence of the enterotomy incisions and postoperative peritonitis; serosal patching at incisional sites may be needed. Thus, when possible, biopsies performed via endoscopy or suction biopsy capsule are preferred over full-thickness biopsies.

With congenital protein-losing enteropathy and lymphangiectasia, carrier dogs may be subclinically affected well into breeding age. A developed fecal enzyme-linked immunosorbent assay (ELISA) can be used in early screening of potential breeding animals and for puppies as young as 3 months. In testing progeny of affected dogs, results of the fecal ELISA become abnormal well before identifiable hypoalbuminemia occurs. This ELISA measures naturally occurring fecal α_1-protease inhibitor in freshly passed stool samples—three consecutive bowel movements are submitted to the diagnostic laboratory for fecal ELISA testing. The assay quantifies the concentration of α_1-protease inhibitor, the second most abundant plasma protein in dogs. Normal concentrations of this fecal protein are less than 6 $\mu g/g$ of feces.

Treatment. The primary therapy for protein-losing enteropathies is to decrease the intestinal loss of plasma proteins so that normal serum protein levels can be restored and edema and effusions controlled. Dietary manipulation and elimination of the underlying cause of the protein-losing enteropathy are the primary methods used in its treatment (Tams and Twedt, 1981). The preferred diet for young dogs and cats with protein-losing enteropathy should contain minimal fat and provide an ample amount of high-quality protein. Commercial diets formulated for gastrointestinal diseases or commercial diets formulated for weight reduction may be prescribed. These diets should be supplemented with the fat-soluble vitamins and be divided into three or more feedings daily.

Low-fat diets are inherently low in calories; yet another part of therapy is to reverse the weight loss and malnourishment that usually accompany protein-losing enteropathies (Sherding, 1986). As an immediate caloric source, medium-chain triglycerides can be added to the diet to replace the calories lost by removal of fat from the diet. Commercially available medium-chain triglycerides are derived from coconut oil and can be added to the daily diet as an oil (e.g., MCT, Mead Johnson Nutritionals; 8.3 kcal/g; 1 tbsp weighs 14 g and contains 115 kcal, to be given at a dosage of 1 to 2 ml/kg body weight) or as a powdered elemental diet mixture (e.g., Portagen, Mead Johnson Nutritionals; 1 1/2 cups added to water to make 1 quart of mixture with 30 kcal/fl oz). Excessive intake of these medium-chain triglyceride products may contribute to vomiting or aggravate diarrhea.

In addition to dietary manipulation, protein-losing enteropathies often improve with antiinflammatory doses of corticosteroids, such as oral prednisolone at an initial dosage of 2 to 3 mg/kg per day. Once remission has been achieved, this dosage is adjusted to a lower maintenance level. Other measures may need to be considered in the unique enteropathy of the basenji. In addition to dietary management and corticosteroids, reduction of stress and short-term use of antimicrobial agents for the control of bacterial overgrowth of the intestinal tract may be needed. When protein-losing enteropathies occur secondary to an identifiable anatomic lymphatic (malformation) obstruction, surgical intervention for relief of the obstruction should be considered.

Wheat-Sensitive Enteropathy in Irish Setters

A wheat-sensitive enteropathy has been identified in Irish setter dogs that is characterized by poor weight gain or weight loss and bouts of intermittent diarrhea, with an onset of signs typically between 4 and 7 months of age (Batt, 1986). In this disorder, morphologic changes in the mucosa of the small intestine, as determined by mucosal biopsies, are variable; changes appear patchy within individual animals and consist of partial villous atrophy with no remarkable alterations in the cellular components of the lamina propria. Specific activities of important brush-border enzymes of the villus are selectively decreased, and this is probably responsible for hypersensitivity to various components in dietary wheat (Batt et al, 1984). Thus the diarrheal disorder is attributed more to brush-border enzyme abnormalities than to specific morphologic changes in the small intestinal mucosa. Dietary management is the most practical approach to its diagnosis and treatment. A wheat-sensitive enteropathy can usually be determined by a positive response to removal of wheat from the diet and return of signs when wheat is reintroduced.

Selective Cobalamin Malabsorption in Giant Schnauzers and in Border Collie Dogs

A selective cobalamin malabsorption disorder has been identified in giant schnauzer and in border collie dogs that is characterized by poor weight gain or weight loss and bouts of lethargy and inappetence, with an onset of signs typically between 3 and 6 months of age (Fyfe et al, 1989). There is a defect in transport of intrinsic factor/cobalamin complex receptor to the ileal brush-border membrane. All other nutrients are absorbed normally. In addition, a moderate nonregenerative anemia with marked aniso-cytosis, occasional megaloblasts, and moderate poikilocytosis, as well as a neutropenia with occasional hypersegmented neutrophils, are noted. Serum cobalamin levels are low, and urine samples contain large amounts of methylmalonic acid. Parenteral, but not oral, administration of vitamin B_{12} (0.25 to 1 mg weekly for 1 month, then every 3 to 6 months) reverses all hematologic and clinical abnormalities. Serum cobalamin levels should be monitored every 6 to 12 months or if signs occur. Affected animals should not be bred.

Enteropathy of Chinese Shar-Peis

Enteropathy has been identified in Chinese shar-pei dogs that is characterized by poor weight gain or weight loss and bouts of intermittent diarrhea, with an onset of signs typically between 2 and 6 months of age. Small intestinal biopsy samples are necessary for diagnosis; most severe cases show eosinophilic and lymphocytic-plasmacytic infiltrates of the intestine. Determination of serum cobalamin and folate concentrations may also be helpful in identifying bacterial overgrowth problems. Elimination diets and immunosuppressive therapy are the most practical approach to treatment. A guarded prognosis is always warranted.

Intestinal Obstruction

Partial and complete luminal obstructions of the intestine, particularly of the small intestine, are frequently seen in dogs and cats younger than 6 months. Ingested foreign object(s) and intussusception are the most frequent causes of these luminal obstructions.

Ingested Foreign Objects. Foreign object(s) ingested by a dog or cat may pass through the pylorus but have difficulty in passing aborally through the intestinal tract, commonly lodging in the jejunum. Foreign objects that are likely to be ingested include stones, coins, pecans, plastic and rubber objects, and jewelry. Whether partial or complete luminal obstruction occurs depends on the shape and size of the foreign object and on whether the object is stationary or is slowly progressing aborally. Once an object is able to pass through the ileocolic junction into the large intestine, signs of obstruction usually abate, and the object passes without complication.

Sharp objects (e.g., pins, tacks, needles, wooden or plastic splinters, and even fishhooks) may pass aborally through the intestine of a young dog or cat without evidence of piercing the intestinal wall or lodging within its lumen. If the owner or veterinarian elects not to surgically remove a sharp intestinal foreign object, the animal should be monitored continually for progression of obstructive signs via serial abdominal radiographs to ensure uncomplicated passage of the object. If the foreign object ceases to move, perforation should be suspected, and immediate surgical intervention is warranted. Passage of a sharp object through the ileocolic junction into the large intestine does not necessarily ensure that the object will be eliminated without complications because penetration of the colon or rectum may still occur.

Linear foreign objects present as a peculiar problem because they can cause extensive damage to the intestine (Basher and Fowler, 1987; Felts et al, 1984). Large sections of small intestine may be involved, and perforation and secondary peritonitis may occur. Linear foreign objects that are commonly ingested include elastic string, elastic binding from a golf ball, fishing line, cord, shoelaces, dental floss, pantyhose, fabric, and Christmas tree decorations. For a linear foreign object to cause problems, it must become fixed at some cranial site within the alimentary tract. Usually the object is either looped around the base of the tongue (Fig. 10–26) or lodged at the pylorus. Intestinal motility then propels the rest of the trailing object in an aboral direction through the intestine. Because the object is fixed cranially, motility of the small intestine is unable to move the luminal object into the large intestine. Consequently, the small intestine moves cranially over the fixed object, with resultant pleating or bunching of the intestine over the linear object, creating a partial or complete intestinal obstruction, multiple perforation sites, and either localized or generalized peritonitis (Fig. 10–27). Cats are much more likely than dogs to ingest linear foreign objects.

Diagnosis. Signs associated with the ingestion of foreign objects are variable and may include vomiting, diarrhea, depression and weakness, dehydration, partial or complete inappetence, abdominal distention, and abdomi-

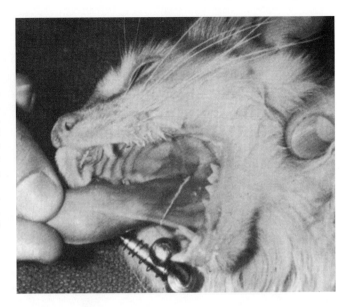

Figure 10–26. Linear intestinal objects such as thread are often looped around the base of the tongue in cats and can be detected by thorough examination under the tongue. The free end of the thread is swallowed and passes into the intestine with resultant pleating or bunching of the intestine over the thread. (From Sherding RG: Diseases of the small bowel. *In* Ettinger SJ [ed]: Textbook of Veterinary Internal Medicine, vol 2, 2nd ed. Philadelphia, WB Saunders, 1983, p 1338.)

nal pain. Usually, vomiting is the primary sign of a foreign object–induced intestinal obstruction. Luminal obstruction of the duodenum and jejunum (cranial to middle jejunal obstruction) results in immediate, frequent vomiting, whereas distal jejunal, ileal, or colonic obstruction results in less frequent vomiting that may be delayed for several days (Strombeck and Guilford, 1990). Complete luminal obstruction produces persistent vomiting, whereas partial obstruction usually causes intermittent vomiting. Vomiting increases in frequency as the obstruction progresses. The presence of bile in vomitus suggests that the obstruction is distal to the point where the bile duct enters into the duodenum. Feculent vomitus is indicative of intestinal stasis and lower intestinal obstructions.

Diarrhea often occurs with partial intestinal obstruction but rarely occurs with a complete obstruction. Abdominal pain that may also be present is evidenced by restlessness, unusual posture, or resistance to abdominal palpation. Many foreign objects are detectable during physical examination by gentle, thorough palpation of the abdomen (Strombeck and Guilford, 1990). It may be possible to repeatedly palpate a foreign object and the distended intestine cranial to the object. Palpation of pleated loops of small intestine warrants a thorough reexamination of the oral cavity, especially at the base of the tongue, for evidence of a linear object being fixed at that site. Occasionally, the linear object may have cut deeply into the base of the tongue, leaving only a reddened ulcerative lesion visible around the frenulum.

Radiopaque foreign objects are easily found on survey abdominal radiographs (Gomez, 1974). Gastric distention is usually evident if an obstruction is present. Linear foreign objects appear as gathered small intestinal segments with foci of asymmetric distention and distinctive gas and fluid interphases (see Fig. 10–27). Any loss of abdominal detail with or without peritoneal free gas accumulation should heighten suspicion of the presence of intestinal wall perforation. At times, especially with a partial obstruction or radiolucent foreign object, a positive contrast study may be required (Kealy, 1987). Caution should be exercised when positive contrast material is used; if intestinal perforation is suspected, a water-soluble contrast medium should be used instead of barium sulfate.

Treatment. The primary treatment of a foreign object–induced intestinal obstruction is removal of the obstructing object. However, animals with obstructions are often metabolically unstable. Immediate management is directed toward correcting fluid, electrolyte, and acid-base imbalances and treating any accompanying septicemia and shock (Richardson, 1981). Intravenous balanced electrolyte fluid therapy, such as lactated Ringer's solution, is started immediately to correct most of the animal's fluid deficits before surgical intervention. At the same time, broad-spectrum antimicrobial agents that are effective against the indigenous intestinal microflora, both gram-positive and gram-negative aerobic and anaerobic organisms, are given with the parenteral fluids. A combination of penicillin derivatives or cephalosporins and aminoglycosides is recommended. In uncomplicated for-

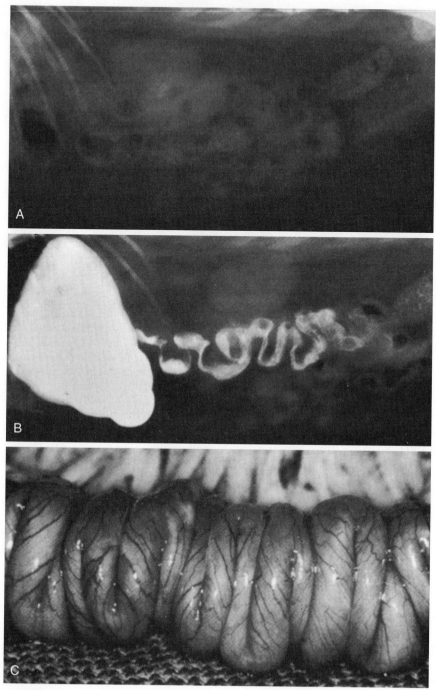

Figure 10–27. A, A lateral abdominal radiograph of a young cat with anorexia, vomiting, and abdominal pain shows bunching of intestinal loops into the midabdomen and eccentrically located gas bubbles in the lumen. These findings suggest a radiolucent linear foreign object. **B,** The diagnosis is confirmed by a contrast study showing characteristic gathered small intestinal segments. **C,** The bunching or pleating caused by the linear foreign object is seen at surgery. (From Sherding RG: Diseases of the small bowel. *In* Ettinger SJ [ed]: Textbook of Veterinary Internal Medicine, vol 2, 2nd ed. Philadelphia, WB Saunders, 1983, p 1339.)

eign object–induced intestinal obstruction with minimal vascular compromise and surgical contamination, antimicrobial therapy is generally required for only the immediate perioperative period, the first 12 to 24 hours. If the obstruction is complicated by shock, devitalized intestine, and peritonitis, however, a longer period of antimicrobial therapy is required.

The method used for surgical relief of an intestinal obstruction caused by foreign object(s) depends on several factors (Bojrab, 1986). Small objects can usually be removed through a single enterotomy. The enterotomy should be performed caudal to the obstructing object in healthy tissue to decrease the possibility of postoperative complications due to dehiscence at the enterotomy site. Large foreign objects may require intestinal resection and anastomosis, especially if the intestine is dark and friable (Bojrab, 1986). When possible, the first step should be to remove the foreign object(s) through a caudal enterotomy and suture the incision. The involved intestinal segment can then be wrapped in a warm, saline-moistened sponge for 3 to 5 minutes. If blood flow and motility do not return to the involved segment after this time, a resection to healthy tissue is warranted.

A short linear foreign object may be removed through a single enterotomy (Richardson, 1981). If the linear object is long, it should be removed through several small enterotomies along the antimesenteric border. A long linear foreign object should never be removed through a single enterotomy site. While the linear object is being pulled through the single enterotomy, it frequently cuts through the mesenteric border of the intestinal wall. Small perforations must then be debrided and closed and subsequently checked to ensure that they have been satisfactorily closed. It is always important to thoroughly palpate the stomach and the noninvolved intestinal segments for other foreign object(s) after the primary obstructing object(s) have been removed (Bojrab, 1986).

After the intestinal obstruction is relieved, intravenous fluid therapy is continued until oral alimentation can be reinstituted. Oral alimentation is usually started during the first postoperative day. Small amounts of water are offered initially. If vomiting does not occur, a highly digestible food is offered three or four times daily in small amounts. Intestinal motility usually returns to near-normal state by the first or second postoperative day. As oral intake increases, fluid therapy support is gradually decreased. Fluid therapy is not terminated until

the animal is adequately maintaining itself by oral alimentation and obstructive signs have ceased. Evidence of dehiscence at the enterotomy or anastomosis site usually becomes apparent by the second to fourth postoperative day. Failure to eat and other signs of peritonitis such as fever, vomiting, and abdominal pain are suggestive of intestinal dehiscence (Richardson, 1981). With debilitated animals, serial postoperative CBCs and determinations of blood glucose levels and blood gas and electrolyte determinations should be done. The heart should be monitored daily for the first week after surgery, as cardiac arrhythmias of ventricular origin are not uncommon after intestinal obstruction (Bojrab, 1986).

Intussusception. Intussusception is also commonly seen as a cause of intestinal obstruction in the young dog and occasionally in the young cat (Wilson and Burt, 1974; Wolfe, 1978). In addition, an intussusception may occur in a recently born puppy or kitten and contribute to the fading puppy or kitten syndrome. The ileocolic junction is the most common site of intussusception, which also occurs in decreasing frequency in the ileum, jejunum, cecum, and duodenum.

Causes. Abnormal intestinal motility is thought to lead to the development of an intussusception. Irritation of the intestinal mucosa due to disorders such as intestinal parasitism, virus-induced or bacteria-induced enteritis, and acute inflammatory disorders or to orally administered drugs and anthelmintics may contribute to abnormal intestinal motility and the intussusception.

Diagnosis. The presence of a palpable cylindric mass together with abdominal pain, vomiting, and passage of mucus and/or blood in the stool are usually diagnostic. Tenesmus may also occur with the diarrhea. If the intussusception has prolapsed through the anus, it must be differentiated from a rectal prolapse; this is done by passing a finger or blunt probe into the rectum between the mass and rectal wall. If the mass is a prolapsed intussusception, the probe or finger may be inserted a considerable distance. An intussusception is confirmed with abdominal radiographs (Kealy, 1987). Results of survey radiographs depend on whether the intussusception is causing a complete or a partial obstruction. If the obstruction is complete, dilated gas-filled and fluid-filled loops of intestine are seen cranial to the intussusception, and the colon is void of feces. If the obstruction is partial, there is little, if any, distention of the intestine, and feces are usually present in the colon. The intussusception itself may not be seen owing to its fluid density and to the overlapping density of fluid-filled intestine. Probably the better method of demonstrating a nonopaque intussusception is via barium enema (Fig. 10–28) (Kealy, 1987) or abdominal ultrasonography.

Treatment. When an intussusception is diagnosed, surgical intervention is warranted. It is also important to determine the inciting cause of the intussusception and to eliminate it, if possible. If the intussusception is due to altered motility secondary to parasite-induced enteritis, the appropriate anthelmintic should be administered. The ability to manually reduce an intus-

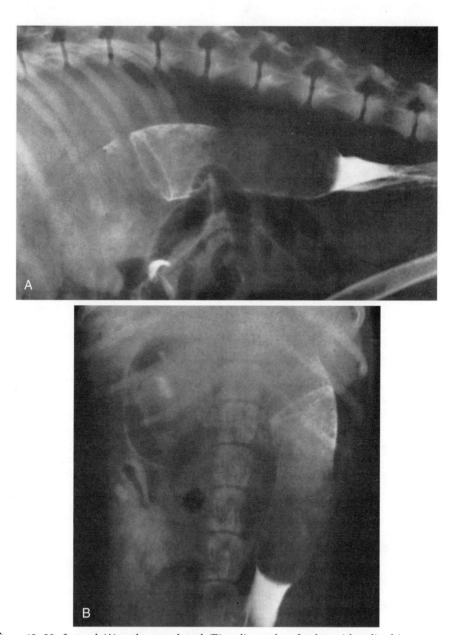

Figure 10–28. Lateral **(A)** and ventrodorsal **(B)** radiographs of a dog with a distal intussusception. The intussusception is demonstrated by barium enema, which is the most satisfactory method of diagnosing this condition. (From Kealy JK: Diagnostic Radiology of the Dog and Cat, 2nd ed. Philadelphia, WB Saunders, 1987, p 93.)

susception at surgery depends on its duration (Fig. 10–29). One hand is used to hold the ensheathing layer (intussuscipiens), while the other hand pushes the apex of the invaginating layer (intussusceptum) cranially and exerts gentle traction on the intestine cranial to the intussusception (Bojrab, 1986). After manual reduction of the intussusception, the intestine and mesentery are carefully checked for viability. If the involved segment is nonviable, then that segment should be resected and the remaining ends anastomosed. In intussusceptions of longer duration, manual reduction may be impossible. Adhesions often develop as a result of vascular damage and production of a fibrinous exudate

from the serosal surfaces. With time, the compromised circulation causes an ischemic necrosis and often a localized peritonitis. In those cases in which manual reduction is impossible because of adhesions or if the segment of intestine is no longer viable, resection and anastomosis are warranted (Bojrab, 1986).

The most frequent postoperative complication, barring intestinal dehiscence and peritonitis, is the recurrence of the intussusception because of existing intestinal irritation and/or altered motility (Bellenger et al, 1982; Wolfe, 1977). This may occur whether manual reduction or intestinal resection was performed. If the intussusception recurs, it may be helpful to

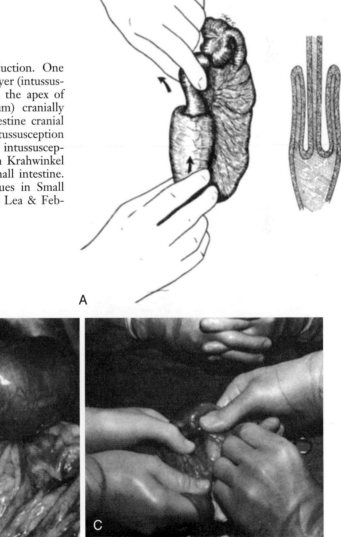

Figure 10–29. A, Intussusception reduction. One hand is used to hold the ensheathing layer (intussuscipiens) while the other hand pushes the apex of the invaginating layer (intussusceptum) cranially and exerts gentle traction on the intestine cranial to the intussusception. B, Actual intussusception found on celiotomy. C, Reduction of intussusception by technique shown in A. (From Krahwinkel DJ Jr, Richardson DC: Surgery of small intestine. In Bojrab MJ [ed]: Current Techniques in Small Animal Surgery, 2nd ed. Philadelphia, Lea & Febiger, 1983.)

double the intestine upon itself so that the portion causing the problem lies at the turn of a U-shaped segment (Engen, 1983). The serosa of the segments cranial and caudal to the site of the intussusception is sutured together at the antimesenteric border with absorbable suture material. Three loops of plicated bowel should be used cranial and caudal to the intussusception (Fig. 10–30).

Fecal Impaction

Causes. Fecal impactions resulting from a mixture of feces and nondigestible hair or bones are the most common cause of infrequent defecation in dogs and cats younger than 6 months. Other causes of fecal impaction may include ingested foreign objects, narrowed pelvic canal after traumatically induced fractured pelvis, collapsed pelvic canal associated with pathologic fractures due to nutritional imbalances, and congenital defects and inflammatory disease of the rectum and anus. Of these, foreign objects and fractured pelvis are the more likely causes of fecal impaction.

Diagnosis. Animals with fecal impaction

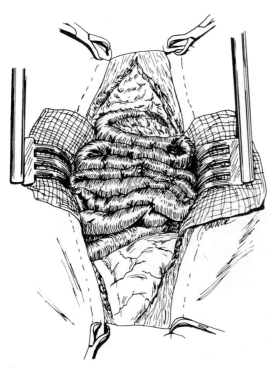

Figure 10–30. Bowel plication after resection of anastomosis to prevent recurrent intussusception. (From Engen MH: Bowel plication for preventing recurrent intussusception. *In* Bojrab MJ [ed]: Current Techniques in Small Animal Surgery, 2nd ed. Philadelphia, Lea & Febiger, 1983.)

usually have a history of failure to defecate for days. The owner may have observed the animal making frequent, unsuccessful attempts to defecate and, in some cases, straining to pass small amounts of liquid feces, often containing blood or mucus. Some animals have the misleading complaint of diarrhea. The disruption and irritation of the intestinal mucosa promote secretion and accumulation of fluid that cannot penetrate the densely packed fecal materials and thus produce diarrhea. If defecation has not been observed, the animal may be brought to the veterinarian because it is depressed, listless, inappetent or anorexic, and vomiting intermittently (Burrows, 1986).

Animals presenting with fecal impaction are generally dehydrated. Cats may assume a crouching, hunched attitude indicative of abdominal pain, and obvious abdominal distention is observed occasionally. Abdominal palpation typically reveals hard fecal mass(es) that may fill the entire length of the large intestine. Rectal examination combined with abdominal palpation is useful in determining the amount of feces retained and compressibility of the material present and possibly in identifying the underlying cause of the fecal impaction, such as foreign object(s) or a narrowed pelvic canal. Survey abdominal radiographs confirm the presence of fecal impaction and any opaque foreign object(s).

Treatment. The treatment of fecal impaction consists of gentle removal of impacted fecal material and, if possible, identification and removal of the underlying cause (Burrows, 1986). The animal with mild to moderate fecal impaction can generally be treated with oral laxatives and frequent small-volume enemas. The animal with more severe fecal impaction is often dehydrated and requires fluid replacement therapy for dehydration and electrolyte imbalances before correction of the fecal impaction is attempted. Breakdown and removal of the impacted fecal mass(es) should be accomplished as slowly and gently as possible. It is less traumatic for the young animal if the fecal mass(es) are softened and removed over 2 or 3 days than if removal of all the fecal impaction is attempted at one time. In dogs and cats older than 4 months with mild to moderate fecal impaction, after fluid replacement therapy has been accomplished, oral administration of a colon electrolyte lavage preparation such as Colyte (Reed & Carnrick) or NuLytely (Braintree Laboratories), about 20 to 30 ml/kg body weight every 12 hours, can be used for completing the removal of residual feces.

Laxatives. Laxatives are mild in their effects and usually cause elimination of formed feces. Their effects depend on dosage; major drugs and dosages are presented in Table 10–4. The dioctyl sodium sulfosuccinate and dioctyl calcium sulfosuccinate laxatives act as detergents to alter the surface tension of liquids and promote emulsification and softening of the feces by facilitating the mixture of water and fat. The animal should be well hydrated before compounds containing these substances are administered (Burrows, 1986). They should not be administered in conjunction with mineral oil, because they aid in the absorption of the mineral oil.

Mineral oil (liquid petrolatum) and white petrolatum are nondigestible and poorly absorbed laxatives. They soften feces by coating them to prevent colonic absorption of fecal water and promote easy evacuation. A small amount of oil absorption does occur, but the primary danger of giving mineral oil is laryngotracheal aspiration. Bulk-forming laxatives such as psyllium and bran increase the frequency of evacuation of the upper large intestine via stimulation produced by added bulk or volume. They soften feces by the retention of water (Burrows, 1986). Metamucil, which contains natural psyllium and generic bran, is best given with moistened food to ensure a high degree of water intake.

Another useful laxative is bisacodyl; this compound exerts its action on colonic mucosa and intramural nerve plexuses (Burrows, 1986). It should be given only to well-hydrated animals older than 4 months and is contraindicated when obstruction is present. Lactulose, a synthetic disaccharide of galactose and fructose, may be used for its laxative effects in the young dog and cat. After oral administration, lactulose is metabolized to organic acids by intestinal bacteria and promotes an osmotic catharsis of feces. The dose is individualized on the basis of stool consistency and is titrated until a semiformed stool is obtained, two to three soft bowel movements per day. Overdosage may induce intestinal cramping (colic signs), profuse diarrhea, flatulence, dehydration, and acidosis.

Enemas. Enemas act by softening feces in the distal region of the large intestine, stimulating colonic motility and the urge to defecate. The enema fluid used should be at room temperature or tepid. Tap water, normal saline solution, and sodium biphosphate solution add bulk; petrolatum oils soften, lubricate, and promote the evacuation of hardened fecal material; and soap-sud solutions promote defecation by their irritant action (Burrows, 1986). Tepid normal saline solution and tap water (about 5 ml/kg body weight) are generally preferred for enemas in animals younger than 6 months. If these are ineffective, a soapy water solution can be used after ensuring that the animal is well hydrated. About 5 ml/kg body weight of a mild soap solution is slowly instilled through a lubricated enema tube. In general, better results with normal saline solution, tap water, or soapy water enemas are obtained if the enema is repeated several times using small volumes. Small volumes are retained for longer periods, allowing time to soften and break down fecal impactions. Sodium phosphate retention enemas are convenient preparations for the relief of fecal impaction. Their use in young dogs and cats is absolutely contraindicated, however, in that they cause marked hyperphosphatemia, hypernatremia, and hypocalcemia (Atkins, 1986).

Prevention. After the successful relief of fecal impaction, attention is directed to the prevention of recurrence. If possible, nondigestible materials should be eliminated from the diet, regular grooming instituted, and the opportunity for regular defecation provided. In all instances, the goal should be to have the animal pass soft, formed feces and to defecate regularly. Commercial veterinary laxatives containing petrolatum as their active ingredient are useful for preventing minor hair impaction in cats.

Rectal Prolapse

Cause. Rectal prolapse is the protrusion of one or more layers of the rectum from the anal orifice. The degree of rectal prolapse can vary, from protrusion of the mucosal layer at the anal orifice to full-thickness extrusion of several centimeters of the rectum through the anal orifice. Rectal prolapse commonly occurs in dogs and cats that are experiencing habitual or continual straining; therefore, obvious causes of straining to void feces or urine should be evaluated. Any defect in the supporting structures of the anorectum or disturbance of the anal sphincters such as innervation disorders will predispose the dog or cat to a rectal prolapse. In dogs and cats younger than 6 months, rectal prolapses of only the mucosal layer are most often associated with severe diarrhea. Soiling of the perianal area and diarrhea may create considerable straining to void feces and result in a rectal prolapse of the mucosa. Foreign objects, such as needles or bones, that lodge in the rectum may also contribute to severe straining, leading to rectal prolapse of the mucosa. If the underlying cause of a rectal prolapse is not eliminated, the prolapsed mucosa may quickly convert into a full-thickness extrusion of the rectum.

Diagnosis. A rectal prolapse of only the mucosal layer assumes a swollen donut shape as it protrudes from the anal orifice. If all the layers are involved, the prolapsed rectum takes on a more cylindric shape. A rectal prolapse can be mistaken for a rare intussusception of a more cranial section of the intestine that has prolapsed through the anal orifice. Differentiation between rectal prolapse and intussusception is made by attempting to insert a finger or blunt probe between the mucocutaneous junction of the anus and protruding bowel. If the finger or blunt probe is easily passed, an intussusception is present; if resistance is met, a rectal prolapse has occurred (Seim, 1986).

Treatment. A rectal prolapse does not occur without cause. Failure to identify and treat the underlying cause of rectal prolapse often results in its unsuccessful treatment. The initial treatment should include fluid replacement therapy for dehydration and electrolyte disturbances, symptomatic control of diarrhea, and administration of appropriate medication in the case of parasitic or bacterial enterocolitis. The rectal prolapse itself can be managed by several methods, including reduction and purse-string suture, amputation, and colopexy (Seim, 1986). The method selected depends on the viability of the prolapsed tissue, the size and reducibility of the prolapse, and recurrence after a previous method has failed. Edematous but viable prolapsed tissue appears moist and varies from pink to dark red. Mucosa that is irreversibly damaged or necrotic appears leather-like and may be purple or black. With the animal under general anesthesia, a minor rectal prolapse of viable mucosa may be reduced manually and maintained by a purse-string suture in the anus for about 7 days, leaving a small orifice for stool passage. The small orifice is created by drawing the purse-string suture closed around a 4-inch rectal thermometer or another object of similar diameter. Desiccants such as hypertonic solutions of glucose or granulated sugar can be applied on the prolapsed tissue to reduce the edema before reduction and placement of the purse-string suture. Topical anesthetic ointment with 1% dibucaine can be instilled in the rectum postoperatively and continued for 2 or 3 days after removal of the purse-string suture (Seim, 1986).

A nonreducible rectal prolapse with necrosis of the mucosa is best managed by full-thickness amputation and anastomosis. A nonreducible viable prolapse or a recurrent rectal prolapse that fails to respond to more conservative treatment may be treated by celiotomy and colopexy (Seim, 1986). For the colopexy, scarified surfaces of the descending colon and the sublumbar body wall are sutured together with several interrupted mattress stitches of nonabsorbable suture material, attaching the submucosal layer of the colon to the muscles of the abdominal wall. Topical anesthetic ointment is instilled rectally after colopexy and continued for 5 or 6 days postoperatively.

THE ANUS

Congenital Anorectal Anomalies

Congenital anorectal anomalies that are infrequently identified in the young dog and cat include imperforate anus, segmental aplasia, rectovaginal fistula, rectovestibular fistula, anovaginal cleft, and rectal urethral fistula (Osborne et al, 1975; Rawlings, 1977; Rawlings and Capps, 1971; Seim, 1986; Wilson and Clifford, 1975). Of these anomalies, imperforate anus, although rarely seen, is the most common. Puppies or kittens with congenital anorectal anomalies usually are presented to a veterinarian because of an absence of defecation, obvious defect in the anatomy of the perineal structures, or voiding of urine or feces through an inappropriate orifice (Chambers, 1986). A distended abdomen often accompanies these anomalies if obstruction is present. The anorectal anomalies occasionally go unnoticed until the animal is several weeks old and may not be readily apparent from the appearance of the perineum.

Imperforate Anus

Often with the imperforate anus, an anal dimple is present ventral to the base of the tail, showing where the anal orifice should have been. The colon is distended with feces and gas if any degree of obstruction is present, and fecal impaction may be severe enough to cause abdominal distention. The presence or absence of voluntary bladder function and an external anal sphincter should be evaluated in the animal presenting with imperforate anus. The presence and function of the external anal sphincter muscle can be evaluated by pinching the bulb of the penis or vulva and watching carefully for an anal wink (bulbourethral reflex) (Oliver and Selcer, 1974). If the sphincter is present and functional, the prognosis for surgical correction is much better.

Imperforate anus encompasses several types of congenital deformity (Seim, 1986). Imperforate anus type 1 results from a failure of perforation of the anal membrane. Treatment consists of simply rupturing the membrane and trimming the excess tissue. A 4-inch rectal thermometer is used to ensure that the anal opening is adequate. Imperforate anus type 2 (also referred to as *atresia ani*) results from failure of the cloacal membrane to rupture, leaving a relatively thick membrane covering the anal orifice (Fig. 10–31). The anal sphincter is usually intact and functional. Treatment is directed at locating the anal dimple, dissecting the membrane to the level of the rectal mucosa, and suturing the mucosa to the subcutaneous tissue and skin. A convenient way of excising the anal membrane and exposing the underlying rectum is to make two incisions at right angles to each other, forming a " + " centered on the anal dimple (Chambers, 1986). The four angled skin flaps thus formed are undermined and excised. The subcutaneous tissue is bluntly separated, and the blind-ended rectum is isolated and gently pulled toward the anus with forceps or stay sutures. The end of the rectum is then incised, and the mucosa is apposed to the skin with simple, interrupted stitches of absorbable suture material.

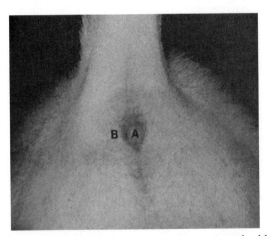

Figure 10–31. Imperforate anus in a 4-week-old puppy. Persistent cloacal membrane (**A**) and bulging perineum (**B**) are shown. (From Greiner TP, Johnson RG, Betts CW: Diseases of the rectum and anus. *In* Ettinger SJ [ed]: Textbook of Veterinary Internal Medicine, vol 2, 2nd ed. Philadelphia, WB Saunders, 1983, p 1500.)

Imperforate anus type 3 (also referred to as *rectal agenesis*) results when the rectum ends blindly at a variable distance from the anal membrane. A lateral abdominal radiograph with the animal's hindquarters slightly elevated will allow visual observation of gas in the termination of the rectum (Seim, 1986). The distance from the rectum to the anal membrane allows differentiation between imperforate anus types 2 and 3. Treatment requires a combined abdominal and perineal surgical approach (Seim, 1986). The distal region of the rectum is exposed abdominally and then delivered through the pelvic canal to an opening made in the anal dimple. Rectal mucosa is then sutured to the subcutaneous tissue and skin in the perianal region. Animals may remain fecal incontinent after surgical correction.

Imperforate anus may be associated with other anorectal anomalies, especially of the genitourinary tract, with the rectum opening into the vagina, urinary bladder, or urethra (Fig. 10–32) (Rawlings and Capps, 1971; Suess et al, 1992). The age and size of a dog or cat with imperforate anus or its combination of concurrent anorectal anomalies make surgical correction difficult because of the complications that may occur postoperatively. The prognosis is good if the animal survives the immediate postoperative period (Greiner, 1972).

Anovaginal and Rectovaginal Fistulas

Correction of anovaginal and rectovaginal fistulas that are predominately cosmetic problems should be delayed until the puppy or kitten is 12 to 16 weeks of age (Chambers, 1986). Contrast radiography is needed to establish the presence and position of fistulas between the anorectum and urogenital tract before surgical correction is attempted. Fistulas require lengthy dissection procedures and general anesthesia. Most of these fistulas can be isolated through a vertical midline perineal incision from the ventral region of the anus to the vulva (Chambers, 1986). Gentle blunt dissection is used to separate the supporting tissue between the rectum and urogenital tract. Once isolated, the fistula is excised, and the lumina of the anorectum and urogenital tract are closed separately with simple interrupted stitches of 4-0 or 5-0 synthetic absorbable suture material. If the anorectum is malpositioned, it is relocated in the center of the external anal sphincter muscle, and the mucosa is sutured to the skin circumferentially with simple interrupted stitches of the same suture material. The fecal impaction is relieved manu-

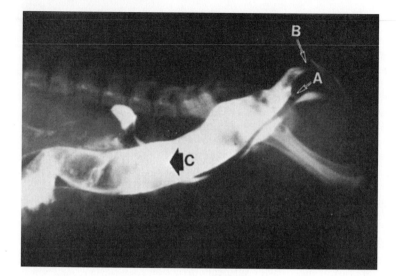

Figure 10–32. Lateral radiograph of vaginogram of a 4-week-old Chihuahua with imperforate anus and dribbling of liquid stool from the vulva. Note the rectovaginal fistula **(A)**, imperforate anus **(B)**, and megacolon **(C)**. (From Chambers JN: Surgical diseases of the anorectum. *In* Jones BD, Liska WD [eds]: Canine and Feline Gastroenterology. Philadelphia, WB Saunders, 1986, p 291.)

ally and with judicious use of enemas. The large intestine often is atonic and may require intermittent evacuation until normal defecation is established.

References and Supplemental Reading

Ader PL: Phycomycosis in fifteen dogs and two cats. J Am Vet Med Assoc 174:1216, 1979.

Alexander JW, Hoffer RE, MacDonald JM, et al: Hiatal hernia in the dog: A case report and review of literature. J Am Anim Hosp Assoc 11:793, 1975.

Arnall L: Some aspects of dental development in the dog. II. Eruption and extrusion. J Small Anim Pract 1:259, 1961a.

Arnall L: Some aspects of dental development in the dog. III. Some common variations in the dentitions. J Small Anim Pract 1:195, 1961b.

Atkins CE: Hypertonic sodium phosphate enema intoxication. *In* Kirk RW (ed): Current Veterinary Therapy IX. Philadelphia, WB Saunders, 1986, p 212.

Atkins CE, Johnson RK: Clinical toxicities of cats. Vet Clin North Am 5:623, 1975.

Baldwin S: Feline enteric diseases. *In* Kirk RW (ed): Current Veterinary Therapy VIII. Philadelphia, WB Saunders, 1983, p 1168.

Basher AWP, Fowler JD: Conservative versus surgical management of gastrointestinal linear foreign bodies in the cat. Vet Surg 16:135, 1987.

Batt RM: Wheat-sensitive enteropathy in Irish setters. *In* Kirk RW (ed): Current Veterinary Therapy IX. Philadelphia, WB Saunders, 1986, p 893.

Batt RM, Carter MW, McLean L: Morphological and biochemical studies of a naturally occurring enteropathy in the Irish setter dog: A comparison with coeliac disease in man. Res Vet Sci 37:339, 1984.

Bedford PGC: Unilateral parotid hypersialism in a dachshund. Vet Rec 107:557, 1980.

Bellenger CR, Middleton DJ, Ilkiw JE, et al: Double intussusception followed by reintussusception in a kitten. Vet Rec 110:323, 1982.

Bennett IC, Law DB: Incorporation of tetracycline into developing dog enamel and dentin. J Dent Res 44:780, 1965.

Berman E: The time and pattern of eruption of the permanent teeth of the cat. Lab Anim Sci 24:929, 1974.

Boehringer BT: Pyloric stenosis in a kitten. Feline Pract 3:12, 1973.

Bojrab MJ: Surgery of the small intestine. *In* Jones BD, Liska WD (eds): Canine and Feline Gastroenterology. Philadelphia, WB Saunders, 1986, p 203.

Boudrieau RJ, Rogers WA: Megaesophagus in the dog: A review of 50 cases. J Am Anim Hosp Assoc 21:33, 1985.

Bredal WP, Thoresen SI, Rimstad E, et al: Diagnosis and clinical course of canine oral papillomavirus infection. J Small Anim Pract 37:138, 1996.

Breitschwerdt EB, Ochoa R, Barta M, et al: Clinical and laboratory characterization of the basenji dog with immunoproliferative small intestinal disease. Am J Vet Res 45:267, 1984.

Brizzee KR, Vitale D: Functional development of the emetic apparatus in the cat. Am J Physiol 196:1189, 1959.

Burrows CF: Constipation. *In* Kirk RW (ed): Current Veterinary Therapy IX. Philadelphia, WB Saunders, 1986, p 904.

Chambers JN: Surgical diseases of the anorectum. *In* Jones BD, Liska WD (eds): Canine and Feline Gastroenterology. Philadelphia, WB Saunders, 1986, p 279.

Cheville NF: The gray collie syndrome. J Am Vet Med Assoc 152:6, 1968.

Clifford DH, Soifer FK, Wilson CF, et al: Congenital achalasia of the esophagus in four cats of common ancestry. J Am Vet Med Assoc 158:1554, 1971.

Cox VS, Wallace LJ, Anderson VE, et al: Hereditary

esophageal dysfunction in the miniature schnauzer dog. Am J Vet Res 41:326, 1980.

Coyler F: Variations and Diseases of the Teeth of Animals. London, John Bale Sons and Danielsson, 1936.

Davis LE: Pharmacologic control of vomiting. J Am Vet Med Assoc 176:241, 1980.

DeHoff WD: Surgery of the stomach. In Jones BD, Liska WD (eds): Canine and Feline Gastroenterology. Philadelphia, WB Saunders, 1986, p 134.

DeNovo RC Jr: Therapeutics of gastrointestinal diseases. In Kirk RW (ed): Current Veterinary Therapy IX. Philadelphia, WB Saunders, 1986, p 862.

Diamant N, Szczepanski M, Mui H: Idiopathic megaesophagus in the dog: Reasons for spontaneous improvement and possible method of medical therapy. Can Vet J 15:66, 1974.

Dillon AR: The oral cavity. In Kirk RW (ed): Current Veterinary Therapy VII. Philadelphia, WB Saunders, 1980, p 855.

Dillon AR: The oral cavity. In Jones BD, Liska WD (eds): Canine and Feline Gastroenterology. Philadelphia, WB Saunders, 1986, p 1.

Dubielzig RR, Goldschmidt MH, Brodey RS: The nomenclature of periodontal epulides in dogs. Vet Pathol 16:209, 1979.

Dubielzig RR, Higgins RJ, Krakowka S: Lesions of the enamel organ of developing dog teeth following experimental inoculation of gnotobiotic puppies with canine distemper virus. Vet Pathol 18:684, 1981.

Ellison GW: Surgical correction of persistent right aortic arch. In Bojrab MJ, Ellison GW, Slocum B (eds): Current Techniques in Small Animal Surgery, 4th ed. Baltimore, Williams & Wilkins, 1998, p 659.

Engen MH: Bowel plication for preventing recurrent intussusception. In Bojrab MJ (ed): Current Techniques in Small Animal Surgery, 2nd ed. Philadelphia, Lea & Febiger, 1983, p 183.

Evermann JF, McKeirnan AJ, Smith AW, et al: Isolation and identification of caliciviruses from dogs with enteric infections. Am J Vet Res 46:218, 1985.

Felts JF, Fox PR, Burk RL: Thread and sewing needles as gastrointestinal foreign bodies in the cat: A review of 64 cases. J Am Vet Med Assoc 184:56, 1984.

Figueiredo C, Barros HM, Alvares LC, et al: Composed complex odontoma in a dog. Vet Med Small Anim Clin 69:268, 1974.

Flesja K, Torstein YRI: Protein-losing enteropathy in the lundehund. J Small Anim Pract 18:11, 1977.

Foil CSO, Short BG, Fadok VA, et al: A report of subcutaneous pythiosis in five dogs and a review of the etiologic agent Pythium spp. J Am Anim Hosp Assoc 20:959, 1984.

Fukata T: Esophageal diverticulum-like pouch in a cat with allergic bronchitis. Vet Med Small Anim Clin 79:175, 1984.

Fyfe JC, Jezyk PF, Giger U, et al: Inherited selective malabsorption of vitamin B_{12} in giant schnauzers. J Am Anim Hosp Assoc 25:533, 1989.

Gaillard ET, Hargis AM, Prieur DJ, et al: Pathogenesis of feline gastric chlamydial infection. Am J Vet Res 45:2314, 1984.

Gaskell CJ, Gibbs C, Pearson H: Sliding hiatus hernia with reflux esophagitis in two dogs. J Small Anim Pract 15:503, 1974.

Geake CI: Odontogenic cyst in a puppy. Vet Med Small Anim Clin 77:1626, 1982.

Glenn BL, Glenn HG, Omtvedt IT: Congenital porphyria in the domestic cat (Felis catus): Preliminary investigations on inheritance pattern. Am J Vet Res 29:1653, 1968.

Gomez JA: The gastrointestinal contrast study. Methods and interpretation. Vet Clin North Am 4:805, 1974.

Gourley IN, Leighton RL: Surgical treatment for cricopharyngeal achalasia in the dog. Pract Vet 44:11, 1972.

Greene CE: Infectious Diseases of the Dog and Cat. Philadelphia, WB Saunders, 1990.

Greiner TP: Surgery of the rectum and anus. Vet Clin North Am 2:167, 1972.

Harpster NK: The cardiovascular system. In Holzworth J (ed): Diseases of the Cat: Medicine and Surgery. Philadelphia, WB Saunders, 1987, p 820.

Harris WF: Clinical toxicities in dogs. Vet Clin North Am 5:605, 1975.

Harvey CE: Parotid gland enlargement and hypersialosis in a dog. J Small Anim Pract 22:19, 1981.

Harvey CE: Oral, dental, pharyngeal, and salivary gland disorders. In Ettinger SJ (ed): Textbook of Veterinary Internal Medicine, vol 2. Philadelphia, WB Saunders, 1989, p 1203.

Harvey CE, O'Brien JA, Durie VR, et al: Megaesophagus in the dog: A clinical survey of 79 cases. J Am Vet Med Assoc 165:443, 1974.

Hoffer RE: Primary esophageal neuromuscular diseases. In Jones BD, Liska WD (eds): Canine and Feline Gastroenterology. Philadelphia, WB Saunders, 1986, p 81.

Hooft J, Mattheeuws D, Van Bree P: Radiology of deciduous teeth resorption and definitive teeth eruption in the dog. J Small Anim Pract 20:175, 1979.

Houlton JEF, Herrtage ME, Taylor PM, et al: Thoracic oesophageal foreign bodies in the dog: A review of ninety cases. J Small Anim Pract 26:521, 1985.

Jakowski RM: Duplication of colon in a Labrador retriever with abnormal spinal column. Vet Pathol 14:256, 1977.

Jurkiewicz MJ, Bryant DL: Cleft palate in dogs: A progress report. Cleft Palate J 5:30, 1968.

Kealy JK: Diagnostic Radiology of the Dog and Cat, 2nd ed. Philadelphia, WB Saunders, 1987.

Key DM: Dilation and torsion of the stomach in a cat. Feline Pract 7:38, 1977.

Kipnis RM: Megaesophagus: Remission in two dogs. J Am Anim Hosp Assoc 14:247, 1978.

Kratochvil Z: Oligodonty and polydonty in the domestic and wild cat. Acta Vet Brno 40:33, 1971.

Ladds PW, Anderson NV: Atresia ilei in a pup. J Am Vet Med Assoc 158:2071, 1971.

Lantz GC: Treatment of gastric dilatation-volvulus. *In* Bojrab MJ, Ellison GW, Slocum B (eds): Current Techniques in Small Animal Surgery, 4th ed. Baltimore, Williams & Wilkins, 1998, p 223.

Lantz GC, Bojrab MJ, Jones BD: Epiphrenic esophageal diverticulectomy. J Am Anim Hosp Assoc 12:629, 1976.

Leib MS, Blass CE: Gastroesophageal intussusception in a dog: A review of the literature and a case report. J Am Anim Hosp Assoc 20:783, 1984.

Leipold HW: Nature and causes of congenital defects of dogs. Vet Clin North Am 8:47, 1977.

Lewis LD, Morris ML Jr, Hand MS: Small Animal Clinical Nutrition. Topeka, KS, Mark Morris Associates, 1987.

Lyon KF: Approach to feline oral disease. J Vet Dent 5:11, 1988.

Madewell BR, Stannard AA, Pulley LT, et al: Oral eosinophilic granuloma in Siberian husky dogs. J Am Vet Med Assoc 177:701, 1980.

Martin JE: Atresia jejuni in a puppy. J Am Anim Hosp Assoc 13:728, 1977.

Moraes Barros PS, Alvarenga J, d'Auria E, et al: Ranula in a cat. Mod Vet Pract 66:413, 1985.

Morris EL, Turnwald GH: What is your diagnosis? Gastroesophageal intussusception. J Am Vet Med Assoc 176:361, 1980.

Mullen HS: Atresia of the colon in a 52-day-old puppy. Vet Med Small Anim Clin 77:1621, 1982.

Nold JB, Powers BE, Eden EL, et al: Ameloblastic odontoma in a dog. J Am Vet Med Assoc 185:996, 1984.

Oliver JE Jr, Selcer RR: Neurogenic disorders of the rectum and anal sphincter. Vet Clin North Am 4:551, 1974.

Osborne CA, Clifford DH, Jessen CR: Hereditary esophageal achalasia in dogs. J Am Vet Med Assoc 151:572, 1967.

Osborne CA, Engen MH, Yano BL: Congenital urethrorectal fistula in two dogs. J Am Vet Med Assoc 166:999, 1975.

Patterson DV: Epidemiologic and genetic studies of congenital heart disease in the dog. Circ Res 23:171, 1968.

Pearson H, Gaskell CJ, Gibbs C, et al: Pyloric and oesophageal dysfunction in the cat. J Small Anim Pract 15:487, 1974.

Pearson H, Gibbs C, Kelly DF: Oesophageal diverticulum formation in the dog. J Small Anim Pract 19:341, 1978.

Pedersen NC, Ho EW, Brown ML, et al: Isolation of a T-lymphotropic virus from domestic cats with an immunodeficiency-like syndrome. Science 235:790, 1987.

Poliak SC, DiGiovanna JJ, Gross EG, et al: Minocycline-associated tooth discoloration in young adults. J Am Med Assoc 254:2930, 1985.

Pope ER, Constantinescu GM: Repair of cleft palate. *In* Bojrab MJ, Ellison GW, Slocum B (eds): Current Techniques in Small Animal Surgery, 4th ed. Baltimore, Williams & Wilkins, 1998, p 113.

Potter KA, Tucker RD, Carpenter JL: Oral eosino-philic granuloma of Siberian huskies. J Am Anim Hosp Assoc 16:595, 1980.

Rawlings CA: Anovaginal and rectovaginal fistulas. *In* Bojrab MJ (ed): Current Techniques in Small Animal Surgery. Philadelphia, Lea & Febiger, 1977, p 161.

Rawlings CA, Capps WF: Rectovaginal fistula and imperforate anus in a dog. J Am Vet Med Assoc 159:320, 1971.

Rawlings CA, Wingfield WE, Betts CW: Shock therapy and anesthetic management of gastric dilatation-volvulus. J Am Anim Hosp Assoc 12:158, 1976.

Richardson DC: Intestinal surgery: A review. Compend Contin Educ Pract Vet 3:259, 1981.

Richardson RC, Jones MA, Elliott GS: Oral neoplasms in the dog: A diagnostic and therapeutic dilemma. Compend Contin Educ Pract Vet 5:441, 1983.

Rickards DA: Removal of persistent deciduous teeth in dogs. Canine Pract 6:46, 1979.

Robotham GR: What is your diagnosis; hiatal hernia. J Am Vet Med Assoc 170:1425, 1977.

Rogers WA, Fenner WR, Sherding RG: Electromyographic and esophagomanometric findings in clinically normal dogs and in dogs with idiopathic megaesophagus. J Am Vet Med Assoc 174:181, 1979.

Rosin E, Hanlon GF: Canine cricopharyngeal achalasia. J Am Vet Med Assoc 160:1496, 1972.

Ross DL: Occlusion in the dog. Southwest Vet 28:247, 1975a.

Ross DL: Veterinary dentistry. *In* Ettinger SJ (ed): Textbook of Veterinary Internal Medicine, vol 2. Philadelphia, WB Saunders, 1975b, p 1047.

Rossman LE, Garber DA, Harvey CE: Disorders of teeth. *In* Harvey CE (ed): Veterinary Dentistry. Philadelphia, WB Saunders, 1985, p 79.

Saperstein G, Harris S, Leipold HW: Congenital defects in domestic cats. Feline Pract 6:18, 1976.

Schneck GW: A case of enamel pearls in a dog. Vet Rec 92:115, 1973.

Scott DW, Walton DK, Slater MR, et al: Immune-mediated dermatoses in domestic animals: Ten years after. Part I. Compend Contin Educ Pract Vet 9:424, 1987a.

Scott DW, Walton DK, Slater MR, et al: Immune-mediated dermatoses in domestic animals: Ten years after. Part II. Compend Contin Educ Pract Vet 9:539, 1987b.

Scott FW: Feline respiratory viral infections. *In* Scott FW (ed): Contemporary Issues in Small Animal Practice, Infectious Diseases. New York, Churchill Livingstone, 1986, p 155.

Seim HB III: Diseases of the anus and rectum. *In* Kirk RW (ed): Current Veterinary Therapy IX. Philadelphia, WB Saunders, 1986, p 916.

Sharp NJH, Nash AS, Griffiths IR: Feline dysautonomia (the Key-Gaskell syndrome): A clinical and pathological study of forty cases. J Small Anim Pract 25:599, 1984.

Shelton GD: Swallowing disorders in the dog. Compend Contin Educ Pract Vet 4:607, 1982.

Sherding RG: Intestinal lymphangiectasia. *In* Kirk RW (ed): Current Veterinary Therapy IX. Philadelphia, WB Saunders, 1986, p 885.

Shulze C: Developmental abnormalities of the teeth and jaws. *In* Gorlin RJ, Goldman HM (eds): Thomas' Oral Pathology, 6th ed. St. Louis, CV Mosby, 1970.

Singer A: What is your diagnosis? Intussusception of stomach and spleen into esophagus. J Am Vet Med Assoc 167:951, 1975.

Smart ME, Fletch SM, Black F: Congenital absence of jejunum and ileum in two neonatal Alaskan malamute pups. Can Vet J 19:22, 1978.

Smith DM, Kirk GR, Shepp E: Maturation of the emetic apparatus in the dog. Am J Vet Res 35:1281, 1974.

Sokolovsky V: Cricopharyngeal achalasia in a dog. J Am Vet Med Assoc 150:281, 1967.

Stickle RL, Sparschu G, Love N, et al: Radiographic evaluation of esophageal function in Chinese sharpei pups. J Am Vet Med Assoc 201:81, 1992.

Strating A, Clifford DH: Canine achalasia with special reference to heredity. Southwest Vet 19:135, 1966.

Strombeck DR: Pathophysiology of esophageal motility disorders in the dog and cat. Vet Clin North Am 8:229, 1978.

Strombeck DR, Guilford WG: Small Animal Gastroenterology. Davis CA, Stonegate Publishing, 1990.

Strombeck DR, Troya L: Evaluation of lower motor neuron function in two dogs with megaesophagus. J Am Vet Med Assoc 169:411, 1976.

Suess RP Jr, Martin RA, Moon ML, et al: Rectovaginal fistula with atresia ani in three kittens. Cornell Vet 8:141, 1992.

Suter PF, Watrous BJ: Oropharyngeal dysphagias in the dog. A cinefluorographic analysis of experimentally induced and spontaneously occurring swallowing disorders. Vet Radiol 21:24, 1980.

Tams TR, Twedt DC: Canine protein-losing gastroenteropathy syndrome. Compend Contin Educ Pract Vet 3:105, 1981.

Todoroff RJ: Gastric dilatation-volvulus. Compend Contin Educ Pract Vet 1:142, 1979.

Twedt DG, Grauer GF: Fluid therapy for gastrointestinal, pancreatic and hepatic disorders. Vet Clin North Am 12:463, 1982.

Valentine BA, Lynch MJ, May JC: Compound odontoma in a dog. J Am Vet Med Assoc 186:177, 1985.

van der Gaag I, Tibboel D: Intestinal atresia and stenosis in animals: A report of 34 cases. Vet Pathol 17:565, 1980.

Wallace LJ: Cervical sialocele in a cat. J Am Anim Hosp Assoc 8:74, 1972.

Walter MC, Matthiesen DT, Stone EA: Pylorectomy and gastroduodenostomy in the dog: Technique and clinical results in 28 cases. J Am Vet Med Assoc 187:909, 1985.

Wardrip SJ: Cleft palate repair in a kitten. Vet Med Small Anim Clin 77:227, 1982.

Watrous BJ: Esophageal disease. *In* Ettinger SJ (ed): Textbook of Veterinary Internal Medicine, vol 2, 2nd ed. Philadelphia, WB Saunders, 1983, p 1191.

Watrous BJ, Suter PF: Normal swallowing in the dog. A cineradiographic study. Vet Radiol 20:99, 1979.

Weigel JP, Dorn AS: Diseases of the jaws and abnormal occlusion. *In* Harvey CE (ed): Veterinary Dentistry. Philadelphia, WB Saunders, 1985, p 106.

Wilson CF, Clifford DH: Perineoplasty for anovaginal cleft in a dog. J Am Vet Med Assoc 159:871, 1975.

Wilson GP, Burt JK: Intussusception in the dog and cat: A review of 45 cases. J Am Vet Med Assoc 164:515, 1974.

Wingfield WE, Cornelius LM, DeYoung DW: Experimental acute gastric dilation and torsion in the dog. I. Changes in biochemical and acid-base parameter. J Small Anim Pract 16:41, 1975.

Wingfield WE, Twedt DC: Medical diseases of the stomach. *In* Jones BD, Liska WD (eds): Canine and Feline Gastroenterology. Philadelphia, WB Saunders, 1986, p 101.

Wolfe DA: Recurrent intestinal intussusceptions in the dog. J Am Vet Med Assoc 171:553, 1977.

Wolfe DA: Compound intussusception in a kitten. Vet Med Small Anim Clin 73:455, 1978.

Woods CB, Rawlings C, Barber D, et al: Esophageal deviation in four English bulldogs. J Am Vet Med Assoc 172:934, 1978.

Zontine WJ: Effect of chemical restraint drugs on the passage of barium sulfate through the stomach and duodenum of dogs. J Am Vet Med Assoc 162:878, 1973.

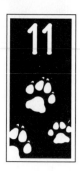

The Liver and Pancreas

Johnny D. Hoskins

THE LIVER AND HEPATOBILIARY DISORDERS

Laboratory Indicators of Hepatic Dysfunction

Liver Enzyme Activities. The serum activities of alanine aminotransferase (ALT) and aspartate aminotransferase (AST) in newborn and growing puppies and kittens are usually within the normal range or slightly higher than those of healthy adult dogs and cats (Keller, 1981). The serum alkaline phosphatase (ALP) and gamma-glutamyltransferase (GGT) activities of 1- to 10-day-old puppies are 20- to 25-fold greater than those of healthy adults. Selected laboratory values used as indicators of hepatobiliary dysfunction in newborn and growing puppies and kittens are listed in Table 11–1. The source of the profound ALP and GGT activity is probably of placental, colostral, and/or intestinal origin. These profound serum ALP and GGT activities after 10 to 14 days postpartum will decrease to moderately increased activities. Although the bone ALP isoenzyme derived from active osteoblast activity may increase the serum ALP activity in growing animals, the magnitude of increase usually is only two- to threefold the normal level (Center et al, 1995). Colostrum is rich in both ALP and GGT activity, and it is possible that these enzymes may be absorbed from the colostrum or intestinal tract during the first days of life. Alternatively, the ingestion of colostrum may stimulate intestinal growth and enzyme production. Therefore, colostrum-deprived puppies can be identified by their serum ALP and GGT activity level, particularly during the first week of life, as an indicator of successful ingestion of colostrum. Thus, increased serum ALP and GGT activities cannot be used in the diagnosis of acute liver dysfunction during the first 10 to 14 days of life. Such increases in serum ALP and GGT activities cannot be used to detect colostrum-deprived kittens.

Serum Bile Acids. Serum bile acids are used to identify hepatic and hepatoportal circulatory dysfunction. The use of the serum bile acid measurement as a test of hepatic dysfunction is of value for the young dog and cat using 12- to 24-hour fasted and 2-hour postprandial serum samples (Center et al, 1985a,b). The normal fasting and 2-hour postprandial values established for adults may be used for puppies and kittens as young as 4 weeks. This test is also reliable for detecting portal circulatory abnormalities (Center et al, 1986a; Meyer, 1986).

Extramedullary Hematopoiesis. Extramedullary hematopoiesis is commonly observed in the livers of the puppy and kitten through 4 months of age. In older puppies and kittens, disorders associated with blood loss and a subsequent need for erythron mass replenishment may also be associated with hepatic extramedullary hematopoiesis.

Developmental Malformations

Congenital Gallbladder Disorders. Congenital division of the gallbladder is the most common anomaly and has been referred to as an *accessory, cleft,* or *diverticular gallbladder* (Bartlett, 1951; Boyden, 1926). These anomalies may develop as an initial subdivision of the

200

	_____		PUPPIES				KITTENS	

Table 11–1 Normal Values for Serum Indicators of Hepatobiliary Disorders in Young Dogs and Cats (Median and Range)

TEST	1–3 Days (N = 30)	2 Weeks (N = 14)	4 Weeks (N = 7)	8 Weeks (N = 8)	Normal Adult Range	2 Weeks (N = 24)	4 Weeks (N = 8)	Normal Adult Range
Bile acids (μM/L)	<15	<15	<15	<15	0–15	ND	<10	0–10
Total bilirubin (mg/dl)	0.5 (0.2–1.0)	0.3 (0.1–0.5)	0 (0–0.1)	0.1 (0.1–0.2)	0–0.4	0.3 (0.1–1.0)	0.2 (0.1–0.2)	0–0.2
ALT (IU/L)	69 (17–337)	15 (10–21)	21 (20–22)	21 (9–24)	12–94	18 (11–24)	16 (14–26)	28–91
AST (IU/L)	108 (45–194)	20 (10–40)	18 (14–23)	22 (10–32)	13–56	18 (8–48)	17 (12–24)	9–42
ALP (IU/L)	3845 (618–8760)	236 (176–541)	144 (135–201)	158 (144–177)	4–107	123 (68–269)	111 (90–135)	10–77
GGT (IU/L)	1111 (163–3558)	24 (4–77)	3 (2–7)	1 (0–7)	0–7	1 (0–3)	2 (0–3)	0–4
Total protein (g/dl)	4.1 (3.4–5.2)	3.9 (3.6–4.4)	4.1 (3.9–4.2)	4.6 (3.9–4.8)	5.4–7.4	4.4 (4.0–5.2)	4.8 (4.6–5.2)	5.8–8.0
Albumin (g/dl)	2.1 (1.5–2.8)	1.8 (1.7–2.0)	1.8 (1.0–2.0)	2.5 (2.1–2.7)	2.1–2.3	2.1 (2.0–2.4)	2.3 (2.2–2.4)	2.3–3.0
Cholesterol (mg/dl)	136 (112–204)	282 (223–344)	328 (266–352)	155 (111–258)	103–299	229 (164–443)	361 (222–434)	150–270
Glucose (mg/dl)	88 (52–127)	129 (111–146)	109 (86–115)	145 (134–272)	65–110	117 (76–129)	110 (99–112)	63–144

ALT = Alanine aminotransferase; AST = aspartate aminotransferase; ALP = alkaline phosphatase; GGT = gamma-glutamyltransferase; ND = not determined.

From Center SA, Hornbuckle WE: New York State College of Veterinary Medicine—1987. Cornell University, Ithaca, NY.

primary cystic diverticulum of the embryo or as a bud from the neck of the embryonic gallbladder. The gallbladder may become trilobed or bilobed (Fig. 11–1). Other anomalies include accessory gallbladders; the development of two separated gallbladders with cystic ducts uniting in a common duct; ductular bladders developing as supernumerary vesicles derived from either hepatic, cystic, or common bile ducts; and trabecular bladders derived from vesicular outgrowths of liver trabeculae. These malformations are infrequently associated with signs of hepatobiliary dysfunction in puppies and kittens.

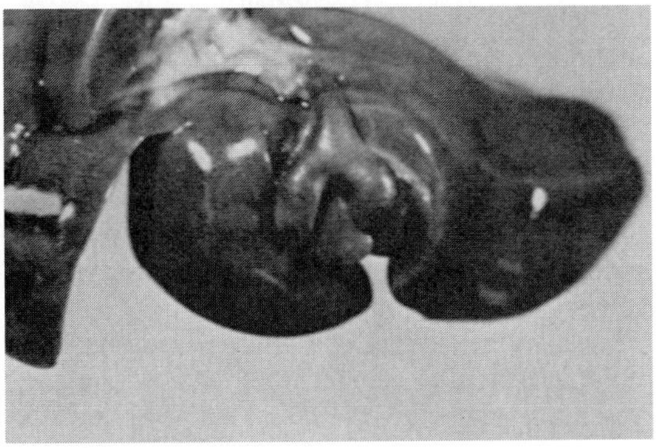

Congenital Hepatic Cysts. Congenital hepatic cysts are infrequently found in the young dog and cat (Black, 1983; Crowell et al, 1979; McKenna and Carpenter, 1980). Cystic lesions may be parenchymal or ductal in origin and may be either solitary or multiple (polycystic). Cystic lesions vary in size from a few millimeters to several centimeters. Congenital hepatic cysts are typically asymptomatic. Rarely, fluid may accumulate in the abdominal cavity as a consequence of cyst rupture or portal hypertension resulting from impingement of major vessels. Cyst contents are usually a clear or modified transudate, although cysts may contain bile or blood. Acquired hepatic cysts are usually solitary, whereas congenital or developmental he-

Figure 11–1. A bilobed gallbladder represents a developmental anomaly in a cat.

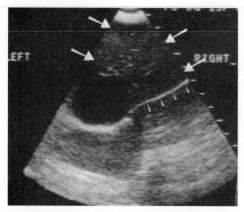

Figure 11-2. Ultrasonographic demonstration of a solitary hepatic cyst in a dog. Arrowheads delineate diaphragm; arrows delineate liver.

patic cysts are commonly multiple. Polycystic hepatic cysts may be associated with cystic lesions in other organs, most notably the kidneys. Polycystic kidneys and liver have been identified in Cairn terrier dogs and Persian cats during the first few months of life (Crowell et al, 1979; McKenna and Carpenter, 1980). Abdominal radiographs may reveal an irregular hepatic margin or focal densities if a few large hepatic or biliary cysts are present. Ultrasonography readily reveals the cystic nature of these lesions and the extent of parenchymal or biliary tract involvement (Fig. 11-2). Treatment is usually not needed for a congenital hepatic cyst unless a large cyst is causing abdominal discomfort or fluid accumulation. If cystic lesions are symptomatic, surgical resection of solitary lesions, partial cyst wall, or a liver lobe may be required.

Congenital Biliary Tract Malformations. Congenital anomalies of the biliary tract are rare in the young dog and cat. One case of suspected biliary atresia in the cat is reported (Blood, 1947).

Congenital Portosystemic Venous Shunts. The hepatic portal system develops from the umbilical and omphalomesenteric systems. The mesenteric portions of the omphalomesenteric veins become the tributaries of the portal vein. Small anastomoses develop between the portal and systemic circulation routes that become the normal portosystemic venous communications (Heath and House, 1970; Khan and Vitums, 1971; Sleight and Thomford, 1969; Vitums, 1959). In the fetus, blood from the umbilical vein flows directly to the caudal vena cava through the ductus venosus, thus bypassing the liver. By passively responding to changes in the

systemic or hepatic circulation, the ductus venosus stabilizes the venous return to the fetal heart as the umbilical venous return fluctuates (Edelstone, 1980). Functional and morphologic closure of the ductus venosus does not occur at the same time after birth (Lohse and Suter, 1977). Functional closure develops gradually during the second and third days after birth in the puppy. Morphologic closure occurs as the ductus atrophies, resulting in the formation of a thin fibrous band, the ligamentum venosum, within the liver. The ductus closure depends on changes in pressure and resistance across the hepatic vasculature that follows the postnatal obliteration of the umbilical circulation. Morphologic closure of the ductus occurs by 1 to 3 months after birth.

Congenital portosystemic venous shunts (PSS) are abnormal vascular connections between the portal and systemic venous circulations (Berger et al, 1986; Boothe et al, 1996; Bostwick and Twedt, 1995; Carr and Thornburg, 1984; Gandolfi, 1984; Scavelli et al, 1986). Several different types of congenital PSS occur in young dogs and cats, including but not limited to (1) persistent patent fetal ductus venosus, (2) direct portal vein to caudal vena cava, (3) direct portal vein to azygos vein, (4) combination of portal vein with caudal vena cava into the azygos vein, (5) left gastric vein to vena caval shunt, (6) portal vein hypoplasia or atresia with secondary anomalous vessel, and (7) anomalous malformation of the caudal vena cava (Center et al, 1995). The most common types of congenital PSS are illustrated in Figure 11-3. In the cat, the most common congenital PSS involves the left gastric vein (Fig. 11-4A).

A congenital PSS in puppies and kittens is usually a single anomalous vessel in extrahepatic or intrahepatic locations, whereas an acquired PSS most commonly occurs as multiple extrahepatic smaller vessels that become patent during sustained portal hypertension. The consequences of the anomalous portal circulation are that the portal blood contains toxins absorbed from the intestines that is delivered directly to the systemic circulation without benefit of hepatic detoxification, contributing to signs of hepatic encephalopathy, and that hepatotrophic factors in the visceral circulation draining the gastrointestinal tract and pancreas do not circulate directly to the liver, causing inadequate liver development and reduced functional liver tissue.

Signs of hepatic dysfunction associated with congenital PSS are usually exhibited at a young age in puppies and kittens. Puppies may exhibit the signs as early as 6 to 8 weeks of age. The

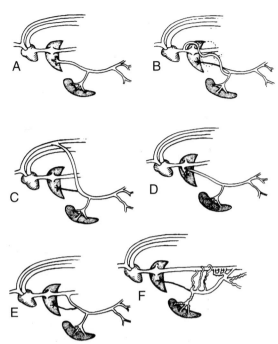

Figure 11–3. Illustrations of the most common forms of portosystemic venous anomalies. **A,** Normal circulation. **B,** Left gastric shunt (most common in the cat). **C,** Portoazygous shunt. **D,** Patent ductus venosus (most common in the dog). **E,** Direct portal to caudal vena caval shunt. **F,** Portal atresia or hypoplasia with secondary portosystemic shunts.

signs in puppies are variable but may include vomiting, diarrhea, anorexia, small body stature, weight loss, intermittent fever, polyphagia, polydipsia, hematuria, hypersalivation, intolerance to anesthetic agents or tranquilizers that require hepatic metabolism or excretion, atypical behavior, and, rarely, ascites or icterus. Intermittent neurologic abnormalities associated with ingestion of protein-laden food or resolving hemorrhage are common and may include episodic aggression, amaurosis, ataxia, incessant pacing, circling, head pressing, and seizures. Some puppies present with ammonium biurate uroliths located in the urinary tract (Marretta et al, 1981).

Most cases of congenital PSS in kittens (by 6 months of age in 75% of affected kittens) occur in Himalayan, Persian, and mixed breed cats, although any breed may have a congenital PSS (Levy, 1997). Kittens may exhibit signs as early as ages 6 to 8 weeks. The signs of congenital PSS are usually hypersalivation, seizures, ataxia, tremors, and depression. Intermittent or permanent blindness and mydriasis are also ob-

served. Other less often noted signs may include vomiting, diarrhea, anorexia, tachypnea, dyspnea, and nasal discharge. Polyuria and polydipsia are observed infrequently. Dysuria may be observed in kittens with ammonium biurate calculi. About two thirds of affected kittens will have small body stature and be thin and unkempt.

A definitive diagnosis of congenital PSS in puppies and kittens is often not possible by routine laboratory evaluations. Complete blood counts (CBCs), serum chemistry profiles, and urinalysis may help rule out other causes of presenting signs such as acute renal failure, electrolyte derangements, hypoglycemia, and urinary tract disorders. The CBC findings may include microcytic, normochromic erythrocytes and/or a mild nonregenerative anemia (Griffiths et al, 1981). Poikilocytosis has been observed in peripheral blood films of some kittens with congenital PSS. Urinalysis may reveal ammonium biurate crystals when viewed under magnification ($\times 400$) to determine their typical color and shape.

Serum chemistry profiles may reveal mild increases in the serum activities of ALT, AST, and ALP. Because of the young age of the animals at initial diagnosis, the serum ALP activity is usually two- to threefold higher than normal. The serum activity levels of the ALT and AST are less frequently increased. In some cases, active liver disease coexists with a congenital PSS, and the animals thus affected have mildly to moderately increased liver enzyme activity and notable hepatic inflammation and/or fibrosis on histopathologic examination. In most animals with congenital PSS, the total bilirubin value is normal. Albumin values may be mildly decreased. Coagulation profiles including prothrombin time, activated partial thromboplastin time, and fibrinogen are usually normal.

Serum glucose values may be normal, mildly reduced, or markedly hypoglycemic. In some cases, the hypoglycemia-produced neuroglycopenia may complicate the recognition of the congenital PSS. Animals with congenital PSS may become hypoglycemic due to insufficient glycogen stores, abnormal responsiveness to glucagon, hyperglucagonemia, or abnormal insulin metabolism (Lickley et al, 1975; Magne and Macy, 1984). These abnormalities, coupled with the metabolic immaturity of the young animal's liver, may cause profound hypoglycemia during the first weeks of life. Toy-breed puppies appear to be at increased risk for profound hypoglycemia. The blood urea nitrogen

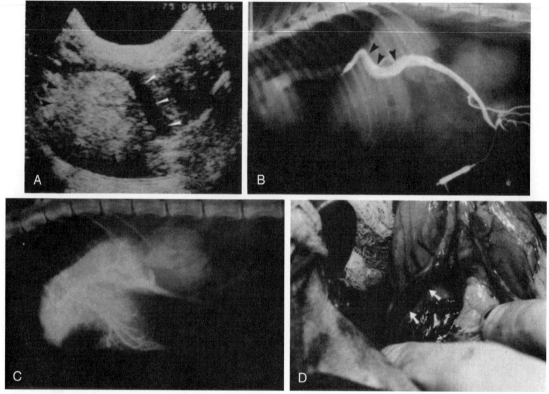

Figure 11–4. Ultrasonography **(A)**, portovenography **(B)**, and gross appearance at surgery **(D)** of a left gastric vein to vena cava shunt in a cat. **C**, Radiograph represents a normal portovenogram from a cat. In **A**, black arrowheads indicate the shunting vessel, and white arrowheads indicate the stomach image. In **B**, arrowheads indicate the shunting vessel. In **D**, arrows identify the shunt. (Courtesy of the Sections of Radiology and Surgery, New York State College of Veterinary Medicine.)

concentration may be low or in the low normal range in any young animal with hepatic dysfunction.

The most reliable and consistent blood test for the detection of liver dysfunction in puppies and kittens with congenital PSS is the 12- to 24-hour fasted and 2-hour postprandial serum bile acid concentrations (Center et al, 1986b; Meyer, 1986).

Diagnostic imaging of a puppy or kitten with abnormal serum bile acid values helps determine if a suspected congenital PSS is present (Table 11–2) (Lamb, 1996; Lamb et al, 1996). Animals with congenital PSS frequently have reduced hepatic size (i.e., rounded contour of the caudal edge of the liver and cranial displacement of the stomach radiographically) (Lamb, 1997). In addition, these animals may have opaque ammonium biurate calculi. Ultrasonographic findings in puppies with congenital PSS include small liver, reduced visibility of intrahepatic portal vasculature, and an anomalous

blood vessel draining into the caudal vena cava or sometimes into the azygos vein (Lamb, 1996).

Two-dimensional, gray-scale ultrasonography is used to image through a ventral abdominal wall; however, in most large puppies the optimal approach to the portal vein is through a lateral abdominal wall using the right intercostal spaces (Lamb, 1997). The portal vein is normally visible by ultrasound imaging as ultrasound waves enter the liver at the porta hepatis, ventral to the caudal vena cava. Lobar branches of the portal vein have echogenic walls.

Congenital intrahepatic portocaval shunts are identified on the basis of their ultrasonographic appearance as left-divisional, central-divisional, or right-divisional intrahepatic shunts (Lamb, 1997). Left-divisional intrahepatic shunts have a relatively consistent bent tubular shape and drain into the left hepatic vein. Central-divisional intrahepatic shunts take the form of a foramen between dilated portions of the intra-

	Table 11–2 Summary of Typical Ultrasonographic Findings in Dogs and Cats with Portosystemic Shunting	
FINDINGS	CONGENITAL PORTOSYSTEMIC SHUNTING	ACQUIRED PORTOSYSTEMIC SHUNTING
Hepatic volume	Usually reduced	Variable
Hepatic parenchyma	Attenuated vessels or reduced numbers of vessels	Diffuse or multifocal echotextural changes
Renal volume	Often increased in dogs (not in cats)	Usually within normal limits
Anomalous vessel	Usually single, may be large, intra- or extrahepatic	Multiple, small, extrahepatic
Portal blood flow velocity	May be increased and variable	Reduced, sometimes hepatofugal
Other potential findings	Urinary calculi	Urinary calculi Dilated abdominal veins Portal vein thrombosis Lesion impinging on portal vein Ascites Pancreatic edema

From Lamb CR: Ultrasonography of portosystemic shunts in dogs and cats. Vet Clin North Am 28:725–753, 1998.

hepatic portal vein and caudal vena cava. Right-divisional intrahepatic shunts appear as large, tortuous vessels that extend far to the right of midline. The morphology of the left-divisional shunts is compatible with patent ductus venosus. The Irish wolfhound and deerhound are predisposed to left-divisional intrahepatic shunts; the Old English sheepdog and Australian cattle dog are predisposed to central-divisional intrahepatic shunts; Labrador and golden retrievers are affected by both left-divisional and central-divisional intrahepatic shunts (Lamb, 1997).

Animals with extrahepatic congenital PSS typically have an anomalous vessel that drains into the caudal vena cava between the right renal vein and the hepatic veins; because of the dorsal location, this anomalous vessel may be visible only through the right dorsal intercostal spaces (Lamb, 1997). Congenital portoazygos shunts may also be visualized using the right dorsal intercostal approach; looking for the shunting vessel at the point where it drains into the caudal vena cava is more accurate than trying to examine the various tributaries of the portal vein (Lamb, 1997). Extrahepatic shunts may be difficult to identify ultrasonographically if access to the relevant structures is hindered by the skill of the person performing the ultrasonographic study, the animal's large body size, a lack of acoustic windows as a result of reduced hepatic size, or the presence of excessive intestinal gas.

Duplex Doppler ultrasonography may be used to measure portal blood flow velocity in puppies with suspected congenital PSS (Lamb and Mahoney, 1994). Normal portal blood flow is relatively uniform and nonpulsatile, average portal blood flow velocity being approximately 15 cm/s in healthy, unsedated puppies. The caudal vena cava normally contains variable blood flow because of the influence of changing right atrial and pleural pressures. In most cases, congenital PSS represents a low resistance pathway for blood to bypass the liver and enter the caudal vena cava. In affected puppies with congenital PSS, the portal vein is exposed to right atrial and pleural pressure changes, and the pattern of portal blood flow may become similar to that noted in the caudal vena cava. Puppies with portal hypertension have reduced mean portal blood flow velocity, which correlates with the presence of multiple extrahepatic anomalous vessels. Puppies with portal hypertension as a result of hepatic arteriovenous fistula have pulsatile hepatofugal flow in the portal vein.

Most extrahepatic and intrahepatic congenital PSSs are detectable using two-dimensional, gray-scale ultrasonography; however, use of color-flow Doppler ultrasonography aids in the detection of small extrahepatic shunting vessels. A congenital extrahepatic PSS usually drains into the caudal vena cava close to the cranial pole of the right kidney, and on color-flow images a localized area of turbulent flow in the caudal vena cava indicates the shunt's location. When two-dimensional gray-scale, duplex

Doppler, and color-flow Doppler modalities are used in combination, the accuracy for ultrasonographic diagnosis of congenital PSS in puppies and kittens can be at least 94% (Lamb, 1997).

Various techniques for opacification of the portal vein and its hepatic branches have been used, including operative mesenteric portography, cranial mesenteric angiography, and percutaneous splenoportography (Suter, 1975). Operative mesenteric portography is the most frequently performed opacification procedure for suspected congenital PSS, where abdominal radiographs are made immediately after injection of contrast medium into a indwelling catheter placed surgically in a mesenteric vein (Fig. 11–4B–C). Obtaining lateral and ventrodorsal portograms usually provides an excellent view of the intrahepatic or extrahepatic shunt. This technique can also be used in combination with surgery, in which case the mesenteric vein catheter is also used to measure portal blood pressure during the congenital shunt ligation or attenuation procedure. Repeating the portogram after shunt ligation or attenuation enables the surgeon to assess the patency of the intrahepatic portal vessel and to check if there is any other congenital shunt(s) present.

Portal scintigraphy with Tc^{99m}-pertechnetate that is absorbed into the portal circulation after administration per rectum is currently being used in puppies and kittens to detect congenital PSS (Forster-van Hijfte et al, 1996; Koblik et al, 1990). By acquiring a dynamic series of gamma camera images of the thorax and cranial abdomen immediately after administration of Tc^{99m}-pertechnetate and comparing the rate of accumulation of Tc^{99m}-pertechnetate activity in the liver and heart, congenital PSS may be detected with a high degree of accuracy. Tc^{99m}-pertechnetate activity in the portal vein normally accumulates first in the liver, but in animals with congenital PSS the distribution of Tc^{99m}-pertechnetate activity is altered as it bypasses the liver, reaching the heart before the liver. The severity of the congenital PSS can be quantified as a shunt index that provides an estimate of the proportion of portal blood that bypasses the liver. Normal puppies have a shunt index of less than 15%; most puppies with congenital PSS have a shunt index greater than 60%.

An alternative technique for portal scintigraphy involves ultrasound-guided injection of a radiochemical directly into a splenic vein (Meyer et al, 1994). This method of injection combined with the use of Tc^{99m}-labeled macroaggregates that are normally trapped in the capillaries or sinusoids of the target organ enables accurate quantification of the degree of congenital shunting. Typical values of a shunt index using this technique are less than 5% for normal puppies and greater than 90% for puppies with congenital PSS. Whether the administration per rectum or splenic vein injection technique is used, portal scintigraphy can provide a comparison between the shunt index before and after surgical treatment (van Vechten et al, 1994). The shunt index is usually markedly decreased after surgery to attenuate or ligate an anomalous vessel, although it may not be in the normal range. A continued high shunt index is a poor prognostic sign.

Surgical ligation or shunt vessel attenuation is the definitive treatment for congenital PSS and is the preferred method of long-term management (Birchard, 1984; Breznock et al, 1983; Vogt et al, 1996; Wrigley et al, 1983). The extrahepatic congenital PSS is more amenable to surgical ligation or shunt vessel attenuation than are intrahepatic congenital PSSs. Medical management should be given to the affected animal before and after surgical correction until improvement in hepatic function is shown. Affected animals undergoing surgery should have their body temperature stabilized and should receive intravenous fluids supplemented with 2.5% or 5.0% dextrose solution and with potassium chloride. In addition, owners should be cautioned that any animal with a congenital PSS probably would have a shortened life expectancy despite satisfactory surgical correction and their conscientious care.

Manometric determination of baseline portal blood pressure should be completed before shunt vessel ligation (Hardie, 1997). After visual observation of the anomalous vessel, a ligature is temporarily placed while manometric determination of the portal blood pressure is made. Equilibration of the manometer pressure usually takes several minutes. If the relative change in portal pressure exceeds 10 cm H_2O or the postligation pressure exceeds 20 cm H_2O, the ligature should be loosened. Assessment of visceral perfusion by color change (cyanosis and/or injection) or of arterial vasospasm causing a throbbing of the mesenteric circulation is not a reliable method of determining the safe tautness of the shunt vessel ligature. In many cases, only a partial surgical ligation, or shunt vessel attenuation, can be completed. Further ligation may be possible in several weeks or months. Incomplete ligation of a congenital PSS can result in marked clinical improvement of the animal and owner satisfaction. Partial shunt vessel ligation may result in eventual complete shunt closure within 6 months in some animals.

Complications after shunt vessel ligation or attenuation are frequent and may lead to the animal's death (Hardie, 1997). It is important that the owner understand the potential complications before surgery is attempted because many times the financial and emotional costs of complications are great. The immediate complication rate for performing a laparotomy on puppies and kittens with congenital PSS is between 14% and 25%. Because many of the complications are life threatening, it is reasonable to tell the owner that this surgery carries a 15% risk of death due to unexpected complications. Intrahepatic shunt ligation requires longer surgery times than does extrahepatic shunt ligation, but the risk of death is no higher than with extrahepatic shunt ligation when performed by a experienced surgeon.

In the immediate postoperative period, the animal is closely monitored for signs of portal hypertension, as indicated by acute abdominal swelling, abdominal pain, shock, vomiting, or bloody diarrhea (Holt, 1994). If portal hypertension is suspected, shock therapy is initiated and the animal is returned to surgery for immediate ligature removal. Feeding may precipitate portal hypertension, and animals should be given small amounts of food and monitored closely after each feeding. If thrombosis of the shunt vessel or the portal vein occurs, signs of portal hypertension may occur up to several days after surgery, and treatment is usually futile. Bleeding after surgery can also result in abdominal distention and signs of shock. At reoperation these animals are usually found to have diffuse hemorrhage. Conservative treatment with packed red blood cells, fresh frozen plasma, or whole blood may be a more appropriate treatment than reoperation, if bleeding is suspected (Hardie, 1997).

Serious complications encountered in animals undergoing congenital PSS surgery include intraoperative cardiac arrest, life-threatening hemorrhage, portal hypertension, seizures that usually start 2 to 3 days after surgery and may progress to status epilepticus, hyperthermia, gastric dilation-volvulus, acute pulmonary edema, and biliary pseudocyst formation (Hardie, 1997). The more manageable complications include abdominal distention, hypotension, hypothermia, hypoglycemia, mild gastrointestinal disturbances, and postoperative pain. Predictor signs of immediate postoperative complications include low packed cell volume before surgery, absence of arborizing intrahepatic vasculature during the mesenteric portogram, partial shunt vessel ligation, and hypothermia in the postoperative period. Kittens are especially prone to developing seizures after shunt vessel ligation and should be administered phenobarbital at therapeutic serum concentrations for the entire perioperative period (Hardie, 1997). Seizures usually occur 12 hours to 4 days after surgery. Kittens that have no evidence of seizures in the perioperative period are weaned off the phenobarbital 1 month after surgery.

Long-term complications are encountered in animals whose congenital PSS is not completely ligated and in animals that are older than 2 years of age at the time of surgery (Hottinger et al, 1995). Approximately 50% of the single shunts cannot be completely ligated at the first surgery because complete occlusion results in portal pressures greater than 20 cm H_2O or a rise in portal pressure greater than 10 cm H_2O. Within this group of partial vessel ligation, recurrence of PSS signs may occur in as many as 40% of animals if a further vessel ligation is not performed. Multiple extrahepatic shunts may form even with partial vessel ligation and are often associated with recurrence of PSS signs. For animals with multiple extrahepatic shunts due to portal hypertension, the 2-year survival rate is 50% regardless of whether they are treated medically or surgically (Hardie, 1997).

Postoperative improvement is apparent from observation of the animal's activity at home but should always be followed by assessment of serum chemistry profile and serum bile acid concentrations for hepatic dysfunction (Hardie, 1997). Medical management should be maintained until postoperative improvement has been unequivocally demonstrated. If serum bile acid values remain increased and the shunt index is greater than 15% at 60 to 90 days after surgery, reoperation is indicated. Reoperation, however, has its own complications, mostly associated with the risk of inadvertently cutting a structure surrounded by scar tissue. Reoperation of congenital intrahepatic shunts can be extremely difficult. If a mattress suture was placed across the anomalous vessel, the long ends of the suture material can be identified and the mattress suture tightened further. In some instances, it is necessary, however, to place additional sutures.

To avoid the risks associated with reoperation of congenital intrahepatic shunts, a new technique has been developed in which an extrahepatic shunt is created between the portal vein and the vena cava using a jugular vein graft (White et al, 1996). This shunt is created at the time of the first surgery, and the intrahepatic shunt is completely closed. The venous graft prevents portal hypertension from developing at the time of the first surgery. The venous graft may slowly occlude, resulting in a normal shunt index 60 to 90 days after surgery. If the shunt index is still high, reoperation is simply a matter of either ligating or placing an ameroid constrictor band on the vein graft.

In some cases, serum bile acid values remain abnormal despite a remarkable improvement in the animal's signs (Hardie, 1997). If serum chemistry profile and serum bile acid concentrations indicate ongoing hepatic dysfunction, then medical management should be continued. Medical management is directed at minimizing the signs of hepatic encephalopathy and includes manipulation of dietary proteins and intestinal flora and avoidance of medications or substances capable of inducing encephalopathic signs. A restricted protein diet (2.0 to 2.5 mg/kg) composed of proteins rich in branched-chain amino acids with comparatively smaller amounts of aromatic amino acids is recommended. Foods containing milk protein (dried milk or cottage cheese) are best. The bulk of the caloric intake should consist of simple carbohydrates such as boiled white rice. Meals should be frequent and in small amounts to maximize digestion and absorption so that minimal residue is passed into the colon, where intestinal anaerobic bacteria degrade nitrogenous compounds to ammonia. Commercial diets formulated for liver or renal dysfunction and a diet formulated for intestinal disease are used with success in most puppies and kittens with congenital or acquired PSS.

Manipulation of intestinal flora with antimicrobial agents and lactulose also produces marked clinical improvement. For animals presenting in encephalopathic crisis, intravenous isotonic electrolyte solutions supplemented with 2.5% or 5.0% dextrose solution and potassium chloride, cleansing enemas with warmed 0.9% saline solution, or enemas with added neomycin (15 to 20 ml of 1% solution three to four times daily), lactulose (5 to 10 ml diluted 1:3 with water three to four times daily), or betadine solution (10% solution, rinse after 10 minutes with warm water) are recommended. For long-term medical management of encephalopathic signs, lactulose is given orally at a dosage of 0.25 to 1.0 ml per 4.5 kg body weight, the dose adjusted to the frequency and consistency of the stools passed each day. Two to three soft or pudding-consistency stools indicate an optimal dose. Too great a dose may result in flatulence,

severe diarrhea, dehydration, and acidemia. To further manipulate the intestinal flora, neomycin (22 mg/kg orally two to three times daily), metronidazole (7.5 mg/kg orally two to three times daily), ampicillin (5 mg/kg orally two to three times daily), or amoxicillin (2.5 mg/kg orally two times a day) may be used intermittently for several weeks.

Congenital Hepatic Arteriovenous Fistulas. Congenital hepatic arteriovenous fistulas between the hepatic artery and portal vein occur in both puppies and kittens (Easley and Carpenter, 1975; Legendre et al, 1976; Moore and Whiting, 1986; Rogers et al, 1977). These congenital malformations are the result of failure of the common embryologic anlage to differentiate into arteries and veins. Congenital hepatic arteriovenous fistulas are associated with portal hypertension and shunting of blood through multiple portosystemic venous collaterals (Table 11–3). Increased pressure in the portal vein, hepatic vein, and hepatic sinusoids is caused by arterialization of the portal circulation. Arteriovenous fistulas located in other areas of the body increase cardiac output and produce signs of heart failure (Gomes and Bernatz, 1970; Moore and Whiting, 1986). The interposition of the hepatic sinusoids between the heart and fistula cushions the hemodynamic effects, influencing heart function in animals with congenital hepatic arteriovenous fistulas. Animals with congenital hepatic arteriovenous fistulas have multiple portosystemic shunts and ascites. Portal venography by splenic pulp injection or mesenteric vein catheterization demonstrates multiple anomalous shunts but does not show the fistulas. Diagnosis is made by nonselective jugular venography (Fig. 11–5), selective celiac angiography, technetium scintigraphy, ultrasonography, or observation of an abnormal liver lobe during laparotomy. Affected liver lobes are large and may have numerous pulsating surface vessels. Unaffected liver lobes are small. A continuous murmur accentuated during systole may be auscultated near the lesion. Palpation of the area may reveal a thrill. Ultrasonographically, congenital hepatic arteriovenous fistulas are identified on the basis of finding multiple large, tortuous, and pulsatile hepatic vessels and enlargement of the celiac and common hepatic arteries.

Congenital Hepatoportal Microvascular Dysplasia. Hepatoportal microvascular dysplasia is characterized by the presence of multiple microscopic intrahepatic shunts (Phillips et al, 1993; Schermhorn et al, 1996). The microvas-

| | Table 11-3 | Summary of Hepatic Disorders That Potentially Cause Portal Hypertension in Young Dogs |

DISORDER	SIGNALMENT AND CLINICAL PROFILE	HISTOPATHOLOGIC FINDINGS AND OUTCOME
Arteriovenous fistula	4–8 mo, purebred, female; feel reasonably well; ascites, vague GI signs, encephalopathic signs; laboratory analysis: hepatic dysfunction	Bile duct proliferation, parenchymal atrophy, arteriolar proliferation; greatly improved after surgery
Veno-occlusive disease	10–19 mo, American cocker spaniel, female	Prominent smooth muscle, dilated central and portal veins, prenchymal atrophy, variable fibrosis; poor quality of life
Hepatoportal fibrosis	4–6 mo, purebred, female	Bile duct proliferation, periportal fibrosis, arteriolar proliferation, hypoplastic and distended portal veins; variable responses to treatment
Idiopathic fibrosis	4 mo to 7 yr, German shepherd, no gender predilection	Three patterns of fibrosis: central perivenous, diffuse pericellular, and periportal; variable responses to treatment
Lobular dissecting hepatitis	3–14 mo, purebred, female	Hyperplastic nodules, diffuse mixed cell inflammatory infiltrate, lobular disruption, portal tracts difficult to recognize; variable responses to treatment
Noncirrhotic portal hypertension	4–7 mo, Doberman pinschers, no gender predilection; vague GI signs, ascites, encephalopathic signs; laboratory analysis: hepatic dysfunction	Bile duct proliferation, parenchymal atrophy, arteriolar proliferation, scant fibrosis around large portal triads, absence of inflammation, intrahepatic cholestasis; variable responses to treatment
Portal vein hypoplasia	1–18 mo, purebred, no gender predilection	Underdeveloped extrahepatic portal vein, hypoplastic intrahepatic portal veins, arteriolar and bile duct proliferation, parenchymal atrophy, portal fibrosis; most die naturally or are euthanized

GI = Gastrointestinal.
Modified from Bunch SE: Noncirrhotic portal hypertension in young dogs. Proc Am Coll Vet Intern Med 15:42, 1997, with permission.

cular dysplasia occurs in the same dog breeds that have congenital PSS, possibly being an inherited disorder in Cairn terriers. Most dogs with microvascular dysplasia are asymptomatic, probably because only a small amount of blood is being shunted away from the liver. When signs are present, they are similar to those seen in dogs with congenital extrahepatic and intrahepatic PSS, with the exception that most dogs with microvascular dysplasia usually present at an older age. The most prominent laboratory abnormality is increased serum bile acid concentrations. There is no ultrasonographic, sur-

gical, or portographic evidence of a congenital PSS, and the rectal portal scintigraphy is normal. Medical treatment is the same as for any suspected congenital PSS. Asymptomatic dogs with increased serum bile acids as their only detectable abnormality do not require treatment.

Hepatic Storage Disorders

Congenital Storage Disorders. Congenital storage disorders affecting the function or availability of lysosomal enzymes or effector proteins

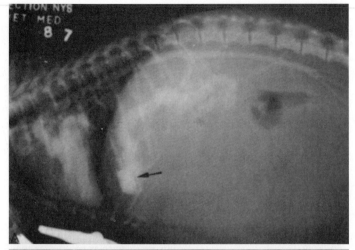

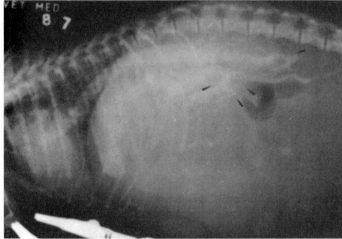

Figure 11–5. Nonselective jugular venography in a dog with an intrahepatic arterioportal fistula. **A,** Early arterial phase after contrast injection demonstrating the arterialization of the hepatic circulation (*arrow* indicates major fistula location). **B,** Late portal phase demonstrating retrograde flow of contrast due to arterialization and subsequent hypertension in the portal circulation. Ascites and enlarged, tortuous portosystemic communications (*arrowheads*) are typical features of intrahepatic arterioportal fistulae. (Courtesy of the Section of Radiology, New York State College of Veterinary Medicine.)

essential for catabolism of glycoproteins, glycolipids, glycosaminoglycans (mucopolysaccharides), gangliosides, and glycogen have been identified in puppies and kittens. These disorders are characterized by tissue accumulation of undegraded storage products. Signs are usually progressive in association with tissue accumulation of storage material. Hepatomegaly may develop from the undegraded storage product accumulating in hepatocytes and Kupffer cells.

Mannosidosis resulting from a deficiency in acid mannosidase activity that causes the intralysosomal accumulation of a mannoside oligosaccharide occurs in kittens (Jezyk et al, 1986; Vendevelde et al, 1982). Clinical findings include hepatomegaly, neurologic dysfunction (including tremors, ataxia, hypermetria, and/or weakness), stunted growth, facial dysmorphia, and early death. Histopathologic examination reveals extensive cytoplasmic vacuolation in hepatocytes and neurons and the presence of unusual axonal spheroids.

The mucopolysaccharide storage disorders are caused by a defect in lysosomal enzymes responsible for the degradation of dermatan sulfate, heparan sulfate, or keratan sulfate—normal constituents of the connective tissue matrix. These disorders are clinically progressive and are associated with tissue accumulation of glycosaminoglycans. Clinical features vary with the specific enzyme deficiency. Hepatosplenomegaly may develop from the accumulation of incompletely degraded mucopolysaccharides in parenchymal and reticuloendothelial cells. Clinical findings may include facial dysmorphia (rounded broad forehead, small ears, and dished face), corneal opacity, bone and joint lesions (including odontoid hypoplasia, intervertebral disk degeneration, spinal canal and vertebral exostoses, osteoporosis, coxofemoral luxation, lytic areas in long bones and vertebrae, joint effusions, and degenerative joint disease), cardiac murmurs, stunted growth, metachromatic granules in leukocytes, neurologic abnormalities (mental slowness, cervical or thoracolumbar myelopathy), and early death. Mucopolysaccharidosis I (α-L-iuronidase deficiency) has been described in a kindred of Plott hounds and in domestic short-haired cats (Haskins et al, 1983; Shull et al, 1984). Mucopolysaccharidosis VI (arylsulfatase B deficiency) has been described in Siamese and domestic short-haired cats (Breton et al, 1983; Haskins et al, 1980, 1981). Mucopolysaccharidosis VII has been described in a dog (Haskins et al, 1984). A presumptive diagnosis of mucopolysaccharidosis can be made by a positive urine toluidine blue spot test. Definitive diagnosis is made by measurement of the activity of specific enzymes in fresh serum, cultured dermal fibroblasts, or leukocytes. Treatment with bone marrow transplantation has been reported to result in clinical improvement (Dial et al, 1985; Gasper et al, 1985).

Gangliosidosis occurs from incomplete catabolism of certain gangliosides and glycolipids and retention of these substrates within lysosomes. Gangliosidosis has been reported in the puppy and kitten (Alroy et al, 1985; Baker and Lindsey, 1974; Barnes et al, 1981; Cork et al, 1977, 1978; Neuwelt et al, 1985; Read et al, 1976; Wenger et al, 1980). Affected animals develop neurologic signs as early as 2 or 3 months of age. Progressive, fine generalized muscle tremors, ataxia, and paresis are the usual clinical findings. Gangliosides accumulate in the central nervous system and in visceral organs, including the liver. Membrane-bound cytoplasmic bodies are observed in cells from affected individuals.

Glycogen storage disorder associated with hepatomegaly has been diagnosed in a kindred of Lapland dogs and in a German shepherd dog (Rafizuzzaman et al, 1976; Walvoort et al, 1982, 1984). Affected animals showed signs as early as 2 months of age that were slowly progressive over many months. Signs included weakness, weight loss, and gradual abdominal distention associated with profound hepatomegaly. Glycogen is freely dispersed in the hepatocellular cytoplasm. A deficiency of amylo-1,6-glucosidase was demonstrated in a German shepherd dog (Ceh et al, 1976), and a deficiency of α-glucosidase was demonstrated in a Lapland dog (Walvoort et al, 1982).

Copper Storage Disorders of the Bedlington Terrier. A chronic active liver disease associated with an age-related accumulation of hepatic copper occurs in Bedlington terrier dogs (Hultgren et al, 1986). An autosomal recessive mode of inheritance is involved; only individuals homozygous for the recessive gene develop the excess copper accumulation in hepatic lysosomes. The adverse effects of retained copper are not noted during the first few years of life in affected Bedlington terrier dogs by the protective lysosomal sequestration of copper. Once lysosomal storage is overwhelmed, a progressive hepatopathy and clinical evidence of chronic active liver disease ensue. In affected dogs, copper accumulation begins before 1 year of age and continues for at least 5 or 6 years. Hepatic copper concentrations exceeding 2000 μg/g dry tissue are consistently associated with morphologic and functional evidence of the progressive hepatopathy that over time progresses to chronic active hepatitis and cirrhosis (Fig. 11–6A) (Hultgren et al, 1986; Twedt et al, 1979). Affected dogs can be identified at 6 months of age on the basis of hepatic biopsy results (Johnson et al, 1984).

Liver tissue can be qualitatively and quantitatively evaluated for copper accumulation. Routine staining with hematoxylin and eosin reveals dark cytoplasmic granules in hepatocytes of affected dogs early in the disease. Tissue-bound copper can be stained with rubeanic acid, rhodanine, or Timm's stain for qualitative and semiquantitative estimation of the degree of copper retention (Fig. 11–6B) (Johnson et al, 1984; Thornburg et al, 1985). Tissues should be stored embedded in paraffin blocks rather than formalin solution if examination is delayed for several months, because copper staining is reduced after prolonged storage in formalin solution (Thornburg et al, 1985). Quantitative assessment of hepatic copper is accomplished by atomic absorption spectroscopy of tissue previously preserved in formalin or paraffin block or frozen. Normal dog liver has less than 400 μg copper per gram of dry tissue (Thornburg et al, 1985; Twedt et al, 1979). Affected Bedlington dogs may develop hepatic copper content up to 2000 μg/g during the first year of life before developing histopathologic evidence of hepatocellular injury. Dogs showing evidence of abnormal copper storage in hepatic biopsy material by 1 year of age should not be used for breeding. Affected Bedlington dogs may have evidence of increased hepatic copper as early as 8 to 12 weeks of age.

Diagnosis of copper-associated hepatopathy in Bedlington terriers can be made by examination of hepatic tissue for excessive copper storage or by performing genetic tests on DNA samples collected from suspected dogs. An autosomal recessive mode of inheritance is in-

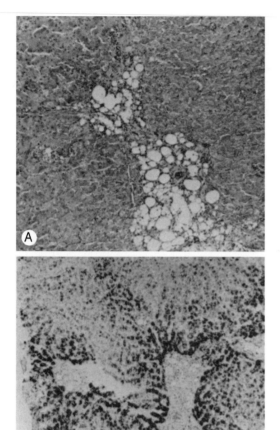

Figure 11–6. Photomicrographs of a liver biopsy specimen from a Bedlington terrier with copper storage hepatopathy. **A,** Routine hematoxylin and eosin staining demonstrating chronic active hepatitis. **B,** Rhodanine staining reveals dark copper-laden storage granules (lysosomes). (×75.) (Courtesy of the Department of Pathology, New York State College of Veterinary Medicine.)

volved in copper-associated hepatopathy in Bedlington terriers. The frequency of the recessive gene in Bedlington terriers is estimated to be as high as 50% in the United States, with a similar frequency in England. This means that more than 25% of Bedlington terriers are "affected," and another 50% are "carriers." The DNA samples can be collected with a soft cheek brush that is provided by a commercial genetic laboratory (VetGen, 3728 Plaza Drive, Suite 1, Ann Arbor, MI 48108; 1–734–669–8440, Toll Free: 1–800–4–VETGEN, Fax: 1–734–669–8441; or see their web site: www.vetgen.com). By gently brushing the inside of the dog's cheek, cells containing DNA are removed. The collected DNA samples then are analyzed to determine the genetic status of the suspect dog. Useful for dogs of any age, the DNA sample collection and analysis activities can be completed before puppies are purchased at 6 to 10 weeks. The results of the DNA testing also can be formally registered with the Orthopedic Foundation for Animals. (For further information about the Orthopedic Foundation for Animal's Registry for Copper Toxicosis in Bedlington Terriers, contact Orthopedic Foundation for Animals, 2300 E. Nifong Boulevard, Columbia, MO 65201–3856 or telephone 1–573–442–0418.)

D-penicillamine, a copper chelator, is recommended for the treatment of the copper-associated hepatopathy in Bedlington terriers as soon as the disorder is confirmed. The recommended dose of D-penicillamine is 125 to 250 mg/day (adult dogs), given 30 minutes before feeding (Hardy, 1983). The most common adverse effects from D-penicillamine administration are vomiting and anorexia. Vomiting may be manageable by dividing the daily dose into two or three doses. If D-penicillamine is not tolerated, another copper chelator, 2,3,2-trientine, administered at 10 to 15 mg/kg orally one to two times daily or zinc acetate administered at 50 to 200 mg orally once a day, decreases intestinal absorption of copper and may be used. In addition to the decopper drugs, vitamin C and prednisolone have been recommended. Vitamin C is known to facilitate the excretion of copper in urine, and large doses may reduce the intestinal absorption of copper. Dosages of 500 to 1000 mg/day have been suggested (Hardy, 1983). Prednisolone at 0.5 to 1.0 mg/kg per day is recommended only for those dogs showing evidence of active hepatic necrosis. Limitation of the dietary intake of copper is usually not possible. Most dog foods contain 5 to 10 mg/kg of copper, which may result in a higher copper intake per kilogram than is appropriate.

Other Copper-Related Hepatopathies.
Hepatopathies associated with increased concentrations of hepatic copper have been recognized in young dogs and cats with chronic active hepatitis, cirrhosis, and chronic bile duct obstruction (Rolfe and Twedt, 1995). Copper may aggravate the underlying pathologic process in these disorders by direct injury to cellular organelles or by promotion of fibrogenesis (Hultgren et al, 1986). The decreased ability to excrete biliary copper probably underlies abnormal hepatic copper retention when a primary cholestatic disease exists. Primary hepatobiliary disease associated with an increased accumulation of hepatic copper, albeit smaller amounts of tissue copper than in Bedlington

terriers, has been described in Doberman pinscher, Skye terrier, West Highland white terrier, and American and English cocker spaniel dogs (Crawford et al, 1985; Thornburg and Rottinghaus, 1985; Thornburg et al, 1986). The chronic active hepatitis associated with an increased liver copper content in Doberman pinschers occurs primarily in middle-aged females. Although the youngest dog reported with this disorder was 1.5 years old, it is unknown whether younger dogs are symptomatic. It is suspected that affected dogs could be identified at a younger age on the basis of routine screening serum chemistry profiles revealing increased liver enzyme activity.

A familial copper-associated liver disease occurs in West Highland white terrier dogs (Thornburg et al, 1986). Increased hepatic copper concentrations are detected in asymptomatic dogs as young as 7 months of age. In three affected dogs younger than 9 months of age, the hepatic copper concentration ranged between 1500 and 1750 μg/g dry weight. Hepatic copper concentrations in affected dogs have ranged as high as 3500 ppm, considerably lower than the maximal values recorded for Bedlington terriers. In an attempt to decrease the perpetuation of this disorder, it has been recommended that relatives of West Highland white terrier dogs dying of liver disease be evaluated by hepatic biopsy before 1 year of age. Those animals with increased hepatic copper content should not be used for breeding purposes. Liver disease has also been observed with unexpected frequency in American and English cocker spaniel dogs (Thornburg and Rottinghaus, 1985). Dogs as young as 9 months have been diagnosed as having chronic active hepatitis. The liver disease appears to be progressive, and dogs dying of cirrhosis have had hepatic copper concentrations three to five times normal.

Abnormal Urate Metabolism

A genetic defect in the Dalmatian dog's liver results in an inability to convert uric acid into allantoin, the soluble excretory product of purine metabolism in non-Dalmatian dogs (Briggs, 1985; Briggs and Harley, 1986; Giesecke and Tiemeyer, 1984). This genetic defect is transmitted by homozygosity for a recessive trait. Serum uric acid concentrations in Dalmatian dogs are consistently increased, and urinary excretion of uric acid is markedly greater than in non-Dalmatian dogs. Typical serum uric acid concentrations in Dalmatian dogs range between 2 and 4 mg/dl versus less than 1 mg/dl

in other breeds of dogs (Kruger and Osborne, 1986; Schaible, 1986). Urine excretion of uric acid in Dalmatians ranges between 400 and 600 mg in 24 hours versus 10 to 60 mg in 24 hours in non-Dalmatians (Kruger and Osborne, 1986). Urine uric acid-to-creatinine values have ranged between 0.3 and 0.6 for normal puppies and 1.3 and 4.6 for pedigree Dalmatian puppies at 3 to 7 weeks of age and between 0.2 and 0.4 for normal dogs and 0.6 and 1.5 for purebred adult Dalmatians (Schaible, 1986). The increased urinary excretion of uric acid puts the Dalmatian at increased risk for the formation of urate uroliths, although not all affected dogs develop uroliths.

Selected Hepatobiliary Disorders

Hepatic Lipidosis. Most puppies and kittens that present with hepatic lipidosis have primary disease in other organ systems or an infectious disease, and therefore it is possible that the hepatic lipidosis was the consequence of acquired nutritional inadequacies. A variety of metabolic disorders can disturb the mobilization of triglycerides from the liver. Whenever intrahepatic lipid synthesis or the hepatocellular uptake of fat exceeds the dispersal of triglycerides from the liver, hepatic lipidosis develops (Fig. 11–7) (Miettinen, 1981; Pulito et al, 1976). Severe hepatic lipidosis occurs most commonly in toy-breed puppies, which become hypoglycemic and die after prolonged anorexia or fasting (van Toor et al, 1991). Clinically, kittens appear to be more susceptible to hepatic triglyceride accumulation than puppies. Any serious medical problem in the kitten can be associated with excessive hepatic lipid accumulation characterized by cytoplasmic vacuole formation that adversely influences hepatic function. Nutritional management that ensures adequate intake of calories, essential amino acids, and essential fatty acids is the best recommended symptomatic therapy. In addition, nutritional management for the mother during pregnancy can be important in possibly preventing hepatic lipidosis in the newborn.

Neonatal Icterus. Neonatal icterus often occurs in puppies and kittens as a result of immunohemolytic anemia (Cain and Suzuki, 1985; Giger et al, 1991; Young et al, 1951). Icterus often occurs in kittens within 3 days of birth with hemolysis from neonatal isoerythrolysis (see Chapter 3).

Noncirrhotic Portal Hypertension in Young Dogs. Most young dogs with noncir-

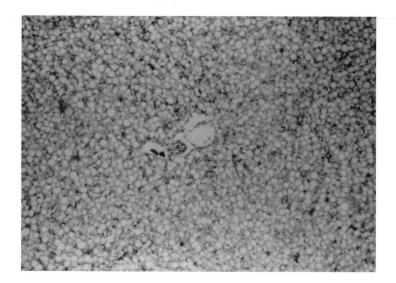

Figure 11–7. Photomicrograph of a liver biopsy specimen from a cat with hepatic lipidosis. (Hematoxylin and eosin stain; ×63.) (Courtesy of the Department of Pathology, New York State College of Veterinary Medicine.)

rhotic portal hypertension are younger than 19 months old, pedigree dogs, and female (see Table 11–3) (Bunch, 1997; DeMarco et al, 1998; Rand et al, 1988; Rutgers et al, 1993; van den Ingh and Rothuizen, 1994; van den Ingh et al, 1995). Typical signs are apathy, ascites, vague gastrointestinal upset (anorexia, vomiting, diarrhea), neurologic derangements, and polydipsia/polyuria. The affected dogs typically have small-sized livers, acquired PSS, and splenomegaly. Common trends in serum chemistry profiles are increased liver enzyme activities and evidence of hepatic dysfunction (e.g., hypoalbuminemia, increased serum bile acid content, and hyperammonemia). Microcytosis is a consistent finding. Liver biopsy is required for an accurate diagnosis in the affected dog. Histopathologic findings include preserved to altered liver architecture, portal hypoperfusion, and variable degrees of fibrosis; there are usually no cytopathic indications of destructive processes such as necrosis or inflammation.

Responses to symptomatic and specific hepatic treatment of affected dogs vary with the degree of portal hypertension present and the length of time hypertension has existed. Symptomatic measures to decrease ascites and signs of hepatic encephalopathy are indicated. Colchicine (0.025 mg/kg orally once daily) and/or prednisone (0.5 to 1.0 mg/kg orally daily initially, then every other day) have been the medications reported to be useful in a small number of cases (Rutgers et al, 1990). It seems that affected dogs have the potential to have a good quality of life for an indefinite period of time.

Feline Inflammatory Liver Disease. Inflammatory liver diseases of young cats is proba-

bly best referred to as feline cholangitis/cholangiohepatitis syndrome (CCHS) (Center, 1997). This syndrome can then be described as being either a suppurative CCHS or a nonsuppurative CCHS. Affected cats with suppurative CCHS usually are 3 months and older and usually are males. A sudden-onset history of vomiting and diarrhea is common. Older cats are icteric, febrile, lethargic, and dehydrated on initial presentation. Less than 50% of cats have hepatomegaly. The most common organisms associated with suppurative CCHS are *Escherichia coli*, *Staphylococcus*, α-hemolytic *Streptococcus*, *Bacillus*, *Actinomyces*, *Bacteroides*, *Enterococcus*, *Enterobacter*, and *Clostridium* species.

Most cats with suppurative CCHS show a moderate increase in serum ALT, AST, ALP, and GGT activities. Some cats have left-shifted leukograms with an accompanying leukocytosis. On ultrasonography, severe ascending cholangitis associated with thickening of the extrahepatic biliary system and inflammation within the lumen of the intrahepatic bile ducts may be observed. Ultrasonography also may show coexisting extrahepatic bile duct obstruction (enlarged gallbladder, distended and tortuous common bile duct, and obvious intrahepatic bile ducts), cholecystitis (thickened, laminar appearance of the gallbladder wall, adjacent fluid accumulation), and pancreatitis (prominent, easily visualized enlarged pancreas with adjacent hyperechoic fat). Cytologic evaluation of liver aspirates or imprints may reveal suppurative inflammation.

Most cats with nonsuppurative CCHS are 1 year of age or older and have been ill for several months (Center, 1997). Clinical signs are subtle and may include only episodic vomiting, diarrhea, and anorexia. Most cats have hepatomegaly, are icteric, and may have ascites. Concurrent disorders frequently include inflammatory bowel disease, low-grade lymphocytic pancreatitis, and cholecystitis. Cats with lymphoplasmacytic inflammation tend to have greater magnitudes of increased serum ALT, AST, ALP, and GGT activities than cats with just lymphocytic inflammation. Cats with lymphocytic inflammation may develop a lymphocytosis (total lymphocyte counts greater than 14,000/μl) without other evidence of malignant lymphoproliferative disease. Similar to cats with suppurative CCHS, abdominal radiographs rarely show important diagnostic information. In most cats with nonsuppurative CCHS, a multifocal hyperechoic pattern is recognized ultrasonographically, which represents peribiliary inflammation and fibrosis. In some cats, ultrasonography may fail to show any abnormalities. Cytologic preparations from liver aspirates may lack evidence of inflammation or may disclose only a few inflammatory cells. A wedge biopsy of the liver for histopathology is preferable for a definitive diagnosis because it more reliably demonstrates whole acinar units and portal triads (Center, 1997).

Treatment of suppurative CCHS incorporates appropriate antimicrobial therapy based on identification of infectious organisms. If bacteria are cytologically observed, a Gram's stain facilitates selection of antimicrobial agents. Cats with extrahepatic bile duct obstruction should have their biliary occlusion decompressed, if possible. If biliary tract decompression cannot be accomplished, the biliary pathway may be rerouted by a cholecystoenterostomy. Biliary diversion is a vital early therapeutic intervention in the prevention or control of sepsis in obstructive suppurative cholangitis. Aerobic and anaerobic bacterial cultures should be collected from bile, tissue adjacent to any focal lesion, gallbladder wall, and liver tissue.

Any icteric cat suspected of having suppurative or nonsuppurative CCHS should be evaluated for coexistent extrahepatic bile duct obstruction, pancreatitis, and inflammatory bowel disease as well as coexistent hepatic lipidosis. If lipid vacuolation is detected, nutritional support with a commercially prepared feline diet should be included in the treatment plan.

Immunosuppressive therapy for cats with nonsuppurative CCHS includes a combination of prednisolone (initial dose of 2 to 4 mg/kg orally once a day or divided twice daily), with titration to the lowest effective dose over the next several months, and metronidazole (7.5 mg/kg orally two to three times daily) (Center, 1997). Supplementation with L-carnitine 250 mg/cat per day, water-soluble vitamins (two times the normal maintenance dose), and vitamin K$_1$ (0.5 to 1.5 mg/kg) subcutaneously or intramuscularly for three doses at 12-hour intervals and then once a week for 1 or 2 additional weeks may be provided. Oral vitamin E can also be added as a supplement to ensure its adequacy as a free radical scavenger; a dose of 100 to 200 IU per day is used. Ursodeoxycholic acid (10 to 15 mg/kg orally per day) is given to all cats with CCHS once extrahepatic bile duct obstruction is corrected. Monthly serum liver enzyme activities and total bilirubin concentrations may be used to monitor treatment response as well as how well the cat is doing at home.

Selected Infectious Diseases

Hepatic Abscessation. Hematogenous, omphalogenic, biliary, and peritoneal extension are sources of infecting organisms that cause hepatic abscesses to appear in puppies and kittens (Hargis and Thomassen, 1980; Valentine and Porter, 1983). Postpartum umbilical infection appears to be the most common cause of hepatic abscessation. Once clinical signs develop, animals deteriorate and die within 2 to 4 weeks. Occasionally, seemingly healthy puppies die unexpectedly, the cause being discovered on histopathologic examination. Most affected puppies are between 3 and 70 days of age and are from large litters (Hargis and Thomassen, 1980). Organisms frequently isolated from hepatic abscesses in puppies and kittens include *Escherichia coli* and *Staphylococcus*, *Streptococcus*, and *Salmonella* species. Puppies and kittens with hepatic abscesses are usually stunted, emaciated, and dehydrated and may have enlarged abdomens due to hepatomegaly and peritonitis. Unaffected liver lobes usually show multifocal necrosis on histopathologic examination. Suspected hepatic abscesses in puppies and kittens should be managed with antimicrobial drugs and other supportive care (see Chapter 5).

Hepatic Parasitism. Hepatic trematode infection may be diagnosed in kittens as young as 4 months of age. The most common liver fluke in cats in North America is *Platynosomum concinnum*. Other species of flukes that may infect cats include *Amphimerus pseudofelineus*, *Opisthorchis tenuicollis*, *Metorchis albidus*, and *Metorchis conjuctus*. Cats acquire *Platynosomum con-*

cinnum infection by the ingestion of the second intermediate hosts: a land snail (*Subulina octona*) and a lizard or marine toad. Once ingested, the infective stage of the parasite migrates up the common bile duct into the gallbladder and bile ducts, where in 8 to 12 weeks it matures into the adult fluke. Embryonated eggs are passed in the feces and are the basis for diagnosis. Clinical signs are noted by 7 to 16 weeks after infection and may include inappetence, lethargy, weight loss, hepatomegaly, emaciation, mucoid diarrhea, depression, vomiting, and abdominal tenderness. Many naturally infected cats show no clinical signs. In heavy infections, clinical signs may develop before the fecal shedding of ova, which occurs as early as 8 weeks after infection. Concentration of eggs in feces by sedimentation is the most reliable diagnostic test. Transient increases in the serum AST and ALT activities develop during fluke migration through the liver. The serum ALP activity may remain normal or may increase. Cats with heavy fluke infection may become jaundiced. Persistent fluke infections and bile duct obstruction may result in biliary cirrhosis. Treatment with praziquantel (20 to 40 mg/kg daily for at least 3 days) is clinically effective.

Hepatobiliary lesions produced by ascarid larval migration are commonly observed during necropsy of young dogs and cats. These lesions are usually not associated with clinical signs or laboratory abnormalities. Severe hepatic and peritoneal migration, gallbladder rupture, and bile peritonitis may, however, occur in a few puppies. In young dogs and cats, after ingesting eggs, the larval forms of *Toxocara canis* and *Toxocara cati* penetrate the wall of the alimentary canal and pass by way of lymphatics or the portal circulation to the liver. Ascarids may also migrate from the gastrointestinal tract directly through the peritoneal cavity to the liver.

Viral-Induced Hepatic Diseases. Canine herpesvirus infection is an acute, rapidly fatal disease that is associated with hepatic necrosis. Puppies acquire canine herpesvirus in utero, during passage through the birth canal, by exposure to infected littermates, or from oronasal secretions of the dam. Abortions and stillbirths may occur if infection is acquired in utero (Poste and King, 1971). Generalized, fatal infections develop in puppies during the first 3 weeks of life. Puppies infected when older than 3 weeks are comparatively resistant and develop mild or inapparent infection. An incubation period of 4 to 6 days follows initial exposure. A diffuse necrotizing vasculitis and spread of virus

into parenchymal organs, including the adrenals, kidneys, lungs, spleen, and liver, results in multifocal organ necrosis. Meningoencephalitis that causes seizure activity is common in canine herpesvirus infections. In survivors, permanent neurologic deficits may persist, most common of which are cerebellar vestibular defects. Ocular involvement causing panuveitis, cataracts, keratitis, retinitis, and subsequent blindness may occur.

Clinical signs of canine herpesvirus infection in puppies may include depression, diminished suckling response, persistent crying, yellow-green diarrhea, abdominal pain, and incoordination. Petechial hemorrhages may be notable on mucous membranes. Cutaneous lesions may include an erythematous rash with red papules progressing to vesicles. Papular or vesicular lesions may develop in the vulvovaginal orifice, prepuce, and/or oral cavity. Neurologic signs may occur during the terminal stages of the disease. Death frequently occurs within 24 to 48 hours after onset of clinical signs in infected puppies.

Definitive diagnosis of canine herpesvirus infection in puppies is made on the basis of history, clinical signs, histopathologic changes, and virus isolation. Hematologic and biochemical abnormalities are nonspecific and variable. Thrombocytopenia may be present in ill puppies. Widespread hepatic necrosis causes increased serum activities of ALT and AST. Icterus does not occur. Gross pathologic findings include disseminated multifocal petechial hemorrhages (Fig. 11–8) and areas of necrosis that are distinctly circumscribed in the liver, kidney, and lungs (Greene and Kakuk, 1984). Hepatomegaly, splenomegaly, and lymphadenopathy are common. Histopathologic lesions are characterized by perivascular necrosis associated with a mild neutrophil and lymphocyte infiltration, hemorrhages, and occasional intranuclear inclusions (Fig. 11–9). Treatment for canine herpesvirus infection is usually unrewarding owing to its rapidly fatal progression. Rectal temperature elevation to about 37.7° C (100° F) and adequate nutritional support may improve puppy survival during an outbreak.

Focal hepatitis and hepatic cord disorganization may develop in puppies and kittens infected with canine or feline parvovirus. Two- to five-fold increases in serum activities of ALT and AST may develop. In some cases, hepatic involvement is progressive, resulting in icterus. Seemingly, a poor prognosis is warranted when hepatic involvement becomes clinically apparent.

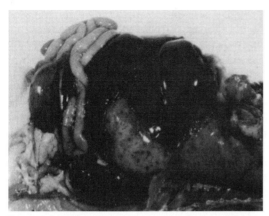

Figure 11–8. Photograph of petechial hemorrhages on visceral surfaces in a puppy with canine herpesvirus infection. Note the hepatomegaly and diffusely mottled appearance of the liver associated with multifocal hepatic necrosis. (Courtesy of Dr. Fred Quimby, Center for Research Animal Resources, New York State College of Veterinary Medicine.)

Coronavirus infection causing feline infectious peritonitis (FIP) most often affects cats between 6 months and 2 years of age. Coronavirus infection has been diagnosed as a cause of stillborn kittens and fading kittens and as an effusive disease in kittens younger than 4 weeks of age. Clinical signs of FIP usually develop in several siblings in a litter, and death losses may span a 6- to 12-month interval. Cats with liver involvement may demonstrate cranial abdominal pain and hepatomegaly. Serum ALT and AST activities are usually increased from 2- to 10-fold in cats with liver involvement. Icterus may develop in those cats with severe, diffuse hepatic lesions. A coagulopathy and thrombocytopenia develop in cats with diffuse vascular injury, in those with severe inflammation and subsequent activation of clotting factors, or in severe hepatic involvement (Weiss et al, 1980). Immunosuppression may help prolong the survival of some cats. Unfortunately, kittens showing signs of hepatic involvement are usually poor candidates for immunosuppressive therapy.

Infection of kittens with feline leukemia virus or feline immunodeficiency virus may occur by horizontal or vertical transmission. By virtue of their oncogenic potential and ability to immunologically compromise the host, these viruses may be associated with neoplastic conditions and infectious diseases involving the liver. Lymphosarcoma and myeloproliferative disease can develop in infected cats within weeks or months of exposure. Affected kittens demonstrate hepatomegaly when they have liver involvement. Icterus develops with diffuse hepatic involvement, periportal infiltration, or major bile duct occlusion. Serum chemistry profile abnormalities are variable, depending on the extent of hepatic involvement.

Bacterial-Induced Hepatic Diseases. Enteric organisms such as *Salmonella* species and *Escherichia coli* can be a source of hepatic parenchymal and biliary tract infections in young dogs and cats (Greene, 1984). *Salmonella* species may exist in young dogs and cats as a part of the normal enteric flora. Transmission of *Salmonella* species from carrier animals to susceptible hosts may result in gastroenteritis, bacteremia, parenchymal organ or lymph node colonization or abscessation, endotoxemia, stillbirths, or a fading puppy or kitten syndrome. Signs of gastrointestinal infection may develop after 3 to 5 days of exposure or after some unusual environmental or physical stress.

Figure 11–9. Photomicrograph of intranuclear inclusions (arrow) in hepatocytes from a puppy with canine herpesvirus infection. (Hematoxylin and eosin stain; ×400.) (Courtesy of Dr. Fred Quimby, Center for Research Animal Resources, New York State College of Veterinary Medicine.)

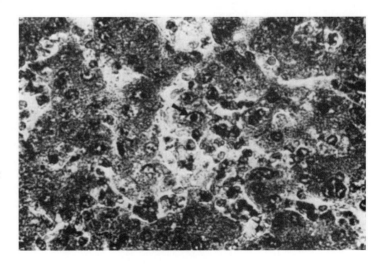

Initial signs may include fever (104° to 106° F), malaise, anorexia, vomiting, abdominal pain, and diarrhea. Diarrhea can be voluminous and usually contains mucus and fresh blood. Further signs may develop, including weight loss, severe dehydration, weakness, hypotension, pale mucous membranes, and, in some cases, evidence of neurologic involvement. Icterus may develop as a result of endotoxemic effects on the liver, hepatic infarction, or bacterial colonization of hepatic tissue. Serum chemistry profile evidence of liver involvement includes increases in the serum activities of ALT, AST, and ALP. Hyperbilirubinemia is an inconsistent finding.

Multifocal necrosis is the most common histopathologic lesion of salmonellosis. A necrotizing pneumonia may also occur in puppies with hepatic involvement. Definitive diagnosis of salmonellosis relies on culture of the organism from involved tissues or body fluids that are normally free of this organism. Positive culture of fecal specimens does not confirm the causal relationship of the organism to the animals' clinical disease. Successful treatment requires attention to supportive nursing care, plasma transfusion for severe hypoproteinemia, and selection of an appropriate antimicrobial agent. The prognosis for puppies and kittens with salmonellosis is generally poor. Efforts to improve kennel or cattery sanitation, to improve nutrition, and to reduce stress on puppies and kittens may curtail further infection.

Bacillus piliformis, the causative agent of Tyzzer's disease, is a gram-negative, spore-forming, obligate intracellular bacterium that can cause enteric and hepatic infections in young dogs and cats, most commonly seen at the time of weaning. Animals subject to infection develop necrotizing enteritis and multifocal hepatitis. Infection in most young dogs and cats is thought to occur by their ingestion of bacterial spores passed in rodent feces. Signs of natural disease in young dogs and cats include a sudden onset of lethargy, depression, anorexia, diarrhea, and abdominal tenderness. Icterus may occur in some affected kittens. Within 24 to 48 hours after the onset of illness, affected animals become hypothermic and severely depressed. Death rapidly follows. Identification of the bacterium is aided by the use of special stains such as Giemsa's stain or Gomori's methenamine silver stain (Greene, 1984). Isolation of the causative agent cannot be accomplished on routinely used bacterial culture media.

Toxoplasmosis. The signs associated with *Toxoplasma gondii* infections vary depending on the chronicity of infection, immune status of the host, mode of infection, and target organs affected. Young dogs and cats are particularly at risk when immunocompromised and debilitated. In utero infection can occur and lead to stillbirths or neonatal disease and death. Affected puppies and kittens may appear normal at birth but become depressed, inappetent, and dyspneic and develop a mucopurulent oculonasal discharge and progressive neurologic disease; they eventually die. Dissemination to multiple organs usually occurs. Hepatic lesions are typified as a multifocal necrotizing hepatitis. Hepatic inflammation may be associated with cranial abdominal pain and peritoneal effusion and is usually associated with vomiting, diarrhea, and inappetence. Animals may become icteric owing to the diffuse nature of the hepatic necrosis.

Laboratory abnormalities associated with toxoplasmosis are variable, depending on the target organs affected and the chronicity of infection. Early hematologic features may include a panleukopenia with a degenerative left shift. A leukocytosis may follow during the recovery period (Greene and Prestwood, 1984). Serum chemistry profile abnormalities indicating hepatic involvement include marked increases in serum ALT, AST, and ALP activities and hyperbilirubinemia. Definitive diagnosis of toxoplasmosis is made on the basis of tissue examination for *Toxoplasma gondii* organisms or demonstration of a rising serologic antigen and/or antibody titer. Recommended treatments for toxoplasmosis include the use of pyrimethamine, trimethoprim-sulfonamide, and clindamycin (Greene and Prestwood, 1984).

THE PANCREAS

Inflammatory Pancreatic Disease

The pancreas is a unique organ possessing both exocrine (digestive) and endocrine (hormonal) functions. Inflammatory pancreatic disease affecting only the exocrine portion is extremely uncommon in young dogs and cats (Strombeck and Guilford, 1990). Consequently, inflammatory pancreatic disease, that is, acute pancreatitis or relapsing pancreatitis that more commonly affects older dogs and cats, has been rarely identified in dogs and cats younger than 6 months of age. The likely causes of inflammatory pancreatic disease in the young dog and cat are abdominal trauma and infectious agents. Abdominal trauma may induce pancreatitis in dogs that are traumatized by motor vehicles and in cats that have fallen or jumped from high places (high-rise syndrome) (Drazner, 1986). In addition, abdominal surgery may result in acute pancreatitis due to traumatic injury to the pancreas (spearing the pancreas with a surgical instrument) or excessive manipulation of the pancreas.

Infectious agents can occasionally contribute to inflammatory pancreatic disease. Pancreatic necrosis can be found on postmortem examination of an occasional dog afflicted with canine parvovirus infection (Drazner, 1986). It is not known whether the canine parvovirus is directly cytotoxic to the pancreatic tissue or pancreatitis occurs secondary to the invasion of enzymes and bacteria of the intestinal tract into the pancreas. In cats, pancreatitis may be associated with the effusive form of FIP (Barlough and Weiss, 1983). Other infectious agents directly associated with inflammatory pancreatic disease in the young dog and cat would be extremely unusual and most likely a one-time occurrence.

Although seldom required, laboratory confirmation of inflammatory pancreatic disease includes a complete blood count, serum chemistry profile, serum amylase and lipase determinations, serum trypsin-like immunoreactivity (TLI) assay, and survey radiographs and/or ultrasonography of the abdomen. Normal values for serum amylase and lipase activities in dogs and cats younger than 6 months of age are generally indicative of normal adult values. Hyperamylasemia and hyperlipasemia combined with typical clinical features of inflammatory pancreatic disease, as seen in adult animals, establish the diagnosis of inflammatory pancre-

atic disease until proved otherwise. The serum TLI assay may be increased—TLI values of more than 35 μg/L in young dogs and more than 50 μg/L in young cats are consistent with pancreatitis. Its treatment is entirely supportive and is managed in a manner similar to that for the afflicted older dog or cat.

Congenital Pancreatic Hypoplasia

By far the most common cause of noninflammatory pancreatic disease in the young dog is congenital pancreatic hypoplasia (Harris, 1985; Jubb, 1983; Sherding, 1979). This disorder of young dogs is characterized by generalized reduction in pancreatic exocrine (acinar) cells, but the islets of Langerhans remain intact (Fig. 11–10). The disorder is more common in large breeds of dogs, that is, German shepherd (Alsatian), Doberman pinscher, Irish setter, Labrador retriever, and Saint Bernard, but has also been seen in the beagle (Hill et al, 1971; Prentice et al, 1980). There may be a sex predilection favoring females (Anderson and Low, 1965), and young dogs that are symptomatic generally present before 1 year of age. Congenital pancreatic hypoplasia has not been recognized in the young cat.

Most dogs affected with congenital pancreatic hypoplasia present with signs of weight loss or failure to gain adequate weight and poor physical appearance (i.e., dull, dry haircoat and excessive shedding) despite exhibiting a good to voracious appetite (Sherding, 1979). Varying degrees of frequent (6 to 10 stools per day), foul-smelling, bulky, greasy, loose stools are de-

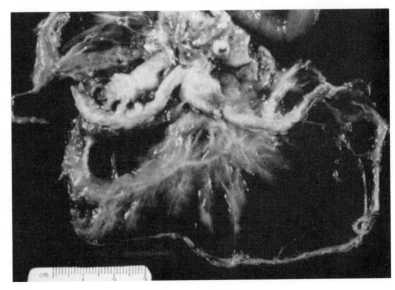

Figure 11–10. Photograph of the pancreas from a young dog with congenital pancreatic hypoplasia. Note the generalized reduction in amount of pancreatic tissue present and the absence of any inflammatory pancreatic disease.

scribed by the dog owner. Often, coprophagia is noted. Affected dogs commonly eat their stools because of their high fat content and because of a dietary energy deficit. The diarrheic stools contain undigested sugars and fats that are being altered by intestinal bacteria to become osmotically active particles (Drazner, 1983). The marked increase in osmotically active particles and the subsequent efflux of water into the lumen of the intestinal tract result in the colon's inability to resorb the increased volume, and diarrhea ensues. The volume of unabsorbed intraluminal water produces marked intestinal distention and altered motility, which may be severe enough to cause intestinal and colonic bacterial overgrowth (Drazner, 1983). Unabsorbed fatty acids may also impair the absorptive capacity of the small intestine by damaging the brush border, blunting the villi, and inhibiting colonic water absorption.

The diagnostic evaluation of dogs suspected to have congenital pancreatic hypoplasia differentiates this disorder from intestinal mucosal malabsorption. Diagnosis of congenital pancreatic hypoplasia is usually not difficult because the presenting signs are rather characteristic and the laboratory test results are helpful in its diagnosis. The serum TLI assay values are classically decreased—TLI values are consistently less than 2.5 μg/L in affected dogs. When the diagnosis is still in question or serum TLI assay results are not available, an exploratory laparotomy can be used for confirmation.

Treatment of dogs with congenital pancreatic hypoplasia depends mainly on dietary management and supplementation with pancreatic digestive enzymes (Lewis et al, 1987). Efforts to treat these dogs are usually rewarded with a favorable response. The expense of treatment and an unconscientious owner, rather than the ineffectiveness of the treatment regimen itself, are most often the reasons that successful treatment is not accomplished. The most effective dietary management for dogs with congenital pancreatic hypoplasia is a highly digestible, low-fiber, moderate-fat diet supplemented with pancreatic enzymes (Lewis et al, 1987). Commercial diets formulated for gastrointestinal disease may be fed. The dog's daily food intake is divided into two or three feedings or is fed free choice. The dietary replacement of pancreatic digestive enzymes is given orally with each meal. Various pancreatic enzyme products are commercially available for this purpose (Sherding, 1979). Reliable commercial products are available in both powder and tablet form. The usual effective dosage of the powder preparation is 1 to 2 tsp per meal for each 20 kg body weight. The pancreatic enzyme product is mixed with the commercially prepared canned or well-moistened dry dog food and fed without necessarily any preincubation time. When diarrhea is in remission and the animal is gaining weight, the pancreatic enzyme product should be titrated to the minimum effective maintenance dose per feeding.

When pancreatic digestive enzymes are given orally, a high percentage of them are inactivated by gastric acid. Even though only a fraction of the pancreatic enzymes administered reach the small intestine in an active state, they are still effective because only a slight increase in duodenal digestive enzyme activity is needed to achieve marked improvement in nutrient assimilation (Drazner, 1986). In some dogs, antimicrobial agents may be a helpful adjunctive therapy for the bacterial overgrowth of the small intestine that often accompanies malassimilation in congenital pancreatic hypoplasia (Drazner, 1986). Medium-chain triglycerides may be added to the dog's diet if additional dietary energy is needed to increase weight gain or maintain condition in the dog that fails to respond otherwise. The medium-chain triglycerides can be used to provide up to 25% of the dog's caloric need and, when fully utilized, provide 8 kcal/ml (Lewis et al, 1987).

The dog's body weight, general condition, and stool character should be monitored weekly during the treatment of congenital pancreatic hypoplasia. Stool volume should decrease precipitously, and gains in body weight should begin soon after initiation of dietary management and the supplementation of pancreatic digestive enzymes (Sherding, 1979). The dietary replacement of pancreatic digestive enzymes is generally required for the rest of the dog's life.

References and Supplemental Reading
THE LIVER AND HEPATOBILIARY DISORDERS

Alroy J, Orgad U, Ucci AA, et al: Neurovisceral and skeletal GM1-gangliosidosis in dogs with beta-galactosidase deficiency. Science 229:470, 1985.

Baker HJ, Lindsey JR: Animal model of human disease: Feline GM1 gangliosidosis. Am J Pathol 74:649, 1974.

Barnes IC, Kelly DF, Pennock CA, et al: Hepatic beta galactosidase and feline GM1 gangliosidosis. Neuropathol Appl Neurobiol 7:463, 1981.

Bartlett LM: A divided intrahepatic gallbladder in a cat. Anat Rec 109:715, 1951.

Berger B, Whiting PG, Breznock EM, et al: Congenital feline portosystemic shunts. J Am Vet Med Assoc 188:517, 1986.

Birchard SJ: Surgical management of portosystemic shunts in dogs and cats. Compend Contin Educ Pract Vet 6:795, 1984.

Black AP: A solitary congenital hepatic cyst in a cat. Aust Vet Pract 13:166, 1983.

Blood DC: Suspected congenital atresia of the hepatic bile ducts in a cat. Aust Vet J Aug:193, 1947.

Boothe HW, Howe LM, Edwards JF, et al: Multiple extrahepatic portosystemic shunts in dogs: 30 cases (1981–993). J Am Vet Med Assoc 208:1849, 1996.

Bostwick DR, Twedt DC: Intrahepatic and extrahepatic portal venous anomalies in dogs: 52 cases (1982–1992). J Am Vet Med Assoc 206:1181, 1995.

Boyden EA: The accessory gall-bladder: An embryological and comparative study of aberrant biliary vesicles occurring in man and the domestic mammals. Am J Anat 38:177, 1926.

Breton L, Guerin P, Morin M: A case of mucopolysaccharidosis VI in a cat. J Am Anim Hosp Assoc 19:891, 1983.

Breznock EM, Berger B, Pendray D, et al: Surgical manipulation of intrahepatic portocaval shunts in dogs. J Am Vet Med Assoc 182:798, 1983.

Briggs OM: Serum urate concentrations in the Dalmatian coach hound. J Comp Pathol 95:301, 1985.

Briggs OM, Harley EH: The fate of administered purines in the Dalmatian coach hound. J Comp Pathol 96:267, 1986.

Bunch SE: Noncirrhotic portal hypertension in young dogs. Proc Am Coll Vet Intern Med 15:42, 1997.

Cain GR, Suzuki Y: Presumptive neonatal isoerythrolysis in cats. J Am Vet Med Assoc 187:46, 1985.

Carr SH, Thornburg LP: Congenital portacaval shunt in two kittens. Feline Pract 14:43, 1984.

Ceh L, Hauge JG, Svenkerud R, et al: Glycogenosis type III in the dog. Acta Vet Scand 17:210, 1976.

Center SA: The jaundiced cat. Proc Feline Med Symp 1997, p 41.

Center SA, Baldwin BH, Erb HN, et al: Bile acid concentrations in the diagnosis of hepatobiliary disease in the dog. J Am Vet Med Assoc 188:935, 1985a.

Center SA, Baldwin BH, Erb HN, et al: Bile acid concentrations in the diagnosis of hepatobiliary disease in the cat. J Am Vet Med Assoc 187:507, 1985b.

Center SA, Baldwin BH, de Lahunta A, et al: Evaluation of serum bile acid concentrations for the diagnosis of portosystemic venous anomalies in the dog and cat. J Am Vet Med Assoc 186:1090, 1986a.

Center SA, Hornbuckle WE, Hoskins JD: The liver and pancreas. In Hoskins JD (ed): Veterinary Pediatrics: Dogs and Cats from Birth to Six Months, 2nd ed. Philadelphia, WB Saunders, 1995, p 189.

Center SA, Hornbuckle WE, Scavelli TD: Congenital portosystemic shunts in cats. In Kirk RW (ed): Current Veterinary Therapy IX. Philadelphia, WB Saunders, 1986b, p 825.

Center SA, Randolph JF, ManWarren T, et al: Effect of colostrum ingestion on gamma-glutamyltransferase and alkaline phosphatase activities in neonatal pups. Am J Vet Res 52:499, 1991.

Cork LC, Munnell JF, Lorenz MD, et al: GM2-ganglioside lysosomal storage disease in cats with beta-hexosaminidase deficiency. Science 196:1014, 1977.

Cork LC, Munnell JF, Lorenz MD: The pathology of feline GM2 gangliosidosis. Am J Pathol 90:723, 1978.

Crawford MA, Schall WD, Jensen RK, et al: Chronic active hepatitis in 26 Doberman pinschers. J Am Vet Med Assoc 187:1343, 1985.

Crowell WA, Hubbell JJ, Riley JC: Polycystic renal disease in related cats. J Am Vet Med Assoc 175:286, 1979.

DeMarco J, Center SA, Dykes N, et al: A syndrome resembling idiopathic noncirrhotic portal hypertension in 4 young Doberman pinschers. J Vet Intern Med 12:147, 1998.

Dial SM, Thrall MA, Gasper PW, et al: Cerebral arylsulfatase B activity in normal and arylsulfatase B–deficient cats prior to and following allogeneic bone marrow transplantation. Vet Clin Pathol 14:12, 1985.

Easley JC, Carpenter JL: Hepatic arteriovenous fistula in two Saint Bernard pups. J Am Vet Med Assoc 166:167, 1975.

Edelstone DI: Regulation of blood flow through the ductus venosus. J Dev Physiol 2:219, 1980.

Gandolfi RC: Hepatoencephalopathy associated with patent ductus venosus in a cat. J Am Vet Med Assoc 185:301, 1984.

Forster-van Hijfte MA, McEvoy FJ, White RN, et al: Per rectal portal scintigraphy in the diagnosis and management of feline congenital portosystemic shunts. J Small Anim Pract 37:7, 1996.

Gasper PW, Thrall MA, Wenger DA, et al: Bone marrow transplantation for correction of feline arylsulfatase B–deficiency (mucopolysaccharidosis VI). Vet Clin Pathol 14:13, 1985.

Giesecke D, Tiemeyer W: Defect of uric acid uptake in Dalmatian dog liver. Experientia 40:1415, 1984.

Giger U, Bucheler J, Patterson DF: Frequency and inheritance of A and B blood types in feline breeds of the United States. J Hered 82:15, 1991.

Gomes MMR, Bernatz PE: Arteriovenous fistulas: A review and ten-year experience at the Mayo Clinic. Mayo Clin Proc 45:81, 1970.

Greene CE: Enteric bacterial infections. In Greene CE (ed): Clinical Microbiology and Infectious Diseases of the Dog and Cat. Philadelphia, WB Saunders, 1984, p 617.

Greene CE, Kakuk TJ: Canine herpesvirus infection. In Greene CE (ed): Clinical Microbiology and Infectious Diseases of the Dog and Cat. Philadelphia, WB Saunders, 1984, p 419.

Greene CE, Prestwood AK: Coccidial infections. In Greene CE (ed): Clinical Microbiology and Infectious Diseases of the Dog and Cat. Philadelphia, WB Saunders, 1984, p 824.

Griffiths GL, Lumsden JH, Valli VEO: Hematologic and biochemical changes in dogs with portosystemic shunts. J Am Anim Hosp Assoc 17:705, 1981.

Hardie EM: Complications following portosystemic shunt ligation. Proc Am Coll Vet Intern Med 15:531, 1997.

Hardy RM: Copper-associated hepatitis in Bedlington terriers. In Kirk RW (ed): Current Veterinary Therapy VIII. Philadelphia, WB Saunders, 1983, p 834.

Hargis AM, Thomassen RW: Hepatic abscesses in beagle puppies. Lab Anim Sci 30:689, 1980.

Haskins ME, Aguirre GD, Jezyk PF, et al: The pathology of the feline model of mucopolysaccharidosis VI. Am J Pathol 101:657, 1980.

Haskins ME, Aguirre GD, Jezky PF: The pathology of the feline model of mucopolysaccharidosis I. Am J Pathol 112:27, 1983.

Haskins ME, Desnick RJ, DiFerrante N, et al: Beta-glucuronidase deficiency in a dog: A mode of human mucopolysaccharidosis VII. Pediatr Res 18:980, 1984.

Haskins ME, Jezyk PF, Desnick RJ, et al: Mucopolysaccharidosis VI Maroteaux-Lamy syndrome, arylsulfatase B–deficient mucopolysaccharidosis in the Siamese cat. Am J Pathol 105:191, 1981.

Heath T, House B: Origin and distribution of portal blood in the cat and the rabbit. Am J Anat 127:71, 1970.

Holt D: Critical care management of the portosystemic shunt patient. Compend Contin Educ Pract Vet 16:879, 1994.

Hottinger HA, Walshaw R, Hauptman JG: Long-term results of complete and partial ligation of congenital portosystemic shunts in dogs. Vet Surg 24:331, 1995.

Hultgren BD, Steven JB, Hardy RM: Inherited, chronic, progressive hepatic degeneration in Bedlington terriers with increased liver copper concentrations: Clinical and pathologic observations and comparison with other copper-associated liver diseases. Am J Vet Res 47:365, 1986.

Jezyk PF, Haskins ME, Newman LR: Alpha-mannosidosis in a Persian cat. J Am Vet Med Assoc 189:1483, 1986.

Johnson GF, Gilbertson SR, Goldfischer S, et al: Cytochemical detection of inherited copper toxicosis of Bedlington terriers. Vet Pathol 21:57, 1984.

Keller P: Enzyme activities in the dog: Tissue analyses, plasma values, and intracellular distribution. Am J Vet Res 42:575, 1981.

Khan IR, Vitums A: Portosystemic communications in the cat. Res Vet Sci 12:215, 1971.

Koblik PD, Komtebedde J, Yen CK, et al: Use of transcolonic 99m-technetium-pertechnetate as a screening test for portosystemic shunts in dogs. J Am Vet Med Assoc 196:925, 1990.

Kruger JM, Osborne CA: Etiopathogenesis of uric acid and ammonium urate uroliths in non-Dalmatian dogs. Vet Clin North Am 16:87, 1986.

Lamb CR: Ultrasonographic diagnosis of congenital portosystemic shunts in dogs: Results of a prospective study. Vet Radiol Ultrasound 37:28, 1996.

Lamb CR: Diagnostic imaging of portosystemic shunts in dogs and cats. Proc Am Coll Vet Intern Med 15:524, 1997.

Lamb CR, Forster-van Hijfte MA, White RN, et al: Ultrasonographic diagnosis of congenital portosystemic shunts in fourteen cats. J Small Anim Pract 37:205, 1996.

Lamb CR, Mahoney PN: Comparison of three methods for calculating portal blood flow velocity in dogs using duplex-Doppler ultrasonography. Vet Radiol Ultrasound 35:190, 1994.

Legendre AM, Krahwindel DJ, Carrig CB, et al: Ascites associated with intrahepatic arteriovenous fistula in a cat. J Am Vet Med Assoc 168:589, 1976.

Levy JK: Diagnosis and management of feline portosystemic vascular shunts. Proc Am Coll Vet Intern Med 15:527, 1997.

Lickley HLA, Chisholm DJ, Rabinovitch A, et al: Effects of portocaval anastomosis on glucose tolerance in the dog: Evidence of an interaction between the gut and the liver in oral glucose disposal. Metabolism 24:1157, 1975.

Lohse CL, Suter PF: Functional closure of the ductus venosus during early postnatal life in the dog. Am J Vet Res 38:839, 1977.

Magne ML, Macy DW: Intravenous glucagon challenge test in the diagnosis and assessment of therapeutic efficacy in dogs with congenital portosystemic shunts. Proc Am Coll Vet Intern Med 1984, p 36 (abstract).

Marretta SM, Pask AJ, Green RW, et al: Urinary calculi associated with portosystemic shunts in six dogs. J Am Vet Med Assoc 178:133, 1981.

McKenna SC, Carpenter JL: Polycystic disease of the kidney and liver in the Cairn terrier. Vet Pathol 17:436, 1980.

Meyer DJ: Liver function tests in dogs with portosystemic shunts: Measurement of serum bile acid concentration. J Am Vet Med Assoc 188:168, 1986.

Meyer HP, Rothuizen J, van den Brom WE, et al: Quantitation of portosystemic shunting in dogs by ultrasound-guided injection of Tc-99m-macroaggregates into a splenic vein. Res Vet Sci 57:58, 1994.

Miettinen EL: Effect of maternal canine starvation of fetal and neonatal liver metabolism. Am J Physiol 240:E88, 1981.

Moore PF, Whiting PG: Hepatic lesions associated with intrahepatic arterioportal fistulae in dogs. Vet Pathol 23:57, 1986.

Neuwelt EA, Johnson WG, Blank NK, et al: Characterization of a new model of GM2-gangliosidosis (Sandhoff's disease) in Korat cats. J Clin Invest 76:482, 1985.

Phillips L, Tappe J, Lyman R: Hepatic microvascular dysplasia with demonstrable macroscopic shunts. Proc Am Coll Vet Intern Med 11:438, 1993.

Poste G, King N: Isolation of a herpesvirus from

canine genital tract: Association with infertility, abortion, and stillbirths. Vet Rec 88:229, 1971.

Pulito AR, Santulli TV, Wigger HJ, et al: Effects of total parenteral nutrition and semi-starvation on the liver of beagle puppies. J Pediatr Surg 11:655, 1976.

Rafizuzzaman M, Svenkerud R, Strande A, et al: Glycogenosis in the dog. Acta Vet Scand 17:196, 1976.

Rand JS, Best SJ, Mathews KA: Portosystemic vascular shunts in a family of American cocker spaniels. J Am Anim Hosp Assoc 24:265, 1988.

Read DH, Harrington DD, Keenan TW, et al: Neuronal-visceral GM1 gangliosidosis in a dog with beta galactosidase deficiency. Science 194:442, 1976.

Rogers WA, Suter PF, Breznock EM, et al: Intrahepatic arteriovenous fistulae in a dog resulting in portal hypertension, portacaval shunts and reversal of portal blood flow. J Am Anim Hosp Assoc 13:470, 1977.

Rolfe DS, Twedt DC: Copper-associated hepatopathies in dogs. Vet Clin North Am 25:399, 1995.

Rutgers HC, Haywood S, Batt RM: Colchicine treatment in a dog with hepatoportal fibrosis. J Small Anim Pract 31:97, 1990.

Rutgers HC, Haywood S, Kelly DF: Idiopathic hepatic fibrosis in 15 dogs. Vet Rec 133:115, 1993.

Scavelli TD, Hornbuckle WE, Roth L, et al: Portosystemic shunts in cats: Seven cases (1976–1984). J Am Vet Med Assoc 189:317, 1986.

Schaible RH: Genetic predisposition to purine uroliths in Dalmatian dogs. Vet Clin North Am 16:127, 1986.

Schermhorn T, Center SA, Dykes A, et al: Characterization of hepatoportal microvascular dysplasia in a kindred of Cairn terriers. J Vet Intern Med 10:219, 1996.

Shull RM, Helman RG, Spellacy E, et al: Morphologic and biochemical studies of canine mucopolysaccharidosis I. Am J Pathol 114:487, 1984.

Sleight DR, Thomford NR: Gross anatomy of the blood supply and biliary drainage of the canine liver. Anat Rec 166:153, 1969.

Suter PF: Portal vein anomalies in the dog: Their angiographic diagnosis. J Am Vet Radiol Soc 16:84, 1975.

Thornburg LP, Beissenherz M, Dolan M, et al: Histochemical demonstration of copper and copper-associated protein in the canine liver. Vet Pathol 22:327, 1985.

Thornburg LP, Rottinghaus G: What is the significance of hepatic copper values in dogs with cirrhosis? Vet Med May:50, 1985.

Thornburg LP, Shaw D, Dolan M, et al: Hereditary copper toxicosis in West Highland white terriers. Vet Pathol 23:148, 1986.

Twedt DC, Sternlieb I, Gilbertson SR: Clinical, morphologic, and chemical studies on copper toxicosis of Bedlington terriers. J Am Vet Med Assoc 175:269, 1979.

Valentine BA, Porter WP: Multiple hepatic abscesses and peritonitis caused by eugonic fermenter-4 bacilli in a pup. J Am Vet Med Assoc 183:1324, 1983.

van den Ingh TSGAM, Rothuizen J: Lobular dissecting hepatitis in juvenile and young adult dogs. J Vet Intern Med 8:217, 1994.

van den Ingh TSGAM, Rothuizen J, Meyer HP: Portal hypertension associated with primary hypoplasia of the hepatic portal vein in dogs. Vet Rec 137:424, 1995.

van Toor AJ, van der Linde-Sipman JS, van den Ingh TSGAM, et al: Experimental induction of fasting hypoglycaemia and fatty liver syndrome in three Yorkshire terrier pups. Vet Q 13:16, 1991.

van Vechten BJ, Komtebedde J, Koblik PD: Use of transcolonic portal scintigraphy to monitor blood flow and progressive postoperative attenuation of partially ligated single extrahepatic portosystemic shunts in dogs. J Am Vet Med Assoc 204:1770, 1994.

Vendevelde M, Fankhauser R, Bichsel P, et al: Hereditary neurovisceral mannosidosis associated with alpha-mannosidase deficiency in a family of Persian cats. Acta Neuropathol 58:64, 1982.

Vitums A: Portosystemic communications in the dog. Acta Anat 39:271, 1959.

Vogt JC, Krahwinkel DJ, Bright RM, et al: Gradual occlusion of extrahepatic portosystemic shunts in dogs and cats using the ameroid constrictor. Vet Surg 25:495, 1996.

Walvoort HC, Slee RG, Koster JF: Canine glycogen storage disease type II: A biochemical study of an acid alpha-glucosidase deficient Lapland dog. Biochem Biophys Acta 715:63, 1982.

Walvoort HC, van Nes JJ, Stokhof AA, et al: Canine glycogen storage disease type II: A clinical study of four affected Lapland dogs. J Am Anim Hosp Assoc 20:279, 1984.

Weiss RC, Dodd WJ, Scott FW: Disseminated intravascular coagulation in experimentally induced feline infectious peritonitis. Am J Vet Res 41:663, 1980.

Wenger DA, Sattler M, Kudoh T, et al: Niemann-Pick disease: A genetic model in Siamese cats. Science 208:1471, 1980.

White RN, Trower ND, McEnvoy FJ, et al: A method for controlling portal pressure after attenuation of intrahepatic portocaval shunts. Vet Surg 25:407, 1996.

Wrigley RH, Macy DW, Wykes PM: Ligation of ductus venosus in a dog using ultrasonographic guidance. J Am Vet Med Assoc 183:1461, 1983.

Young LE, Christran RM, Ervin DM, et al: Hemolytic disease in newborn dogs. Blood 6:291, 1951.

THE PANCREAS

Anderson NV, Low DG: Juvenile atrophy of the canine pancreas. Anim Hosp 1:101, 1965.

Barlough JE, Weiss RC: Feline infectious peritonitis. In Kirk RW (ed): Current Veterinary Therapy VIII. Philadelphia, WB Saunders, 1983, p 1186.

Drazner FH: Mechanisms of diarrheal disease. *In* Kirk RW (ed): Current Veterinary Therapy VIII. Philadelphia, WB Saunders, 1983, p 773.

Drazner FH: Diseases of the pancreas. *In* Jones BD, Liska WD (eds): Canine and Feline Gastroenterology. Philadelphia, WB Saunders, 1986, p 295.

Harris FM: Juvenile pancreatic atrophy in a dog. Mod Vet Pract 66:341, 1985.

Hill FWG, Osborne AD, Kidder DE: Pancreatic degenerative atrophy in dogs. J Comp Pathol 81:321, 1971.

Jubb JC: Juvenile pancreatic atrophy (pancreatic hypoplasia) in dogs. Vet Med Small Anim Clin 78:1841, 1983.

Lewis LD, Morris ML Jr, Hand MS: Small Animal Clinical Nutrition III. Topeka KS, Mark Morris Associates, 1987.

Prentice DE, James RW, Wadsworth PF: Pancreatic atrophy in young beagle dogs. Vet Pathol 17:575, 1980.

Sherding RG: Canine exocrine pancreatic insufficiency. Compend Contin Educ Pract Vet 1:816, 1979.

Strombeck DR, Guilford WG: Small Animal Gastroenterology, 2nd ed. Davis CA, Stonegate Publishing, 1990.

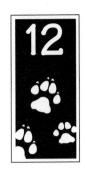

The Skin and Claws

Johnny D. Hoskins

Skin disease and skin-associated appendages represent significant clinical problems in puppies and kittens younger than 6 months. Because of these animals' susceptibility to infectious diseases and because of the identification of congenital and hereditary dermatoses in young puppies and kittens, dermatologic problems commonly occur in this young age group.

CONGENITAL, HEREDITARY, AND DEVELOPMENTAL DERMATOSES

Owners of young dogs and cats frequently ask questions about their animal's haircoat color or the general or specific appearance of the haircoat in relation to existing skin pigmentation or condition. To clarify the medical and veterinary literature, certain dermatologic definitions are needed. *Congenital dermatoses* are abnormalities of the skin that are present at birth. The cause of such congenital dermatoses is usually not known, but most congenital dermatoses are due to genetic defects that arise spontaneously. Hereditary developmental dermatoses, which are not present at birth but are exhibited later in life, are the most common. Some of the reported congenital, hereditary, and developmental dermatoses that occur in young dogs and cats are briefly described in Table 12–1. Specific reference citations for the dermatoses presented in Table 12–1 are provided in the References and Supplemental Reading section.

By definition, hereditary alopecia is the absence of hair at sites where it normally should be, and hypotrichosis is less hair than normal. Although most clinical conditions in dogs and cats are truly hypotrichoses, some of these conditions progress to true alopecias. Hereditary alopecia may include faulty growth and development (dysplasia) or involution (atrophy) of some or all of the hair follicles. Hairlessness may result from the relative lack of hair follicles; from the conversion of follicles producing mature primary and secondary hair shafts to those producing miniaturized hairs; from having no primary or no secondary hairs or no hairs at all; or from the formation of abnormal hair shafts that may be more fragile or may impart an abnormal quality to the haircoat. Such hairlessness problems may be localized, regionalized, generalized, or confined to a certain pigmentation pattern in multicolored dogs and cats. Many affected animals exhibit a widespread hypotrichosis that is less severe on the face and distal regions of the extremities. Hereditary alopecias may be present at birth or may develop days to months after birth (Foil, 1995).

INFECTIOUS DISEASES OF THE SKIN

Viral, rickettsial, bacterial, fungal, and parasitic diseases may affect the skin of puppies and kittens.

Viral and Rickettsial Diseases

Viral diseases that affect the skin of kittens include poxvirus diseases related to cowpox virus, the upper respiratory tract viruses (feline calicivirus and feline herpesvirus), papillomaviruses, feline immunodeficiency virus (FIV), and feline leukemia virus (FeLV). In puppies, canine dis-

Text continued on page 230

Table 12-1	Guide to Congenital, Hereditary, and Developmental Dermatoses	
CONDITION	BREEDS AFFECTED	REMARKS
Acantholytic genodermatosis	English setter, setter-beagle cross	Skin disease with crusting, alopecia, and hyperplastic changes that mimics demodicosis or dermatophytosis; lesions develop as early as 4–9 wk of age
Acral mutilation syndrome	German short-haired and English pointers	Sensory neuropathy that results in progressive mutilation of distal extremities; begins as biting and licking at paw(s), with hindlimbs being most severely involved; initial signs of the syndrome are apparent at 3–5 mo of age
Acrodermatitis	American bull terrier	At birth, affected individuals have skin pigmentation lighter than normal and are physically weak; puppies cannot chew or swallow well and have retarded growth; by 6 wk of age, skin lesions appear on footpads, ears, and muzzle and around all body orifices
Albinism, partial or complete	White bull terrier, Sealyham terrier, white and merle collie, Dalmatian, Persian	Defects that are linked to pigmentary attributes; may be linked to congenital deafness, ocular defects, and hematologic abnormalities
Alopecia universalis	American hairless terrier, beagle, Siamese, hairless Sphinx cat, Canadian hairless cat	Offspring are born with sparse haircoat and lose it within 5–8 wk of birth; generalized lack of hair coverage
Black hair follicular dysplasia	Black and white mixed breeds, bearded collie, basset hound, papillon, saluki, beagle, cocker spaniel, pointer, Gordon setter, Portuguese water dog, schipperke, dachshund	Defective haircoat found only in black haircoat regions; includes hypotrichosis; fractured, stubby hairs lacking normal sheen; and periodic scaliness of skin
Collagen disorder of the footpads	German shepherd	All footpads are softer than normal, often tender; discrete ulcers may develop on one or more pads, especially the carpal and tarsal pads; lesions contain multifocal areas of collagenolysis and neutrophilic inflammation
Color mutant alopecia	Doberman pinscher, Irish setter, chow chow, dachshund, standard poodle, Great Dane, Italian greyhound, whippet, basset hound, Boston terrier, saluki, Yorkshire terrier, miniature pinscher, Chihuahua	Individuals are born with a normal haircoat but after a period of time develop progressive alopecia; affected individuals are characterized by partial alopecia, dry lusterless haircoat, scaliness, and papules; defects in melanization and cortical structure of affected hairs also occur
Congenital hypothyroidism	See Chapter 16 for further details	
Cutaneous asthenia (Ehlers-Danlos syndrome, dominant collagen dysplasia, dermal fragility syndrome, dermatosparaxis)	Beagle, dachshund, boxer, Saint Bernard, German shepherd, English springer spaniel, greyhound, Australian kelpie, Manchester terrier, Welsh corgi, Persian, Himalayan, domestic short-haired cat	Connective tissue disease characterized by loose, hyperextensive, and abnormally fragile skin easily torn by minor trauma

Table 12–1	Guide to Congenital, Hereditary, and Developmental Dermatoses *Continued*	
CONDITION	**BREEDS AFFECTED**	**REMARKS**
Cutaneous mucinosis	Chinese shar-pei	Produces peculiar puffed-face appearance favored in some breed lines and contributes to thickness of multiple skin folds; diagnosis is made by an intradermal fine-needle prick, which causes a thick clear fluid to exude from the puncture site; condition responds somewhat to corticosteroid administration
Cutaneous vasculopathy	German shepherd	Vasculitis and collagenolysis of nose, ear margins, footpads, and tail tips; other possible signs include anorexia, pyrexia, lymphadenopathy, and lameness; inherited as autosomal recessive trait; some affected puppies recover spontaneously
Dermatomyositis	Collie, Shetland sheepdog, Pembroke Welsh corgi, Australian cattle dog, chow chow, German shepherd	Idiopathic inflammation of skin and muscles; family history of syndrome exists; early skin lesions favor locations over bony prominences that are especially exposed to trauma; almost all individuals with skin lesions have some degree of muscle involvement; skin lesions usually develop between 7 wk and 6 mo of age
Dermoid sinus (dermoid cyst)	Rhodesian ridgeback, Shih Tzu, boxer	Neural tube defect resulting from incomplete separation of skin and neural tube during embryonic development; dermoid sinus is tubular indentation of skin extending from dorsal midline as blind sac ending in subcutaneous tissue or extending through spinal canal to dura mater; surgical excision is curative except in cases of neurologic deficits
Digital hyperkeratosis	Irish terrier, Dogues de Bordeaux	Hyperkeratosis of the footpads of all four paws develops at an early age; affected pads tend to fissure, become secondarily infected, and painful; management includes antimicrobial therapy as needed and frequent 50% propylene glycol in water soaks
Ectodermal defect	Miniature poodle, whippet, cocker spaniel, Belgian shepherd, Lhasa apso, Yorkshire terrier, French bulldog, Rottweiler	Affected individuals are born with two thirds of normally haired parts of body exhibiting hairlessness; hairless skin is extremely thin and contains no cutaneous appendages
Epidermal dysplasia	West Highland white terrier	Familial defect in keratinization that first exhibited as erythema and pruritus of extremities and ventrum; progresses to severe hyperpigmentation and seborrhea
Epidermolysis bullosa syndromes	Collie, Shetland sheepdog, toy poodle, Beauceron	*Epidermolysis bullosa simplex* of collie and Shetland sheepdog probably is a mild form of canine familial dermatomyositis in which muscle lesions are inapparent; *junctional epidermolysis bullosa* of toy poodle characterized by vesicles and bullae of the footpads, oral mucous membranes, and trauma points of the skins; *epidermolysis bullosa syndrome* in Beauceron characterized by alopecia, erosion, and crusting around mucocutaneous junctions and pressure points
Epitheliogenesis imperfecta	Many dog and cat breeds	Discontinuity of squamous epithelium; present at birth as glistening red, well-demarcated defect in skin; defect is covered with one to three layers of flat to cuboidal epithelium and a stroma devoid of all adnexa; defect is lethal if extensive

Table continued on following page

Table 12–1	Guide to Congenital, Hereditary, and Developmental Dermatoses *Continued*	
CONDITION	BREEDS AFFECTED	REMARKS
Follicular dysplasia syndromes	Siberian husky, English springer spaniel, Airedale terrier, Alaskan malamute, German short-haired and wire-haired pointer, Irish water spaniel, Portuguese water dog, curly-coated retriever, Chesapeake Bay retriever, miniature schnauzer	Defective haircoat exhibited by regional or truncal alopecia; includes hypotrichosis, fractured stubby hairs lacking normal sheen, and periodic scaliness of skin; *familial seasonal flank alopecia* in boxer, English bulldog, and French bulldog occurs as a form of follicular dysplasia
Hypotrichosis	Beagle, Yorkshire terrier, Labrador retriever, Lhasa apso, Irish water spaniel, silver miniature poodle, French bulldog, basset hound, Rottweiler, cocker spaniel, whippet, Belgian shepherd, schipperke, Sphinx, Cornish Rex, Devon Rex, Mexican hairless, Siamese, Birman	Incomplete ectodermal defect in that affected individuals have remnants of hair follicles and other epidermal appendages in skin; in some cases, may be confined to certain hair color pattern; hypotrichosis may also develop after birth as a delayed-onset trait
Ichthyosis	West Highland white terrier, Irish terrier, collie, Labrador retriever, Jack Russell terrier, American pit bull terrier, Boston terrier, Doberman pinscher	Extreme hyperkeratosis on all or part of skin and exaggerated thickening of digital, carpal, and tarsal pads; present at birth and becomes progressively more severe with age; management includes hydrating, antiseborrheic, and emollient therapies applied almost on daily basis; incurable condition
Lethal acrodermatitis	English bull terrier	Characterized by growth retardation, acrodermatitis, pyoderma, paronychia, diarrhea, pneumonia, and abnormal behavior that results in death usually before 15 months of age
Lichenoid-psoriasiform dermatosis	Springer spaniel	Asymptomatic, generally symmetric, erythematous, lichenoid papules and plaques initially noted on pinnae and in external ear canal and inguinal region; with time, lesions become more hyperkeratotic and spread to face, ventral trunk, and perineal area; symptomatic management of skin lesions
Lupoid dermatosis	German short-haired pointer	Scale and crusting with keratin fronds and thickened skin are first seen on the head and back, then become generalized; typically first appears at 5–7 mo of age; histopathologic lesions similar to systemic lupus erythematosus
Nasal vasculopathy	Scottish terrier	Idiopathic pyogranulomatous inflammation and leukocytoclastic vasculitis of the nasal planum, nostrils, and nasal mucosa; may first appear at 3–4 wk of age as bilateral nasal discharge
Nevi	German shepherd, miniature poodle and schnauzer, Shetland sheepdog, Chinese pug, Welsh terrier	Circumscribed developmental defect in skin; when nevus forms a hyperplastic mass, it is referred to as hamartoma; various other types include sebaceous, hyperpigmented epidermal, comedonicus, follicular, mucocutaneous angiomatous, and regional collagenous nevi

Table 12-1	Guide to Congenital, Hereditary, and Developmental Dermatoses *Continued*	
CONDITION	**BREEDS AFFECTED**	**REMARKS**
Partial alopecia	Chinese crested dog, Mexican hairless dog, Chihuahua, Abyssinian sand dog, Turkish naked dog, Peruvian hairless dog, Xoloitzcuintli	These breeds are bred specifically for varying degrees of alopecia and as such become accepted standard
Pituitary dwarfism (see Chapter 16 for further details)	German shepherd, Carnelian bear-dog, spitz, toy pinscher, weimaraner	Signs not noticed until 2–3 mo after birth; failure to replace the puppy coat with normal adult coat after 2–3 mo of age; thereafter puppy coat becomes worn and epilated, progressing to symmetric alopecia; skin may show progressive hyperpigmentation, thinness, and pityriasis; affected dogs lack normal growth hormone levels and are also usually hypothyroid; early management includes both growth hormone and thyroid hormone replacement therapy before normal closure of the epiphyses to obtain more normal skin, haircoat, and skeletal growth
Rex mutant	Cornish Rex, Devon Rex	Kittens have wavy, wooly hair; adults develop short, curly plush hair; guard hairs and vibrissae are absent or normal
Sebaceous adenitis	Standard poodle, Akita, Samoyed, vizsla	Characterized by changes in haircoat quality, seborrhea that is progressive and severe and alopecia; onset of signs in early adulthood but skin biopsy results confirm at 4 mo of age; in standard poodle most likely autosomal recessive skin disease
Seborrhea, congenital	English springer spaniel, Persian	Affected individuals born with dry skin and discolored hair; patches of hyperkeratosis and scale then develop, and adherent scale and debris accumulate on hair shafts; ceruminous otitis develops at an early age
Tricolor coats	Tricolored cats	Tricolored cats possess white, black, and orange hairs blended together (tortoise-shell) or in large patches (calico)
Tyrosinase deficiency	Chow chow	Changes in color of tongue, buccal mucosa, and portions of hair shaft are result of deficiency of tyrosinase, the enzyme necessary in chemical reactions that produce melanin
Tyrosinemia	German shepherd	Early-age onset of eye and skin lesions with mental retardation; serum tyrosine levels are elevated because of deficiency of cytosolic hepatic tyrosine aminotransferase; inflammatory response to tyrosine crystals deposited in tissue results in eye and possibly skin lesions
Vitiligo	Doberman pinscher, Rottweiler, Belgian shepherd, Tervuren and German shepherds, Old English sheepdog, dachshund, Siamese	Loss of skin pigment, especially around nose, lips, buccal mucosa, and facial skin; footpads and nails, as well as haircoat, may be affected

temper virus, canine herpesvirus, and papillo-mavirus infections are important, and canine pseudorabies has been reported. Rocky Mountain spotted fever (RMSF) and canine and feline ehrlichial infections are rickettsial diseases that may cause skin lesions, as well as systemic signs.

The most common poxvirus infection in domestic cats is cowpox, caused by an *Orthopox-virus* (Bennett et al, 1990), but infections with *Parapoxvirus* (Hamblet, 1993) and uncharacterized poxviruses have been identified. Feline cowpox is seen mostly in rural cats that hunt rodents. Cat-to-cat transmission does not appear to be important. The usual route of *Orthopoxvirus* infection in cats is skin inoculation, probably through a bite or other skin wound. The disease begins with a primary skin lesion, usually located on the head, neck, or forelimb. After a few days, widespread secondary skin lesions develop that are small circular plaques that soon become encrusted. Sloughing or removal of crusts leaves a moist red flat ulcer. Most cats show no clinical signs other than skin lesions. If cats do develop systemic signs of illness, they may exhibit pyrexia, tachypnea, conjunctivitis, or diarrhea. Cats with FeLV or FIV infection exhibit more severe signs. Most cats recover fully from the infection within 3 to 4 weeks. Diagnosis may be made by the demonstration of typical poxvirus inclusions in skin biopsy material or in sloughed crusts using either light or electron microscopy or by virus isolation.

Footpad swelling and ulceration and skin ulceration occur infrequently with feline calicivirus and feline herpesvirus virus infections in kittens (Cooper and Sabine, 1972; Flecknell et al, 1979; Johnson and Sabine, 1971). The skin lesions have been seen in cats with no signs of upper respiratory infection, but more commonly accompany oral and nasal ulcerative disease.

Feline leukemia virus–associated skin disease is variable and reflects the immunosuppressive nature of the virus. Some of the FeLV-infected cats may be simultaneously infected with FIV. Feline immunodeficiency virus infection is associated with stomatitis, chronic abscesses, and cellulitis (Fleming et al, 1991). Feline papillomavirus-induced skin lesions are generally seen in immunosuppressed aged and FIV-infected adult cats (Egberink et al, 1992; Lozano-Alarcon et al, 1996) and might be expected to be observed in FIV-infected kittens. Multiple fibrosarcomas in young cats may be feline sarcoma virus induced, and these skin tumors are more anaplastic and more invasive than solitary fibrosarcoma tumors of older cats.

Canine distemper may be associated with a pustular dermatitis resembling impetigo during the acute illness or nasal and/or digital (hardpad disease) hyperkeratosis. Papillomatosis is a contagious disease of young dogs caused by the canine papillomavirus. Lesions are most common around the mouth and within the oral cavity. Individual lesions are usually white and verrucous. Most tumors regress spontaneously without leaving a trace after the development of cell-mediated immunity. Dogs as young as 5 months are infected with pseudorabies from association with swine and ingestion of uncooked pork (Monroe, 1989). Extreme pruritus is common, but death ensues within 96 hours of the onset of signs.

Typically, rickettsial diseases such as canine and feline ehrlichial infections and RMSF do not have specific dermatologic signs other than accompanying petechiation of the skin and mucous membranes and, in the case of RMSF, vasculitis lesions, and rear limb and scrotal swellings.

Bacterial Diseases

Although there is no true dermatologic entity known as *puppy pyoderma*, superficial bacterial infections are common in puppies younger than 6 months. Most are surface pyodermas, and *impetigo* is a poorly chosen term often used to describe the superficial pustular dermatitis found on the ventrum of young puppies. Some superficial pustular dermatitis cases may just be manifestations of urine scalding of the sensitive glabrous skin in the ventrum region, whereas others reflect opportunistic bacterial infections in mildly immunocompromised individuals. Many common bacterial skin diseases, especially of young dogs, are associated with the coagulase-positive staphylococci, specifically *Staphylococcus intermedius*.

In newborn animals, neonatal dermatitis, impetigo, and superficial pustular dermatitis of kittens are important. In the older puppy, superficial folliculitis and acne may develop. Young dogs may develop furunculosis, pododermatitis, or cellulitis as bacterial complications of demodicosis. *Neonatal dermatitis* or acute moist dermatitis of neonates and *impetigo* may actually describe the same skin disease. In most young puppies, very superficial yellow pustules develop on the ventral abdomen and inguinal fold. In very young, immunocompromised, or, occasionally, in thick-coated older puppies, these pustules become coalescent and form the spreading weeping and crusted lesions of acute moist dermatitis (Foil, 1995). Most cases are diagnosed by their physical appearance. Cytologic evaluation of the contents of a large pustule usually reveals degenerate neutrophils and cocci. In severe cases care should be taken not to confuse this with juvenile cellulitis, which typically involves facial edema and swollen lymph nodes. Superficial pustular dermatitis of kittens is similar to puppy impetigo, although much less common.

Most cases may be treated with mild antiseptic cleansers or antibacterial shampoos. The animal's environment should be cleaned if it is contaminated. Severe crusted lesions in the thick haircoat should be clipped off to facilitate cleansing. Rarely, systemic antimicrobial agents may be required. Most puppies will spontaneously overcome the skin problem after reaching 16 weeks of age. Occasionally, the skin problem will progress into bacterial folliculitis.

Older puppies may develop the papular, pustular, occasionally pruritic rash of superficial bacterial folliculitis, although the skin disease is more common in the pubertal and young adult dog. Once again, the bacterium isolated is *Staphylococcus intermedius*. The primary lesions can usually be visually observed on the ventral abdomen region and on the inner thigh. On the trunk, a patchy alopecia or a scattered tufting of the haircoat may be evident. The head and distal regions of the extremities are rarely affected in uncomplicated bacterial folliculitis. This problem should be distinguished from demodicosis and dermatophytosis. Bacterial folliculitis seems to be more common and more difficult to treat in short-coated, large-breed puppies and in the Chinese shar-pei puppy. In short-coated, large-breed puppies, the lesions may be more papular and may be confined mostly to pressure points (Foil, 1995). In the Chinese shar-pei, the clinical manifestation is often patchy alopecia with or without pruritus; one should always rule out concurrent demodicosis and dermatophytosis. Folliculitis may be prominent in dogs with follicular dysplasia, color mutant alopecia, and some of the other hereditary alopecias discussed earlier. Bacterial folliculitis, furunculosis, and cellulitis of German shepherd dogs, which is a chronic, relapsing to intractable form of the disease that some have described as unique to the breed, can have an onset as early as 3 months of age (Krick and Scott, 1989).

The diagnosis of bacterial folliculitis may be made presumptively, based on the clinical signs, once the aforementioned alternatives have been ruled out of the differential diagnosis. Bacterial culture and sensitivity testing of ruptured intact pustules as well as cytologic examination of discharged exudate may be warranted in recurrent or unresponsive cases.

Therapy should include antibacterial shampooing (benzoyl peroxide, ethyl lactate, triclosan, or chlorhexidine), general health maintenance, and a 2-week course of an appropriate systemic antimicrobial agent (Table 12–2). Recurrent or complicated cases should be treated for 3 or 4 weeks. Any tendency toward the development of furunculosis or cellulitis warrants reevaluation for the presence of parasitic or fungal infection. If the face is involved, juvenile cellulitis should be considered.

Deeper bacterial infections of the skin and underlying tissues include infections with the *Actinomyces*, *Nocardia*, and *Dermatophilus* organisms, the mycobacterial diseases, and subcutaneous abscess secondary to bite wounds or foreign bodies or associated with immunodeficiency.

Percutaneous abscesses are the most common bacterial skin diseases of kittens. *Pasteurella* species and *Rhodococcus equi* are the most common isolates from bite wound abscesses, although a variety of anaerobic organisms, such as *Porphyromonas* species, *Fusobacterium* species, and *Peptostreptococcus anaerobius*, and facultatively aerobic organisms are isolated. The aerobic organisms involved are usually, but not uniformly, susceptible to the penicillin derivatives, such as penicillin G, amoxicillin, and ampicillin. In treating anaerobic infections, chloramphenicol can be substituted for penicillin derivatives. Chloramphenicol can be hazardous to people. If anaerobic infection is suspected, second- or third-generation cephalosporins, clindamycin, and metronidazole can be administered. Certain *Fusobacterium* species also are susceptible to erythromycin and doxycycline. *Rhodococcus* infections are primarily susceptible to aminoglycosides, chloramphenicol, and erythromycin.

Mycoplasma-like organisms or bacterial L-forms may be associated with abscesses that fail to respond to routine antimicrobial therapy. Infections with *R. equi* have been implicated in granulomatous lymphadenitis and subcutaneous abscess in young kittens and cats (Elliot et al, 1986; Higgins and Paradis, 1980). The presence of numerous gram-positive rods on cytologic examination may cause the veterinarian to worry about the possibility of mycobacterial disease (Foil, 1995). These distinctions may be readily made in the microbiology laboratory. There is also some public health risk of expo-

Table 12–2	Suggested Antimicrobial Therapy for Bacterial Skin Diseases	
THERAPEUTIC AGENT	**DOSAGE AND ROUTE***	**COMMENTS**
Amoxicillin-clavulanate	10–20 mg/kg bid–tid PO	Label dose may be too low; broad antimicrobial spectrum of activity
Cefadroxil	20–30 mg/kg bid PO	Rapid and complete absorption even with food
Cefoxitin sodium	20–30 mg/kg tid IV, IM	Particularly effective against anaerobes
Cephalexin	20–30 mg/kg tid PO, SC, IV	Less active against *Staphylococcus*
Chloramphenicol	50 mg/kg IV, IM, SC, PO tid for dogs, bid for cats	Broad antimicrobial spectrum of activity; can be hazardous to people
Clindamycin	11 mg/kg bid PO, IV, IM	Label dose may be too low; effective against anaerobes
Erythromycin	10–15 mg/kg tid PO	May cause anorexia and vomiting
Gentamicin	2 mg/kg tid IM, SC	Maintain adequate hydration; evaluate renal function often
Metronidazole	7.5–10 mg/kg bid–tid PO	Effective in anaerobic infections and abscesses
Ormetroprim-sulfonamide	27.5 mg/kg sid PO	Side effects less than those of trimethoprim-sulfadiazine
Oxacillin	10–15 mg/kg tid–qid PO	Some gastrointestinal disturbance
Penicillin G	20,000–40,000 U/kg bid–tid IV, IM, SC, PO	Two times the dose if given orally because of gastric degradation; effective against *Actinomyces* species and *Dermatophilus congolensis*
Sulfadiazine	80 mg/kg bid–tid PO	Effective for *Nocardia* infection
Trimethoprim-sulfadiazine	15 mg/kg bid SC, IM, PO	Drug eruptions, arthropathies, keratoconjunctivitis sicca

*PO = Oral administration; SC = subcutaneous administration; IV = intravenous administration; IM = intramuscular administration; sid = once daily; bid = twice daily; tid = three times daily; qid = four times daily.

sure to *Rhodococcus* organisms, as there is for some mycobacteria, so that active cases should be treated with care, especially until tuberculosis is ruled out.

A geographic-restricted cause of subcutaneous abscess formation and lymphadenitis in cats and kittens that is also of serious public health concern is *Yersinia pestis*, the agent of bubonic plague (Carlson, 1996; Eidson et al, 1991). In kittens these skin lesions usually accompany signs of systemic illness, and the infection is usually fatal.

Subcutaneous abscesses in puppies are less common than in kittens and are often associated with staphylococci or streptococci. Multiple subcutaneous abscesses in a 2-month-old puppy were shown to be caused by *Peptostreptococcus tetradius* (Price, 1991). The organism is an anaerobic gram-positive coccus that is part of the normal oral flora of human beings.

Infections of the skin caused by *Actinomyces* species, *Nocardia* species, or *Dermatophilus congolensis* may be seen rarely in puppies and kittens. The typical cutaneous lesion caused by *Actinomyces* species is a soft or boggy nodule, either on the thoracic wall or on an extremity, that may be associated with lameness. The nodule may be associated with one or more fistulous tracts or deep purpuric pustules that may rupture to produce thick yellow or red-yellow pus. In puppies, the purulent exudate usually contains soft whitish sulfur granules. Such lesions often overlie body cavity infection or osteomyelitis. *Nocardia* cutaneous lesions may be similar, may involve lymph nodes, and are unlikely to discharge sulfur granules in the puppy and kitten. *Dermatophilus congolensis* infection may cause proliferative ulcerating masses in the oropharynx of cats that resemble squamous cell carcinoma (Baker et al, 1972). It may produce superficial crusting and ulcerative disease resembling dermatophilosis in large animals and subcutaneous pyogranulomatous nodules (Carakostas et al, 1984; Chastain et al, 1976). In most cases, the diagnosis is made on the basis of cytologic and histopathologic recognition of the distinctive railroad track appearance of the gram-positive filamentous coccobacillus. Cultural identification has been difficult. Treatment consists of cleansing or débridement and administration of systemically acting penicillin, ampicillin, or amoxicillin.

A presumptive diagnosis may be reached when *Actinomyces* species lesions are examined cytologically. If sulfur granules are being discharged, these may be collected and crushed on a slide for Gram staining. All *Actinomyces* species are gram-positive filamentous coccobacilli. When there are no granules to examine, cytology may be less rewarding. In addition, it is preferable to obtain tissue surgically, both for histopathologic examination with special stains and for cultural studies. Also, exudate, when it is available in good quantity, should be submitted in a sealed container for cultural examination. *Nocardia* species may be acid-fast cytologically, histologically, and in young culture. *Actinomyces* species are anaerobic. *Dermatophilus congolensis* requires selective agars but may be identified cytologically.

The mycobacterial disease that may affect the skin in young puppies and kittens is tuberculosis. The atypical mycobacterial granuloma and feline leprosy are more likely to be seen in older animals. Any of three organisms may cause systemic tuberculosis in young dogs and cats: *Mycobacterium tuberculosis*, *M. bovis*, or *M. avium-intercellulare*. The human tuberculosis organism is more often identified from dogs with the disease. Cats are most likely to have gastrointestinal or pharyngeal tuberculosis caused by *M. bovis*. Either dogs or cats may be sporadically infected with *M. avium-intercellulare*, which may have either an avian or an environmental source.

The clinical signs that young dogs and cats with tuberculosis show are quite varied, ranging from severe disseminated disease to chronic focal granulomatous processes (Clercx et al, 1992). When the skin is involved it is by way of spread from infected superficial lymph nodes that rupture. The cervical lymph nodes are most likely to be involved. Here, a typical cutaneous lesion would be a chronic or relapsing fistulous tract with underlying lymphadenopathy, and such a presentation has been described in a 5-month-old puppy with *M. tuberculosis* infection (Foster et al, 1986). Diagnosis is made with cytologic and cultural examination, as well as by histopathologic examination of biopsy material. Cultural identification is performed with the use of special agar and may be slow. Cultural identification is necessary for determination of the public health consequences of individual cases. Treatment of *M. tuberculosis* or *M. bovis* infections in young dogs and cats is not recommended. Because infection with *M. avium-intercellulare* may have an environmental source and be of no public health consequence, specific identification of cases not associated with known sources of infection may prevent unnec-

essary euthanasia of a dog or cat. Treatment should be based on specific identification and, in the case of saprophytic mycobacteria, on sensitivity testing.

Fungal Diseases

Young dogs and cats may be afflicted with candidiasis, *Malassezia* dermatitis, and dermatophytosis. *Candidiasis* is an uncommon disease of the oral mucous membranes, gastrointestinal tract, or urinary tract caused by various species of *Candida* yeasts, most often *Candida albicans* (Kral and Uscavage, 1960). *Candida* infections may follow severe debilitating and immunosuppressive illnesses. Many afflicted animals also have a history of receiving broad-spectrum antimicrobial therapy. Lesions consist of whitish plaques or verrucous papules; shallow, necrotic ulcers; or vesicular eruption associated with ragged ulceration. Oral mucous membranes, lips, nose, nail beds, and perianal skin may be affected. The *Candida* organisms are easily demonstrated cytologically by preparing a Gram-stained smear of exudate. Treatment consists of correcting underlying causes if possible and using daily antifungal agents. Systemically acting ketoconazole, fluconazole, or itraconazole therapy should be curative. There are no definitive guidelines for the earliest age at which it might be safe to use the systemically acting ketoconazole, fluconazole, and itraconazole agents in young dogs or cats; however, these agents have been used safely in puppies and kittens as young as 8 weeks. If used, the animal's appetite and liver function should be closely monitored.

Malassezia dermatitis may be a primary or secondary dermatopathy that is characterized by erythema, hyperkeratosis and seborrhea, pruritus, alopecia, and an increased number of *Malassezia* yeasts in the stratum corneum and within the hair follicles (Bruner and Blakemore, 1999; Mason and Evans, 1991). The diagnosis is most readily made with impression smears or tape strip preparations of the skin surface taken from erythematous seborrheic sites (Bond and Sant, 1993; Plant et al, 1992). These slides are then heat fixed and slides or tape strips stained with modified Wright's stain. An average of more than two yeast forms seen per high-power field ($\times 450$) is considered abnormal; dogs with *Malassezia* dermatitis often have very high numbers observed, with counts per oil immersion field ($\times 1000$) as high as 190. Treatment is most readily accomplished with systemically acting ketoconazole or itraconazole. Topical treatment with selenium disulfide, chlorhexidine, 2% ketoconazole, or 2% miconazole shampoos may be useful, especially for long-term maintenance (Mason, 1993; Bruner and Blakemore, 1999).

Dermatophytosis is most common in dogs and cats younger than 6 months (Lewis et al, 1991). Many agents have been associated with ringworm lesions in puppies and kittens, but most cases are caused by one of three species of keratinophilic fungi: *Microsporum canis*, *M. gypseum*, or *Trichophyton mentagrophytes*. *Microsporum gypseum* is acquired from the soil, usually organically rich soil. *T. mentagrophytes* infections may be acquired directly from other animals, usually rodents, or from soil that is heavily contaminated with infected hair and scale such as occurs in and around rodent burrows or farm barns.

Microsporum canis infections are more complex and of greater importance as dogs and cats of all ages are major sources of human infections with this type of ringworm organism. The cats and, more rarely, dogs are inapparent carriers of *M. canis* (van Cutsem et al, 1985; Woodgyer, 1977). Long-haired kittens are especially likely to harbor the *M. canis* organisms (Quaife and Womar, 1982). In addition, kittens from multiple cat households have many predisposing factors for acquiring dermatophytosis; therefore, they are important sources for animal and human cases. Families and animal handlers exposed to cats that harbor *M. canis* are at great risk and often acquire the infection on direct contact with the animal or from the contaminated environment. As a veterinarian, one should always protect oneself, one's employees, and one's clients from this potentially serious infection.

In addition to the typical ringworm lesion of a circular patch showing hair loss and scaliness, an entire spectrum of clinical manifestations of dermatophytosis may be extremely diverse, such as concurrent papular pustular dermatitis, patchy alopecia, onychomycosis, boggy abscessed nodule, and nodule with ulceration and draining tract formation. Also, there are other skin conditions that may mimic the typical ringworm lesions, such as staphylococcal folliculitis, acute moist dermatitis, drug eruption, demodicosis, and zinc-responsive dermatitis. Singular ringworm lesions often occur on the face or extremities. In young dogs, generalized dermatophytosis is seen with some regularity. In homeless puppies, it is not uncommon to find dermatophytosis, demodicosis, and sarcoptic mange on one unfortunate puppy. Lesions in kittens most often start as scaly patches of hair loss on ear tips, chin, bridge of the nose, upper lips, and the preauricular skin. They may be-

come covered with thin, dry, grayish crusts, or, if secondarily infected with bacteria, a thicker crust with exudate (Foil, 1998; Carney and Moriello, 1993). In long-haired breeds of kittens, lesions often spread from the head to the forelimbs and may become generalized.

Diagnosis can be accomplished easily using appropriate culturing techniques (Foil, 1998). Culture techniques should be designed to maximize chances of obtaining infected hairs for placement on culture growth media and should minimize contamination of the culture growth media by bacteria and saprophytic fungi. The growth of contaminates may be inhibited by the use of selective agar, such as the dermatophyte test medium. Clipping hair to 0.5 cm in areas to be sampled will reduce carriage of contaminant spores onto the dermatophyte test medium. Gently patting the area to be sampled with a sponge slightly dampened with isopropyl alcohol, and then patting it dry, greatly reduces contamination without reducing successful inoculation of dermatophytes. It is always important to maintain a high index of suspicion for dermatophytosis, especially when examining kittens—meaning that every kitten is considered to have dermatophytosis until it is cultured negative. It would not be overly cautious to perform survey brush culturing on every new long-haired kitten presented for routine examination, especially if the new home will have young children or persons who are immunosuppressed (Foil, 1998).

Topical treatment should be instituted in every case of dermatophytosis. The primary reason for this recommendation is to reduce ongoing environmental contamination and human exposure. Lesions should be clipped widely, or whole-body clipping should be done when lesions are numerous, especially in long-haired cats. Clipping of the entire haircoat should be done with a number 10 blade. It should be noted, however, that clipping may cause the lesions to become more inflamed and appear more numerous (Moriello, 1994). Various topical preparations are available for use on local or widespread dermatophytosis (Table 12–3). Currently, lime sulfur rinses, miconazole and ketoconazole shampoos, and enilconazole rinses are recommended as most likely to be effective (Foil, 1998). Caution should be exercised in using the topical imidazoles on kittens or very young puppies, as irritant dermatitis may develop.

Systemic therapy needs to be used only in selected cases (see Table 12–3). Systemically acting griseofulvin or itraconazole is the treatment

Table 12–3 Topical and Systemic Therapy for Dermatophytosis

PRODUCT	AVAILABLE FORMULATIONS	COMMENTS
Topical Therapy		
Enilconazole	As a rinse, fogger	Apparently safe for cats
Clotrimazole	Apply twice a day as cream, lotion	Not formulated to penetrate infected hair; for localized disease
Miconazole	Apply twice a day as cream, shampoo	For localized disease
Ketoconazole	Apply twice a day as cream, shampoo	Cream not formulated to penetrate infected hair
Captan	Apply as rinse, shampoo	Use as 2% (2 tbsp/gal) solution every 5–7 d
Lime sulfur	Apply as rinse	Use as 2% solution every 5–7 d
Chlorhexidine	Apply as shampoo, rinse	Use as 2% solution rinse daily; shampoo every 5–7 d
Sodium hypochlorite	Apply as rinse	Use as 1:20–1:30 dilution in water after shampooing
Povidone-iodine	Apply as shampoo, rinse, ointment	Use as 1:4 dilution in water daily
Systemically Acting Therapy		
Griseofulvin		
Microsized	125-mg, 250-mg, 500-mg tablet; 125-mg, 250-mg capsule; 125 mg/5 ml suspension	Administer at 25–50 mg/kg twice a day orally for at least 4–8 wk; for small kittens, usually culture negative at 8 wk and cured at 10 wk
Ultramicrosized	125-mg, 165-mg, 250-mg, 330-mg tablet	Administer at 5–10 mg/kg twice a day orally for at least 4–8 wk; dose is approximately two-thirds that of microsized preparation; some preparations contain polyethylene glycol
Ketoconazole	200-mg tablet	Administer at 10–20 mg/kg once a day orally for at least 3–4 wk; cats often receive 50 mg total dose daily; with side effects, every other day treatment is used
Itraconazole	100-mg capsule, 100 mg/10 ml solution	Administer at 5–10 mg/kg once a day orally for at least 3–4 wk; capsules may be opened and contents divided to administer recommended dose

Modified from Foil CS: Dermatophytosis. *In* Greene CE (ed): Infectious Diseases of the Dog and Cat, 2nd ed. Philadelphia, WB Saunders, 1998, p 362.

of choice for *Microsporum canis* infections (Foil, 1998). Griseofulvin is teratogenic, however, when given in the first two thirds of pregnancy. Griseofulvin can be used safely in young puppies and kittens once they are eating on their own, but the dose should be calculated carefully according to weight, and the lower end of the dose range given in Table 12–3 should be used. If the ultramicrosized form of griseofulvin is used, the lower dose range given should be strictly observed. It is not necessary to give this preparation with fatty meals as it is for the older griseofulvin formulations. Puppies should be treated for at least 4 to 8 weeks, at which time treatment may be stopped if all clinical signs have resolved. Treatment of kittens should be monitored with culture, using a sterile toothbrush to sample the haircoat. It may be very difficult to clear the infection from a long-haired cat. The veterinarian should check for bone marrow suppression with the aid of complete blood count monitoring for long-term or high-dose treatment of kittens. The haircoat should be kept clipped short until dermatophyte test medium cultures are negative. The most common side effects of griseofulvin therapy are anorexia, vomiting, and diarrhea. Bone marrow suppression and neurologic signs have occurred, probably as idiosyncratic reactions. Bone marrow suppression may be irreversible and fatal.

Systemically acting itraconazole is generally well tolerated by young dogs and cats (see Table 12–3). If itraconazole is administered orally at 5 to 10 mg/kg daily for 3 to 4 weeks, high levels of itraconazole are detected in the hair for at least 4 weeks after treatment has stopped. A variety of adverse reactions have been observed with itraconazole therapy, the most serious of which are increased serum liver enzymes, icterus, and/or cutaneous drug eruptions. The most common side effect, however, is anorexia and occasional vomiting. Histamine blockers and other antacids should not be administered during itraconazole therapy.

Elimination of dermatophytosis from multiple cat households is of concern to breeders of long-haired cats. An ideal treatment plan for elimination of dermatophytes from a multiple cat household is labor intensive and expensive (Carney and Moriello, 1993). One approach is to isolate kittens immediately after weaning and treat them as outlined previously until their cultures are negative. Another approach is to begin griseofulvin or itraconazole treatment of queens who repeatedly produce infected kittens during the last week of pregnancy and continue treatment of the queen until weaning. Thereafter, the kittens should be isolated and treated individually until cultures are negative. Once again, the treatment of young kittens should be based on a very careful weight/dose assessment.

There has been some interest in the use of a *Microsporum canis* vaccine to treat kittens born into infected catteries. To date, a killed *M. canis* vaccine (Fel-O-Vax MC-K, Fort Dodge Animal Health, Kansas City, Kansas) to treat kittens and cats is approved for use. The killed *M. canis* vaccine may reduce the severity and even the incidence of clinical ringworm. The vaccine, however, does not protect individual cats from infection upon subsequent exposure. Local reactions may occur at the site of vaccination in some cats.

Parasitic Skin Diseases

Skin diseases in young dogs and cats may be caused by protozoal, nematode, or arthropod parasites (Foil, 1995). The arthropod parasites are certainly very important causes of skin disease in puppies and kittens. Protozoal skin diseases are uncommonly reported in North America. Leishmaniasis and coccidia have been reported as causing nodular granulomatous skin lesions (Sangster et al, 1985). A sporozoan, *Caryospora* species, was shown to be associated with severe pyogranulomatous dermatitis and lymphadenitis in a 2-month-old puppy (Dubey et al, 1990). Skin lesions have been described in canine babesiosis in about 3% of cases (Carlotti et al, 1993). Lesions include mucosal or cutaneous purpura, petechiae, urticaria/angioedema, and necrosis of extremities, the latter presumably secondary to cutaneous vasculitis. Of the nematode parasites that may cause skin disease (i.e., *Rhabditis*, *Strongyloides*, *Anatrichosoma*, and *Lagochilascaris* organisms and hookworms), only hookworm dermatitis is seen with any regularity in young dogs. A boxer puppy with nodular skin lesions was reported to be harboring within the nodules the nematode parasite *Anatrichosoma* species (Hendrix et al, 1987). *Lagochilascaris* organisms have been associated with purulent draining tracts (Craig et al, 1982). *Rhabditis strongyloides* may cause a severe pruritic erythroderma with folliculitis and furunculosis in the parts of the body in contact with infested bedding (Willers, 1970). *Strongyloides stercoralis* infection may cause a pruritic and exfoliative erythroderma or hemorrhagic pododermatitis as well as systemic signs in puppies in heavily infested environments (Malone et al, 1980).

Hookworm dermatitis may affect young dogs housed on or exercised in an area heavily infested with hookworm larvae. The disease is seasonal, being confined to the warm months in climates with cold winters. Older dogs may be more likely to develop severe or persistent dermatologic disease from hookworm larval penetration because hypersensitivity contributes to the development of clinical signs (Smith and Elliot, 1969). Infection with *Uncinaria stenocephala* is more likely to be associated with dermatologic disease than is infection with the *Ancylostoma* species.

Skin disease is predominantly confined to the interdigital webs and the edges of the footpads. Severe cases may involve the ungual folds. Occasionally, other parts of the body that come into contact with the ground may be affected (Baker and Grimes, 1970). Lesions consist of erythematous patches and papules. Pruritus and hair loss, followed by scaly crusting, are seen at the edges of the footpads, which become soft and spongy. The footpads may slough in sheets. With chronic infections, the feet may become swollen and painful and the footpads hardened and fissured. Nail beds may be swollen and nails become deformed. The differential diagnoses in puppies would include canine distemper hardpad disease, bacterial paronychia, *Trichophyton* dermatophytosis, *Rhabditis* dermatitis, zinc-responsive dermatosis, and hereditary footpad hyperkeratosis.

Diagnosis is made on the basis of skin lesions, fecal examination of the affected dog and other in-contact dogs, and the history of contaminated environment, such as the housing and bedding. Larvae are uncommonly found on skin scrapings of the lesions and are also not reliably found in biopsy specimens. Treatment consists of cleaning up or changing the living environment and use of effective anthelmintic products. Salt or borate or organophosphate-based spray may be used to kill infective larvae when the animal cannot be removed from the premises. Constructing kennels with concrete surfaces rather than housing kennel dogs on gravel or bare ground is preferable for control of hookworms. Cutaneous lesions may take weeks to resolve after exposure has ceased (Smith and Elliot, 1969). Control of secondary bacterial infection and the use of topical corticosteroids may hasten resolution.

CANINE DEMODICOSIS

Canine demodicosis occurs in two forms—localized and generalized (Foil, 1995). The mite *Demodex canis* is a normal inhabitant of facial hair follicles of dogs. The factors that allow the mite to proliferate and cause skin lesions are still not understood. As a disease, canine demodicosis is not usually contagious; it is familial—at least in the case of generalized demodicosis. A defect in cellular immunity plays a role in the initiation of generalized demodicosis (Scott et al, 1976; Wilkie et al, 1979), but characterization of the immunologic defect is still incomplete.

Localized demodicosis is extremely common in puppies and is not associated with a familial pattern of occurrence. It is commonly stated that greater than 90% of cases of localized demodicosis in prepuberal dogs will resolve spontaneously in 3 to 8 weeks. There is no difference in rate or time of resolution in treated and untreated cases (Scott, 1979). Many cases of generalized demodicosis, however, begin as a localized form. Besides investigating the dog's family history and whether the puppy belongs to an at-risk breed for demodicosis, it is difficult to predict the outcome for the individual puppy with localized disease.

Generalized demodicosis is a familial disease and, as such, occurs more frequently in pedigreed dogs. Some individual breeds of dogs are more frequently affected than other breeds (Table 12–4). Generalized demodicosis may resolve spontaneously. It is estimated that 30% to 50% of cases in dogs younger than 1 year will resolve without specific miticidal therapy. When evalu-

Table 12–4	Dog Breeds with Familial Predilection to Develop Generalized Demodicosis

Old English sheepdog
Collie
Afghan hound
German shepherd
Cocker spaniel
Shih Tzu
Lhasa apso
Staffordshire and pit bull terrier
Doberman pinscher
Rottweiler
Dalmatian
Great Dane
English bulldog
Boston terrier
Dachshund
Chihuahua
Boxer
Chinese pug
Chinese shar-pei
Beagle
German short-haired pointer

ating the prognosis for an individual puppy, the veterinarian should take into account whether the dog belongs to an at-risk breed, whether closely related dogs have developed generalized disease, whether there is an associated health problem such as parasitism, malnutrition, or use of corticosteroids, and whether there is widespread and/or deep secondary bacterial infection. The presence of any such factor will make spontaneous resolution unlikely and will indeed reduce the prognosis for a favorable outcome with therapy (Foil, 1995).

The clinical signs of localized demodicosis are familiar to all veterinarians. A focal or periocular patch of hair loss is associated with varying degrees of erythema, scaling, and papular or pustular eruption (Foil, 1995). Occasionally, furunculosis and cellulitis may develop in localized disease. Localized demodicosis in poodles and other breeds of dogs with long hair growth cycles may cause no alopecia. Most lesions occur on the face; the next most common site is a distal region of extremity. Localized demodicosis can be defined as five or fewer individual lesions affecting not more than one body region, such as the head or the extremities (Foil, 1995). Any dog with more extensive disease is at least suspect for having demodicosis that may be passed on to offspring. It has also been stated that any dog with localized demodicosis that develops regional or widespread lymphadenopathy is likely to develop generalized disease.

Generalized demodicosis in puppies may be squamous (uncomplicated by secondary bacterial infection) or pustular (complicated by secondary bacterial infection) (Foil, 1995). Pododemodicosis unaccompanied by widespread disease is extremely uncommon in young puppies. Either form may develop in multifocal patches consisting of erythema, scaling, follicular plugging, postinflammatory hyperpigmentation, and hair loss. Such lesions may be regional or generalized. Pustular disease may occur in the form of superficial folliculitis or may be manifested as furunculosis or regional cellulitis (Fig. 12–1). Long-haired dogs may have generalized demodicosis with minimal alopecia. Puppies with cellulitis may show signs of systemic illness; indeed, this is a life-threatening form of canine demodicosis (Fig. 12–2).

Diagnosis requires thoroughly performed skin scraping techniques. *Demodex canis* mites are intrafollicular, so skin should be pinched to extrude mites from hair follicles and comedones before scraping. Scrapings should be deep enough to produce capillary bleeding. Care should be taken not to scrape scarred lesions because no follicles will be present in scars. The preferred sites for scraping are newer lesions with erythema, papules, or prominent plugging of follicles. Puppies with apparent localized dis-

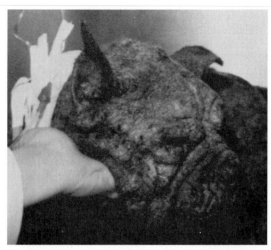

Figure 12–2. Severe cellulitis in a fatal case of generalized demodicosis in a boxer puppy.

ease should be scraped in lip folds and plantar interdigital webs, as well as inspected for inapparent lesions so that generalized disease may be recognized early. Young puppies with localized or generalized demodicosis should be checked for and treated for intestinal parasitism. Because it is possible for young dogs to have more than one skin disease, dermatophyte cultures should be obtained. If the young dog is extremely pruritic, sarcoptic mange may accompany demodicosis. Recognition of concomitant disease that may be treated will enhance the possibility of spontaneous resolution of demodicosis.

Treatment of localized demodicosis is not always necessary (Foil, 1995; Kwochka, 1993). At times, the veterinarian may be forced to treat to appease the concerned owner. In such cases, ointments or shampoos containing rotenone, benzoyl peroxide, or chlorhexidine may be employed. Treatment will make skin lesions appear worse initially. Skin lesions complicated by cellulitis or furunculosis should be treated with systemically acting antimicrobial agents. Usually, the secondary invader is *Staphylococcus intermedius*, so antimicrobial agents appropriate to that organism should be used (see Table 12–3). Systemically acting or topical corticosteroids should not be used in a puppy with localized demodicosis. In cases of localized demodicosis that remain active for more than 8 weeks, the veterinarian may find it prudent to treat as for generalized demodicosis. In such cases, treatment should be rigorous and follow all recommended aspects of the treatment protocol. In particular, recommendations about whole-body

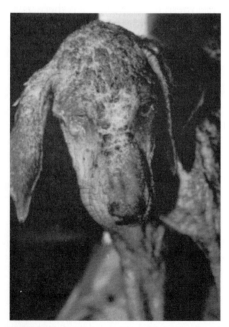

Figure 12–1. Doberman puppy with generalized pustular demodicosis and cellulitis.

clipping should be followed. In these cases, subsequent breeding should then be discouraged, because any propensity for developing generalized demodicosis will have been masked.

Not every case of generalized demodicosis in young puppies should be treated. The financial status of the owner and their willingness to appropriately treat the puppy should be taken into account before treatment of generalized demodicosis is initiated. Unless severe furunculosis or cellulitis accompanies demodicosis or unless the puppy has no value to the owner except as a potential breeder, it is not recommended to perform euthanasia on a puppy younger than 6 months because of generalized demodicosis. As in localized demodicosis, puppies with generalized disease should be checked for and treated for other health problems. Pyoderma should always be treated with appropriate antimicrobial agents (see Table 12–3). If the demodicosis has not resolved shortly after the onset of puberty or if the demodicosis is progressing rapidly, specific treatment should be recommended.

The preferred treatment for generalized demodicosis is amitraz (Mitaban, Pharmacia-Upjohn, Kalamazoo, Michigan). A suggested treatment algorithm for juvenile-onset demodicosis is outlined in Figure 12–3. The efficacy of amitraz therapy as it is labeled for use in the United States has been reported to have long-term cure rates of 25% to 50% or less (Kwochka et al, 1985; Scott and Walton, 1985). Kwochka and associates (1985) have shown that the efficacy is improved by weekly treatments with amitraz. The veterinarian will find that dogs in the at-risk group are rarely negative on scrapings before the fourth month of treatment, so the owner should be prepared for a long course of amitraz therapy (Foil, 1995).

Other factors that may influence treatment and potential adverse reactions to amitraz should be mentioned (Foil, 1995). Occasionally, a puppy with demodicosis is pruritic. This is also recognized as an adverse reaction during treatment in a small percentage of cases. Some of these cases will resolve with successful antimicrobial treatment of secondary bacterial infection. In other cases, systemically acting antihistamines may be helpful (diphenhydramine, 2.2 mg/kg twice a day; chlorpheniramine, 2 to 4 mg, total dose twice a day) (Kwochka, 1993). In such cases, the administration of an antihistamine on the day of amitraz therapy may exacerbate the most common adverse reactions to amitraz, which include central nervous system depression accompanied by bradycardia, hypothermia, and hyperglycemia. It is advisable to have an in-hospital observation period for several hours after amitraz dipping. Corticosteroids should not be used to control pruritus in canine demodicosis. Central nervous system depression and bradycardia are often seen even without the use of concomitant antihistamine therapy and may begin shortly after and continue for several hours after amitraz dipping. These adverse reactions are more common and more severe in small toy breed dogs, especially the Chihuahua and the Maltese. This undesirable side effect may be treated with yohimbine (Garvey, 1993; Hsu and Hopper 1986); yohimbine is used at a dose of 0.01 mg/kg subcutaneously every 3 hours, as needed, after amitraz dipping or 0.03 mg/kg subcutaneously as a pretreatment antidote. Another problem that may be encountered is the owner's desire to bathe the animal or allow it to swim between treatments. Because amitraz action is persistent for many days after application, bathing and swimming should not be allowed. If an owner insists on weekly bathing, then weekly treatment should be applied. A final principle is that dogs should be kept closely clipped throughout the course of treatment (Foil, 1995).

Ivermectin is an effective therapy for generalized demodicosis in young dogs that do not respond to bimonthly or weekly amitraz therapy or that experience severe adverse reactions to amitraz therapy. Oral ivermectin dosages generally vary between 400 and 600 $\mu g/kg$ daily. Because of the large daily dose to be administered, it is best to begin the dog with 50 $\mu g/kg$ on day 1 and increase the daily dose by 50 $\mu g/kg$ until the final dose of 400 $\mu g/kg$ is reached on day 8. If any signs of possible ivermectin toxicity are observed, ivermectin therapy is immediately stopped. It is also preferred to restrict the final dose of daily ivermectin to the lower end of the dosage range, such as 400 $\mu g/kg$ in young dogs. Daily ivermectin therapy is continued until there are at least two successive negative skin scrapings obtained 1 month apart. The dog is closely monitored for any signs of ivermectin toxicity for 1 year. If relapse of demodicosis were to occur, most dogs would relapse within the first year—about 70% of dogs will achieve two negative skin scrapings on alternate-day therapy with dosages varying between 400 and 600 $\mu g/kg$. Daily administration of ivermectin for generalized demodicosis in the cat is not usually done.

For dogs and cats of all ages, off-label use of ivermectin formulations (ivermectin formulations are not currently approved for this use)

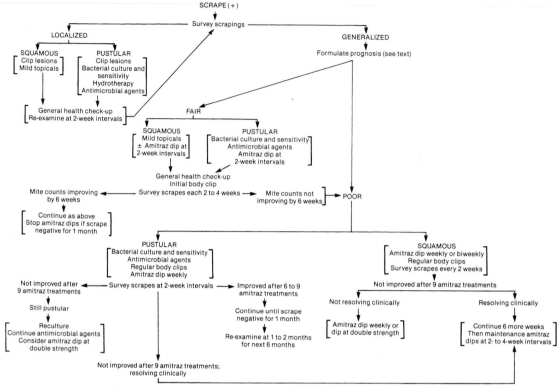

Figure 12–3. Treatment algorithm for juvenile-onset demodicosis.

can provide broad-spectrum activity against mites (i.e., *Demodex canis, Sarcoptes scabiei, Notoedres cati, Otodectes cynotis, Cheyletiella* species, and *Pneumonyssus caninum*). The ivermectin formulation most often used is the 1% nonaqueous injectable solution. The 0.5% alcohol-based pour-on solution has been shown to be an effective and practical formulation to use in some mite infestations in dogs and cats. Collies, Australian shepherds, Shetland sheepdogs, Old English sheepdogs, and other dog breeds are more susceptible to ivermectin toxicity. Toxicity reactions include ataxia, behavior disturbances, tremors, mydriasis, weakness/recumbency, apparent blindness, hypersalivation, depression, and, in severe cases, coma and death. Although the margin of safety appears to be narrower in cats than in dogs, idiosyncratic reactions are uncommon. The no-effect level for ivermectin in adult cats is approximately 500 μg/kg. In general, ivermectin is more effective against ectoparasitic arthropods when it is given parenterally than when it is given orally. Oral ivermectin is typically administered once every 7 days, whereas subcutaneous or topical (pour-on) ivermectin is given once every 14 days.

Milbemycin has also been used to success-

fully treat generalized demodicosis in young dogs—oral daily dosage usually ranges from 0.5 to 3.8 mg/kg. Milbemycin is not currently approved for this use. Success rates are from 70% to 90% and are higher with the higher dose; however, central nervous system signs of stupor, tremors, and ataxia are more likely to be seen in a few dogs at the higher doses. Treatment with milbemycin is continued until there are at least two successive negative skin scrapings obtained. The dog is then monitored closely for 1 year. It is best to begin treatment with 0.5 to 1 mg/kg daily and increase to 1 to 2 mg/kg daily if clinical improvement is not seen within 1 to 2 months.

FELINE DEMODICOSIS

Feline demodicosis is much less common than is canine demodicosis. The mites *Demodex cati* (a long, slender follicular mite) and other *Demodex* species (dwells superficially within the stratum corneum and is short and broad morphologically) are normal inhabitants of the feline skin (Morris and Beale, 2000). Clinical demodicosis usually occurs in adult cats rather than in kittens. It does appear that the superficial *Demo-*

dex species is a more common cause of dermatitis. It is also believed that cases of localized and generalized demodicosis in cats will resolve spontaneously as occurs in dogs; however, evidence sufficient to support a homologous situation in cats is still lacking. Both broad, superficial scrapings and concentrated, deep scrapings should be obtained in all cases of suspected feline demodicosis. The treatment of choice is 2% sulfurated lime dips every 5 to 7 days for six treatments. Adverse effects will be noted with the sulfurated lime dip if the cat ingests the dip. An Elizabethan collar should be used to prevent grooming until the dip has dried on the body. Dips are stopped only when repeated skin scrapings are completely free of eggs, mites, and mite fragments.

OTHER MITE-RELATED INFESTATIONS

Miscellaneous cutaneous mite infestations of young dogs and cats include chiggers or harvest mites; various mites that are parasitic on other species, such as poultry mites; and cat fur mites (Foil, 1995). Other than the cat fur mite *Lynxacarus radovsky*, these are not particularly problematic for young animals. The cat fur mite is an uncommon parasite of adult and immature cats (Craig et al, 1993). Infested cats show mild pruritus and unkempt appearance with mild pityriasis.

The mites that are important ectoparasites of puppies and kittens include *Sarcoptes scabiei*, *Notoedres cati*, *Otodectes cynotis*, and *Cheyletiella* species (Foil, 1995). Canine scabies is a sporadically and locally common disease of young and adult dogs caused by *Sarcoptes scabiei* var. *canis*. Sarcoptic mange is a highly contagious and extremely pruritic dermatosis. It is also an important zoonosis because it causes a pruritic although self-limiting dermatosis in 10% to 50% of persons who are exposed to affected pets (Griffin, 1993). It is unusual to recognize signs of scabies in puppies younger than 6 weeks, which may be a result of poorly developed scratch reflexes in young puppies, as well as a manifestation of an incubation period that usually exceeds 3 weeks. Also, it has been postulated that clinical signs may result from the development of hypersensitivity to the mite infestation (Griffin, 1993).

Clinical signs in young dogs afflicted with scabies are characteristic. Pruritus is marked and is exhibited by scratching at the head and elbows and head shaking. The scratch reflex may be easily elicited in dogs, especially with manipulation of the pinnae of the ear. The head, the margins of the pinnae, the elbows, and the hocks generally show lesions first. There is a papular eruption that may be obscured by excoriations and by scaling and crusting. If left undiagnosed and untreated, the scabies may become generalized and result in widespread hair loss, scaling, hyperkeratosis, lichenification, and ongoing excoriation. Weight loss may also be a result of the severe incessant pruritus (Griffin, 1993).

The diagnosis is established by demonstrating the mite, mite eggs, or mite fecal material in skin scrapings (Foil, 1995). Occasionally the mite may be demonstrated in fecal flotation examination. When the clinical signs are characteristic, the diagnosis should be pursued with therapeutic trials. Treatment may be accomplished using a variety of parasiticidal agents (Table 12–5), although the treatment of choice is considered by many to be the systemically acting ivermectin or milbemycin. Ivermectin is not currently approved for this use. Ivermectin is usually administered at a dose of 200 to 400 μg/kg once every 7 days orally or once every 14 days subcutaneously for four to six treatments. The 0.5% alcohol-based pour-on ivermectin formulation is efficacious at treating dogs 3 months of age and older when applied at 500 μg/kg on the dorsum at day 1 and day 14. The same dog breed precautions, 1% nonaqueous injectable ivermectin solution, should be used with this formulation. Milbemycin has been successfully used to treat scabies in young dogs. Dosage regimens range from 0.5 to 1 mg/kg daily for 2 months to 1 mg/kg on alternate days for 16 days. Dogs as young as 6 weeks may be treated; mild lethargy may be observed in this age group. Others have recommended using 2 mg/kg on days 0, 7, and 14. Topically applied selamectin is also effective in the prevention of canine scabies.

When topical agents are chosen, there should be an initial clipping of long-haired or dense-haired dogs and use of a therapeutic shampoo aimed at removal of scales and crusts. For puppies younger then 12 weeks and for breeds of dogs in which ivermectin is not recommended (i.e., collies, Australian shepherds, Shetland sheepdogs, and Old English sheepdogs), the treatment of choice is sulfurated lime dips at 4% to 8% every 5 to 7 days for six treatments. An alternative topical treatment is amitraz at regular label strength applied two to four times at 2-week intervals. No matter what the choice of treatment, all in-contact dogs should be treated. All bedding should be cleaned thor-

Table 12–5	Parasiticidal Therapy for Puppies and Kittens			
PRODUCT	FLEAS	LICE	MITES	TICKS
Allethrin (many trade names)	+	−	−	−
Amitraz (Mitaban)	−	−	+	−
Carbaryl (many trade names)	+	+	+	+
Chlorpyrifos (many trade names)	+	+	+	+
Cythioate (Proban)	+	−	−	−
D-Limonene (many trade names)	+	+	−	−
Diazinon (many trade names)	+	+	−	+
Fenthion (Pro-Spot)	+	−	−	−
Fipronil (Frontline)	+	+	−	+
Imidacloprid (Advantage)	+	+	−	−
Ivermectin (many trade names)	−	−	+	−
Lime-sulfur (many trade names)	−	−	+	−
Lindane (many trade names)	+	+	+	+
Linalool (many trade names)	+	−	−	−
Lufenuron (Program)	+	−	−	−
Malathion (many trade names)	+	+	−	+
Methylcarbamate (many trade names)	+	+	−	+
Permethrin (many trade names)	+	+	−	+
Phosmet (Paramite)	+	+	+	+
Pyrethrins (many trade names)	+	+	−	+
Resmethrin (many trade names)	+	+	−	−
Rotenone (many trade names)	+	+	−	+
Selamectin (Revolution)	+	−	+	+

All topical products should be administered or applied exactly according to label directions, as it is not legally permissible to use or recommend the use of such products beyond label restrictions. + = Indicated for use; − = not indicated for use.

oughly. Control of pruritus with judicious use of corticosteroids may be warranted for the older puppy.

Notoedric mange of cats is similar to sarcoptic mange of dogs and is caused by a similar, closely related mite. Like sarcoptic mange, the disease is highly contagious and may involve exposed persons in self-limiting pruritic dermatitis. The common name for the infestation is *head mange*, which illustrates the primary site of cutaneous involvement. The ear margins are first affected, but the disease rapidly progresses to involve the entire head and neck. Notoedric mange is highly pruritic and may cause severe self-mutilation, especially in the older kitten. Diagnosis is easy to establish with the scraping of superficial scale and crust and microscopic examination. The mites are similar in appearance to canine scabies mites, with the short legs each bearing long pedicles with distal suckers, so they are easily distinguished from ear mites that reside outside the external ear canals. Treatment is readily accomplished with either 2% sulfurated lime dips or with the use of ivermectin at 200 μg/kg administered every 7 days orally or every 14 days subcutaneously for

six to eight treatments. Ivermectin is not approved for this use in the cat. It should not be given to kittens less than 6 weeks old. All in-contact animals should be treated. Amitraz, also unapproved for this use in cats, is efficacious in head mange. Adverse reactions may occur with the use of amitraz in cats.

Otodectes cynotis infestation is a very common cause of ear problems in puppies and kittens and may occasionally be implicated in more widespread dermatitis as the cause of otodectic mange, especially in cats (Foil, 1995). The mite should be routinely searched for in all cases of existing ear problems and head pruritus in puppies and kittens. The ear exudate in a typical case is dark gray to reddish brown and waxy or granular. In secondary bacterial or yeast infection, the exudate may be yellow-brown or purulent. The mite may easily be demonstrated with mineral oil preparations of earwax and debris. Occasionally, *Otodectes* mites may be demonstrated in skin scrapings from the head or body. There are numerous proprietary preparations available for treating ear mite infestations. The important principles include thorough cleansing of affected ears initially and during the first stages of treatment and extending time of treatment adequately to span the life cycle of 3 weeks. Any treatment plan should include all in-contact dogs and cats. Also, at least one whole-body parasiticidal treatment should be applied.

Another approach for the treatment and control of *Otodectes* mites may include the use of systemically acting ivermectin and selamectin. Ivermectin, at a total dose of 500 μg, is applied to each ear canal 7 to 14 days apart for an average of five treatments to control the infestation in most cats. The subcutaneous route of ivermectin administration at 200 to 400 μg/kg every 14 days for two treatments or three oral treatments 7 days apart result in faster elimination of the ear mites and decrease the recurrence rate. The 0.5% alcohol-based pour-on formulation of ivermectin at a dose of 500 μg/kg applied between the shoulder blades can be used and is about 96% effective. Topically applied selamectin is effective in the prevention of ear mite problems.

Cheyletiella infestation is contagious and is an important, unrecognized zoonosis (Foil, 1995). Puppies may first develop disease after the first trip to the groomer. Affected puppies and kittens are scurfy, showing mild to severe dorsally distributed scale. Pruritus is variable and usually mild to nonexistent in young animals. With pruritus, crusting and hair loss may develop. The dorsal lumbar area and the top of the head and neck are usually most severely affected in puppies. Kittens may show a dorsal miliary dermatitis. Exposed persons may develop a pruritic papular eruption, generally on the forearms and upper chest. Diagnosis is usually easily established in young animals. Long-haired animals should be clipped with scissors over selected lesions or areas of scale. Thereafter one of several techniques may be employed to demonstrate the mites. Clear acetate tape may be impressed on the skin to collect dander and debris. A broad superficial skin scraping using mineral oil on the scalpel blade may collect sufficient material. The debris may be examined in a drop of mineral oil on low power of the microscope. Alternatively, a flea comb may be used to comb dander and debris onto a large piece of dark paper or collected into a Petri dish. The combings may be examined with a magnifying lens or under a dissecting microscope. Fecal flotation examinations may also reveal mites that have been ingested by the animal.

Treatment should involve all in-contact animals and include environmental treatments (Foil, 1995). Adult female mites may survive and be infective off the host for several days, so the home or kennel should be cleaned and sprayed or treated with an aerosol fogger. Kittens may be treated with pyrethrin-containing or rotenone-containing shampoos. Treatments should be repeated on a monthly basis. Puppies may be treated with virtually any insecticidal preparation that is labeled for the age group involved (see Table 12–5). Very young puppies may be treated successfully with sulfurated lime dips or pyrethrin-containing products. Topical treatment should be preceded by the use of a keratolytic shampoo, and long-haired animals should be clipped. Ivermectin is very effective for cheyletiellosis and has been used safely in kittens and puppies younger than 6 weeks at a dosage of 200 to 300 μg/kg every 7 days orally or every 14 days subcutaneously for six to eight treatments. The 0.5% alcohol-based pour-on formulation of ivermectin may be used successfully to treat cheyletiellosis in the cat at 500 μg/kg applied down the back for two treatments 2 weeks apart.

LICE

Lice are host specific and do not survive well off the specific hosts. Puppies may be infested with *Linognathus setosus*, a sucking louse, or *Trichodectes canis* or *Heterodoxus spiniger*, which are biting lice. The cat louse, *Felicola subrostratus*, is a biting louse. Infestations are contagious and may be spread by fomites. Clinical features are variable, and more often pruritus along the dorsal midline leads to excoriation and secondary dermatitis (Foil, 1995). The diagnosis may often be made by physical examination or by acetate tape impressions of the haircoat. Both lice and nits are readily visible. Treatment may be accomplished with any insecticidal topical preparation approved for use on the puppy or kitten (see Table 12–5). All in-contact animals should be treated, and the bedding should be cleaned. Treatments should be repeated in 10 to 14 days.

FLEAS AND FLIES

Flea infestation is an important health problem of most puppies and kittens. Knowing about the life cycle of the flea that commonly infests dogs and cats of all ages is a tremendous aid in the battle against the ubiquitous flea (Dryden and Rust, 1994; Rust and Dryden, 1997). There are four stages in the life cycle of the flea: egg, larva, pupa (cocoon), and adult. When environmental conditions are favorable, the adult flea has a great reproductive potential. Fleas thrive at low altitudes in temperature ranges of 65° to 80°F. Under these conditions, the flea life cycle can be completed, from hatching of an egg to the laying of the next generation of eggs, in as little as 16 days. Adult fleas are long-lived and can survive several months without being fed. The female flea does need a meal of blood to lay eggs and to feed her young. Each fertilized female flea may lay as many as 25 eggs per day.

The female flea lays her eggs in the fur of a dog or cat or any fur-bearing animal. The eggs are not sticky; they tend to fall out of the fur and survive in the protected places where a dog or cat or another fur-bearing animal sleeps or plays. The eggs will hatch into very small worm-like larvae. The larvae feed on organic debris, especially the dried blood droppings (flea dirt) left by adult fleas. Therefore, larvae depend on the animal to return time after time to the places where the eggs dropped off. The larvae molt and form pupae that spin cocoons and then emerge as young and hungry adults in about 3 weeks. Adult fleas hatch from the cocoons when proper stimulation is present. Such stimuli include vibration, increased carbon dioxide levels, heat, and motion. The adult can emerge from the cocoon in a very short time period, less than a few seconds, and immediately jump to find an appropriate host. Once on the host, they feed on blood obtained by biting through the skin.

The newly emerging fleas can be hard to find on the host; however, fleas do often produce evidence of their visit in the form of "flea dirt" and/or the animal, and certainly human, scratching. Flea dirt can be seen on the animal even when no fleas are readily visible. By combing or brushing the animal's fur, tiny dark dots or comma-shaped pieces of debris can be found. If these particles are combed onto a piece of wet white paper, they will dissolve and stain the paper red because the flea dirt is partially digested blood.

Effective flea control requires removal of fleas from the animal, removal of fleas from the environment, and control of the life cycle of the flea (see Table 12–5). To control fleas on the puppy or kitten, it is important to remember that flea control should be applied to all animals in the household or environment. Any newly acquired puppy or kitten that is in reasonable health may be immediately bathed in a pyrethrin-based shampoo, so the fleas may be washed down the drain instead of establishing their life cycle in a new home. It is important that long-haired animals be combed out with a fine-toothed comb as they are drying, as fleas may revive after pyrethrin shampoo exposure, especially if the shampoo contact time is less than 5 minutes. If the puppy is still nursing, it should be immediately combed free of fleas with a fine-toothed flea comb and not bathed with a pyrethrin-based shampoo.

Once fleas have had a chance to establish their life cycle in a new home, no control program will be successful that does not emphasize environmental control. In general, the same environmental control methods may be used for young animals as for adults. Care should always be taken that animal and people are not directly exposed to insecticides used in flea extermination. All effective in-house or in-building programs should take advantage of new technologies in flea control. There are new insecticides that have long residual activity, such as synthetic pyrethroids and microencapsulated products, and there are insect growth regulators, such as methoprene, fenoxycarb, and pyriproxifen, employed for preadult flea control.

Advances in environmental flea control have been less remarkable. Several yard sprays that contain organophosphate compounds, such as malathion, chlorpyrifos, or diazinon, will kill fleas on contact, have residual activity, or both. Problem areas in a yard may include areas under porches, under stairs, in sheds or doghouses (which should be treated like the house), and areas under or around shade trees or bushes. Organic material may protect fleas from exposure to the active ingredient. At present, the use of organophosphate compounds labeled for outdoor flea control is still the best and most economical approach. Such approaches will have to incorporate repeated applications at 2-week intervals throughout the flea season where temperature and humidity are favorable for flea reproduction. In areas with lawn, gravel, or sand, biologic control can be effected with specially developed nematodes such as *Steinernema carpocapsae*.

The newer flea control products available are safe and are applied topically on the skin or administered orally on a monthly basis. These products contain such active ingredients as lufenuron, fipronil, imidacloprid, or selamectin (see Table 12–5). In general, any flea control product containing lufenuron, fipronil, imidacloprid, or selamectin as its active ingredient should not be administered or applied to nursing animals. Pyrethrin-based products are generally safe for frequent application; the most effective products are synergized pyrethrin sprays. Very small animals and nursing animals sprayed with alcohol-based or other volatile organic solvents may be severely chilled as the solvent evaporates. Water-based sprays are preferable, and small animals and nursing animals should never be thoroughly saturated with a spray. Most sprays are now pump sprays, not aerosol sprays. These can be quite effective as flea control agents, depending on the active ingredient of the flea control product. Sprays should be applied once to twice weekly or, in some endemic areas, every day after the animal returns to the house from the outdoors. It is not necessary to totally soak the animal. One or two sprays over the tail base, one on the rear aspect of each hind leg, one on the stomach area, and one or two around the neck or back are generally sufficient. The spray may be applied to a cotton ball and the moistened cotton ball used to wipe the spray around the eyes and ears to avoid getting the product in the animal's eyes. The safest and most effective spray products contain microencapsulated pyrethrins. Flea collars or medallions that are safe for use on puppies and kittens are not effective in most environments. Topical treatments should be coordinated with in-house environmental flea control.

Cutaneous myiasis may develop in young puppies and kittens when fly eggs are deposited on open wounds or macerated skin. Areas of the body affected usually are the perineum, eyes, nose, and mouth (Fadok, 1980). Lesions may develop into extensive subcutaneous pockets overlaid by punched-out holes as the fly larvae enlarge the wound. Lesions should be clipped off and cleaned and maggots flushed from the wounds.

The parasitic fly of the genus *Cuterebra* causes another form of myiasis that affects young puppies and especially kittens (Foil, 1995). Larvae have the ability to penetrate the skin directly and develop within subcutaneous cysts with a central breathing pore. Lesions are nodular and inflamed and contain central pores; most develop on the head and ventral region of the neck. Young puppies and kittens are exposed to these parasites of rodents and rabbits when near the burrows of the normal host. Treatment consists of manually removing the grub and flushing the resultant wound.

A related parasitic fly, *Dermatobia hominis*, afflicts humans, cattle, and dogs in Latin America. A case affecting a fila Brasileiro puppy exported from Brazil to the Netherlands has been reported (Roosje et al, 1992). Lesions were similar to those associated with *Cuterebra* infestation.

TICKS

Ticks not only rob a puppy or kitten of its blood but are also likely to transmit disease. In fact, ticks can transmit many diseases, including ehrlichiosis, borreliosis, babesiosis, cytauxzoonosis, hemobartonellosis, RMSF, coxiellosis, and tularemia. Whereas many species of ticks parasitize dogs and cats, hard ticks of the genera *Rhipicephalus*, *Ixodes*, and *Dermacentor* species are the most commonly encountered. There is certain urgency in detecting ticks early because they can consume much blood in a relatively short period and can transmit diseases in as little as 24 hours after attachment. The goal is therefore to recognize and remove them before they can do much damage. In tick-infested areas, this means that owners should closely examine their puppies and kittens after each outing. Owners encountering embedded ticks should dab the tick with isopropyl alcohol and carefully remove it with forceps that are commercially available for this purpose and dispose of the ticks in a jar of alcohol or by flushing them down the toilet. Bare fingers should not be used to grasp ticks because if the tick's body bursts during extraction any organisms or toxins it is carrying are placed in direct contact with the skin and could result in infection. At the least, owners should use plastic wrap to protect themselves from direct exposure to the ticks.

Tick dipping with organophosphates was once considered to be routine for tick control, but safer products have greatly reduced the need for such activity. In general, a pyrethrin spray is used to achieve a rapid knockdown effect on existing ticks. Pyrethroids can be used on dogs but not cats for this process and have a longer residual effect. Products such as fipronil can be used even for relatively young puppies and kittens; fipronil lasts approximately 1 month. Amitraz tick collars cause ticks to voluntarily withdraw often before there is time for disease transmission. In areas with heavy tick infestations, combinations of these products or using them together with organophosphate dips is needed for effective tick control. Products designed for humans that contain the insect repellant DEET should not be used on puppies and kittens and are considered too toxic for routine use.

Environmental control depends on the species of tick encountered, but keeping the yard free of underbrush, leaf litter, and the like removes the cover and food sources for the small animals that serve as hosts for ticks. For those living in grassy and wooded areas, organophosphates such as chlorpyrifos and tetrachlorvinphos may be needed to provide additional control. Because *Rhipicephalus sanguineus* can infest houses, professional extermination services are usually warranted when this parasite becomes an indoor pest.

IMMUNE-MEDIATED AND INFLAMMATORY DISEASES

Immune-Mediated Disorders

Immune-mediated disorders are extremely uncommon in young dogs and cats. The various immune-mediated skin diseases, such as pemphigus complex, bullous pemphigoid, or lupus erythematosus, would only be a diagnosed clinical problem, at the earliest age, in puppies and kittens older than 3 months. The symptomatology and diagnosis do not differ from those in adult dogs and cats.

Allergic Disorders

Allergic skin disease is again more likely to become symptomatic in young adult animals. Allergic dermatoses that are seen in young cats or dogs are food allergy, drug eruption, flea allergy, and possibly atopy (MacDonald, 1993a; Reedy and Miller, 1989). A hypersensitivity-type dermatitis secondary to the presence of intestinal parasites has also been reported (Scott, 1978).

Food allergy dermatitis is difficult to define, and many cases of purported food allergy may represent food intolerance, being mediated by nonimmunologic—metabolic, toxic, or pharmacologic—effects of ingestants (Guilford, 1992; Halliwell, 1992; MacDonald, 1993a). In cats, food allergy dermatitis is seen in adults, not in kittens younger than 5 months. Food allergy dermatitis is often, however, seen in young dogs. In retrospective studies of food allergy in dogs, the percentage of cases with onset at an age less than 1 year has ranged from 10% to 52%, with the youngest puppy being 3 months of age (Carlotti et al, 1990; Harvey, 1993; White, 1986).

Clinical findings are variable and nonseasonal, but pruritus and erythema are the most common signs (Foil, 1995). Papular eruptions, urticaria, or, rarely, eosinophilic pustules may also be seen. Skin lesions may be localized to very specific sites on the body, regional, or generalized; the distribution pattern often mimics atopy, and ear pruritus and recurrent ear problems are common manifestations (Rosser, 1990). Some puppies may have gastrointestinal signs—most commonly increased numbers of soft stools and flatulence.

Diagnosis of food allergy dermatitis is problematic to the veterinarian and the owner. Other possible causes of pruritic dermatitis should be ruled out before investigation of food allergy is begun (Foil, 1995). Most puppies are allergic to a single substance in the diet, multiple sensitivities being uncommon at such a young age. The allergen is generally one that the puppy has been eating throughout its life. Cereal grains and cow's milk have been the most commonly reported allergens (August, 1985). Diagnosis consists of feeding a food allergy elimination diet until signs and symptoms are resolved. Because dermatologic signs may be slow to resolve, especially when complicated by secondary bacterial, fungal, or parasitic infection, it is recommended to feed the restricted test diet for up to 12 weeks or until signs have subsided. An appropriate elimination diet could be the commercially prepared or home-prepared elimination diets that are fed to adult dogs with similar allergic problems. For young puppies, these elimination diets may not be nutritionally adequate because their mineral content is far from ideal (Roudebush and Cowell, 1992). All chewable treats, supplements, and medications should be avoided for the test period. Once signs and symptoms have subsided and the puppy has been successfully maintained without antiinflammatory medications for 2 weeks, the puppy should be reexposed to the original diet to confirm the diagnosis. In most cases, exacerbation will occur within 5 to 7 days, although some will take up to 2 weeks. After relapse, the puppy is returned to the test diet until asymptomatic again. Thereafter, individual foodstuffs or single-source protein commercial diets may be introduced at 2-week intervals to find a suitable balanced diet for the puppy. Furthermore, neither intradermal skin testing nor in vitro allergy testing is very useful for the diagnosis of food allergy (Halliwell, 1992; Jeffers et al, 1991).

Skin eruptions from drugs administered or applied may occur at any age but would be expected to be uncommon in puppies and kittens because prior exposure to the offending drug is usually necessary. Clinical manifestations of drug-induced skin eruption are highly variable and can occur with virtually any drug, whether given topically or systemically. Skin eruptions may be pruritic and often consist of erythematous, exfoliative, or purpuric lesions. The more serious types of drug eruption are erythema multiforme, toxic epidermal necrolysis, and syndromes mimicking immune-mediated dermatoses.

Atopy refers to an inherited tendency to develop reaginic antibodies to environmental allergens. Although atopy is both inherited and common, it is not usually seen in puppies and kittens. Most atopic dogs do not show clinical signs before 6 months of age, and most are symptom-free until at least 1 year of age. The primary symptom of atopy is pruritus. Affected dogs lick and chew at their feet, may rub their face, and tend to develop rashes in the region of the axillae and groin. Problems with excessive keratinization and pyoderma are secondary. In cats, in addition to pruritus, eosinophilic granuloma complex and symmetric alopecia are other manifestations (Chalmers et al, 1995). The diagnosis is confirmed by allergy testing. Intradermal allergy testing has been used for many decades and is still considered to be the diagnostic test of choice over the newer in vitro serum assays. Monoclonal antibody tests are superior to polyclonal antibody tests, and combinations of monoclonal antibodies that could recognize different epitopes on the same molecule might enhance the sensitivity of the detection system of in vitro serum assays (Derer et al, 1998). The treatment of atopy includes residual topical therapies, antihistamines, fatty acids, immunotherapy, and corticosteroids, alone or in combination.

Allergy to intestinal parasites has been reported to cause pruritic dermatitis in dogs and cats of all ages. It is diagnosed by fecal examination and by observing resolution of dermatologic signs subsequent to treatment with an appropriate anthelmintic agent. The incidence of this poorly understood syndrome is entirely unknown, but, because it is easily treated, it should be considered in young animals with nonspecific pruritic skin disease.

Inflammatory Diseases

Several inflammatory skin diseases seen in puppies and kittens include juvenile pustular dermatosis, juvenile cellulitis, urticaria and angioedema, cutaneous vasculitis, juvenile polyarteritis syndrome, toxic epidermal necrolysis, idiopathic nodular panniculitis, and feline collagenolytic granuloma.

Juvenile pustular dermatosis resembles a bacterial skin disease but responds to corticosteroid administration, such as triamcinolone acetonide

at 0.1 mg intramuscularly or subcutaneously daily for 5 days. It occurs in Chinese shar-pei, pointers, and Labrador retrievers 3 days to 3 weeks of age (Foil, 1995). Clinical signs begin with pustules that evolve into brown crusts on the head and trunk. Puppies may be mildly or severely affected. Depression and anorexia may lead to death, although the dermatosis does not produce a fever. Because the syndrome may be difficult to differentiate from staphylococcal pyoderma, systemically acting antimicrobial agents should be administered.

Juvenile cellulitis is also known as *puppy strangles*, *juvenile pyoderma*, and *lymphadenitis apostematosa* (Reimann et al, 1989; White et al, 1989). Juvenile cellulitis is a common disease of dachshund, Labrador and golden retriever, and pointer puppies from 3 weeks to 12 months of age, although it can occur in any dog breed (Foil, 1995). Most cases occur in puppies younger than 16 weeks. Often, several individuals in a litter are affected. Enlargement of the mandibular lymph nodes is the most consistent finding, but cutaneous lesions are usually noticed first by the owner. The signs begin with rapidly developing edema and papules and pustules of the head and neck, particularly involving the lips, the eyelids, and the pinnae of the ears. A mucopurulent ocular discharge and purulent otitis externa develop within a short time. Affected skin becomes progressively indurated and erythematous, and serous to purulent exudate may be produced (Fig. 12–4). Lymph nodes of the head and neck enlarge and may become adherent to the swollen skin. Occasionally, a lymph node may rupture and discharge hemorrhagic purulent exudate. Genital and perianal skin and paws may be affected in some cases,

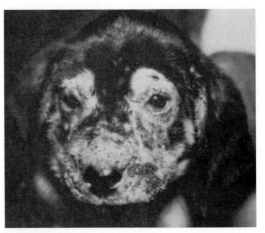

Figure 12–4. Mixed-breed puppy with advanced juvenile cellulitis (puppy strangles).

and generalized lymphadenopathy or cellulitis of the limbs may develop. Fever and anorexia may accompany the cellulitis. In the rare case, the head and neck may not be affected, but it may be restricted to another region such as a hind leg. When juvenile cellulitis occurs in atypical locations, skin and/or lymph node biopsies are needed to confirm the diagnosis. Histopathologic findings typically indicate a pyogranulomatous cellulitis and lymphadenitis with no causative agent identified.

Leukocytosis with neutrophilia and nonregenerative anemia are found in some puppies affected with juvenile cellulitis. The disease may be fatal if left untreated, but in treated dogs the outcome is usually favorable. Most veterinarians will feel obliged to treat such cases with broad-spectrum systemically acting antimicrobial agents, but the juvenile cellulitis lesions will not resolve until corticosteroids, such as prednisone given at a dose of 2 mg/kg orally for 10 to 14 days, are administered. Resolution of signs is usually rapid thereafter. Occasionally, a severely affected puppy will relapse after withdrawal and require longer therapy. Gentle topical therapy to remove purulent exudate is also helpful. Abscessed lymph nodes may be surgically drained to give symptomatic relief. Whether affected puppies should later be used for breeding is not known.

Urticaria and angioedema can result from allergic and nonallergic mechanisms (Foil, 1995; Noxon, 1991). The skin lesions consist of dermal edema and are generally short lived. In puppies, such syndromes are most often seen as reactions to vaccination or to stinging insects (Fig. 12–5). In kittens, this reaction may be a sequela to routine vaccinations. Recurrent urticaria may be more common in the English bulldog, bull terrier, boxer, and Chinese shar-pei. In short-coated dogs, folliculitis may be misdiagnosed as urticaria. Angioedema could be confused with the early stages of juvenile cellulitis or snakebite. Therapy involves elimination and avoidance of the inciting cause if it is known. Acute reactions that are deemed to interfere with a patent airway or to be progressing to systemic anaphylaxis may be treated with epinephrine diluted 1:1000 and administered subcutaneously or intramuscularly (0.01 ml/kg) (Noxon, 1991). Persistent cases with concomitant pruritus may be relieved by corticosteroids. Antihistamines are useful as preventive medications if exposure is thought to be unavoidable.

Cutaneous vasculitis is characterized by cutaneous hemorrhage or purpura, ulceration, and necrosis usually of acral sites (footpads, ear mar-

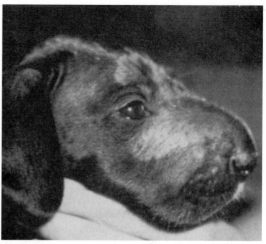

Figure 12–5. Great Dane puppy with facial angioedema.

gins, lips, tongue, and tail tip) (Halliwell and Gorman, 1989). Superficial vasculitis may be seen as a manifestation of a drug eruption or in association with acute febrile infectious illness, which would be the most common expected finding in young puppies. Of the infectious diseases, rickettsial organisms are most frequently associated with cutaneous vasculitis. Occasionally, vasculitis lesions develop on the extremities of large-breed puppies in association with hypertrophic osteodystrophy.

Juvenile polyarteritis syndrome, also known as *beagle pain syndrome*, is seen in 4- to 10-month-old beagles; the usual manifestations include intermittent fever, cervical pain, and anorexia, but facial edema and skin ulceration may also be noted (Scott-Moncreiff, 1992). The idiopathic cutaneous and renal glomerular vasculopathy commonly referred to as "Alabama rot," which is seen mostly in greyhounds, but occasionally in other dog breeds, is seen occasionally in dogs as young as 6 months (Carpenter et al, 1988). Skin lesions begin as dusky erythematous or purpuric, tender swellings on the tarsus, stifle, inner thigh, or forelimb. These lesions progress to sharply demarcated, deep ulcerations that are slow to heal. The skin lesions may be associated with signs of systemic inflammation and azotemia or may be followed by renal failure. Another cause of vasculopathy affecting the skin in the dog or cat is cold agglutinin disease. A 12-week-old puppy has been described with infarction of toes, ears, and tail tip due to cold agglutinins after treatment of lead poisoning with calcium EDTA and oral penicillamine (Dickson, 1990).

Toxic epidermal necrolysis is an uncommon dermatosis that is often secondary to an underlying systemic disease or may represent a drug eruption. It may occur in dogs or cats of any age (Scott et al, 1979). Affected puppies may exhibit painful skin followed by erythroderma and then blistering over large areas of the body. These skin lesions will rapidly progress to ulceration, crusting, and scaling and quickly become infected and purulent. There may be lesions on the oral mucosa and the mucocutaneous junctions of the lips and prepuce. The diagnosis should be established by multiple skin biopsies. Therapy is entirely predicated on identifying and removing the underlying disease or drug. Left untreated, toxic epidermal necrolysis may be rapidly fatal.

Idiopathic nodular panniculitis is also known as *sterile nodular panniculitis*. In dogs, idiopathic nodular panniculitis may occur at any age (Scott and Anderson, 1988), although it has been stated that it is more common in puppies between 2 and 6 months of age (Baker and Stannard, 1975). The youngest affected puppies and kittens have been 10 weeks old. It occurs most commonly in the dachshund, and other breeds at risk reportedly include the toy and miniature poodle, Manchester terrier, collie, and wirehaired fox terrier (Scott and Anderson, 1988). Panniculitis appears as a singular or as multiple subcutaneous nodules on the trunk, neck, or proximal regions of the extremities. The nodules vary from firm to soft and fluctuant. Some nodules may develop adhesions to the overlying skin or may rupture, discharging hemorrhagic purulent exudate (Fig. 12–6). Some affected puppies will exhibit intermittent lethargy, anorexia, and fever (Scott and Anderson, 1988).

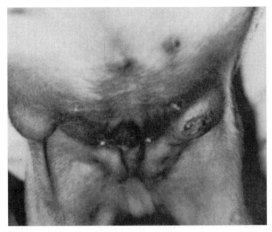

Figure 12–6. Idiopathic nodular panniculitis in an English mastiff puppy.

Almost all cases are idiopathic and have a good prognosis.

Lesion diagnosis should be confirmed by histopathology, and appropriate samples should be cultured to rule out infectious agents that may cause granulomatous panniculitis in young dogs. Another important consideration in the differential diagnosis is injection site reaction from vaccines or drugs (Hendrick and Dunagan, 1991). In cats being fed a largely fish-based diet, pansteatitis should be considered (see discussion of nutritional problems in Chapter 21). Treatment of sterile nodular panniculitis in the young dog is readily accomplished in most cases with a 2-week course of corticosteroids, such as prednisone given at a dosage of 1 to 2 mg/kg daily. Most puppies will have permanent remission with one course of therapy. In relapsing cases, the use of vitamin E, at 400 IU twice a day, may have a positive effect.

Feline collagenolytic granuloma in kittens usually occurs in the form of a linear plaque on the caudal thighs. Kittens and cats 6 months of age or older are affected more often than young kittens. Female cats are affected more often than male cats (Power, 1990). Well-circumscribed firm yellow-pink linear alopecic plaques that may be up to 10 cm long characterize lesions. In addition to occurring on the caudal thigh regions, lesions may be seen on the forelimb or ventral region of the neck, in the oral cavity, on the upper lip, on the bridge of the nose, the chin, the pinna, perirectally, or on the footpads and paws. The lesions may be diagnosed reliably by histopathology, although the clinical appearance may be adequate. Treatment with glucocorticoids is usually successful, and in this form of the eosinophilic granuloma complex remission is often permanent. Lesions that are recurrent or persistent should be evaluated for underlying disease, especially involving insect hypersensitivities.

CUTANEOUS NEOPLASIA

Cutaneous neoplasia may be epithelial or mesenchymal in origin (Goldschmidt and Shofer, 1992). The only epithelial tumor very common in puppies is canine viral papillomatosis. Other uncommon epithelial tumors in young dogs include basal cell tumors, squamous cell carcinomas, sebaceous gland tumors, apocrine gland tumors, perianal adenomas, intracutaneous cornifying epitheliomas, and hair follicle tumors. In kittens, the most common epithelial tumors are sebaceous adenomas and ceruminous gland adenomas. Mesenchymal tumors that occur in young dogs and cats are canine fibromas and fibrosarcomas, feline giant cell tumors, feline malignant nerve sheath tumors, feline hemangiomas and hemangiosarcomas, canine cutaneous histiocytomas, feline mast cell tumors, and cutaneous lymphosarcomas. Urticaria pigmentosa-like disease has also been described in puppies (Gross and Schick, 1993).

Canine cutaneous histiocytoma often occurs in dogs between 4 months and 6 years of age. English bulldogs, terriers, greyhounds, boxers, flat-coated and Labrador retrievers, cocker spaniels, Rottweilers, Chinese pugs, and Chinese shar-pei have an increased incidence. Cutaneous histiocytomas are characteristically round, well circumscribed, and raised with an attenuated or ulcerated epithelial surface (Fig. 12–7). Rapid growth is characteristic of the tumor (Bostock, 1986). Most tumors occur on the head or legs. Untreated histiocytomas regress spontaneously within a few weeks and leave no scar. Surgical excision is, consequently, curative.

Cutaneous mast cell tumors in young cats may be benign and self-limiting (Buerger, 1986; Chastain and Turk, 1987). The incidence is increased in the Siamese breed (Carpenter et al, 1987; Goldschmidt and Shofer, 1992). These mast cell tumors usually occur as firm, exophytic dermal nodules less than 1 cm in diameter. The overlying epidermis is alopecic. The lesions may or may not be pruritic. Such lesions should be excised and submitted for histopathologic examination to rule out the possibility of basal cell tumor or granulomatous disease.

Urticaria pigmentosa–like disease was described in a Newfoundland puppy beginning at 2 months of age (Gross and Schick, 1993). Le-

sions consisted of multiple mast cell–containing papules and plaques. Lesion manipulation caused erythema and edema. Lymph node involvement was noted. Lesions may spontaneously regress, whereas others may progress to mast cell leukemia or lymphoma.

Tumor-like lesions that occur in puppies or kittens include idiopathic calcinosis circumscripta in large and giant dog breeds, focal mucinosis in the young Chinese shar-pei, epidermal cysts, canine follicle cysts, canine apocrine cysts, and feline ceruminous cysts (Foil, 1995).

Calcinosis circumscripta may occur in dogs younger than 1 year, with the youngest puppy reported to be 2 months old (Scott and Buerger, 1987). German shepherd dogs are most commonly affected along with other large and giant dog breeds. Lesions are usually solitary, firm to cystic dermal masses occurring on the lateral surfaces of the limbs or the face. Surgical excision is curative.

Cutaneous mucinosis is common in the Chinese shar-pei and may be generalized, regional, or focal. When focal papules or plaques develop, the syndrome may resemble a neoplastic or inflammatory condition. Papular and plaque-like mucinosis has been described in a young chow chow–cross puppy, with similarities to the human diseases discrete papular mucinosis and juvenile cutaneous mucinosis (Beale et al, 1991). Affected puppies may exhibit noncorticosteroid-responsive pruritus, crusting, and mucocutaneous ulcerations in addition to widely distributed papules and plaques, with depigmentation of the lips and footpads. Focal mucinosis has also been described in adult Doberman pinschers (Dillberger and Altman, 1986). Lesions consist of asymptomatic rubbery papules, nodules, or plaques, or circumscribed areas of alopecia. They consist of an excess accumulation of dermal mucin, which may be so striking that the appearance may resemble a vesicle or cyst. The diagnosis is easily established by histopathology. The lesions are benign and may regress spontaneously. Excision is curative.

Cutaneous cysts may be secondary to trauma or may be a developmental defect. In kittens and puppies, they are solitary, soft, well-circumscribed intradermal nodules. The overlying epidermis may contain a pore, appear normal, or be hyperplastic and hyperpigmented. Excision is curative.

Feline ceruminous cysts occur in the external ear canal and are usually small and multiple. They are often pigmented and may be associated with inflammation. Excision can be diffi-

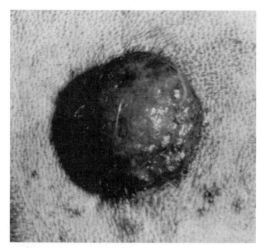

Figure 12–7. Canine cutaneous histiocytoma.

cult. Some may respond to topical cortico-steroid applications.

DEWCLAW, TAIL, AND EAR SURGERY

Dewclaw Removal

The dewclaw represents the first digit of the hindlimb and is often referred to as the first digit of the forelimb as well. Dewclaws of the hindlimbs are absent in most dogs, although single and double dewclaws are a breed standard for some breeds, such as Great Pyrenees and briard. Because dewclaws are attached by skin only, they are predisposed to trauma. Dewclaws of the forelimbs usually have three phalanges and are firmly attached to the limb. Because of their predisposition to trauma, dewclaws are usually removed from the very young puppy at the owner's request; from breeds that require frequent grooming, such as poodles, schnauzers, and fox terriers; or from the hunting breeds (Table 12–6). Occasionally, dewclaws may re-

Table 12–6	Guidelines for Dewclaw Removal

Dog breeds in which dewclaw removal is acceptable
  Alaskan malamute
  Belgian malinois
  Belgian sheepdog
  Belgian Tervueran
  Bernese Mountain dog
  Boxer
  Chesapeake Bay retriever
  Dalmatian
  Dandie Dinmont terrier
  Kerry blue terrier
  Komondor
  Lakeland terrier
  Large Munsterlander
  Norwegian elkhound
  Papillon
  Pointer (front dewclaws only)
  Shetland sheepdog
  Siberian husky
  Saint Bernard
  Vizsla
  Weimaraner
  Welsh corgi and Cardigan corgi
Dog breeds in which dewclaw removal may be
    acceptable
  Basset hound
  Puli
Dog breeds in which dewclaw removal is
    unacceptable
  Briard
  Great Pyrenees

quire amputation from older puppies after traumatic injury.

Dewclaws are best removed at 3 to 5 days of age. For puppies 1 week old, local infiltrative anesthesia should be used. Dewclaw removal from puppies older than 1 week should be postponed until they are 12 to 16 weeks old and performed under general anesthesia. For puppies less than 1 week old, the dewclaws are amputated using scissors. The dewclaw and the web of skin between the dewclaw and the metatarsus (or the metacarpus) is cleansed with antiseptic solution, and it is simply removed as close to the limb as possible. If first and second phalanges are present, the dewclaw is abducted so that the scissors can be slid up to the first/second phalangeal joint. All of the second phalanx should be removed. Cutting through the diaphysis of the second phalanx or inadvertently cutting through the first phalanx may expose the medullary cavity to infection and may result in osteomyelitis.

Hemostasis is rarely a problem in young puppies, especially those with only skin attachments. Any bleeding can be controlled by pressure or topical application of styptics or silver nitrate sticks. Skin sutures are rarely required but may facilitate hemostasis. A single cruciate suture of monofilament nonabsorbable suture can be placed, or chromic catgut can be used. For older puppies, general anesthesia is required. The limbs are clipped and prepared for aseptic surgery. Use of a tourniquet may facilitate surgery. An elliptic incision is made around the dewclaw. Dissection is performed to expose the first/second phalangeal joint. Disarticulation of the joint is performed using a scalpel blade. The tourniquet can then be loosened so that the dorsal common and axial palmar digital arteries can be identified and ligated. The subcutaneous tissue and skin are closed. Bandages are not required for young puppies; however, a soft bandage is usually placed on the limbs of older dogs and left in place for 1 to 2 days postoperatively. Suture removal is performed at 7 to 10 days.

Canine and Feline Onychectomy

Onychectomy is an elective procedure performed mostly on cats and usually is done at 8 to 12 weeks of age. Hemorrhage tends to be less of a problem when performed on animals at a younger age as opposed to mature animals. The ethics of whether to perform canine or feline onychectomy varies by veterinarian and from one country to another. Careful consideration of the animal's activity and its environment, whether an indoor and/or outdoor animal, should be made before the procedure is performed and particularly before both forelimb and hindlimb onychectomy are performed. Rarely is canine and feline onychectomy done on all four limbs.

Surgical techniques used in performing canine and feline onychectomy are only acceptable if they result in complete excision of the third phalanx. It should be remembered that the ungual crest of the third phalanx surrounds the nail bed, with the ungual process extending into the claw. Onychectomy may be performed with either nail clippers or with a scalpel blade. For example, using the forelimb, a tourniquet is placed above the elbow to avoid pressure on the median and ulnar nerves. The paw is not usually clipped but is cleansed with an antiseptic solution. The nail clipper is placed over the claw and over the top of the extensor process of the third phalanx. The blade of the nail clippers is partially closed so that it engages the tissue. Using forceps attached to the nail, the veterinarian extends the claw so that the nail clippers can be slid over the bottom of the flexor process, taking care to push the footpad back with the nail clipper. This maneuver is imperative to excise the flexor process of the third phalanx. The nail clipper is then completely closed and the third phalanx severed. Failure to fully extend the claw will result in a significant portion of the third phalanx remaining, with potential for regrowth, osteomyelitis, or significant postoperative pain. Alternatively, the entire procedure can be performed with a scalpel blade, again starting at the back of the extensor process.

Thereafter, the wound is examined for any remnants of the third phalanx. Any remnants should be completely excised with the scalpel blade. Overzealous use of the nail clippers can result in removal of a portion of the second phalanx. This should be avoided because exposure of the medullary canal of the second phalanx will increase the risk of osteomyelitis and postoperative complications. The wound is then closed, regardless of the age of the animal, with absorbable sutures, such as 3-0 or 4-0 chromic catgut. The sutures are placed so that wound closure is side to side. Tissue adhesives could also be used for the wound closure. Tissue adhesives should be applied sparingly on the outer skin edge rather than within the wound, whereas wound healing only occurs around the dried adhesive. Also, the wound should be completely dry for tissue adhesives to be effective.

A firm bandage is then placed on the distal region of the forelimb before the tourniquet is released. The foot bandage should be left on no longer than 24 hours. If bleeding occurs at the time of bandage removal, a second bandage should be placed and removed 12 hours later. At bandage removal, the toes should be inspected. One should avoid cleansing the paw because this may only stimulate bleeding. Postoperative antimicrobial agents are generally unnecessary. Shredded paper may be used in the litter tray for the first week after surgery. Suture removal is usually unnecessary. Potential complications reported after onychectomy include persistent pain and reluctance to walk, osteomyelitis, infection and granuloma formation that may be associated with use of tissue adhesives, nail regrowth associated with inadequate amputation of the third phalanx, ischemic necrosis of the feet that is associated with poor bandage care, palmagrade stance, and protrusion of the second phalanx (Tobias, 1994). Regrowth and abscess formation require surgical exploration, débridement, and excision of any remnants of the third phalanx and appropriate antimicrobial therapy.

Deep digital flexor tendonectomy is an effective alternative to the classic onychectomy in the cat (Rife, 1988). This procedure, by excising a portion of the deep digital flexor tendon, renders the cat unable to flex the deep digital flexor tendon and expose its claw. The claw should be kept trimmed—the cat will still be able to scratch, and the untrimmed nail may grow into the digital pad. The paw is prepared as for the classic onychectomy. A skin incision is made on the ventral aspect of the digit, just proximal to the digital pad. The tendon is located underneath the skin and undermined using small curved scissors or hemostats, and the tendon is then elevated and exteriorized from the wound. A 5-mm section of tendon is removed. The skin incision is closed with absorbable sutures or tissue adhesive. Tissue adhesive appears to reduce postoperative hemorrhage more effectively than suturing and obviates the need for postoperative bandages. Postoperative considerations are as for the classic onychectomy. It is imperative that the owner is made aware of the need for regular trimming of the nails.

Tail Docking

The amputation of tails for cosmetic purposes and compliance with breed standards is referred to as *tail docking*. The tail docking procedure should be performed with the first few days of life (Table 12–7). Surgery of puppies older than 5 days requires general anesthesia and may be associated with increased postoperative pain, bleeding, and wound dehiscence. The tail can be removed without anesthesia from puppies younger than 5 days. The tail is cleansed with antiseptic solution, and the puppy is restrained. A piece of gauze or umbilical tape is wrapped firmly at the base of the tail to act as a temporary tourniquet. The amputation site is selected. No attempt is made to cut between vertebrae because the bones are soft. The skin is pushed toward the head, and a pair of angled cuts is made with scissors or a scalpel blade to create a dorsal and ventral tail flap. The flaps are closed with a single cruciate suture of absorbable material such as chromic catgut. The tourniquet is then released, and pressure over the tail is applied until bleeding stops. Complications are uncommon when the tail docking procedure is performed properly. Premature removal of the suture by the dam may result in exposure of the caudal vertebrae and predispose to infection and scar formation. Failure to push the skin toward the head to create adequate tissue coverage of the tail end may result in excessive scar formation.

Canine Otoplasty

Canine otoplasty, or ear cropping, is performed to meet breed standards for some dogs as requested by owners or breeders (Table 12–8). The otoplasty is performed preferably in puppies about 9 to 10 weeks old, unless otherwise indicated. These puppies should have been started on their routine vaccination program and should be screened for congenital coagulopathies. This is particularly important for Doberman pinscher puppies, which have a high incidence of von Willebrand's disease. Ear cropping is not technically difficult to perform but is an exacting procedure with a high propensity for complications that cause owners to consider the results unacceptable.

Position Statements on Tail Docking and Ear Cropping

Worldwide professional organizations and breed associations have encouraged veterinarians and dog enthusiasts to abandon the traditional practice of doing cosmetic tail docking and ear cropping procedures. Canine and feline declawing procedures are also being attacked as being inhumane and cruel. Position statements

of selected organizations as of October 1999 are as follows:

The *European Convention for the Protection of Pet Animals*, a member of the Council of Europe, adopted Article 10 in 1987 stating that surgical operations for the purpose of modifying the appearance of a pet animal or for other noncurative purposes shall be prohibited and, in particular, docking of tails, cropping of ears, devocalization, declawing, and defanging.

The *Council of the Royal College of Veterinary Surgeons* resolved in 1992 that docking of dogs' tails is an unjustified mutilation and unethical unless done for therapeutic or acceptable prophylactic reasons. Tail amputation is now banned in the United Kingdom and many European countries. Ear cropping is not performed in the United Kingdom.

The *Canadian Veterinary Medical Association* (CVMA) opposes surgical alteration of any animal for purely cosmetic purposes. The CVMA believes that cosmetic surgery is unnecessary, except in injury or for reasons of health. Examples of cosmetic procedures include tail docking in the equine, bovine, or canine species; tail nicking/setting in the equine species; ear cropping; and onychectomy in species other than the domestic cat. The CVMA encourages breed associations to change their breed standards so that cosmetic procedures are not required.

A law has been proposed in *Germany* that will, if passed, forbid the docking of tails of most breeds, including Rottweilers, Doberman pinschers, and boxers. A few hunting breeds will still be allowed to have their tails docked.

Australian Veterinary Association (AVA) policy states that cosmetic tail docking and ear cropping are unnecessary, unjustified surgical alterations and are detrimental to the animal's welfare. The AVA therefore recommends that Kennel Control Councils throughout Australia phase tail docking requirements out of the relevant breed standards, and federal and state authorities and animal welfare organizations have declared tail docking illegal in all states and territories except where performed for therapeutic reasons. The AVA has produced 20,000 color brochures that argue the case against tail docking. The brochures have been sent to the AVA's 4500 members for distribution to the public. The AVA recommends that the docking of dogs' tails be made illegal in Australia except for professionally diagnosed therapeutic reasons, and only then by suitably qualified persons under conditions that minimize pain and stress. The AVA says there is strong evi-

Table 12–7 **Guidelines for Tail Docking**

BREED	LENGTH FOR PUPPIES YOUNGER THAN 1 WK
Affenpinscher	Dock close to body; leave 1/3 in (8–9 mm)
Airedale terrier	Leave two-thirds to three-fourths tail; tip of the docked tail should be even with the top of the skull when the puppy is in show position
American cocker spaniel	Leave one-third tail; approximately 3/4 in (19 mm)
Australian cattle dog	Tails are not docked
Australian kelpie	Tails are not docked
Australian silky terrier	Leave one-third tail; approximately 1/2 in (12–13 mm)
Australian shepherd	Leave four to five vertebrae
Australian terrier	Leave two-thirds tail; cut 1/16 in (1–2 mm) beyond tan hair on ventral surface of tail
Boston terrier	Naturally docked; if tail is too long, dock to natural length; may be naturally docked
Bouvier des Flandres	Leave 1/2 to 3/4 in (12–19 mm)
Boxer	Leave 3/4 in (19 mm)
Brittany spaniel	Leave 3/4 to 1 in (19–25 mm); may be naturally docked
Brussels griffon	Leave one-fourth to one-third tail
Cavalier King Charles spaniel	Optional; leave at least two-thirds tail; always leave white tip in broken-colored puppies
Clumber spaniel	Leave one-quarter to one-third tail; dock at point of natural tail taper; tail should be 4 in long in adult
Doberman pinscher	Leave one-half to three-fourths tail or two vertebrae
English bulldog	May be naturally docked
English cocker spaniel	Leave one-third tail or four to five vertebrae
English toy spaniel	Leave one-third tail
Field spaniel	Leave one-third tail
Fox terrier, smooth and wire-haired	Leave two-thirds to three-fourths tail; tip of the dock should be even with the top of the skull when the puppy is in show position
French bulldog	May be naturally docked
German short-haired pointer	Leave two-thirds tail
German wire-haired pointer	Leave two-thirds tail
Irish terrier	Leave two-thirds to three-fourths tail; tip of the dock should be even with the top of the skull when the puppy is in show position
Kerry blue terrier	Leave one-half to two-thirds tail; tip of the dock should be even with the top of the skull when the puppy is in show position
Lakeland terrier	Leave two-thirds tail; tip of the dock should be even with the top of the skull when the puppy is in show position
Miniature pinscher	Leave 1/2 in (12–13 mm) or two vertebrae; tail must cover anus
Norwich terrier	Leave one-fourth to one-third tail; tail should be long enough to grasp and pull dog from foxhole
Old English sheepdog	May be naturally docked; if necessary, dock as close to body as possible or leave one vertebra
Poodle, miniature	Leave one-half to two-thirds tail; approximately 1 1/8 in (28–29 mm)
Poodle, standard	Leave one-half to two-thirds tail; approximately 1 1/2 in (38 mm)
Poodle, toy	Leave one-half to two-thirds tail; approximately 1 in (25 mm)
Rottweiler	May be naturally docked; if necessary, dock as close to body as possible or leave one vertebra
Schipperke	Dock close to body such that there is no tail left; may be naturally docked
Schnauzer, giant	Leave 1 1/4 in (32 mm) or two or three vertebrae
Schnauzer, miniature	Leave approximately 3/4 in (19 mm); tail should be less than 1 in (25 mm); tail is docked at demarcation of white and gray hair on ventral tail; tail must cover anus

Table continued on opposite page

Table 12–7	Guidelines for Tail Docking *Continued*	
BREED	**LENGTH FOR PUPPIES YOUNGER THAN 1 WK**	
Schnauzer, standard	Leave 1 in (25 mm) or two vertebrae; dock just beyond light markings on ventral tail surface	
Sealyham terrier	Leave one-third to one-half tail	
Soft-coated wheaten terrier	Leave one-half to three-fourths tail	
Spino Italiani	Leave three-fifths tail	
Springer spaniel, English	Leave one-third tail	
Springer spaniel, Welsh	Leave one-third to one-half tail	
Sussex spaniel	Leave one-third tail	
Vizsla	Leave two-thirds tail	
Weimaraner	Leave three-fifths tail; approximately 1 1/2 in (38 mm); tail tucked between legs must cover genitalia	
Welsh Pembroke corgi	May be naturally docked; if necessary, dock as close to body as possible or leave one vertebra	
Welsh terrier	Leave two-thirds to three-fourths tail; tip of the dock should be even with the top of the skull when the puppy is in show position	
Wire-haired pointing griffon	Leave one-third tail	
Yorkshire terrier	Leave 1/2 in (12–13 mm); leave one-third tail; if hair clipped, dock 1/4 in (6–7 mm) beyond tan hair; if not clipped, dock 1/8 in (2–4 mm) beyond tan hair	

Because opinions vary as to the most desirable length of tails in some breeds, it is always advisable for owners to seek advice from experienced breeders and handlers in their part of the country.

dence that the procedure is painful for puppies. Ear cropping has been banned in Australia.

The *Parliament of New Zealand* is considering revising the current animal welfare law. The new bill promotes the duty of care toward animals, better provision for the welfare of animals from ill treatment and neglect, and the prevention of unreasonable pain and distress of animals. Conditionally prohibited acts in this bill include tail docking and debarking dogs and declawing cats unless the procedure is carried out by a veterinarian who is of the opinion, on reasonable grounds, that the operation is necessary for the welfare of the animal.

Adopted July 9, 1999, the *American Veterinary Medical Association* position reads (Scott, 1999):

"Ear cropping and tail docking in dogs for cosmetic reasons are not medically indicated nor of benefit to the patient. These procedures cause pain and distress, and, as with all surgical procedures, are accompanied by inherent risks of anesthesia, blood loss, and infection. Therefore, veterinarians should counsel dog owners about these matters before agreeing to perform these surgeries."

The *Australian National Kennel Council* (ANKC) and its Member Bodies abhor the practice of cropping of ears of all breeds of dogs. The act of ear cropping is an offense under the Rules and Regulations of the Australian National Kennel Council and its Member Bodies. Dogs imported into Australia with

Table 12–8	Guidelines for Canine Otoplasty		
BREED	**AGE**	**LENGTH OF EAR TRIM**	
Boston terrier	6 mo	As long as possible	
Boxer	9 wk	2 1/2 in (63–64 mm) to 2 3/4 in (70 mm)	
Doberman pinscher	9 wk	2 3/4 in (70 mm)	
Great Dane	9 wk	3 1/2 in (89 mm) to 3 3/4 in (95 mm)	
Miniature pinscher	12 wk	1 3/4 in (44–45 mm)	
Schnauzer, miniature	12 wk	2–2 1/2 in (51–64 mm)	
Schnauzer, standard	9 wk	2 1/2 in (63–64 mm)	

cropped ears shall not be permitted to compete in Conformation breed classes but may compete in official trials (Obedience and Field). Such dogs with cropped ears may be displayed only at Conformation Classes. Any dogs with ears that have been cropped in Australia are not allowed to participate in any recognized ANKC activity (including training). This applies to dogs born after January 1, 1993.

The *American Kennel Club* recognizes that ear cropping, tail docking, and dewclaw removal, as described in certain breed standards, are acceptable practices integral to defining and preserving breed character and/or enhancing good health. Appropriate veterinary care should be provided.

References and Supplemental Reading

Congenital, Hereditary, and Developmental Dermatoses

Andresen E, Willeberg P: Pituitary dwarfism in German shepherd dogs: Additional evidence of simple, autosomal recessive inheritance. Nord Vet Med 28:481, 1976a.

Andresen E, Willeberg P: Pituitary dwarfism in Carnelian bear-dogs: Evidence of a simple, autosomal recessive inheritance. Hereditas 84:232, 1976b.

Antin IP: Dermoid sinus in a Rhodesian ridgeback dog. J Am Vet Med Assoc 157:961, 1970.

Arnold U, Opitz M, Grossere I, et al: Goitrous hypothyroidism and dwarfism in a kitten. J Am Anim Hosp Assoc 20:753, 1984.

August JR, Chickering WR, Rikihisa Y: Congenital ichthyosis in a dog: Comparison with the human ichthyosiform dermatoses. Compend Contin Educ Pract Vet 10:40, 1988.

Austin VH: Congenital seborrhea of the springer spaniel. Mod Vet Pract 59(4):53, 1973.

Austin VH: Blue dog disease. Mod Vet Pract 56:31, 1975.

Baber KP, Grimes TD: Cutaneous lesions in dogs associated with hookworm infestation. Vet Rec 87:376, 1970.

Barnett KC, Cottrell BD: Ehlers-Danlos syndrome in a dog: Ocular, cutaneous, and articular abnormalities. J Small Anim Pract 28:941, 1987.

Bettenay SV: Acrodermatitis of bull terriers: Long-term management. Proceedings of First World Congress of Veterinary Dermatology, Dijon, France, Sept 1992, p 69.

Briggs OM, Botha WS: Color mutant alopecia in a blue Italian greyhound. J Am Anim Hosp Assoc 22:611, 1986.

Brignac MM, Foil CS, Al-Bagdadi FAK, et al: Microscopy of color mutant alopecia. Proc Am Acad Vet Dermatol Am Coll Vet Dermatol Annu Mg, Washington, DC, 1988, p 14.

Calderwood-Mays MB, Bellah JR, Pohlenz-Zertuche HO: Regional collagenous nevi in three dogs: Nevus, nodular dermatofibrosis, or something new? In Ihrke PJ, Mason IS, White SD (eds): Advances in Veterinary Dermatology, vol 2. Oxford, England, Pergamon Press, 1993, p 315.

Carlotti DN: Canine hereditary black hair follicular dysplasia and colour mutant alopecia: Clinical and histopathological aspects. In von Tscharner C, Halliwell REW (eds): Advances in Veterinary Dermatology, vol 1. London, Balliére Tindall, 1990, p 43.

Chastain CB: Unusual hypothyroidism and hypothyroidism in the unusual. Proc Am Coll Vet Intern Med Forum 7:126, 1989.

Chastain CB, McNeel SV, Graham CL, et al: Congenital hypothyroidism in a dog due to an iodide organification defect. Am J Vet Res 44:1257, 1983.

Chastain CB, Swayne DE: Congenital hypotrichosis in male basset hound litter mates. J Am Vet Med Assoc 187:845, 1985.

Collier LL, Leathers CW, Counts DF: A clinical description of dermatosparaxis in a Himalayan cat. Feline Pract 10(5):25, 1980.

Conroy JD, Rasmusen BA, Small E: Hypotrichosis in miniature poodle siblings. J Am Vet Med Assoc 166:697, 1975.

Crawford MA, Foil CS: Vasculitis: Clinical syndromes in small animals. Compend Contin Educ Pract Vet 11:400, 1989.

Cummings JF, deLahunta A, Winn SS: Acral mutilation and nociceptive loss in English pointer dogs. Acta Neuropathol (Berl) 53:119, 1981.

DeLack JB: Hereditary deafness in the white cat. Compend Contin Educ Pract Vet 6:609, 1984.

Dunstan RW, Rosser EJ Jr: Newly recognized and emerging genodermatoses in domestic animals. Curr Probl Dermatol 17:216, 1987.

Dunstan RW, Sills RC, Wilkinson JE, et al: A mechanobullous disease (junctional epidermolysis bullosa) in a toy poodle. Proc Am Acad Vet Dermatol Am Coll Vet Dermatol Annu Mtg, Phoenix, 1987, p 10.

Engstrom D: Tyrosinase deficiency in the chow chow. In Kirk RW (ed): Current Veterinary Therapy. Philadelphia, WB Saunders, 1966, p 352.

Ferrer L, Durall I, Closa J, et al: Colour mutant alopecia in Yorkshire terriers. Vet Rec 122:360, 1988.

Foil CS: Comparative genodermatoses. Clin Dermatol 3(1):175, 1985.

Fontaine J, Charlier G, Henroteaux M: Anomalie du collagène dermique: Dermatosparaxie chez un chat européen. Pointe Vet 24:67, 1992.

Freeman LJ, Hegreberg GA, Robinette JD: Ehlers-Danlos syndrome in dogs and cats. Semin Vet Med Surg (Small Anim) 2:221, 1987.

Freire-Maia N: Ectodermal dysplasias. Hum Hered 21:309, 1971.

Freire-Maia N: Ectodermal dysplasias revisited. Acta Genet Gemellol 26:121, 1977.

Fyfe JC, Jezyk PF, Giger U, et al: Inherited selective malabsorption of vitamin B_{12} in giant schnauzers. J Am Anim Hosp Assoc 25:533, 1989.

Geary MR, Baker KP: The occurrence of pili torti

in a litter of kittens in England. J Small Anim Pract 27:69, 1986.

Genodermatosis Research Foundation: SA test litter status. Prog SA Res Winter/Spring, p 4, 1994.

Gething MA: Suspected Ehlers-Danlos syndrome in the dog. Vet Rec 89:638, 1971.

Gosselin Y, Papageorges M, Teuscher E: Black hair follicular dysplasia in a dog. Canine Pract 9(2):8, 1982.

Greco DS, Feldman EC, Peterson ME, et al: Congenital hypothyroid dwarfism in a family of giant schnauzers. J Vet Intern Med 5:57, 1991.

Grieshaber RL, Blakemore JC, Yaskulski S: Congenital alopecia in a bichon frise. J Am Vet Med Assoc 188:1053, 1986.

Gross TL, Halliwell RE, McDougal BJ, et al: Psoriasiform lichenoid dermatitis in the springer spaniel. Vet Pathol 23:76, 1986.

Gross TL, Ihrke PJ, Walder EJ: Veterinary Dermatopathology: A Macroscopic and Microscopic Evaluation of Canine and Feline Skin Disease. St. Louis, Mosby-Year Book, 1992.

Guaguere E, Alhaidari Z: Pigmentary disturbances. In von Tscharner C, Halliwell REW (eds): Advances in Veterinary Dermatology, vol 1. London, Balliére Tindall, 1990, p 395.

Gupta BN: Epitheliogenesis imperfecta in a dog. Am J Vet Res 34:443, 1973.

Gwin RM, Wyman M, Lim DJ, et al: Multiple ocular defects associated with partial albinism and deafness in the dog. J Am Anim Hosp Assoc 17:401, 1981.

Hargis AM, Brignac MM, Al-Bagdadi FAK, et al: Black hair follicular dysplasia in black and white Saluki dogs: Differentiation from color mutant alopecia in the Doberman pinscher by microscopic examination of hairs. Vet Dermatol 2:69, 1991.

Hargis AM, Haupt KH, Prieur DJ, et al: A skin disorder in three Shetland sheepdogs: Comparison with familial canine dermatomyositis of collies. Compend Contin Educ Pract Vet 7:377, 1985.

Hargis AM, Mundell AC: Familial canine dermatomyositis. Compend Contin Educ Pract Vet 14:855, 1992.

Harper RC: Congenital black hair follicular dysplasia in bearded collie puppies. Vet Rec 102:87, 1978.

Haupt KH, Prieur DJ, Hargis AM, et al: Familial canine dermatomyositis: Clinicopathologic, immunologic, and serologic studies. Am J Vet Res 46:1870, 1985a.

Haupt KH, Prieur DJ, Moore MP, et al: Familial canine dermatomyositis: Clinical, electrodiagnostic, and genetic studies. Am J Vet Res 46:1861, 1985b.

Hegreberg GA, Padgett GA, Gorham JR, et al: A heritable connective tissue disease of dogs and mink resembling the Ehlers-Danlos syndrome of man. II. Mode of inheritance. J Hered 60:249, 1969.

Hegreberg GA, Padgett GA, Henson JB: A heritable connective tissue disease of dogs and mink resembling the Ehlers-Danlos syndrome of man. III. Histopathologic changes of the skin. Arch Pathol 90:159, 1970a.

Hegreberg GA, Padgett GA, Ott RL, et al: A heritable connective tissue disease of dogs and mink resembling Ehlers-Danlos syndrome in man. I. Skin tensile strength properties. J Invest Dermatol 54:377, 1970b.

Hegreberg GA, Padgett GA, Page RC: The Ehlers-Danlos syndrome of dogs and mink. Symposium Proceedings III, Animal Models for Biomedical Research, New York, National Academy Science, 1970c.

Hendy-Ibbs PM: Hairless cats in Great Britain. J Hered 75:506, 1984.

Hewitt MP, Mills JHL, Hunter B: Epitheliogenesis imperfecta in a black Labrador puppy. Can Vet J 16:371, 1975.

Ihrke PJ, Mueller RS, Stannard AA: Generalized hypotrichosis in a female Rottweiler. Vet Dermatol 4:65, 1993.

Jezyk PF, Haskins ME, MacKay-Smith WE, et al: Lethal acrodermatitis in bull terriers. J Am Vet Med Assoc 188:833, 1986.

Keep JM: Cutis hyperelastica in a dog. Aust Vet J 45:593, 1969.

Koch H, Walder E: Epidermolysis bullosa dystrophica in beaucerons. In von Tscharner C, Halliwell REW (eds): Advances in Veterinary Dermatology, vol 1. London, Balliére Tindall, 1990, p 441.

Kunkle GA: Congenital hypotrichosis in two dogs. J Am Vet Med Assoc 185:84, 1984.

Kunkle GA: Hereditary alopecias and haircoat abnormalities of the dog. Dermatol Rep 4(1):6, 1985.

Kunkle GA, Chrisman CL, Gross TL, et al: Dermatomyositis in collie dogs. Compend Contin Educ Pract Vet 7:185, 1985.

Kunkle GA, Jezyk PF, West CS, et al: Tyrosinemia in a dog. J Am Anim Hosp Assoc 20:615, 1984.

Kunkle GA, Schmeitzel LP: Canine dermatomyositis. Compend Contin Educ Pract Vet 13:866, 1992.

Langeback R: Variation in hair coat and skin texture in blue dogs. Nord Veterinaermed 38:383, 1986.

Letard E: Hairless Siamese cats. J Hered 29:173, 1938.

Mann GE, Stratton J: Dermoid sinus in the Rhodesian ridgeback. J Small Anim Pract 7:631, 1966.

Marks A, van den Broek AHM, Else RW: Congenital hypotrichosis in a French bulldog. J Small Anim Pract 33:450, 1992.

Mason KV, Halliwell REW, McDougal BJ: Characterization of lichenoid-psoriasiform dermatosis of springer spaniels. J Am Vet Med Assoc 8:897, 1986.

McEwan NA: Confirmation and investigation of lethal acrodermatitis of bull terriers in Britain. In Ihrke PJ, Mason IS, White SW (eds): Advances in Veterinary Dermatology, vol 2. Oxford, England, Pergamon Press, 1993, p 151.

Melman SA, Campbell K, Small E, et al: Lamellar ichthyosis-like syndrome in a dog. Proc Am Acad Vet Dermatol Am Coll Vet Dermatol Annu Mtg, Phoenix, 1987, p 23.

Miller WH: Colour dilution alopecia in Doberman pinschers with blue or fawn coat colours: A study of the incidence and histopathology of this disorder. Vet Dermatol 1:113, 1990a.

Miller WH: Follicular dysplasia in adult red and black Doberman pinschers. Vet Dermatol 1:181, 1990b.

Miller WH: Alopecia associated with coat color dilution in two Yorkshire terriers, one Saluki, and one mix-breed dog. J Am Anim Hosp Assoc 27:39, 1991.

Minor RR, Lein DH, Patterson DF, et al: Defects in collagen fibrillogenesis, causing hyperextensible, fragile skin in dogs. J Am Vet Med Assoc 182:142, 1983.

Muller GH: Ichthyosis in two dogs. J Am Vet Med Assoc 169:1313, 1976.

Munday BL: Epitheliogenesis imperfecta in lambs and kittens. Br Vet J 126:47, 1970.

O'Neill CS: Hereditary skin disease in the dog and the cat. Compend Contin Educ Pract Vet 3:791, 1981.

O'Shea G: Introducing the American hairless terrier. Dog World 70:146, 1985.

Paradis M, Scott DW: Naevi récemment reconnus chez le chien: Naevus comédonien, naevus organoïde linéaire et naevus du follicule pileux. Pointe Vet 21:489, 1989.

Paradis M: Footpad hyperkeratosis in a family of dogues de Bordeaux. Vet Dermatol 3:75, 1992.

Patterson DF, Minor RR: Hereditary fragility and hyperextensibility of the skin of cats. Lab Invest 37:170, 1977.

Pedersen K, Scott DW: Idiopathic pyogranulomatous inflammation and leukocytoclastic vasculitis of the nasal planum, nostrils and nasal mucosa in Scottish terriers in Denmark. Vet Dermatol 2:85, 1991.

Plotnick A, Brunt JE, Reitz B: Cutaneous asthenia in a cat. Feline Pract 20:9, 1992.

Post K, Dignean MA, Clark EG: Hair follicle dysplasia in a Siberian husky. J Am Anim Hosp Assoc 24:659, 1988.

Robinson R: The Canadian hairless or sphinx cat. J Hered 64:47, 1973.

Robinson WF, Shaw SE, Stanley B, et al: Congenital hypothyroidism in Scottish deerhound puppies. Aust Vet J 65:386, 1988.

Roudebush P, MacDonald JM: Mucocutaneous angiomatous hamartoma in a dog. J Am Anim Hosp Assoc 20:168, 1984.

Scott DW, Schultz RD: Epidermolysis bullosa simplex in the collie dog. J Am Vet Med Assoc 171:721, 1977.

Scott DW, Yager-Johnson JA, Manning TO, et al: Nevi in the dog. J Am Anim Hosp Assoc 20:505, 1984.

Selcer EA, Helman RG, Selcer RR: Dermoid sinus in a Shih Tzu and a boxer. J Am Anim Hosp Assoc 20:634, 1984.

Selmanowitz VJ, Kramer KM, Orentreich N: Congenital ectodermal defect in miniature poodles. J Hered 61:196, 1970.

Selmanowitz VJ, Kramer KM, Orentreich N: Canine hereditary black hair follicular dysplasia. J Hered 63:43, 1972.

Selmanowitz VJ, Markofsky J, Orentreich N: Blackhair follicular dysplasia in dogs. J Am Vet Med Assoc 171:1079, 1977.

Smits B, Croft DL, Abrams-Ogg ACG: Lethal acrodermatitis in bull terriers: A problem of defective zinc metabolism. Vet Dermatol 2:91, 1991.

Sponenberg DP, Scott E, Scott W: American hairless terriers: A recessive gene causing hairlessness in dogs. J Hered 79:69, 1988.

Stogdale L, Botha WS, Saunders GN: Congenital hypotrichosis in a dog. J Am Anim Hosp Assoc 18:184, 1982.

Thomsett LR: Congenital hypotrichia in the dog. Vet Rec 73:915, 1961.

Weir JAM, Yager JA: Familial cutaneous vasculopathy of German shepherd dogs. Proc Am Acad Vet Dermatol Am Coll Vet Dermatol Annu Mtg, San Diego, 1993, p 95.

White SD, Batch S: Leukotrichia in a litter of Labrador retrievers. J Am Anim Hosp Assoc 26:321, 1990.

White SD, Rosychuk RAW, Scott KV, et al: Inflammatory linear verrucous epidermal nevus in four dogs. Vet Dermatol 3:107, 1993.

Other Dermatologic Disorders

August JR: Dietary hypersensitivity in dogs: Cutaneous manifestations, diagnosis, and management. Compend Contin Educ Pract Vet 7(6):469, 1985.

Baker GT, Breeze RG, Dawson CO: Oral dermatophilosis in a cat: A case report. J Small Anim Pract 13:649, 1972.

Baker BB, Stannard AA: Nodular panniculitis in the dog. J Am Vet Med Assoc 167:752, 1975.

Beale KM, Calderwood-Mays MB, Buchanon B: Papular and plaque-like mucinosis in a puppy. Vet Dermatol 2:29, 1991.

Bennett M, Gaskell RM, Baxby D: Feline cowpox virus infection. J Small Anim Pract 31:167, 1990.

Bond R, Sant RE: The recovery of Malassezia pachydermatis from canine skin. Vet Dermatol News 15:25, 1993.

Bostock DE: Neoplasms of the skin and subcutaneous tissues in dogs and cats. Br Vet J 142:1, 1986.

Bruner SR, Blakemore JC: Malassezia dermatitis in dogs. Vet Med 94:613, 1999.

Buerger RG: Cutaneous mast cell neoplasia in the cat: A retrospective evaluation and histomorphologic grading of fourteen cases. Proc Am Acad Vet Dermatol Am Coll Vet Dermatol Annu Mtg, 1986, p 15.

Carakostas MC, Miller RI, Woodward MG: Subcutaneous dermatophilosis in a cat. J Am Vet Med Assoc 185(6):675, 1984.

Carlotti DN, Pages J-P, Sorlin M: Skin lesions in canine babesiosis. In Ihrke PJ, Mason IS, White SW (eds): Advances in Veterinary Dermatology, vol 1. Oxford, England, Pergamon Press, 1993, p 229.

Carlotti DN, Remy I, Prost C: Food allergy in dogs and cats. A review and report of 43 cases. Vet Dermatol 1:55, 1990.

Carlson ME: *Yersinia pestis* infection in cats. Feline Pract 24:22, 1996.

Carney HC, Moriello KA: Dermatophytosis: Cattery management plan. *In* Griffin CE, Kwochka KK, MacDonald JM (eds): Current Veterinary Dermatology: The Science and Art of Therapy. St. Louis, Mosby-Year Book, 1993, p 34.

Carpenter JL, Andelman NC, Moore FM, et al: Idiopathic cutaneous and renal glomerular vasculopathy of greyhounds. Vet Pathol 25:401, 1988.

Carpenter JL, Andrews LK, Holzworth J, et al: Tumors and tumor-like lesions. *In* Holzworth J (ed): Diseases of the Cat: Medicine and Surgery, vol 1. Philadelphia, WB Saunders, 1987, p 406.

Chalmers SA, Medleau L, Rakich P: Atopic dermatitis in cats: Review and case reports. J Vet Allerg Clin Immunol 3:7, 1995.

Chastain CB, Carithers RW, Hogle RM, et al: Dermatophilosis in two dogs. J Am Vet Med Assoc 169:1079, 1976.

Chastain CB, Turk MAM: Benign cutaneous mastocytomas in litters of Siamese kittens. Proc Am Acad Vet Dermatol Am Coll Vet Dermatol Annu Mtg, 1987, p 41.

Clercx C, Coignoul F, Jakovljevic S, et al: Tuberculosis in dogs: A case report and review of the literature. J Am Anim Hosp Assoc. 28:207, 1992.

Cooper LM, Sabine M: Paw and mouth disease in a cat. Aust Vet J 48:644, 1972.

Craig TM, O'Quin BO, Robinson RM, et al: Parasitic nematode (*Lagochilascaris major*) associated with a purulent draining tract in a dog. J Am Vet Med Assoc 181(1):69, 1982.

Craig TM, Teel PD, Dubuisson LM, et al: *Lynxacarus radovsky* infestation in a cat. J Am Vet Med Assoc 202:613, 1993.

Derer MM, Morrison-Smith G, de Weck AL: Monoclonal anti-IgE antibodies in the diagnosis of dog allergy. Vet Dermatol 9:185, 1998.

Dickson NJ: Cold agglutinin disease in a puppy associated with lead intoxication. J Small Anim Pract 31:105, 1990.

Dillberger JE, Altman NH: Focal mucinosis in dogs: Seven cases and review of cutaneous mucinoses of man and animals. Vet Pathol 23:132, 1986.

Dryden MW, Rust MK: The cat flea: Biology, ecology and control. Vet Parasitol 52:1, 1994.

Dubey JP, Black SS, Sangster LT, et al: *Caryospora*-associated dermatitis in dogs. J Parasitol 76:552, 1990.

Egberink HF, Berrocal A, Bax HAD, et al: Papillomavirus associated skin lesions in a cat seropositive for feline immunodeficiency virus. Vet Microbiol 31:117, 1992.

Eidson M, Thelsted JP, Rollag OJ, et al: Clinical, clinicopathologic and pathologic features of plaque in cats: 119 cases (1977–1985). J Am Vet Med Assoc 199:1191, 1991.

Elliott G, Lawson GHK, MacKenzie CP: *Rhodococcus equi* infection in cats. Vet Rec 118:693, 1986.

Fadok VA: Miscellaneous parasites of the skin, part I. Compend Contin Educ Pract Vet 2:782, 1980.

Flecknell PA, Orr CM, Wright AI, et al: Skin ulceration associated with herpesvirus infection in cats. Vet Rec 104:313, 1979.

Fleming EJ, McCaw DL, Smith JA, et al: Clinical, hematologic, and survival data from cats infected with feline immunodeficiency virus: 42 cases (1983–1988). J Am Vet Med Assoc 199:913, 1991.

Foil CS: The skin. *In* Hoskins JD (ed): Veterinary Pediatrics: Dogs and Cats from Birth to Six Months, 2nd ed. Philadelphia, WB Saunders, 1995, p 227.

Foil CS: Dermatophytosis. *In* Greene CE (ed): Infectious Diseases of the Dog and Cat, 2nd ed. Philadelphia, WB Saunders, 1998, p 362.

Foster ES, Scavelli TD, Greenlee PG, et al: Cutaneous lesion caused by *Mycobacterium tuberculosis* in a dog. J Am Vet Med Assoc 188:1188, 1986.

Garvey MS: Commentary on amitraz toxicosis associated with ingestion of an acaricide collar in a dog. J Am Vet Med Assoc 203:56, 1993.

Goldschmidt MH, Shofer FS: Skin Tumors of the Dog and Cat. Oxford, England, Pergamon Press, 1992.

Griffin CE: Scabies. *In* Griffin CE, Kwochka KK, MacDonald JM (eds): Current Veterinary Dermatology: The Science and Art of Therapy. St. Louis, Mosby-Year Book, 1993, p 85.

Gross TL, Schick RO: Dermatopathology of newly described skin diseases. *In* Ihrke PJ, Mason IS, White SW (eds): Advances in Veterinary Dermatology, vol 2. Oxford, Pergamon Press, 1993, p 417.

Guilford WG: Adverse reactions to food. *In* Kirk RW, Bonagura JD (eds): Current Veterinary Therapy XI. Philadelphia, WB Saunders, 1992, p 587.

Halliwell REW: Management of dietary hypersensitivity in the dog. J Small Anim Pract 33:156, 1992.

Halliwell REW, Gorman NT: Veterinary Clinical Immunology. Philadelphia, WB Saunders, 1989.

Hamblet CN: Parapoxvirus infection in a cat. Vet Rec 132:144, 1993.

Harvey RG: Food allergy and dietary intolerance in dogs: A report of 25 cases. J Small Anim Pract 34:175, 1993.

Hendrick MJ, Dunagan CA: Focal necrotizing granulomatous panniculitis associated with subcutaneous injection of rabies vaccine in cats and dogs: 10 cases (1988–1989). J Am Vet Med Assoc 198:304, 1991.

Hendrix CM, Blagburn BL, Boosinger TR, et al: *Anatrichosoma* sp. infection in a dog. J Am Vet Med Assoc 191:984, 1987.

Higgins R, Paradis M: Abscess caused by *Corynebacterium equi* in a cat. Can Vet J 21:63, 1980.

Hsu WH, Hopper DL: Effect of yohimbine on amitraz-induced CNS depression and bradycardia in dogs. J Toxicol Environ Health 18:423, 1986.

Jeffers JG, Shanley KJ, Meyer EK: Diagnostic testing of dogs for food hypersensitivity. J Am Vet Med Assoc 198:245, 1991.

Johnson RP, Sabine M: The isolation of herpesviruses from skin ulcers in domestic cats. Vet Rec 89:360, 1971.

Kral F, Uscavage JP: Cutaneous candidiasis in a dog. J Am Vet Med Assoc 136:612, 1960.

Krick SA, Scott DW: Bacterial folliculitis, furunculosis, and cellulitis in the German shepherd dog: A retrospective analysis of 17 cases. J Am Anim Hosp Assoc 25:23, 1989.

Kwochka KW: Demodicosis. In Griffin CE, Kwochka KK, MacDonald JM (eds): Current Veterinary Dermatology: The Science and Art of Therapy. St. Louis, Mosby-Year Book, 1993, p 72.

Kwochka KW, Kunkle GA, Foil CO: The efficacy of amitraz for generalized demodicosis in dogs: A study of two concentrations and frequencies of application. Compend Contin Educ Pract Vet 7:8, 1985.

Lewis DT, Foil CS, Hosgood G: Epidemiology and clinical features of dermatophytosis in dogs and cats at Louisiana State University: 1981–1990. Vet Dermatol 2:53, 1991.

Lozano-Alarcon F, Lewis TP, Clark EG, et al: Persistent papillomavirus infection in a cat. J Am Anim Hosp Assoc 32:392, 1996.

MacDonald JM: Flea allergy dermatitis and flea control. In Griffin CE, Kwochka KK, MacDonald JM (eds): Current Veterinary Dermatology: The Science and Art of Therapy. St. Louis, Mosby-Year Book, 1993a, p 57.

MacDonald JM: Food allergy. In Griffin CE, Kwochka KK, MacDonald JM (eds): Current Veterinary Dermatology: The Science and Art of Therapy. St. Louis, Mosby-Year Book, 1993b, p 121.

Malone JB, Breitschwerdt EB, Little MD, et al: Strongyloides stercoralis–like infection in a dog. J Am Vet Med Assoc 176:130, 1980.

Mason KV: Cutaneous Malassezia. In Griffin CE, Kwochka KK, MacDonald JM (eds): Current Veterinary Dermatology: The Science and Art of Therapy. St. Louis, Mosby-Year Book, 1993, p 44.

Mason KV, Evans AG: Dermatitis associated with Malassezia pachydermatis in 11 dogs. J Am Anim Hosp Assoc. 27:15, 1991.

Monroe WE: Clinical signs associated with pseudorabies in dogs. J Am Vet Med Assoc 195:599, 1989.

Moriello KA: Cheyletiellosis. In Griffin CE, Kwochka KK, MacDonald JM (eds): Current Veterinary Dermatology: The Science and Art of Therapy. St. Louis, Mosby-Year Book, 1993, p 90.

Morris DO, Beale KM: Feline demodicosis. In Bonagura JD (ed): Kirk's Current Veterinary Therapy XIII. Philadelphia, WB Saunders, 2000, p 580.

Noxon JO: Anaphylaxis, urticaria and angioedema. Semin Vet Med Surg (Small Anim) 6:265, 1991.

Plant JD, Rosenkranz WS, Griffin CE: Factors associated with and prevalence of high Malassezia pachydermatis numbers on dog skin. J Am Vet Med Assoc 201:879, 1992.

Power HT: Eosinophilic granuloma in a family of specific pathogen-free cats. Proc Am Acad Vet Dermatol Am Coll Vet Dermatol Annu Mg, 1990, p 45.

Price PM: Pyoderma caused by Peptostreptococcus tetradius in a pup. J Am Vet Med Assoc 198:1649, 1991.

Quaife RA, Womar SM: Microsporum canis isolations from show cats. Vet Rec 110:333, 1982.

Reedy LM, Miller WH Jr: Allergic Skin Diseases of Dogs and Cats. Philadelphia, WB Saunders, 1989.

Reimann KA, Evans MG, Chalifoux LV, et al: Clinicopathologic characterization of canine juvenile cellulitis. Vet Pathol 26:499, 1989.

Rife JN: Deep digital flexor tendonectomy: An alternative to amputation onchyectomy for declawing cats. J Am Anim Hosp Assoc 24:73, 1988.

Roosje PJ, Hendrix ML, Wisselin MA, et al: A case of a Dermatobia hominis infection in a dog in the Netherlands. Vet Dermatol 3:183, 1992.

Rosser EJ: Food allergy in the dog: A prospective study of 51 dogs. Proc Am Acad Vet Dermatol Am Coll Vet Dermatol Annu Mg, 1990, p 47.

Roudebush P, Cowell CS: Results of a hypoallergenic diet survey of veterinarians in North America with a nutritional evaluation of homemade diet prescriptions. Vet Dermatol 3:23, 1992.

Rust MK, Dryden MW: The biology, ecology, and management of the cat flea. Annu Rev Entomol 42:451, 1997.

Sangster LT, Styer EL, Hall GA: Coccidia associated with cutaneous nodules in a dog. Vet Pathol 22:186, 1985.

Scott DW: Immunologic skin disorders in the dog and cat. Vet Clin North Am 8:641, 1978.

Scott DW: Canine demodicosis. Vet Clin North Am 9:79, 1979.

Scott DW, Anderson WI: Panniculitis in dogs and cats: A retrospective analysis of 78 cases. J Am Anim Hosp Assoc 24:551, 1988.

Scott DW, Buerger RG: Idiopathic calcinosis circumscripta in the dog. Proc Am Acad Vet Dermatol Am Coll Vet Dermatol Annu Mg, 1987, p 8.

Scott DW, Halliwell REW, Goldschmidt MH, et al: Toxic epidermal necrolysis in two dogs and a cat. J Am Anim Hosp Assoc 15:271, 1979.

Scott DW, Schultz RD, Baker E: Further studies on the therapeutic and immunologic aspects of generalized demodectic mange in the dog. J Am Anim Hosp Assoc 12:203, 1976.

Scott DW, Walton DK: Experiences with the use of amitraz and ivermectin for the treatment of generalized demodicosis in dogs. J Am Anim Hosp Assoc 21:535, 1985.

Scott-Moncrieff JCR: Clinical syndromes of vasculitis in dogs. Proc Am Coll Vet Intern Med Forum 10:662, 1992.

Scott Nolen R: AVMA adopts position on ear cropping and tail docking. J Am Vet Med Assoc 215:461, 1999.

Smith BL, Elliott DC: Canine pedal dermatitis due to percutaneous Uncinaria stenocephala infection. NZ Vet J 17:235, 1969.

Tobias KS: Feline onychectomy at a teaching institution: A retrospective study of 163 cases. Vet Surg 23:274, 1994.

van Cutsem J, De Keyser H, Rochette F, et al: Survey

of fungal isolates from alopecic and asymptomatic dogs. Vet Rec 116:568, 1985.

Wilkie BN, Markham RJF, Hazlett C: Deficient cutaneous response to PHA-P in healthy puppies from a kennel with a high prevalence of demodicosis. Can J Comp Med 43:415, 1979.

White SD: Food hypersensitivity in 30 dogs. J Am Vet Med Assoc 188:695, 1986.

White SD, Rosychuk RAW, Stewart LJ, et al: Juvenile cellulitis in dogs: 15 cases (1979–1988). J Am Vet Med Assoc 195:1609, 1989.

Willers WB: *Pelodera strongyloides* in association with canine dermatitis in Wisconsin. J Am Vet Med Assoc 156:319, 1970.

Woodgyer AJ: Asymptomatic carriage of dermatophytes by cats. N Z Vet J 25:67, 1977.

The Ear

A.J. Venker-van Haagen

Ear diseases occur at all ages in dogs and cats. The diseases seen in young dogs and cats include congenital deafness, congenital deformations of the external ear, and acute bacterial, viral, and parasitic infections. Because congenital deafness, in particular bilateral deafness, is a severe handicap to the puppy or kitten and has serious consequences for the owner who was looking forward to training the young dog, early testing of hearing in young puppies is accentuated in this chapter.

MANAGEMENT OF EAR DISEASE

As for all other diseases, management of ear disease starts with the taking of the history. For young dogs and cats the history of ear disease might well be short and plainly indicative of an acute problem with a circumscribed localization. Some exceptions are generalized juvenile pyoderma, demodicosis, and, in the cat, viral infections, for in these conditions the disease of the ear may be just a part of the clinical signs. Another aspect of the history in young dogs and cats is the relation between the onset of the disease and the change of environment, separation from litter mates, and starting of solitary life under new and different circumstances. Deafness is often only recognized when the puppy or kitten is separated from its playmates and placed in a new environment. The first steps in socializing with the new owner require communication, in which the human voice is the principal tool. Lack of response to commands may be interpreted as playfulness for awhile, but soon it dawns on the owner that the situation is not normal.

The clinical examination of the young dog or cat begins with a general impression of the animal's alertness and mobility, its body weight, the condition of its coat, and any immediately obvious abnormalities. The general physical examination includes examination of respiratory movements, body temperature, pulse rate, skin and coat, mucous membranes, and lymph nodes, and it is supplemented by auscultation of the heart and lung sounds. Neurologic examination may be indicated when the ear disease involves the vestibular system, the facial nerve, or other cranial nerves.

The examination of the ear starts with inspection of the externally visible parts of the ear and adjacent structures. The pinnae of puppies may differ from those of older dogs in that initially all pinnae hang on the sides of the head, and at around the age of 6 weeks they begin to stand in those dogs in which the final ear carriage is standing. At the age of 4 to 6 months there may, however, be a temporary return to the puppy carriage of the pinnae. In kittens the pinnae stand within the first 2 weeks of life and are then relatively large for the head when compared with the adult cat. In dogs and cats the convex surface of the pinna is covered with hair at the age of 2 weeks. The external ear canal begins to open at the age of 2 weeks in dogs and at about the same age in cats. According to the results of hearing tests that we have performed, however, air-conducted hearing is not demonstrable in puppies before the age of 25 days.

Otoscopic examination of the ear canal and the tympanic membrane is in theory possible from the age of 25 days in dogs but is usually not requested before the age of 3 months or more. In the dog and the cat, examination is almost always possible without sedation or anesthesia. The key to success is gentle handling of the patient and avoidance of pressure on the lining of the ear canal, which is very sensitive. If the dog is not cooperative, an experienced assistant can restrain it in a sternal position; a cat can be taken under the arm and its head stabilized. The veterinarian then grasps the tip of the pinna and pulls it firmly in a lateroventral direction. The ear canal is thereby formed into a long, straight canal, with the axes of the vertical and horizontal parts coming into line with each other. The otoscope is then introduced under visual guidance, following the lumen of the ear canal and avoiding as much as possible any touching of the wall. To complete the examination, the pinna and the ear canal are maneuvered under visual control so that the otoscope, passively following the movements, will illuminate the different parts of the ear canal and the tympanic membrane.

In most cases of external ear canal disease, the ear canal will be found to be filled with cerumen or exudate. Cleaning the ear canal is the most important part of management of otitis externa and is essential in both diagnosis and treatment (Venker-van Haagen, 1983). The cleaning must be complete and yet not irritating to the lining. The most effective way is with a forceful stream of water. This is best done using the Haeberle flusher (Haeberle GmbH Comp & Co, Stuttgart, Germany) designed for the cleaning or caloric testing of the human ear. The instrument is connected permanently to a cold water supply pipe; the water in the reservoir is electrically heated and thermostatically controlled. The instrument produces a forceful stream of water at supply line pressure, and the thermostat is set to body temperature. The kitten or puppy is held in the same way, and its ear is kept in the same position as for otoscopic examination. The hand that held the otoscope now takes the handle of the flusher to introduce the stream of water into the canal. When the returning water is clean the animal is allowed to shake its head. This results in a dry ear canal and a dry tympanic membrane. The procedure can be repeated if necessary. Puppies and kittens do not like the procedure, but they can be calmed by an experienced assistant.

When the ear canal is clean and its lumen is sufficiently wide, the canal and the tympanic membrane can be inspected. The tympanic membrane is a transparent round membrane, but it appears to be oval because it is seen through the otoscope at a 60° angle, the ventral part being farther away from the viewer than the dorsal part. The pars tensa, the tensed part, is transparent and slightly blue or gray with radial striping. The dorsal part, the pars flaccida, is pink, and it bulges slightly when pressure in the middle ear is increased. The manubrium of the malleus is a solid white structure in the pars tensa, bordered by small, bright red blood vessels. These characteristics are especially striking in young animals.

EAR DISEASES IN YOUNG DOGS AND CATS

Diseases of the Pinna

Congenital Deformation of the Pinna. Congenital deformation of the pinna is rare in dogs and cats, and when it occurs correction is not always needed, although faulty ear carriage may be seen as a loss of value of the dog. Veterinarians in the Netherlands do not encourage surgical intervention when the pinnae are in principle healthy, and cropping of the pinnae without medical indication is prohibited. Further information may be found elsewhere (Neer, 1995).

Inflammation. Lesions of the pinna may be part of more generalized skin disease (Roth, 1988). They can be bacterial, fungal, parasitic, immune mediated, or vascular (drug mediated) in origin (Scott et al, 1995). These disorders are not age dependent, and hence young dogs and cats are not excluded. Bacterial folliculitis of the pinna with focal areas of alopecia has been described in dogs, and dermatophytosis of the pinna with focal alopecia and extensive crusts can be found in cats (Angarano, 1988). Nonpruritic areas of alopecia in dogs should be scraped for demodectic mites. Pruritus and crusting of the pinna can be caused by *Sarcoptes* mites in dogs and *Notoedres* mites in cats (Wisselink, 1986).

Trauma. Trauma of the pinna can occur at any age. A tear in the pinna is usually the result of a fight with another dog or cat. The cat's claws and the dog's canine teeth are the sharp instruments that cause this trauma. The resulting bleeding can be impressive, and the veterinarian must act immediately to induce primary wound healing.

In young dogs it is often possible to place several sutures without local or general anesthesia. A small, fresh tear (up to 1 cm in length) can be sutured after cleaning and removal of some of the surrounding hair. The skin on the concave side of the pinna is apposed and sutured with interrupted sutures, starting at the edge of the pinna. Then the skin on the convex side is apposed and sutured in the same way. The cartilage is not included in these sutures. Bleeding stops during suturing, but a resistant artery may have to be ligated separately. The use of delayed-solubility suture material is preferred so that the sutures do not have to be removed.

Most cats will not submit to suturing without severe resistance, and hence they, as well as dogs with larger lacerations, should be anesthetized. When the wound is not fresh and inflammation is apparent, surgical correction is postponed and the inflammation treated first. Surgical correction then begins with debridement of the wound edges. Suturing follows the same procedure as in fresh wounds.

Othematoma. Othematomas occur at all ages. The bleeding occurs between the cartilagenous layers of the pinna and is usually considered to result from trauma, such as caused by shaking the head or scratching. Kuwashara (1986) has suggested an immune-mediated disease as the underlying cause. Surgical intervention is necessary because without treatment the pinna will shrivel, and subsequent ossification of the cartilage will cause continuous irritation. Also, shriveling of the pinna may cause obstruction of the external orifice of the ear canal and thus induce chronic otitis externa.

The purpose of surgery is to remove the blood clot and press the layers of the pinna together long enough to effectuate reunion of the layers. A reliable method consists of suturing through all layers of the pinna, placing sutures over its entire surface. Interrupted mattress sutures of monocryl are excellent for this purpose and should be left in place for 2 weeks.

Abscesses. In cats, a penetrating wound inflicted by the claw of another cat usually causes abscesses of the pinna. The cat is depressed and febrile, and the ear is obviously painful. The skin over the abscess should be opened and the pus removed by gentle compression, followed by flushing with 0.9% sodium chloride solution. A broad-spectrum antimicrobial agent should be administered systemically for 10 days. In the young cat no complications are expected.

Tumors of the Pinna. Tumors of the pinna occur at all ages in dogs and cats but are very rare in young dogs and cats (Venker-van Haagen, 1995).

Diseases of the External Ear Canal

The external ear canal in puppies and kittens is closed during the first days of life. In puppies the external meatus of the ear canal begins to open at the age of 2 weeks. According to our hearing tests in four puppies, the ear canals are functionally open at the age of 25 or 26 days.

Congenital Deformations of the Ear Canal. Congenital deformations of the ear canal (usually atresia) are rare and are usually unilateral and therefore not often detected before fistulas occur. Unilateral deafness is well masked in the kitten and puppy. When atresia of the ear canal is found without clinical signs, it is advisable to refrain from intervention. Abscesses of the middle ear require drainage, followed by antimicrobial therapy for 10 days.

Otitis Externa. In young dogs and cats otitis externa is most commonly caused by the parasite *Otodectes cynotis*. The parasite is common in groups of young cats and dogs and when found in one dog or cat in a litter all animals of the litter and the mother should be examined. The mites appear to irritate the ceruminous glands in particular because excessive thick, brown cerumen always accompanies mite infestation. The mites can be detected on this dark brown background with an otoscope. The mites begin to walk when the light of the otoscope warms them. This way of detecting ear mite infestation is almost foolproof and is more reliable than microscopic examination of a cerumen sample.

Treatment begins with flushing of the ear canal. When all cerumen is washed away, the tympanic membrane is clearly visible. In most cases the wall of the ear canal is slightly irregular. Topical antiparasitic drugs are ototoxic and can only be used when the tympanic membrane is intact, so only the veterinarian should administer them. A single application is usually sufficient when reinfection is prevented. After antiparasitic treatment, the otitis is treated for 5 days by local application of an ointment containing broad-spectrum antimicrobial agents and a corticosteroid. One week after the initial treatment, the ears are reexamined. Further treatment is usually not needed.

Another cause of otitis externa in young dogs is a foreign body. This is usually a grass awn. Detection with the otoscope is easy when the otitis externa is still mild, and the plant part can then be removed via the otoscope.

Cleaning of the ear canal of young dogs and cats as part of the routine care by the owner should be discouraged. The skin of the ear canal is too tender, and regular cleaning can result in otitis externa. It should be explained to the owner that a small amount of cerumen visible at the external opening of the ear canal is normal and quite acceptable.

Diseases of the Tympanic Membrane and the Middle Ear

The tympanic membrane is composed of three layers: the epidermis, which is a continuation of the epidermis of the external ear canal; the lamina propria, or fibrous and vascular layer; and the mucosa, which is a continuation of the mucosa of the middle ear. The pathology of the tympanic membrane is usually related to the pathology of the external ear canal or that of the middle ear. Chronic irritation results in thickening of the tympanic membrane, recognized via the otoscope as a loss of transparency. This may be seen, for example, after a long-standing plug has been removed, and it is usually, especially in young dogs and cats, temporary. Middle ear disease is diagnosed more often in cats than in dogs. Reddening of the tympanic membrane is a common sign of middle ear disease. In dogs spontaneous rupture of the tympanic membrane is rare. We have diagnosed this in young dogs with purulent middle ear disease in the course of juvenile cellulitis (Scott et al, 1995). When the tympanic membrane is ruptured accidentally and no middle ear disease occurs, the perforation heals in 1 to 3 weeks, depending on its size (Venker-van Haagen, 1983; Johnson et al, 1990; Steiss et al, 1992). In cats the most common cause of rupture is a polyp in the middle ear that grows through the tympanic membrane into the external ear canal. Among 64 cats in which middle ear polyps were removed, 14 were 1 year old or younger (Venker-van Haagen, 1995). After removal of the polyp, the tympanic membrane is healed and transparent within 4 weeks, at least in cases in which the middle ear disease is cured.

Otitis media without proliferative disease of the external ear canal is diagnosed by otoscopic examination. The tympanic membrane is not transparent and usually red, and it is sometimes ruptured. The discharge from the middle ear is visible in the external ear canal when there is a rupture and is mucopurulent in acute inflammation, as is the case in young animals. When the tympanic membrane is not visible, diagnosis is difficult because radiographs do not conclusively show acute middle ear inflammation.

In young animals the treatment of otitis media consists of systemic broad-spectrum anti-microbial therapy for at least 2 weeks. The inflammation is resolved when the tympanic membrane appears to be normally colored and transparent.

CONGENITAL DEAFNESS

Deafness that is present at or soon after birth may have either an acquired or a hereditary etiology and may occasionally occur in any puppy whether pure bred or mixed breed. Acquired deafness may be caused by viral infections, anoxia, or the ototoxic side effects of drugs or other materials. Because dogs and cats are born deaf, deafness in a puppy or kitten is not abnormal up to a certain age. In cats the earliest discriminating hearing tests were performed at the age of 7 days. Cochlear potential measurements from a round-window electrode were found to be conclusive about the presence or absence of hearing in cats over 7 days of age (Maïr, 1973). In dogs, hearing tests were performed from the age of 4 weeks (Maïr, 1976; Shelton et al, 1993) by means of cochlear potential measurements from round-window electrodes (Maïr, 1976) or brainstem auditory evoked responses (BAERs) (Shelton et al, 1993).

Testing the Hearing of Young Puppies

In our laboratory, two Irish wolfhound puppies and two beagle puppies were investigated for hearing from the third day after birth. Brainstem auditory evoked potentials (BAERs) were recorded from surface electrodes (Dantec, 9013L0202) on the pinnae and the skin over the parietal bone on the midline. For the recording of air-conducted BAERs, each pup was placed in a plexiglass cage (30 × 40 × 40 cm) with two microphones at opposite ends of the cage. No sedation was used. The puppies were free to move when in the cage. The equipment used was as described previously (Wolschrijn et al, 1997), and the stimulus was a click produced by a rectangular wave of 0.2 ms duration with an intensity of 80 dB SPL and 90 dB SPL, as measured in the center of the cage (Sound Level Meter, Brüel and Kjaer, 2231). The stimulus repetition rate was 10 per second. The sound was delivered via both microphones simultaneously. For subsequent recording of bone-conducted BAERs, the puppies were taken out of the cage while leaving the electrodes in place. The same stimulus was used (80 dB SPL) except that it was now applied via the bone conductor (Bone Vibrator B.71B, Radioear Corporation) placed on the stop (Wolschrijn et al, 1997). The

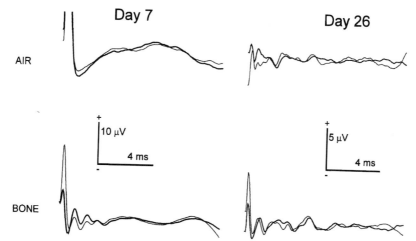

Figure 13–1. Duplicate brainstem auditory evoked potential recordings from one of the two beagle puppies with air-conducted stimuli (AIR) and with bone-conducted stimuli (BONE) at the ages of 7 days and 26 days. At age 7 days, the air-conducted hearing was absent, while the bone-conducted hearing was evident. At age 26 days, both air-conducted and bone-conducted hearing were evident.

bone conductor was pressed against the skull by hand, maintaining the pressure that resulted in the best response signals. The tests were conducted every other day until BAERs for both the air-conducted and the bone-conducted stimuli were recorded.

In both the Irish wolfhound puppies brainstem evoked potentials were first recorded on the 11th day after birth with the bone-conducted stimulus. In both beagle puppies the first brainstem evoked potentials were recorded on the seventh day after birth with the bone-conducted stimulus (Fig. 13–1). The first recording of brainstem evoked potentials with air-conducted stimuli was on the 25th day after birth in both Irish wolfhound puppies and on the 26th day in both beagle puppies (see Fig. 13–1). During the test period (from the 3rd to the 27th day after birth) none of the puppies showed signs of sound perception.

The results indicate that bone-conducted BAERs detected cochlear activity at a younger age than air-conducted BAERs. The method does not discriminate between unilateral and bilateral cochlear activity, but with bone-conducted BAERs bilateral cochlear deafness can be elucidated before 2 weeks of age in dogs.

Congenital Deafness Caused by a Genetic Defect

Congenital deafness caused by a genetic defect has been thoroughly investigated for the white cat (Bosher and Hallpike, 1965; Suga and Hattler, 1970; Maïr, 1973; Pugol et al, 1977) and the Dalmatian dog (Johnsson et al, 1973; Maïr, 1976). These investigations were in part motivated as animal model studies for the Waardenburg syndrome in humans. This syndrome is characterized by hereditary deafness associated with disorders of pigmentation of hair, iris, and skin (Waardenburg, 1951). Congenital deafness associated with disorders of pigmentation was described in the cat (Bosher and Hallpike, 1965; Maïr, 1973) and in the dog (Anderson et al, 1968; Igarashi et al, 1972; Maïr, 1976). In dogs, deafness is associated with merle pigmentation (e.g., Shetland sheepdog, collie, harlequin Great Dane) and carriers of the piebald gene (e.g., bull terrier, Samoyed, Great Pyrenees mountain dog, Sealyham terrier, greyhound, bulldog, Dalmatian dog). In this form of inherited deafness one or both ears are completely deaf.

Most investigators of the histologic development of the cochlea in deaf white cats agree that the primary degeneration of the epithelial and sensory elements occurs in the first weeks after birth, after which secondary degeneration of the neural structures follows (Bosher and Hallpike, 1965; Suga et al, 1970; Maïr, 1973). Normal neural structures were found together with an advanced stage of degeneration of the epithelial elements in deaf white cats (Rebillard et al, 1976). In a later study, however, it was reported that the spiral ganglion neurons in 2 of 11 white kittens (7 and 16 days old) were completely degenerated. It was concluded that the degeneration of the cochlea in white cats may be considered to be a process affecting both sensory and neural structures with a variety of features and a very variable timing (Pugol et al, 1970).

The earliest postnatal histologic events in deaf Dalmatian dogs were studied at the age of 4 weeks. At that age a volume reduction of the saccule and of the cochlear duct had already occurred (Maïr, 1976). This volume reduction is a consequence of the descent of Reissner's membrane toward the organ of Corti and, in a later stage, the covering of the organ of Corti by this membrane. In the cochlear duct, other signs of degeneration were a decrease in thickness of the stria vascularis and of the cellular components of the organ of Corti. In older deaf Dalmatian dogs the degeneration was more severe and was accompanied by loss of ganglion cells (Maïr, 1976). In a histologic study comparing cochleas of hearing and deaf Dalmatian dogs at the age of 6 weeks, the findings of Maïr (1976) were confirmed for the deaf dogs, whereas the cochleas of the dogs with normal hearing were completely normal (Branis and Burda, 1985). The relation between a variance in pigmentation and inner ear dysfunction is recognized in several hereditary syndromes in several species of mammals, including humans. The pigmentation abnormalities are always of the "white spotting" kind, also known as hypopigmentation. When the entire coat is white, the animal must be regarded as having one very large spot rather than as being an albino.

The difference between the two types of whiteness, albinism and hypopigmentation, is fundamental. In the albino, melanocytes can be identified in the hair follicles, but they are incapable of forming melanin due to a biochemical block. In hypopigmented animals or in spotted regions of pigmented animals no melanocytes can be identified (Billingham and Silvers, 1960). In the albino there is no pigmentation at all, whereas in hypopigmented animals pigment is present in the retina, showing that the genetic capacity to produce melanin is not lacking (Deol, 1970). The abnormalities in the inner ear are confined to the cochlea and saccule. There is a severe degeneration of the organ of Corti, stria vascularis, spiral ganglion, and the macula of the saccule. The relation between hypopigmentation and inner ear abnormalities was investigated by Deol (1970) in mice. His main conclusions were that "spotting" of the coat was always associated with hypopigmentation of the stria vascularis in the cochlea, usually a heavily pigmented area. Hypopigmentation of the stria vascularis was always associated with degeneration of the cochlea. There was no correlation between the severity of hypopigmentation of the coat and the hypopigmentation of the stria vascularis of the cochlea (Deol, 1970). These finding may be applicable to the dog and the cat as well.

The relation between the piebald gene and "spotting" was established in mice (Mayer, 1965), and the abnormality was localized in the neural crest. The abnormal parts develop abnormal melanoblasts in the differential areas, resulting in local hypopigmentation. The abnormal areas varied in location and size, as did the pigmentation in the stria vascularis. The degeneration of the cochlea varied in severity within the cochlea. Hearing was not tested in these animals.

From these findings it may be concluded that when an animal with "spotting" or hypopigmentation is born with unilateral or bilateral deafness, the deafness is based on a hereditary defect. Furthermore, when, as in dogs, hypopigmentation is a breed characteristic, deafness will occur in the breed.

Ototoxicity

The labyrinth contains the sensory cells for both hearing and equilibrium. In labyrinthitis and ototoxicity both of these functions are impaired. When the sensory cells are destroyed, they are not replaced, and hence the hearing loss is permanent. The loss of function of the semicircular canals and utricle may be partially compensated by the central nervous system (Gacek et al, 1989, 1992).

The ototoxicity of a drug or any other chemical is its toxic effect on the inner ear, including the cochlea, the vestibule, and the semicircular canals. The toxic materials can reach the inner ear via local application in the middle ear or hematogenously via absorption from the digestive tract, respiratory tract, or wounds or via parenteral administration. In veterinary practice, ototoxic drugs (in young dogs and cats antiparasitic drugs are the most obvious candidates) usually pass a perforated (iatrogenic?) tympanic membrane and enter the perilymph via the membranes of the oval and round windows. There is direct contact between the perilymph and the hair cells.

The toxic effect is the degeneration of the sensory cells within the membranous labyrinth, causing dysfunction of the cochlea (deafness) and vestibular dysfunction (loss of equilibrium). When the ototoxicity is unilateral, the signs of vestibular dysfunction are most impressive (Gallé et al, 1986). In the acute phase there is a head tilt with the affected ear under, horizontal nystagmus with the fast phase away from the affected side, rolling over toward the affected side and inability to stand, nausea, and refusal of food. Within 3 days central compensation results in diminishing and eventual disappearance of the nystagmus, gradual attempts to stand, and beginning efforts to eat and drink, but the head tilt is unchanged. Within 3 weeks the situation improves, but jumping and walking down stairs often result in falling. The compensation is optimal after about 3 months, but the head tilt is then still obvious.

Many substances used for local application in the ear canal contain ototoxic components, including disinfectants, antimicrobial agents, antiparasitics, and even the vehicle in some ear drops. None of these medications should ever be instilled into the external ear canal unless it is certain that the tympanic membrane is intact.

References and Supplemental Reading

Anderson H, Henricson B, Lunquist PG, et al: Genetic hearing impairment in the Dalmatian dog. Acta Otolaryngol (Suppl) (Stockh) 232:1, 1968.

Argakano DW: Diseases of the pinna. Vet Clin North Am Small Anim Pract 18:869, 1988.

Billingham RE, Silvers WK: The melanocytes of mammals. Q Rev Biol 35:1, 1960.

Bosher SK, Hallpike CS: Observations of the histologic features, development, and genesis of the inner ear degeneration of the deaf white cat. Proc R Soc Bil 162:147, 1965.

Branis M, Burda H: Inner ear structure in the deaf and hearing Dalmatian dog. J Comp Pathol 95:295, 1985.

Deol MS: The relationship between abnormalities of pigmentation and the inner ear. Proc R Soc Lond A 175:201, 1970.

Gacek RR, Lyon MJ, Schoonmaker J: Morphologic correlates of vestibular compensation in the cat. Acta Otolaryngol (Suppl) (Stockh) 462:1, 1989.

Gacek RR, Schoonmaker J, Lyon MJ: Ultrastructural changes in contralateral superior vestibulo-ocular neurons one year after vestibular neurectomy in the cat. Acta Otolaryngol (Suppl) (Stockh) 495:1, 1992.

Gallé HG, Venker-van Haagen AJ: Ototoxicity of the antiseptic combination chlorhexidine/cetrimide (Savlon^R): Effects on equilibrium and hearing. Vet Q 8:56, 1986.

Igarashi M, Alford BR, Saito R, et al: Inner ear anomalies in dogs. Ann Otol 81:249, 1972.

Johnson AP, Smallman LA, Kent SE: The mechanism of healing of tympanic membrane perforation. Acta Otolaryngol (Stockh) 109:406, 1990.

Johnsson LG, Hawkins JE, Muraski AA, et al: Vascular anatomy and pathology of the cochlea in Dalmatian dogs. In de Lorenzo AJD (ed): Vascular Disorders and Hearing Defects. Baltimore, University Park Press, 1973, p 249.

Kuwashara J: Canine and feline aural hematomas: Clinical, experimental and clinicopathological observations. Am J Vet Res 47:2300, 1986.

Maïr IWS: Hereditary deafness in the white cat. Acta Otolaryngol (Suppl) (Stockh) 314:1, 1973.

Maïr IWS: Hereditary deafness in the Dalmatian dog. Arch Oto-Rhino-Laryngol 212:1, 1976.

Mayer TC: The development of piebald spotting in mice. Dev Biol 11:319, 1965.

Neer TM: The ears. In Hoskins JD (ed): Veterinary Pediatrics: Dogs and Cats from Birth to Six Months, 2nd ed. Philadelphia, WB Saunders, 1995, p 283.

Pugol R, Rebillard M, Rebillard G: Primary neural disorders in the deaf white cat cochlea. Acta Otolaryngol 83:59, 1977.

Rebillard G, Rebillard M, Carlier R, et al: Histopathological relationships in the deaf white cat auditory system. Acta Otolaryngol 82:48, 1976.

Roth L: Pathologic changes in otitis externa. Vet Clin North Am Small Anim Pract 18:755, 1988.

Scott DW, Miller WH, Griffin CE: Small Animal Dermatology, 5th ed. Philadelphia, WB Saunders, 1995, pp 420, 938.

Shelton SB, Stockard-Pope MS, Chrisman CL, et al: Brain stem auditory-evoked responses to clicks and tone bursts in notched noise in Dalmatian puppies. Prog Vet Neurol 4:31, 1993.

Steiss JE, Boosinger TR, Wright JC, et al: Healing of experimentally perforated tympanic membranes demonstrated by electrodiagnostic testing and histopathology. J Am Anim Hosp Assoc 28:307, 1992.

Suga F, Hattler KW: Physiological and histopathological correlates of hereditary deafness in animals. Laryngoscope 80:80, 1970.

Venker-van Haagen AJ: Management of ear diseases. In Kirk RW (ed): Current Veterinary Therapy VIII. Philadelphia, WB Saunders, 1983, p 47.

Venker-van Haagen AJ: The ear. In Goldston RT, Hoskins JD (eds): Geriatrics and Gerontology of the Dog and Cat. Philadelphia, WB Saunders, 1995, p 209.

Waardenburg PJ: A new syndrome combining developmental abnormalities of eyelids, eyebrows and nose root with pigmentary defects of the iris and head hair and with congenital deafness. Am J Hum Genet 3:195, 1951.

Wisselink MA: The external ear in skin diseases of the dogs and cats: A diagnostic challenge. Vet Q 8:307, 1986.

Wolschrijn CF, Venker-van Haagen AJ, van den Brom WE: Comparison of air-conducted and bone-conducted brain stem auditory evoked responses in young dogs and dogs with bilateral ear canal obstruction. Vet Q 19:158, 1997.

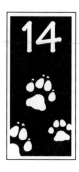

14

The Eye

Johnny D. Hoskins and Mary B. Glaze

THE OPHTHALMIC EXAMINATION

History

A complete ophthalmic history is an essential part of every puppy's or kitten's examination. Owners may be asked questions regarding the animal's signalment, history of the presenting complaint(s), and any pertinent medical or ophthalmic diseases in the animal's family histories. Other historical information that may be included is the animal's vaccination status, diet, environment, and exposure to other animals. Previous therapy should be identified to prevent repetition of an unsuccessful regimen.

Procedure

Ophthalmic examination should be performed in a quiet area. Puppies usually require only gentle but firm restraint of the head. Very young puppies cooperate nicely when held in an assistant's arms. Kittens can also be gently restrained and are less likely to demonstrate the constant ocular motion typical of puppies. Uncooperative puppies or kittens may be placed in a towel or restraint bag. Assessment of ocular abnormalities such as orbital swelling, squinting, or ocular discharge can be done in a well-lighted room, but actual ophthalmoscopic examination should be done with the lights dimmed. A bright source of focal illumination is required; the Finoff transilluminator on a fully charged direct ophthalmoscope handle is ideal.

Vision is assessed by observing the animal's response to a threatening gesture toward the eye, throwing cotton balls across the animal's

visual field, or evaluating maneuverability through an obstacle course. Initial animal responses are most reliable, especially in kittens. The menace reflex is present but poorly developed in puppies and kittens when the eyelids separate at 5 to 14 days; it may not appear to be present until the third or fourth week of life. The cilia of the eyelids are situated on the upper eyelid of the dog and are normally absent in the cat. Active blinking movements of the eyelids are protective of the cornea and disperse the tear film over the corneal surface. Pupillary light responses are typically slow until the retina matures. Other expected ophthalmic features of the puppy and kitten are summarized in Table 14–1.

Corneal or conjunctival cultures and evaluation of tear production using the Schirmer tear test should be completed before any drops are applied to the eyes. For culturing, the lower eyelid is everted and a saline-moistened, sterile, cotton-tipped swab is rolled across the conjunctiva, being careful to avoid the eyelid margin and its contaminants. Conjunctival scrapings are obtained with a heat-sterilized spatula following topical anesthesia, and the sample is collected from the same region as the culture. The sample is gently applied to a clean glass slide and prepared with Wright's or Gram's stain for cytologic examination. Fluorescein dye is used to demonstrate corneal ulcers. To avoid errors in interpretation, excess dye should be flushed from the eye with a sterile saline solution before the corneal surface is viewed.

Examination of the lens and fundus requires that the pupil be dilated with one drop of 1% tropicamide, followed in 5 minutes by a second application. Maximum mydriasis occurs within

270

Table 14–1	Normal Ophthalmic Features of the Puppy and Kitten	
Globe position	Kittens demonstrate a divergent strabismus until the second month of life	
Cornea	Animals are born with mild corneal cloudiness owing to increased water content within the cornea. Corneal cloudiness resolves in 2–4 wk as the level of hydration approximates that of the adult cornea	
Iris	Iris is not heavily pigmented at birth. Blue-gray iris usually changes to the adult coloration within a few weeks	
Lens	Remnants of the hyaloid artery may be seen attached to the posterior lens capsule for a few days after the eyelids completely separate	
Fundus	Tapetum is blue-gray, gradually assuming the adult coloration by 4–7 mo of age. The optic disc may appear slightly smaller and of a different color owing to incomplete myelination, but the caliber and distribution of the retinal vessels are similar to those of the adult	

15 to 20 minutes. Examination of the anterior segment (eyelids, conjunctiva, cornea, anterior chamber, and iris) is best done with a bright-light source and a magnifying loupe. After the pupil is dilated, the penlight or direct ophthalmoscope (set at +8 to +12 diopters) can be used to examine the lens. The retina and optic disc may be evaluated by 3 weeks of age and older at a direct ophthalmoscope setting of −2 to +2 diopters. If the puppy retracts the eye or protrudes the third eyelid, it may help to reduce the intensity of light.

THE EYELIDS

Developmental Abnormalities

Eyelid Agenesis. Eyelid agenesis is a congenital defect of the eyelid margin resulting in absence of varying segments of the eyelid margin, palpebral conjunctiva, and fornices. The agenesis may be unilateral or bilateral, affecting the kitten more often than the puppy. The lateral one third or two thirds of the upper eyelid margin is most frequently involved. Keratitis and ulceration result from direct contact of the cornea with facial hairs and from exposure secondary to imperfect eyelid closure. Small eyelid defects may be successfully managed with ophthalmic lubricant ointments applied three to four times a day to reduce ocular irritation or by performing an entropion procedure to evert the offending hairs. If one third of the eyelid or more is missing, a pedicle graft from the inferior temporal aspect of the lower eyelid can be transposed to the upper eyelid.

Distichiasis. Distichiasis is an extra row of eyelashes (cilia) that protrudes from the orifices of the meibomian glands onto the eyelid margin. The upper, lower, or both eyelids may be involved (Fig. 14–1A). Congenital distichiasis

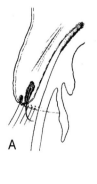 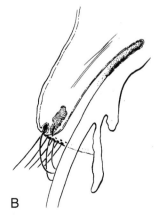 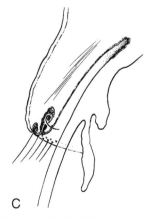

Figure 14–1. A, Abnormally placed eyelash (cilium) protruding from a meibomian gland orifice. **B,** Trichiasis with misdirected eyelashes (cilia) in contact with the cornea. **C,** Ectopic cilium projecting through the conjunctival surface that contacts the cornea.

often occurs in the English bulldog, toy and miniature poodle, American cocker spaniel, golden retriever, Shetland sheepdog, Chesapeake Bay retriever, Lhasa apso, Shih Tzu, and Pekingese dog breeds. Distichiasis is uncommon in kittens but may occur in the Abyssinian. Canine distichiasis may be inherited as an autosomal dominant trait. Surgical treatment is performed on those puppies in which other causes of epiphora, blepharospasm, conjunctivitis, and keratitis have been ruled out. Manual epilation is temporarily effective, but cilia will regrow within 2 to 3 weeks. Electroepilation destroys the follicular tissue within the meibomian gland but is time consuming in puppies with numerous distichia and may require several applications before satisfactory results are obtained. Cryoepilation with application of liquid nitrogen or application of nitrous oxide cryoprobe also appears to be a safe and effective method of managing distichiasis. Tarsoconjunctival resection or lid-splitting is not usually recommended for young puppies due to the potential for postoperative scarring and secondary entropion.

Trichiasis. Trichiasis occurs when otherwise normal eyelashes or facial hairs deviate inward, contacting the surface of the eye (Fig. 14–1B). The resulting irritation may lead to corneal vascularization, pigmentation, or ulceration if untreated. Management of the trichiasis should begin with correction of any primary condition that may be present, such as entropion, redundant facial folds, or eyelid agenesis. Electroepilation or cryoepilation will remove offending cilia. Ophthalmic corticosteroid preparations will reduce corneal vascularization and slow corneal melanosis and scarring in the absence of corneal ulceration.

Ectopic Cilia. Ectopic cilia are hairs that emerge from the meibomian glands through the palpebral conjunctiva of the eyelid, usually 2 to 6 mm from the eyelid margin (Fig. 14–1C). The hair rubs against the corneal surface, often creating an ulcer. If an ulcer in the upper one third of the cornea fails to heal normally, close inspection of the palpebral surface of the upper eyelid is recommended. The ectopic hair frequently appears as a small dark spot at the base of the meibomian gland. En bloc excision of the palpebral conjunctiva and affected meibomian gland is usually curative.

Entropion. Entropion is a defect in which the eyelid margin turns toward the globe. Entropion occurs commonly in various breeds of dogs and infrequently in the cat (Fig. 14–2).

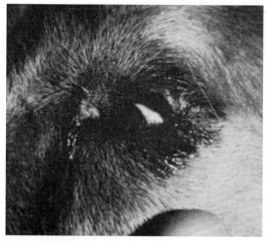

Figure 14–2. Entropion. Note the inversion of the lower eyelid and the associated overflow of tears.

The lower eyelid is more often affected; the tarsal plate of the lower eyelid is poorly formed while the inferior orbicularis oculi muscle segment contracts with greater force. It is likely that several genes that define the eyelid structure, globe-orbit relationship, and facial skin influence the degree of entropion. Entropion often occurs in the narrow palpebral fissure of the chow chow, the deeply set eye of the golden retriever, and the Chinese shar-pei's redundant facial folds. Painful ocular disorders may also cause entropion, with inward deviation of the eyelid secondary to spasm of the orbicularis oculi muscle. Application of a topical ophthalmic anesthetic agent such as 0.5% proparacaine eliminates the spastic component and gives a more reliable representation of eyelid conformation.

Young animals with entropion but without keratopathy may be given palliative treatment with a high-viscosity ophthalmic lubricant ointment until they are 4 to 5 months of age before surgical intervention is attempted. Delaying surgery in the Chinese shar-pei may not be possible because of the severity of the breed's entropion and its potential for causing corneal damage. Affected puppies may benefit from a temporary eyelid correction to forestall corneal vascularization, ulceration, and fibrosis. This "tacking" procedure may be performed with sedation or regional anesthesia in the 3- to 4-week-old puppy. A suture of 6-0 Vicryl is passed through the skin and muscle of the eyelid in a vertical mattress pattern, the base of which should be parallel to and 3 mm above the margin of the offending eyelid (Fig. 14–3A). A permanent correction may then be performed at

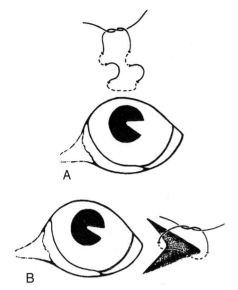

Figure 14–3. Methods for correction of entropion. **A,** A suture of 6-0 Vicryl is passed through the skin of the outer palpebral area in a vertical mattress pattern, the base of which is parallel to and 4 mm above the eyelid margin so as to rotate the inturned portion of the eyelid margin outward. **B,** Canthal entropion is corrected by removing a crescent-shaped or arrowhead-shaped piece of skin from the temporal canthus so as to evert the inturned portion of the temporal canthus outward.

a later time. The conventional procedure for correction of entropion is the Hotz-Celsus procedure. An elliptical section of the eyelid skin is removed, and the skin margins are reapposed using 4-0 silk interrupted sutures. Best eversion is achieved when the incision nearer the eyelid margin is approximately 4 mm from the margin. The sutures may be removed 10 days after surgery.

In some dog breeds, such as the Chinese shar-pei and chow chow, the retractor anguli oculi muscle is poorly developed, allowing inward deviation of the temporal canthus. This may be corrected by performing a temporal canthoplasty. A crescent-shaped or arrowhead-shaped incision is made 3 to 4 mm from the canthal margin (Fig. 14–3B). The incision is then closed with 4-0 silk interrupted sutures to evert the canthus.

Ectropion. The eyelid of the puppy affected with ectropion is everted away from the globe, exposing the underlying bulbar conjunctiva. As a consequence, the conjunctival cul-de-sacs accumulate debris, and the conjunctiva is mildly and chronically inflamed. Ectropion tends to occur with greater frequency in those dog breeds with laxity of the lower eyelids such as the cocker spaniel, bloodhound, basset hound, and Saint Bernard. Temporary relief of ocular signs may be attained with ophthalmic lubricant ointments. The repair of ectropion is usually an elective and cosmetic procedure. Shortening the lower eyelid by means of a wedge resection in its lateral aspect is perhaps the simplest means of correction. Minor forms of ectropion may also be treated surgically by employing the V to Y incision.

Acquired Abnormalities

Lacerations. Eyelid lacerations occur as those that parallel the eyelid margin and those that are perpendicular to the eyelid margin. Meticulous suturing after minimal debridement is indicated in most instances. The perpendicular laceration should be closed in two layers due to the force of the orbicularis muscle pulling the wound margins apart. A layer of absorbable suture in a continuous pattern is used to close the conjunctiva/tarsus, and a second layer of nonabsorbable material is placed in the skin (Fig. 14–4). The eyelid margin should be sutured precisely to avoid the obvious cosmetic and functional defects resulting from poor marginal apposition.

Immunologic Diseases. Allergic and immune-mediated skin diseases may also involve the eyelid and conjunctiva. Immediate hypersensitivity results in severe swelling of the eyelids and conjunctiva with varying amounts of epiphora and pruritus. Reactions to insect bites, food, or medication may initiate an IgE-mediated response that is manageable with antihistamine and/or corticosteroid therapy. Although uncommon in the young dog or cat, delayed hypersensitivity involving the eyelids may present as a component of atopy. The animal will display swelling and congestion of the conjunctiva and serous ocular discharge that becomes more mucoid as the condition progresses. Schirmer's tear test values may be reduced in more advanced cases. Although topical antimicrobial and corticosteroid ophthalmic solutions may provide palliative or transient relief, allergy testing and desensitization are preferred for long-term control of ocular signs.

Bacterial Infections. Young puppies are commonly affected with staphylococcal folliculitis, which may involve the eyelids. Swelling of the eyelids, face, and muzzle, coupled with pustular dermatitis in young dogs, is most likely due to juvenile pyoderma. Topical ophthalmic

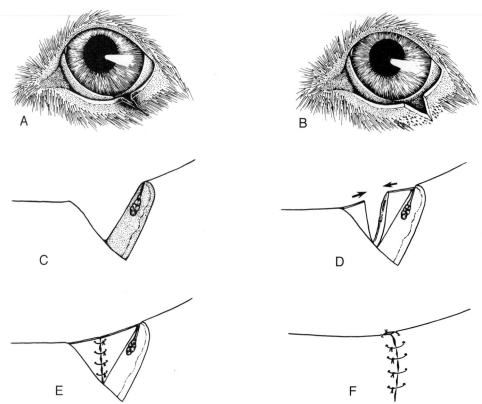

Figure 14–4. Surgical closure of a lower eyelid laceration. **A,** Appearance of the laceration before debridement. **B,** Appearance of the same laceration after adequate cleaning and debridement. **C,** The same laceration before splitting the tarsus from the palpebral conjunctiva. **D,** The tarsus and palpebral conjunctivae are dissected free on both sides of the laceration (arrows) to create a tarsal flap and a conjunctival flap. **E,** The conjunctival flap is approximated with 6-0 absorbable suture in an interrupted suture pattern and the knots externalized. **F,** The tarsal flap and skin are then sutured for final closure of the laceration.

and systemic antimicrobial agents are recommended. Corticosteroids are used in all cases at least initially and is started with the antimicrobial agents, continuing both for a minimum of 2 weeks. Warm compresses assist in establishing local drainage of eyelid pustules. Complete resolution of the juvenile pyoderma may take as long as 6 to 12 weeks.

Parasitic Infestations. Generalized or local infestation with a variety of ectoparasites may result in alopecia, erythema, and pruritus of the eyelids (Fig. 14–5). The more common parasites involved are *Demodex canis*, *Notoedres cati*, *Otodectes cyanotis*, and *Sarcoptes scabiei*. Serial skin scrapings of the affected areas with or without identification of the offending parasite(s) makes the diagnosis. Local treatment of the affected eyelids with a suitable insecticidal ointment is generally indicated. When an effective parasiticide is selected, the possibility of local irritation

involving the conjunctiva or cornea should be considered.

THE CONJUNCTIVA

Developmental Abnormalities

Dermoids. Dermoids are congenital masses of tissue containing skin, hair follicles, and sebaceous glands. They most commonly occur in the temporal perilimbal conjunctiva and may also involve the eyelid margin or the cornea (Fig. 14–6). Dermoids often cause ocular irritation and epiphora. Treatment involves careful dissection of the dermoid from the surrounding conjunctiva and the underlying sclera. If the cornea is involved, a superficial keratectomy is also indicated.

Aberrant Canthal Dermis. Aberrant canthal dermis is characterized by long hairs, which extend from the medial canthal caruncle onto

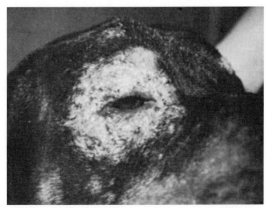

Figure 14–5. Periorbital dermatitis with swollen margin of eyelids in which *Staphylococcus* was cultured. Skin scrapings of the affected area also showed the presence of numerous *Demodex* spp mites. (Courtesy of Dr. Carol S. Foil, Baton Rouge, Louisiana State University.)

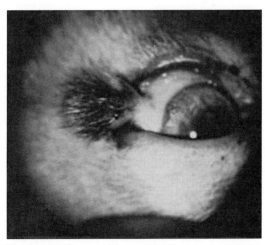

Figure 14–6. Dermoid located in the temporal-limbic region of the conjunctiva that involves the eyelid margins.

the corneal surface. The hairs wick the tears from the eye onto the eyelid, causing facial staining in the puppy or kitten. If the condition is allowed to persist, the cilia may cause corneal pigmentation. The condition is most frequently seen in the Lhasa apso, Shih Tzu, Pekingese, poodle, and Chinese pug dog breeds and infrequently in the Persian cat. Cryotherapy is a simple, effective method of destroying the hair

follicles within the caruncle. The caruncle may also be surgically excised (Fig. 14–7). A sliding conjunctival flap is created by bluntly undermining the surrounding conjunctiva. The flap is then sutured to the medial canthal ligament, closing the surgically created conjunctival defect. In either instance, it is important to avoid damaging the nearby nasolacrimal puncta and canaliculi.

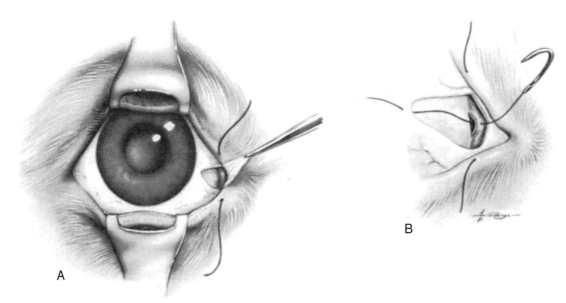

Figure 14–7. Sliding conjunctival flap for treatment of aberrant canthal dermis. **A,** The dermis is dissected off, and a conjunctival flap is created. **B,** The sliding flap is sutured to the edge of the medial palpebral ligament with one or two simple interrupted sutures of 5-0 Vicryl. (From Slatter DH: Conjunctiva. *In* Slatter DH [ed]: Fundamentals of Veterinary Ophthalmology. Philadelphia, WB Saunders, 1981, p 284.)

Acquired Abnormalities

Bacterial Conjunctivitis. Bacterial conjunctivitis occurs unilaterally or bilaterally in the young dog but is seldom seen as a primary entity in the young cat. The conjunctival inflammation results in varying degrees of hyperemia and chemosis that is typically accompanied by a mucopurulent exudate. Ocular hyperemia and discharge may also accompany many external ocular abnormalities, such as distichia, ectopic cilia, hordeolum, foreign object, nasolacrimal disease, and keratoconjunctivitis sicca (KCS). If primary bacterial conjunctivitis is suspected, a Schirmer's tear test should be performed to rule out KCS before continuing with the ocular examination and before washing exudates from the eye. Additional diagnostic methods used in suspected conjunctival disease may include bacterial culture and sensitivity testing, conjunctival cytology, and conjunctival biopsy. Bacterial culture is most frequently employed after poor clinical response to topical ophthalmic antimicrobial agents. The treatment regimen for primary bacterial conjunctivitis should consist of gentle removal of crust or exudates daily from the eyelids using soft gauze sponges moistened with a buffered collyrium. A bactericidal, broad-spectrum antimicrobial ointment is applied four times daily, taking care not to contaminate the tip of the tube applicator. An Elizabethan collar may also be needed to prevent the animal from rubbing the eyes. Most bacterial conjunctivitis responds within 5 to 7 days.

Viral Conjunctivitis. Viral conjunctivitis may occur in the young dog and cat in mild to severe forms and in response to a variety of systemic viral diseases. Canine distemper virus infection produces hyperemia of the conjunctiva and serous ocular discharge in addition to other systemic signs associated with canine distemper. Conjunctival smears from acute canine distemper may yield intracytoplasmic inclusion bodies. As the disease progresses, ocular exudate becomes more copious and mucoid, and a keratitis develops. Schirmer's tear test values diminish, and mucopurulent nasal discharge ensues. Treatment is supportive and consists of administration of systemic and topical ophthalmic broad-spectrum antimicrobial agents and artificial tear preparations to maximize ocular tear volume.

Feline herpesvirus is the most serious of the feline viral diseases that affect the ocular surface. Three stages of ocular disease may occur. The first is a neonatal form, which consists of severe conjunctivitis and, occasionally, corneal perforation in kittens 2 to 4 weeks of age. The second stage consists of severe conjunctivitis accompanied by overt signs of upper respiratory infection in cats around 6 months of age. The third stage involves older cats with keratoconjunctivitis that may or may not be accompanied by signs of upper respiratory infection. Viral inclusion bodies are not easily seen on direct conjunctival smears by the time affected cats are presented to the veterinarian, but an initial lymphocytic response followed by a neutrophilic response as the herpesvirus infection progresses may be seen. A carrier state may develop in most affected cats, resulting in reinitiation of signs when the cat is stressed. Definitive diagnosis may be made by viral isolation via oropharyngeal swab procedures or by conjunctival/corneal biopsy analysis using fluorescent antibody or polymerase chain reaction techniques. Treatment involves the use of topical ophthalmic broad-spectrum antimicrobial agents to control secondary bacterial infection. In cases in which keratitis occurs, topical trifluridine or idoxuridine may be used five times daily for 7 to 10 days. Corticosteroid therapy should not be used because it enhances viral replication.

Feline calicivirus infection also produces a mild conjunctivitis and epiphora. Viral inclusion bodies are not seen on direct conjunctival smears. Virus isolation or fluorescent antibody testing of oropharyngeal swabs is required for definitive diagnosis. Topical ophthalmic antimicrobial agents administered four to five times daily may provide symptomatic relief throughout the overt course of the feline calicivirus infection, which usually lasts for 7 to 10 days. Feline reovirus infection is of least clinical significance and may result in a mild conjunctivitis with epiphora. The clinical course usually lasts for 2 to 3 weeks. Treatment of feline reovirus infection is similar to that of feline herpesvirus or feline calicivirus infections.

Mycoplasmal Conjunctivitis. Mycoplasmal infections have been identified in cats with upper respiratory infection. Initial signs attributed to the agent include epiphora and conjunctival hyperemia with a mucoid ocular discharge. As the disease progresses, the conjunctiva becomes pale, hypertrophic, and chemotic. Pseudomembrane formation in the conjunctival cul-de-sac is common. Giemsa-stained conjunctival smears may exhibit a neutrophilic response and clusters of basophilic staining coccoid organisms on the surface of the epithelial cells. The conjunctivitis has a self-limiting course of 3 to 4 weeks but may become chronic. An ophthalmic broad-spectrum antimicrobial agent applied topically may be helpful in reducing the severity of conjunctival signs. Tetracycline ointment applied four to five times daily is indicated, but the *Mycoplasma* organisms are often sensitive to most of the commonly used antimicrobial agents.

Feline Chlamydial Conjunctivitis. *Chlamydia psittaci* infection is one of the more serious ocular diseases involving the conjunctiva. *Chlamydia* infection begins as a unilateral conjunctivitis that typically becomes bilateral in 5 to 7 days. The conjunctiva may develop a gray coloration with serous discharge progressing to mucopurulent exudation. Conjunctival smears from infected eyes reveal intracytoplasmic inclusion bodies in conjunctival epithelial cells. Early diagnosis and treatment are usually effective and may prevent recurrent infection. Because *Chlamydia* organisms reproduce in epithelial cell cytoplasm, they are resistant to many antimicrobial agents. Infective forms of the organisms are released when the epithelial cell ruptures, and at this time topical tetracyclines and chloramphenicol are effective. Topical antimicrobial therapy must be continued for 28 days to completely cover the life cycle of the organism.

THE NICTITATING MEMBRANE
Prolapse of the Nictitans Gland

Incomplete development of soft tissue attachments will cause the nictitans gland to protrude beyond the leading edge of the third eyelid. Beagles, Boston terriers, cocker spaniels, Lhasa apsos, and English bulldogs and Burmese cats are commonly affected. Exposure of the nictitans gland's surface often contributes to conjunctivitis. A 30% to 57% decrease in tear production can be expected when the nictitans gland is removed. Partial gland resection, leaving a portion of the secretory gland tissue, is effective, but repositioning of the nictitans gland to preserve its tear-producing capabilities is preferred. The prolapsed nictitans gland may be sutured to adjacent tissue such as orbital fascia, extraocular muscle, or sclera, or its overlying conjunctiva may be imbricated to return the nictitans gland to a more normal position.

Eversion of the Cartilage

Eversion of the cartilage is characterized by a scroll-like appearance of the nictitating membrane's leading edge. The junction of the horizontal and vertical arms of the T-shaped cartilage appears to be the weakest segment of the cartilage. Eversion occurs in several dog breeds, including the Great Dane, Saint Bernard, German shepherd, Weimaraner, German short-haired pointer, golden and Labrador retrievers, and English bulldog, as well as the Burmese cat. Clinical signs in affected animals include watery or mucoid ocular discharges and lymphoid hyperplasia in long-standing cases. Removal of the malformed section of cartilage through an incision on the bulbar surface is recommended. The gland of the nictitating membrane may prolapse after the cartilage resection.

THE GLOBE AND ORBIT
Congenital Abnormalities

Microphthalmos. Failure of the eye to develop to normal size is referred to as *microphthalmos*. Complete absence of the eye (anophthalmos) is extremely unusual in puppies and kittens. Microphthalmos is characterized by varying degrees of enophthalmos, with or without other ocular defects. Microphthalmos with multiple colobomas is an autosomal recessive trait linked to coat color in the Australian shepherd. In addition to small globes, affected dogs may have persistent pupillary membranes, cataract, equatorial staphylomas, choroidal hypoplasia, retinal dysplasia and detachment, and optic nerve hypoplasia. Vision is frequently impaired. Other breeds in which multiple ocular defects have been associated with coat color include the Great Dane, collie, Shetland sheepdog, and dachshund. Microphthalmos is also associated with inherited congenital cataracts in the miniature schnauzer, Old English sheepdog, Akita, and King Charles Cavalier spaniel. Microphthalmos occurs with retinal dysplasia in Bedlington and Sealyham terriers, beagles, Labrador retrievers, and Doberman pinschers. Administration of griseofulvin to pregnant cats may produce microphthalmos in their offspring.

Atypical Eye Position. Strabismus is outward or inward deviation of the eye. Kittens are born with an outward or divergent strabismus that is noted after eyelid opening and normally should be corrected by 2 months of age. Divergent strabismus also occurs in brachycephalic dog breeds, notably the Boston terrier. Convergent or inward strabismus (cross-eye appearance) is inherited in the Siamese cat as an autosomal recessive trait. The abnormality is caused by aberrant development of the central visual pathways, particularly the lateral geniculate nucleus. Bilateral ventrolateral strabismus may be seen in puppies and kittens with hydrocephalus because of the enlargement of the calvaria and bony orbits.

A wandering movement of the eyes in young puppies and kittens (ocular nystagmus) is generally associated with congenital blindness. Rapid, repetitive, involuntary movement of the eyes (nystagmus) commonly occurs in Siamese kittens and may be related to the neuroanatomic abnormalities that produce strabismus. Vision is functionally normal. The nystagmus may lessen as the kitten matures. Nystagmus also occurs in some cats with Chediak-Higashi syndrome.

Acquired Abnormalities

Orbital Cellulitis and Abscessation. Orbital cellulitis is usually characterized by an acute-onset unilateral exophthalmos, protrusion of the third eyelid, chemosis, pain on opening the mouth, and fever. In addition, abscessation typically causes a swelling or discoloration in the mouth behind the last maxillary molar. Foreign objects and fight wounds are likely causes in puppies and kittens. *Cuterebra* larvae may occasionally invade the orbit and cause the orbital cellulitis. Response to twice-daily hot compresses and a broad-spectrum systemic antimicrobial agent is generally rapid. If no response is noted within 24 hours, incising the mucous membrane behind the last maxillary molar and inserting a small hypodermic needle into the retrobulbar area establishes ventral drainage. In many cases, only a serosanguinous discharge is seen on withdrawal of the hypodermic needle. Damage to orbital structures occurs when the procedure is performed carelessly. If exophthalmos is extreme, a bland ophthalmic ointment may be applied to the corneal surface to prevent drying.

Orbital Neoplasia. Orbital neoplasia should be considered in any puppy or kitten with gradual, painless exophthalmos. Neoplasia is more common in older animals, although embryonal neoplasia can affect young animals. Orbital involvement with lymphosarcoma and fibrosarcoma may also occur in young cats.

Traumatic Displacement. Complete displacement of the eye from the orbit is most commonly seen in brachycephalic dogs, but cats may also present with proptosis, retrobulbar hemorrhage, or fracture of the bony orbit. A completely displaced eye is an emergency and should be treated as soon as possible. A soft eye, indicating rupture of the fibrous tunic, or one with extensive avulsion of extraocular muscles or optic nerve, should be enucleated. Those with severe intraocular hemorrhage usually shrink over time because of irreparable damage to the ciliary body. A more favorable prognosis accompanies the intact eye with a constricted pupil. Most animals require general anesthesia to replace the eye. The eye should first be irrigated with sterile physiologic saline solution. A blunt probe, such as a strabismus or spay hook, is used to elevate the eyelid margins, and simultaneous gentle counterpressure is applied against the cornea with a moistened cotton ball to push the eye back into place. Preplaced sutures can be used in place of the blunt probe to elevate the eyelid margins. Once the eye is replaced, the eyelids are closed using horizontal mattress sutures of 4-0 nonabsorbable material placed over stents. Sutures should enter the eyelid 5 mm from the margin and exit through the meibomian gland openings to prevent corneal damage.

Broad-spectrum systemic antimicrobial agents and a taping level of corticosteroids are recommended for 7 to 10 days. If the animal allows, topical antimicrobial ointment may be applied three or four times daily between the eyelid margins at the medial canthus. Warm compresses are recommended for 3 to 4 days after the replacement. Sutures should be left in place for at least 10 to 14 days and should be replaced if the animal is unable to close the eyelids after the sutures are removed. Prognosis for vision is not known until after suture removal. Sequelae include lateral strabismus due to rupture of the medial rectus muscle, blindness, low tear production, and postinflammatory atrophy of the eye (phthisis bulbi).

Enophthalmos. Enophthalmos is recession of the eye within the orbit. Saint Bernards, Great Danes, Doberman pinschers, golden retrievers, and Irish setters often appear enophthalmic owing to their large orbits and deeply set eyes. Congenital enophthalmos is most often associated with microphthalmos. Acquired causes may include chronic orbital inflammation, loss of retrobulbar fat in debilitated or slow-growing animals, and phthisis bulbi. Causes of transient enophthalmos include Horner's syndrome, in which loss of sympathetic tone in the orbital fascia results in the eye's sunken appearance, or any painful eye disorder. Enophthalmos may be accompanied by mucoid to mucopurulent discharge, ptosis, and entropion.

THE CORNEA

Congenital Abnormalities

Corneal Opacities. The cornea of the newborn puppy or kitten is a light blue color; or at least the cornea is less clear than that of the adult. In 2 to 4 weeks, corneal clearing is sufficient to permit ophthalmoscopic examination. It is not unusual to observe multifocal or diffuse faint white opacities in the corneas of young puppies and kittens. The opacities represent superficial foci of edema, and most are self-limiting. The cause of these opacities is unknown. Therapy is not necessary unless the opacities are accompanied by a mucopurulent discharge, in which case topical ophthalmic antimicrobial preparations may be applied. Animals born with their eyelids open often have diffuse corneal edema that clears in 14 to 18 days. Because reflex lacrimation is absent at birth, the exposed cornea is subject to desiccation and infection and can be avoided by frequent application of a broad-spectrum antimicrobial ointment every 3 or 4 hours until the animal is 10 to 12 days old.

Cats with lysosomal storage diseases may develop corneal opacities related to the accumulation of polysaccharides within the endothelial cells and fibroblasts of the cornea. Fine granular deposits in the corneal stroma may give the eye a ground-glass appearance as early as 8 weeks of age. Corneal clouding or stippling may occur in kittens with GM_1 gangliosidosis, in cats of Siamese ancestry with mucopolysaccharidosis I and mucopolysaccharidosis VI, and in Persians with α-mannosidosis.

Deep corneal opacities are usually associated with remnants of embryonic pupillary membranes (persistent pupillary membranes) that adhere to the inner corneal surface (Fig. 14–8). The tissue strands, which arise from the anterior iris face, should be differentiated from postinflammatory synechiae extending from the pupillary margin. Therapy is not indicated in most cases, and on occasion the corneal opacity may diminish over several weeks or months.

Dermoid. Owners often notice a skin-like appendage soon after the animal's eyelids separate (Fig. 14–9). The dermoid usually involves the temporal cornea and conjunctiva in both puppies and kittens. Saint Bernards, German shepherds, dachshunds, and Dalmatians and the Birman and Burmese cats have an increased incidence of dermoids. If the dermoid contains no hair, any signs of squinting and ocular discharge may be minimal. Therapy consists of superficial keratectomy, usually performed

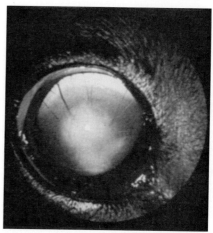

Figure 14–8. Persistent pupillary membranes contact the corneal endothelium, creating a nonprogressive opacity.

around 12 to 14 weeks of age. Complete excision is essential, or regrowth may occur.

Acquired Abnormalities

Symblepharon. An infectious conjunctivitis and keratitis that develop before eyelid separation may result in adhesion of the conjunctiva to the cornea (symblepharon). A similar situation also may follow chronic conjunctivitis associated with upper respiratory infection in cats. Ophthalmic examination shows a thin vascularized membrane overlying the cornea (Fig. 14–10). Occasionally, the overlying tissue can be partially elevated from the corneal surface with topical anesthesia and a small-toothed for-

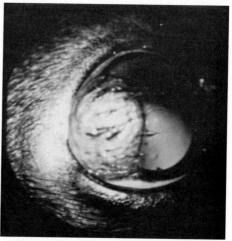

Figure 14–9. A dermoid overlies the temporal conjunctiva and cornea in a dachshund puppy.

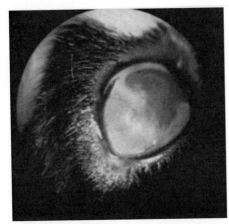

Figure 14–10. Infectious keratoconjunctivitis resulted in extensive symblepharon and corneal opacification in this 8-week-old kitten.

ceps. Prompt medical therapy of external eye disease minimizes symblepharon formation. Surgical repair is difficult, and re-adherence following surgery is common.

Dystrophies. Corneal dystrophies are familial, bilaterally symmetric corneal opacities that can affect any layer of the cornea. Stromal dystrophies in dogs are characterized by deposition of triglycerides, phospholipids, and neutral fat within the cornea; the cat more often demonstrates stromal edema and ulceration. Most stromal dystrophies appear after 1 year of age, but occasionally dogs may demonstrate mild corneal changes before 6 months of age. The Siberian husky dog is best known for its corneal dystrophy, which appears in the central cornea as a round or horizontally oval opacity as early as 5 months of age. The affected corneas ultimately show a homogeneous gray haze but in the early stages may only contain fine, highly refractile crystals in the stroma (Fig. 14–11). The inherited trait is recessive, with variable expressivity. Although the corneal opacities seldom become dense enough to affect vision, the use of affected dogs in breeding programs is not recommended. There is no treatment.

An axial dystrophy occurs in Airedale terriers as early as 6 months of age. Stromal deposition of triglycerides and neutral fats results in marked subepithelial opacification. The terrier's vision deteriorates as the axial dystrophy progresses. Multifocal 1- to 3-mm opacities may occur in the central superficial corneas of Shetland sheepdogs at 6 months of age. These sheepdogs at 3 to 4 years of age develop epithelial erosions overlying the corneal opacities. A progressive corneal dystrophy occurs in stump-tailed Manx cats. Early signs of axial outer stromal edema are noticed at approximately 4 months of age. The cornea progressively deteriorates, with accumulation of fluid-filled vesicles within the stroma (bullous keratopathy). Eventually, breakdown of both the epithelium and stroma occurs. An autosomal recessive pattern of inheritance is suspected.

Melanosis. Superficial corneal pigmentation is common in young brachycephalic dogs, notably the Chinese pug, Shih Tzu, Lhasa apso, and Pekingese. The pigmentation occurs most often in the nasal corneal quadrant, sometimes involving the adjacent conjunctiva. Therapy is directed at correcting adnexal abnormalities such as medial entropion and canthal trichiasis, which promotes additional pigmentation.

Sequestra. A recognizable corneal degeneration occurs in the cat that is characterized by formation of a brown to black superficial plaque in the cornea (Fig. 14–12). A breed predisposition has been identified in the Persian and Siamese. The corneal degeneration is often accompanied by corneal ulceration and superficial vascularization. The discolored plaque should be differentiated from corneal pigmentation by its sparing of the peripheral cornea. The sequestrum is excised by superficial keratectomy.

Injuries. Small corneal perforations are accompanied by pain, perilesional corneal edema, anterior uveitis, and sometimes hyphema. If the depth of the anterior chamber is comparable with that of the unaffected eye, the perforation

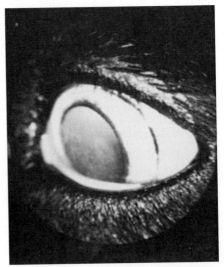

Figure 14–11. A lipid dystrophy appears as a faint, granular opacity in the central cornea of a Siberian husky puppy.

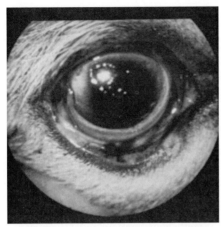

Figure 14–12. A corneal sequestrum appears as a darkly colored plaque in the central cornea of a young Abyssinian cat.

may have sealed itself and require no more than restricted activity, topical and systemic antimicrobial agents, and topical atropine. Ophthalmic ointments should be avoided in the perforated eye because the oil base of the ointment causes a severe reaction when introduced into the anterior chamber. Larger corneal perforations and lacerations require prompt surgical repair. These injuries have more severe corneal edema and uveitis; prolapsed iris tissue may also extend above the corneal surface (Fig. 14–13). Preoperative examination should be minimal to prevent any further damage to the eye. The surgical techniques and reparative capability of the cornea are similar to those in the adult animal.

Foreign Objects. After application of topical anesthesia, superficial corneal foreign objects

may be removed with a moistened sterile cotton-tipped swab, a 25-gauge needle, or a slightly blunted ophthalmic instrument known as a foreign body spud. Deeper foreign objects require general anesthesia and surgical extraction. After removal, a broad-spectrum antimicrobial solution is applied four to six times daily to prevent infection. Topical atropine is used as needed to dilate the pupil.

Ulceration. Corneal ulceration exists when there is a loss of epithelium and some portion of the corneal stroma. Most corneal ulcers are caused by traumatic insult, either from another animal or from such endogenous factors as low tear production or eyelid abnormalities. Secondary bacterial infection may occur once the corneal surface has been disrupted. Although corneal ulcers associated with feline herpesvirus infection are well characterized, such ulcers are uncommon in kittens younger than 6 months of age. The fluorescein dye test can be used to determine epithelial integrity after the eyelids have been completely separated in puppies and kittens. If the epithelium is disrupted, the stroma will absorb the dye and the ulcerated area will appear bright green. Fluorescein staining is to be performed after a Schirmer's tear test and corneal culture have been completed.

Superficial corneal ulcers in which only epithelium and superficial stroma are missing may heal in just a few days. Treatment is summarized in Table 14–2. Corticosteroids are not recommended in the treatment of corneal ulcers because they slow epithelial healing and potentiate destructive enzymatic activity within the corneal lesion. If the animal rubs the eye, use of an Elizabethan collar or other protective device is indicated. When corneal healing is delayed, ectopic cilia or other adnexal abnormalities should be pursued. Tear production should also be evaluated, and corneal culture and cytology should be done to rule out an infectious cause.

Deep corneal ulcers are more likely to have an infectious cause; bacterial culture and sensitivity testing should be performed. Tear production should also be evaluated. Brachycephalic dog breeds are predisposed to the development of deep ulcers and descemetoceles, probably related to traumatic insult or corneal exposure (Fig. 14–14). These dogs also may develop collagenase-associated ulcers that are characterized by a melting, gelatinous appearance in the affected cornea. Epithelial cells, inflammatory cells, and various bacteria, especially *Pseudomonas*, produce the collagenase responsible for the rapid corneal breakdown. An antimicrobial

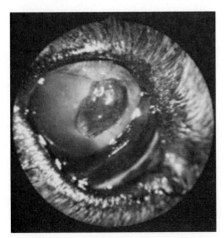

Figure 14–13. A full-thickness corneal laceration is accompanied by uveal tissue prolapse and hyphema.

Table 14–2 Treatment of Superficial Corneal Ulceration

INITIAL THERAPY

Eliminate underlying cause of the ulcer;
bactericidal antimicrobial solution q4h;
1% atropine solution q12–24h (if miotic);
apply protective collar

Reevaluate in 48–72 h

IF IMPROVED	IF NOT IMPROVED
Continue antimicrobial solution; reduce frequency of atropine solution to q24–48h; reevaluate in 3–5 d	Evaluate tear production; rule out misdirected cilia, foreign object; culture/cytology of ulcer, determine adherence of marginal epithelium; continue intial therapy; reevaluate in 24 h

IF FLUORESCEIN STAIN NEGATIVE	IF NOT IMPROVED
Continue antimicrobial solution for 5 more days; discontinue atropine solution	Repeat diagnostic procedures; change antimicrobial solution if antimicrobial sensitivity testing dictates; consider another opinion or referral

agent with activity against *Pseudomonas* species should be instilled hourly until culture results are obtained. Acetylcysteine solution, diluted to 5% to 10% with artificial tears, is also applied hourly until collagenolysis stops. Topical 1% atropine solution is used for the concurrent anterior uveitis. Deep ulcers with impending corneal rupture necessitate surgical intervention, such as a third eyelid flap, temporary apposition of the eyelids (tarsorrhaphy), conjunctival flap, or corneoscleral transposition.

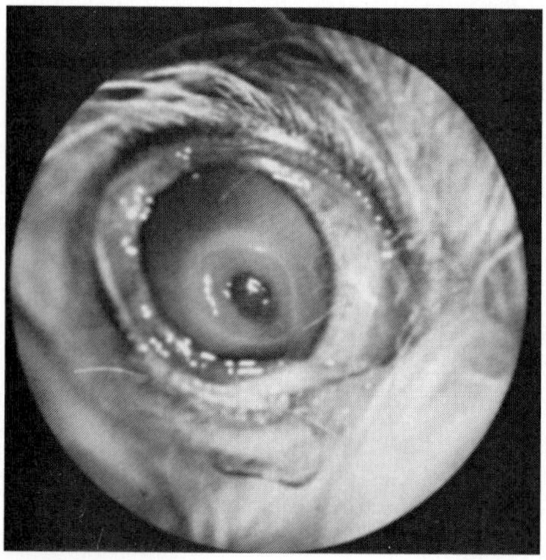

Keratoconjunctivitis Sicca. The early stages of inadequate tear production are frequently characterized by conjunctivitis, varying amounts of tenacious mucopurulent discharge, and a dull, irregular appearance to the cornea. As inadequate tear production persists, gradual vascularization and pigmentation of the cornea occur, and corneal ulcers may appear. Eventually, total corneal pigmentation is noted. Diagnosis is confirmed by determination of tear production using the Schirmer's tear test. A standardized strip of absorbent paper is creased, inserted over the lower eyelid into the conjunctival sac, and left for 1 minute. Values below 10 mm/min are indicative of inadequate tear production, regardless of the animal's age.

The causes of inadequate tear production in puppies and kittens are varied. Congenital lacrimal gland abnormalities may be present, resulting in delayed separation of the eyelids and early signs of corneal disease. Dogs with canine distemper and cats with acute or chronic upper respiratory tract infection may develop inadequate tear production. Traumatic insult to the nictitans gland or its nerve supply also reduces tear production. Tear production may improve

Figure 14–14. A deep corneal ulcer requires surgical correction in this young Shih Tzu dog. The center of the ulcer extends to Descemet's membrane.

with once or twice daily topical application of 2% cyclosporine formulated for ophthalmic use. Alternatively, an artificial tear, broad-spectrum antimicrobial agent, and corticosteroid are combined for topical application as frequently as possible in the nonulcerated eye. A mucolytic such as acetylcysteine may be added at a concentration of 5% if mucopurulent discharge is excessive. The resulting solution requires refrigeration. Artificial tear ointment at bedtime should minimize overnight drying. Improvement should occur within 6 to 8 weeks of applied topical regimen.

THE ANTERIOR UVEA

The irides of the puppy and kitten are often a different color than those of the adult. The blue-gray iris of puppies and kittens usually changes to the adult coloration within a few weeks. Iris color is ultimately related to the degree of stromal pigmentation and is influenced by coat color.

Congenital Abnormalities

Persistent Pupillary Membranes. Persistent pupillary membranes are strands of tissue that arise from the anterior iris surface and represent remnants of an embryonic vascular system. The persistent pupillary membranes may be confined to the iris surface or may extend from the iris to the cornea or lens (see Fig. 14–8). Persistent pupillary membranes are inherited in the basenji.

Iris Cysts. Iris cysts are floating, fluid-filled vesicles that arise from the posterior iris epithelium and are usually found in the anterior chamber. Iris cysts may be unilateral or bilateral and singular or multiple in number.

Pupillary Abnormalities. A notch-like defect (coloboma) is occasionally seen in the ventronasal pupillary border of young dogs and cats, resulting in a keyhole-shaped pupil. An eccentric pupil (corectopia) may accompany multiple ocular defects, as occurs in the Australian shepherd. Eccentric pupils are usually oval and 1 to 2 mm off center (Fig. 14–15).

Heterochromia. Heterochromia is a variation in iris color. Heterochromia may describe zones of different colors in a single iris or may refer to the iris of one eye being different in color from the other. This difference in coloration is commonly seen in subalbinotic animals, including the merle-coated collie, Shetland

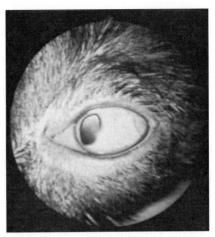

Figure 14–15. An eccentric pupil (corectopia) may signal multiple ocular anomalies.

sheepdog, Australian shepherd, harlequin Great Dane, Siberian husky, malamute, and Dalmatian dogs, and Siamese and white-coated cats. Variations in the degree of pigmentation in the retinal pigment epithelium and choroid may occur simultaneously. In white-coated cats, blue iris color is often associated with unilateral or bilateral deafness. Pale iris coloration may be a distinguishing feature of cats with Chediak-Higashi syndrome. Affected irides are pale yellow-green rather than the bold copper or yellow of the unaffected Persian cat.

Iridocorneal Abnormalities. Congenital mesodermal goniodysgenesis occurs in the iridocorneal angle of the basset hound. This mesodermal goniodysgenesis often forms extensive barriers across the iridocorneal angle, predisposing the animal to impaired aqueous outflow. Despite the presence of the congenital mesodermal goniodysgenesis, the onset of glaucoma does not usually occur in the basset hound until the dog is older than 6 months.

Acquired Abnormalities: Anterior Uveitis

Early recognition and treatment of anterior uveitis are important because the condition is painful and potentially blinding. Traumatic insult, toxicosis, and infectious diseases are common causes of anterior uveitis in young dogs and cats but not neoplastic, metabolic, or degenerative disorders. Anterior uveitis may result from disorders limited to the eye itself or may be secondary to systemic illness. Primary ocular abnormalities resulting in anterior uveitis are generally unilateral. Traumatic insult is probably the most common cause of a unilateral anterior uveitis in the young dog and cat.

The nature of intraocular foreign objects determines the characteristics of the intraocular inflammation. The most reactive materials include iron, steel, copper, and organic matter. Relatively inert materials include lead, glass, plastic, and rubber. Infection of extraocular tissues, such as a corneal ulcer, with breaching of the corneal/scleral barrier by pathogens or their toxins, may result in severe intraocular inflammation. Aberrant intraocular parasites, including *Ancylostoma* species, *Toxocara* species, and *Cuterebra* organisms, can cause anterior uveitis and subsequently endophthalmitis. Although *Dirofilaria immitis* occurs in the anterior chamber of dogs, affected animals are older than 6 months.

Anterior uveitis secondary to systemic illness is generally bilateral. Infectious diseases with secondary ocular effects are numerous. Anterior uveitis associated with canine adenovirus type 2 and canine distemper infections are uncommon, but canine herpesvirus commonly causes a panuveitis in young puppies. Feline infectious peritonitis is associated with prominent ocular signs. Feline leukemia virus and feline immunodeficiency virus infections rarely cause primary ocular disease. Intraocular hemorrhage and anterior uveitis are more likely secondary to severe anemia and metastatic lymphosarcoma, respectively. Ocular manifestations of bacterial infections may arise secondary to localized infections such as osteomyelitis or may represent systemic bacterial diseases such as seen in sepsis, leptospirosis, or brucellosis. Systemic fungal diseases are frequently associated with anterior uveitis but are uncommon in young dogs and cats. Feline toxoplasmosis should be considered in bilateral anterior uveitis. Rickettsial diseases to be considered include Rocky Mountain spotted fever and ehrlichiosis.

Anterior uveitis is often identified at least initially by the presence of lacrimation, blepharospasm, and enophthalmos—immediate indicators of ocular pain. Of the specific findings, conjunctival and episcleral hyperemia is the first to appear. Generalized corneal edema follows. Blood vessels may invade the deep corneal layers, forming a red paintbrush ring around the corneal circumference. The aqueous humor appears cloudy as protein enters the anterior chamber through the disrupted blood-aqueous barrier. Other changes in the anterior chamber include the influx of leukocytes (hypopyon), erythrocytes (hyphema), or fibrin strands. Col-

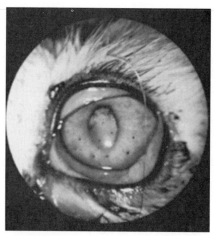

Figure 14–16. Inflammatory cells precipitate onto the corneal endothelium in a cat with feline infectious peritonitis.

lections of inflammatory cells on the inner corneal surface are referred to as keratic precipitates (Fig. 14–16). Changes in the pupil include miosis (Fig. 14–17) and sluggish response to light. Adhesions of the iris to the lens (posterior synechiae) may cause permanent changes in the pupillary shape. Inflammation of the ciliary body causes decreased aqueous production and a decline in intraocular pressure.

Treatment of anterior uveitis is usually symptomatic care (Table 14–3). Corticosteroids are used to reduce inflammation as quickly as possible. Topical application of 0.1% dexamethasone or 1% prednisolone acetate is performed every 2 to 4 hours in the early management of anterior uveitis. Even hourly applications may be

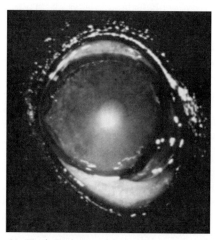

Figure 14–17. Anterior uveitis is characterized by corneal edema, aqueous turbidity, and miosis.

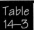

Table 14-3	Treatment of Anterior Uveitis

INITIAL TOPICAL THERAPY

1% prednisolone acetate suspension q4h;
1% atropine solution as needed to dilate pupil

Reevaluate after 24 h

IF IMPROVED

Reduce frequency of prednisolone acetate suspension to q6h; continue atropine solution as needed to maintain mydriasis; reevaluate in 72 h

IF NO IMPROVEMENT*

Recheck for corneal ulcer, continue initial therapeutic regimen; if no mydriasis, add topical 10% phenylephrine solution q6h; consider subconjunctival corticosteroids; reevaluate in 24 h

IF IMPROVED

1% prednisolone acetate suspension q8h; reduce frequency of application of atropine solution to maintain mydriasis; continue therapy 10–14 d beyond resolution of uveitis

IF NO IMPROVEMENT

Reevaluate diagnosis; continue above regimen; consider another opinion or referral

*If infectious disease has been ruled out and topical therapy is ineffective in controlling the uveitis, systemic corticosteroids may be included in the treatment plan.

necessary for severely inflamed eyes. In animals with severe anterior uveitis, subconjunctival corticosteroids may be used. Methylprednisolone and triamcinolone acetonide are generally well tolerated by the eye. The usual volume is 0.2 ml of a 40-mg/ml concentration. For severe anterior uveitis without systemic infectious disease, oral corticosteroids may be considered, especially if the choroid is involved. The dosage of prednisolone, beginning at 1 to 2 mg/kg every 12 hours, should be gradually reduced as soon as ocular response allows. Abrupt cessation may be associated with a rebound of severe inflammation.

Pupillary dilation is accomplished by topical application of a parasympatholytic agent such as 1% atropine applied to effect. The inflamed iris will not respond as well to atropine as the unaffected iris, and the effects may diminish sooner than expected. Atropine reduces pain as uveal muscle spasm is relieved, prevents adhesions between iris and lens, and restores vascular permeability. Cats may salivate following application of atropine when the bitter drug exits the nasolacrimal system and is licked from the nose. If atropine is ineffective, 10% phenylephrine may be used in the regimen for its synergistic sympathetic effect. Therapy should be contin-

ued for 10 to 14 days beyond resolution of ocular signs.

GLAUCOMA

Congenital glaucoma is usually secondary to traumatic insult or inflammation. Normal intraocular pressure in the young dog and cat ranges between 15 and 30 mmHg. Acute glaucoma is painful and accompanied by conjunctival and episcleral hyperemia, generalized corneal edema, pupillary dilation, and vision loss (Fig. 14–18). With prolonged pressure elevations, degeneration of the retina and optic nerve results in permanent blindness. Determination of intraocular pressure confirms the glaucoma diagnosis.

The aim of immediate therapy for glaucoma is to save or return vision through immediate control of intraocular pressure. Decisive treatment should be administered with minimal delay, as marked increases in intraocular pressure result in irreversible damage to the retina and optic nerve in 24 to 48 hours. A combination of agents yields the greatest reduction in intraocular pressure (Table 14–4). A 20% mannitol is administered intravenously at 1 to 2 g/kg early in acute glaucoma management to reduce

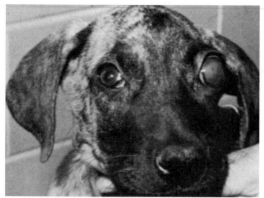

Figure 14–18. Scleral elasticity is responsible for the dramatic buphthalmos that accompanies glaucoma in the puppy or kitten. (Courtesy of Dr. Gretchen M. Schmidt, Wheeling, Illinois.)

intraocular pressure quickly. Pressure begins to decrease within 10 to 15 minutes; the effect lasts for 5 to 6 hours. Reduction in aqueous production is achieved with carbonic anhydrase inhibitors, such as dichlorphenamide administered twice daily at 2.5 to 5 mg/kg orally. Aqueous outflow may be improved by the use of a miotic, such as 2% pilocarpine applied topically three or four times daily. Miotics are not effective at intraocular pressures above 50 mmHg, so it is important to combine them with the other drugs listed previously.

Surgical therapy is indicated if medical therapy cannot lower intraocular pressure sufficiently within 24 to 48 hours, if wide variations in diurnal pressures exist, or if the owner is unwilling to dedicate time to daily therapy. There is no universal acceptance of any of the surgical procedures for glaucoma. Cyclocryotherapy is often used because it is noninvasive and an 80% success rate has been reported by various investigators. By applying a cryoprobe to the sclera overlying the ciliary body, one can damage portions of the secretory epithelium, and aqueous production is reduced.

THE LENS AND VITREOUS

The lens develops rapidly in the early stages of embryogenesis, during which time it is nourished by the hyaloid vessel. The fully developed lens is avascular; by the second week of life, no remnants of the hyaloid system should remain. The normal lens often exhibits minor imperfections that can be easily detected with magnification in dogs and cats younger than 1 year. These include prominent anterior and posterior Y sutures and minute granules in its nucleus and cortex. A mosaic of brown pigment spots is occasionally seen on the anterior lens capsule near the center of the pupil, representing remnants of embryonic mesoderm. Disease of the vitreous would be expected to influence the lens

Table 14–4	Treatment of Early-Onset Primary Glaucoma

ADMINISTER CONCURRENTLY

20% mannitol solution 1 g/kg IV;
dichlorphenamide (50-mg tablets) 2.5 mg/kg PO q12h;
2% pilocarpine ophthalmic solution topically q3h

Reevaluate IOP in 1–2 h

                                    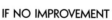

IF IMPROVED	IF NO IMPROVEMENT
Do not repeat mannitol solution; reduce topical pilocarpine solution to q8h; recheck IOP q4h	Repeat mannitol solution, 1 g/kg IV; continue topical pilocarpine solution q3h; recheck IOP in 1–2 h

IF IMPROVED/STABLE	IF NO IMPROVEMENT
Continue dichlorphenamide tablets q12h; continue topical pilocarpine solution q8h; consider cyclocryotherapy for maintenance	Reevaluate diagnosis; increase dichlorphenamide tablets to q8h; continue topical pilocarpine solution q6h; consider immediate referral

IV = Intravenous administration; IOP = intraocular pressure; PO = oral administration.

or retina because of its attachments at the posterior lens surface and the optic disc.

Congenital Abnormalities

Congenital lens abnormalities include alterations in size or shape. Congenital absence of the lens (aphakia) is uncommon. In microphakia, the margin of the abnormally small lens along with elongated ciliary processes may be observed after pupillary dilation. Microphakia occurs along with other ocular defects in the Saint Bernard and beagle and in cats. Luxation of the microphakic lens may cause glaucoma. Lenticonus is a cone-like anterior or posterior protrusion of the lens. Abnormally shaped lenses occur in many dog breeds, with or without associated opacities, and in Persian cats.

The most common vitreous abnormality is the retention of varying amounts of the hyaloid system. Hyaloid remnants are usually bloodless, appearing as a white vermiform structure that extends a short distance into the vitreous from the optic disc or from the posterior lens capsule. Such remnants are not associated with any recognizable visual deficits. Persistent hyperplastic primary vitreous is a congenital abnormality characterized by the presence of a fibrovascular membrane on the posterior lens surface. It usually is manifested by a congenital pupillary opacity (leukocoria), a fibrovascular sheath on the back of the lens with an attached hyaloid stalk, elongated ciliary processes, and secondary cataract (Fig. 14–19). A hereditary basis for persistent hyperplastic primary vitreous is established in Doberman pinschers, Staffordshire

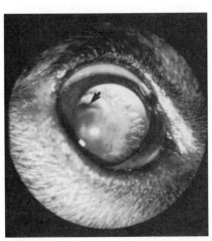

Figure 14–19. In addition to cataracts, this puppy demonstrates intralenticular hemorrhage (arrow) secondary to persistent hyperplastic primary vitreous.

bull terriers, Bouvier des Flandres, and possibly standard schnauzers.

Congenital Cataracts

Cataracts in dogs and cats younger than 6 months are usually congenital or juvenile cataracts. Congenital cataracts are present at birth, although they may be unnoticed until 6 to 8 weeks of age. They may be inherited or secondary to in utero influences, so it is important to question the owner regarding the presence of cataracts in the sire, dam, their previous litters, or their pedigrees. Congenital cataracts occur in Persian cats and are associated with multiple ocular defects in beagles, cocker spaniels, Old English sheepdogs, Australian shepherds, Bedlington terriers, and Sealyham terriers. Cataracts also occur in Labrador retrievers and Samoyeds with retinal dysplasia/detachment and skeletal abnormalities.

Juvenile Cataracts

Juvenile cataracts can develop from birth until 6 years of age. Although inflammatory, metabolic, nutritional, toxic, and traumatic events are considered to cause juvenile cataracts, heredity is the major cause. The development of juvenile cataracts is usually progressive, but their rate of progression varies. Complete opacification of the lens may occur in less than 1 year after recognition. Capsular and nuclear cataracts are usually nonprogressive, whereas cortical and equatorial cataracts are expected to progress.

Uveitis of any cause may precipitate juvenile cataract formation, as inflammatory adhesions disrupt the lens capsule and changes in aqueous humor affect lens metabolism. Metabolic cataracts secondary to diabetes mellitus may occur. Nutritional cataracts may occur in orphaned puppies and kittens fed a commercial milk replacer, presumably due to an imbalance in essential amino acids in the milk replacer. In most instances, the lens opacification is mild and decreases with eating a growth diet. Juvenile cataracts can be caused by various toxic influences, including chemicals, radiation, and electrical shock. Cataracts may occur in dogs given dimethyl sulfoxide. Traumatic insult to the lens may disrupt lens fibers or initiate an inflammatory response that leads to lens opacities. Traumatic insult is the most common cause of cataract in the young cat.

Inherited juvenile cataracts are known to occur in several breeds of dogs and cats (Figs. 14–20 and 14–21). Early recognition of cata-

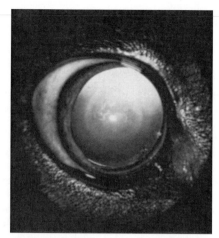

Figure 14–20. A 4-month-old German shepherd puppy demonstrates a nuclear cataract, unchanged from initial examination at 8 weeks of age. The dog also had retinal dysplasia.

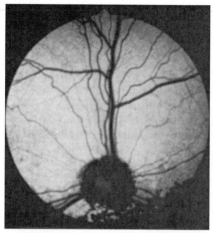

Figure 14–22. The normal canine fundus is characterized by a well-defined optic disc, over which lies a vascular anastomotic ring. Robust, branching vessels are seen throughout the reflective tapetal fundus.

racts is essential in eliminating affected animals from a breeding program (Table 14–5). Congenital or juvenile cataracts are best managed by temporization if functional vision is present because a high percentage may undergo spontaneous resorption within the first year. If uveitis develops, topical mydriatics and corticosteroids are indicated. Surgical lens extraction may be elected, but the effect of the lens opacities on visual pathway development should first be determined. Inadequate light stimulation from the time the eyelids open until approximately 12 weeks of age produces irreversible functional and structural abnormalities in the visual cortex.

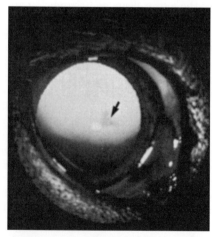

Figure 14–21. A 5-month-old golden retriever puppy demonstrates a triangular posterior polar cataract (arrow), believed to represent the heterozygous genotype for inherited cataract.

It is then possible for a successful lens extraction to be performed without improvement in the animal's visual capabilities.

THE RETINA AND OPTIC NERVE

Tapetal coloration of the fundus of the puppy and kitten is usually gray or blue at 6 to 8 weeks of age, gradually acquiring its adult coloration by 4 to 7 months of age when the tapetum matures. Myelination of the optic disc may also be incomplete in the puppy and kitten, giving the impression of a small, well-defined nerve head that takes on a more fluffy appearance as adult myelination occurs. The normal mature fundus is depicted in Figures 14–22 and 14–23. Both congenital and acquired disorders of the retina and optic nerve are recognized in the young dog and cat. These may be inherited, as with collie eye anomaly, or secondary to postnatal influences, as occurs with canine distemper–induced retinitis. Congenital abnormalities can be diagnosed as early as 6 weeks of age, when the posterior segment is clearly observed. The more common congenital abnormalities of the canine fundus are summarized in Table 14–6. Acquired abnormalities develop with advancing age and in this discussion are limited to those in dogs and cats younger than 6 months of age.

Congenital Anomalies of the Posterior Segment

Collie Eye Anomaly. An autosomal recessive trait affecting about 80% of the breed,

Table 14-5	Selected Inherited Cataracts of Young Dogs and Cats		
BREED	MODE OF INHERITANCE	LOCATION	PROGRESSION
Afghan hound	Not defined	Equatorial	Progressive
Akita	Not defined	Nuclear and cortical	Variable progression
Alaskan malamute	Not defined	Posterior subcapsular	Variable progression
American cocker spaniel	Autosomal recessive	Cortical	Progression
Australian shepherd	Not defined	Nuclear and cortical	Nonprogressive
Basenji	Not defined	Anterior capsular	Nonprogressive
Beagle	Not defined	Anterior capsular	Nonprogressive
Boston terrier	Not defined	Nuclear and cortical	Progressive
King Charles Cavalier spaniel	Not defined	Nuclear and cortical	Progressive
Chesapeake Bay retriever	Not defined	Posterior subcapsular	Variable progression
Chow chow	Not defined	Nuclear and cortical	Variable progression
Collie	Not defined	Nuclear and cortical	Unknown
Doberman pinscher	Dominant with incomplete penetrance	Posterior subcapsular	Variable progression
English cocker spaniel	Not defined	Anterior capsular	Nonprogressive
Flat coated retriever	Not defined	Posterior subcapsular	Nonprogressive
German shepherd	Autosomal dominant	Nuclear	Nonprogressive
Golden retriever	Not defined	Perinuclear	Progressive
		Posterior subcapsular	Nonprogressive
Labrador retriever	Incomplete dominance	Nuclear and cortical	Variable progression
	Not defined	Perinuclear	Progressive
		Posterior subcapsular	Nonprogressive
Miniature schnauzer	Autosomal recessive	Nuclear and cortical	Variable progression
Old English sheepdog	Not defined	Nuclear and cortical	Progressive
Poodle, toy and miniature	Not defined	Cortical	Progressive
Poodle, standard	Not defined	Equatorial	Progressive
Rottweiler	Not defined	Posterior subcapsular and cortical	Nonprogressive
Samoyed	Autosomal recessive	Nuclear and cortical	Variable progression
Siberian husky	Not defined	Posterior subcapsular equatorial	Variable progression
Staffordshire terrier	Not defined	Nuclear and cortical	Progressive
		Posterior subcapsular	Nonprogressive
Welsh springer spaniel	Autosomal recessive	Cortical	Progressive
West Highland white terrier	Autosomal recessive	Nuclear and cortical	Progressive
	Not defined	Posterior Y suture	Nonprogressive
British short-haired cat	Autosomal recessive	Nuclear	Unknown
Himalayan	Autosomal recessive	Cortical	Progressive

Table 14-6	Congenital Abnormalities of the Canine Fundus*	
DISORDER	BREED	CHARACTERISTIC FEATURES
Collie eye anomaly	Collie, Shetland sheepdog, border collie, Australian shepherd	Chorioretinal hypoplasia, optic disc coloboma, retinal detachment
Retinal dysplasia	Springer spaniel, Labrador retriever	Multifocal retinal folds, retinal detachment
	Cocker spaniel, beagle	Multifocal retinal folds
Hemeralopia	Alaskan malamute	Day blindness, normal fundus
Night blindness	Tibetan terrier, briard	Night blindness, normal fundus
Optic nerve hypoplasia	Any breed	Visual deficit, small optic disc

*Diagnosed as early as 6–8 wk of age.

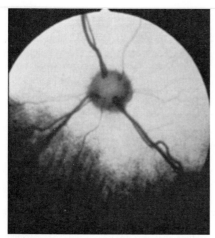

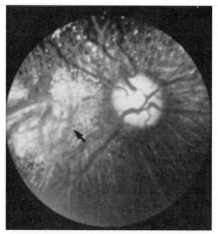

Figure 14–23. The normal feline fundus is characterized by a small, well-defined optic disc, several paired vessels that enter and leave the disc at its periphery, and a brightly reflective tapetum. Choroidal vessels are visible as dark streaks in the nontapetum due to a normal variation in pigmentation.

Figure 14–24. A common lesion of collie eye anomaly is chorioretinal hypoplasia in which anomalous choroidal vessels are visualized against the scleral background (arrow).

collie eye anomaly is characterized by an array of posterior segment abnormalities. Both smooth-coated and rough-coated collies are affected, regardless of color pattern. The disorder is usually nonprogressive and can be easily diagnosed in the 6- to 8-week-old puppy. Bilateral ophthalmoscopic lesions, in order of increasing severity, include choroidal hypoplasia, optic nerve and scleral colobomas, and retinal detachment. Affected eyes may demonstrate one or more of these lesions, although rarely symmetrically. Choroidal hypoplasia is a common finding in affected animals and appears to have minimal effect on functional vision. The lesion appears as a focal abnormality temporal to the optic disc, usually at the junction of the tapetal and nontapetal fundus (Fig. 14–24). Mildly affected puppies may demonstrate choroidal hypoplasia at 4 to 6 weeks of age, only to have the lesion masked by pigmentation as the eyes mature.

A coloboma occurs in about 20% to 30% of the breed. When the optic disc is affected, its surface appears excavated; overlying retinal vessels change course abruptly (Fig. 14–25). Scleral colobomas (also known as ectasias or staphylomas) produce similar excavations in the fibrous tunic and alterations in the course of the overlying vessels (Fig. 14–26). Visual field defects probably accompany large colobomas, but vision is functionally unimpaired. About 5% to 10% of affected animals experience retinal detachments. These may be congenital or may

occur in dogs up to 1 year of age with extensive colobomas.

Because of the high prevalence of collie eye anomaly, breeders have continued to breed affected animals. Owners should be warned that the breeding of mildly affected collies may produce offspring with more serious ocular defects than their parents. The Shetland sheepdog, border collie, and Australian shepherd also have a congenital ocular anomaly similar to that of the smooth-coated and rough-coated collie. The

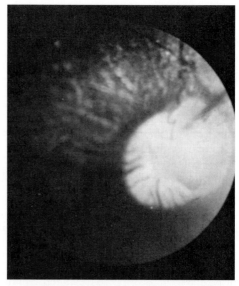

Figure 14–25. A pit-like depression or coloboma of the optic disc of a young collie dog may cause no recognizable defect in vision.

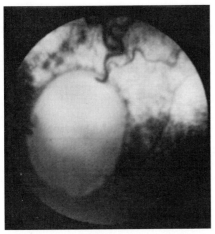

Figure 14–26. A peripapillary scleral defect (ectasia) gives the impression of an enlarged optic disc in a dog with collie eye anomaly.

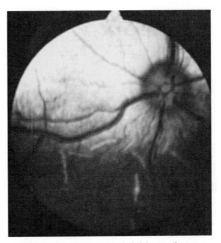

Figure 14–27. Multiple retinal folds in the nontapetal area of a collie puppy appear as white streaks against the pigmented background.

prevalence in the Shetland sheepdog is less than 20%, and its mode of inheritance is not known.

Microphthalmia with Colobomas. Large equatorial staphylomas occur in Australian shepherds with multiple ocular anomalies. These areas of thin, stretched sclera are up to 20 diopters deep. Associated ocular defects include retinal detachment, retinal dysplasia, pupillary abnormalities, and cataracts. The disorder is inherited as an autosomal recessive trait with incomplete penetrance. Affected dogs are homozygous merles and have a predominantly white haircoat. A similar syndrome occurs in merled Shetland sheepdogs, merled rough-coated collies, and harlequin Great Danes.

Retinal Folds. Retinal folds predominantly in the nontapetal portion of the fundus are seen frequently in young collies and occasionally in other breeds of dog. They appear as vermiform streaks because of their rod-like shape and pale color (Fig. 14–27). Retinal folds should be differentiated from the retinal disorganization that occurs in retinal dysplasia.

Heritable Retinal Dysplasia. Retinal dysplasia is characterized by folds in the outer retinal layers and by retinal rosettes, in which variably differentiated retinal cells are arranged around a central lumen. Severe forms of retinal dysplasia may demonstrate retinal detachment due to subretinal fluid accumulation. The diagnosis is easily made in the 6- to 8-week-old puppy or kitten. Many breeds of dog have retinal dysplasia alone or in association with other congenital ocular defects. Retinal dysplasia is uncommon in the cat.

English springer spaniels inherit retinal dysplasia as an autosomal recessive trait. Affected animals exhibit bilaterally nonprogressive, multifocal lesions that appear as round or linear areas of discoloration in the tapetal fundus (Fig. 14–28). As the tapetum matures, the margins of the dysplastic foci appear hyperreflective, while their centers are darkly pigmented. Vision is usually spared. Blindness results when retinal tears or detachment accompany severe disorganization of the retina.

Several types of retinal dysplasia occur in Labrador retrievers. One form closely resembles that of the English springer spaniel, with

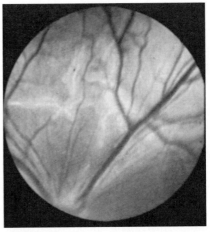

Figure 14–28. Retinal dysplasia in an 8-week-old springer spaniel puppy appears as branching folds overlying the immature tapetum. As the eye matures, these folds often appear hyperreflective with pigmented centers.

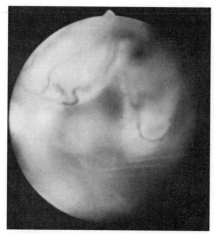

Figure 14–29. Severe forms of retinal dysplasia are characterized by blindness due to total retinal detachment, as in this young Labrador retriever dog.

multifocal folds and rosettes within the tapetal portion of the fundus. Another form is characterized by totally detached dysplastic retinas and blindness (Fig. 14–29). Both forms are recessively transmitted. Severe retinal dysplasia also occurs in association with short-limbed dwarfism. The gene has recessive effects on the skeleton and incompletely dominant effects on the eye. Affected animals demonstrate retinal detachments, corneal opacification, cataracts, and vitreal degeneration.

In vitreoretinal dysplasia of the Bedlington terrier, most affected dogs have a complete retinal detachment and are blind at initial examination. Sealyham terriers also present with totally detached dysplastic retinas and blindness, as well as microphthalmia. Multifocal retinal dysplasia is detected in American cocker spaniels. In the tapetal fundus, dysplastic foci appear as small linear or branching folds that are less reflective than adjacent unaffected tissue. In the nontapetal fundus, the folds appear white or gray in comparison with the normally pigmented background. Blindness or other apparent visual deficits have not been observed in these affected animals. A recessive mode of inheritance is likely. Beagles have multifocal retinal dysplasia that is similar to that of the American cocker spaniel. Other dog breeds in which retinal dysplasia are reported either singly or in association with multiple ocular defects include the Akita, Australian shepherd, Doberman pinscher, Old English sheepdog, Rottweiler, and Yorkshire terrier.

Nonheritable Retinal Dysplasia. The retina continues to mature until 6 to 8 weeks of age in both the puppy and kitten. Infectious agents incriminated in the dog to cause retinal dysplasia are canine herpesvirus, canine parvovirus-2, and canine adenovirus-1. In the kitten, irregular areas of atrophy in the tapetal fundus and pigment mottling in the nontapetal area follow in utero or postnatal feline parvovirus infection. Feline leukemia virus infection may also induce retinal dysplasia.

Tapetal Hypoplasia. Beagles with no visible tapetum and a uniform reddish brown fundus reflex are occasionally seen. The lack of tapetal development is inherited as an autosomal recessive trait. Lack of visible tapetum may occur infrequently in other breeds of dog and appears to have no discernible effect on vision. Cats affected with Chediak-Higashi syndrome may also have a reddish fundic reflection due to decreased tapetal development and fundic hypopigmentation.

Congenital Night Blindness. Night blindness is first evident by 6 weeks of age in the briard and Tibetan terrier. The fundus of the briard appears normal, whereas low-level illumination shows an increased tapetal granularity in the Tibetan terrier. Electroretinographic (ERG) studies confirm the presence of congenital retinal dysfunction. The inheritance pattern is not known, but an autosomal recessive mode is suspected.

Hemeralopia. Day blindness occurs in Alaskan malamutes, with onset of behavioral changes as early as 8 to 20 weeks of age. Hemeralopia also occurs in the miniature poodle by 3 months of age. Dogs are visually impaired in daylight but function well at night and on overcast days. The fundus appears normal in affected animals. Diagnosis is confirmed on ERG evidence of abnormal cone response.

Feline Retinal Degeneration. Hereditary retinal degeneration is uncommon in the cat. Diffuse outer segment retinal atrophy occurs in Persian kittens with signs of tapetal hyperreflectivity and retinal vessel attenuation. An autosomal recessive trait is suspected. Photoreceptor degeneration also occurs in domestic short-haired cats with visual impairment as early as 14 weeks of age and fundic signs similar to those in Persian cats. A dominant inheritance pattern is suspected.

GM$_1$ Gangliosidosis. Fundic lesions occur in 3-month-old kittens with lysosomal storage disease, although the progressive ataxia and tremors demonstrated by affected mixed-breed and Siamese cats are far more impressive. Accu-

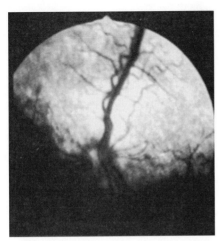

Figure 14–30. Optic nerve hypoplasia is characterized by a small optic disc, normal retinal vasculature, and poor vision.

mulations of glycolipid within retinal ganglion cells appear as small dark spots in the tapetum and pale gray spots in the nontapetal fundus. The disorder is transmitted as an autosomal recessive trait in the Siamese cat.

Optic Nerve Hypoplasia. Unilateral or bilateral optic nerve hypoplasia occurs infrequently in various breeds of dog, including the beagle, dachshund, collie, Russian wolfhound, German shepherd dog, Great Pyrenees, and Saint Bernard. Optic nerve hypoplasia is inherited in the miniature poodle. Unilateral lesions are often incidental findings because the dog compensates with the nonaffected eye. Poor vision is the usual presenting complaint in bilaterally affected animals, although owners may fail to recognize the vision problem when the animal is with its siblings. Affected eyes exhibit sluggish to absent direct pupillary light reflexes. Resting pupil size may be larger than normal. The affected optic disc is often less than half its normal size, its center is depressed, and the periphery is pigmented (Fig. 14–30). The retinal vasculature is usually normal. Complete aplasia of the optic nerve is uncommon.

Optic Nerve Colobomas. Colobomas of the optic disc are most often associated with collie eye anomaly. Colobomas also occur as one of a multitude of ocular anomalies found in the Australian shepherd and basenji and occasionally in the cocker spaniel. Choroidal and optic nerve colobomas are occasionally seen in domestic cats, including the domestic short-haired and Persian cats.

Acquired Disorders of the Posterior Segment

Progressive Retinal Atrophy. Progressive retinal atrophy (PRA) is an inherited disorder affecting the retinal photoreceptor layer. Early-age onset PRA occurs in the collie, Irish setter, and Norwegian elkhound and possibly also in the miniature schnauzer, Tibetan terrier, Cardigan Welsh corgi, and miniature long-haired dachshund. Dogs with PRA first demonstrate their visual deficit in dim lighting. Progressive loss of day vision occurs, followed by total blindness. The pupils dilate as PRA advances, and the owners may comment on the bright green or yellow tapetal reflection from the eyes. Total blindness usually occurs in 6 to 18 months after the onset of night blindness. If the dog's environment is changed suddenly, owners may mistake the dog's disorientation for acute vision loss. Progressive retinal atrophy is characterized by bilateral attenuation of the retinal vessels, involving first the peripheral arterioles and later the retinal veins. Altered tapetal reflectivity also occurs; as the retina thins and absorbs less light, the tapetum appears increasingly granular and hyperreflective (Fig. 14–31). Optic disc pallor and total absence of retinal vessels typify the most advanced cases of PRA.

Several types of PRA occur in the dog. The PRA in the collie, Irish setter, and Cardigan Welsh corgi is characterized as rod-cone dysplasia. Dysplastic abnormalities are evident as early as 24 days of age. Affected animals may demonstrate night blindness by 6 weeks, although the first detectable fundic evidence occurs at 14 to

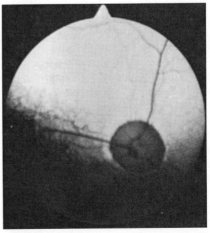

Figure 14–31. Night blindness, tapetal hyperreflectivity, and retinal vessel attenuation are characteristic of generalized progressive retinal atrophy.

16 weeks. Total blindness occurs by 1 year of age. The PRA is inherited as an autosomal recessive trait. A blood-based DNA test is available to identify the gene mutation responsible for rod-cone dysplasia in the Irish setter and Cardigan Welsh corgi. Two progressive retinopathies occur in the Norwegian elkhound: rod dysplasia and early retinal degeneration. Dogs affected with rod dysplasia show night blindness at 6 months of age but may retain some vision until 3 to 5 years of age. An ERG may detect rod dysplasia as early as 6 weeks of age, but only subtle changes in tapetal granularity are seen in the 6-month-old dog. Easily detectable fundic signs occur at 1 to 3 years of age. The signs of early retinal degeneration occur much earlier than those of rod dysplasia. Affected puppies are night blind by 6 weeks of age and totally blind by 1 year of age. Fundic changes are detectable at 6 months of age and advanced by 1 year. The mode of inheritance is autosomal recessive. A progressive retinal degeneration that differs from classic PRA occurs in the borzoi and papillon as early as 6 months of age. Initial lesions may be unilateral, with focal areas of hyperreflectivity in the extreme peripheral tapetum. These areas eventually coalesce into a diffuse retinal degeneration.

Hereditary retinal degeneration is uncommon in young cats. Signs of tapetal hyperreflectivity and retinal vessel attenuation are similar to those in affected dogs. An early-age onset rod-cone dysplasia occurs in the Abyssinian cat, inherited as an autosomal dominant trait. An increase in pupil size between 2 and 3 weeks of age is followed by changes in tapetal reflectivity by 8 weeks of age. Progressive vascular attenuation results in an avascular retina by 1 year of age. The ERG is unrecordable as early as 17 days of age.

Nonheritable Retinopathies. Primary retinitis is uncommon in the young dog and cat. More often, evidence of active retinitis accompanies choroidal disease and consists of cellular infiltration, exudation, edema, or hemorrhage. The retinitis appears as ill-defined areas of diminished tapetal reflectivity or nontapetal discoloration (Fig. 14–32). Inflammatory exudate from the choroid or the retina may separate the inner neural retina from the underlying pigment epithelium, causing a retinal detachment. Inactive retinitis lesions are well marginated, appearing hyperreflective in the tapetal region and depigmented in the nontapetal area (Fig. 14–33). Pigment clumping may be seen at the center of inactive inflammatory foci. Infectious causes of chorioretinitis in the young dog in-

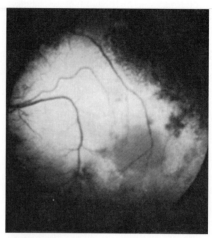

Figure 14–32. An exudate associated with active chorioretinitis creates a poorly marginated area of tapetal hyporeflectivity.

clude canine distemper, toxoplasmosis, bacterial septicemia, and intraocular larval migrans by *Toxocara canis*. Causes in the young cat include toxoplasmosis, lymphosarcoma, feline infectious peritonitis, and ophthalmomyiasis. Noninfectious causes range from toxins such as ethylene glycol to embryonic neuroepithelial tumors such as medulloepithelioma. Treatment is generally directed at the underlying systemic disease, remembering that topical medication does not reach therapeutic levels in the retina or the choroid.

Posterior segment hemorrhage may occur as a nonspecific component of chorioretinitis or may accompany one of several bleeding disor-

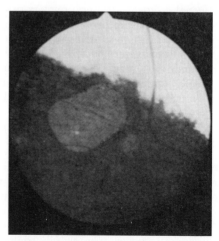

Figure 14–33. A well-demarcated zone of depigmentation in the nontapetal fundus suggests an inactive chorioretinitis. A similar lesion in the tapetal area would appear hyperreflective with a pigmented center.

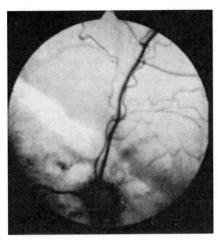

Figure 14–34. An early lesion of feline taurine deficiency appears as a hyperreflective band across the tapetal fundus. If not corrected, the dietary deficiency can lead to total blindness.

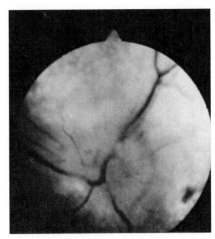

Figure 14–35. Optic neuritis is characterized by optic disc swelling, peripapillary retinal edema, hemorrhage, and sudden blindness.

ders, including anemia, immune-mediated disease, thrombocytopenia, or polycythemia. Retinal vascular congestion may occur with congenital heart defects, such as atrioventricular septal defects and tetralogy of Fallot, and secondary to systemic hypertension. Retinal hemorrhage and venous engorgement may occur in a cat with thiamine deficiency. Classically, taurine deficiency is seen in cats maintained on a taurine-poor diet. Retinal changes usually require several months to develop, but lesions have been identified within 18 weeks of beginning a taurine-poor diet. A bilaterally symmetric, hyperreflective ellipse develops temporal to the optic disc. This progresses to a horizontal band-shaped lesion across the posterior pole (Fig. 14–34). Progression results in generalized retinal atrophy and irreversible blindness.

Optic Neuritis. Optic neuritis is characterized by blindness during active inflammation. Bilateral cases show fixed, dilated pupils. The affected optic disc appears enlarged and hyperemic, with indistinct margins, peripapillary retinal elevation, and adjacent hemorrhage (Fig. 14–35). The causes of optic neuritis are varied and in the young dog or cat usually include infectious diseases and traumatic insult. Treatment is directed at the underlying cause. Systemic corticosteroids are indicated to minimize the amount of nerve damage. Oral prednisolone (1 to 2 mg/kg) is administered daily for 14 days, then gradually decreased in dosage over 2 to 3 weeks until an alternate-day maintenance dose is reached. In general, if medical therapy is successful, improvement will be seen within 7 to 10 days. Optic atrophy and permanent blindness are common sequelae.

Optic Nerve Edema. Papilledema may mimic optic neuritis on fundic examination; vision and pupillary light responses are usually intact. Papilledema may be associated with increased cerebrospinal fluid pressure in congenital hydrocephalus or may be secondary to orbital inflammation. The treatment of papilledema is directed at the primary cause and, in general, has a better prognosis than does optic neuritis.

Optic Nerve Atrophy. Progressive degeneration of the optic nerve may follow optic neuritis, chronic papilledema, traumatic insult, advanced retinal degeneration, glaucoma, or demyelinating disease. The optic disc appears depressed, shrunken, and pale, and there is diminished blood supply (Fig. 14–36). The affected

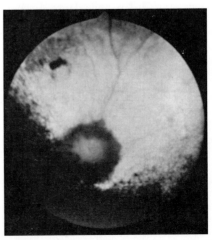

Figure 14–36. This atrophic optic disc is small and discolored; the affected eye is blind.

eye is blind. Optic atrophy is an irreversible process that does not respond to therapy.

References and Supplemental Reading

Acland GM, Aguirre GD: Retinal degenerations in the dog. IV. Early retinal degeneration (erd) in Norwegian elkhounds. Exp Eye Res 44:491, 1987.

Aguirre GD: Retinal degeneration associated with the feeding of dog foods to cats. J Am Vet Med Assoc 172:791, 1978a.

Aguirre GD: Retinal degeneration in the dog. I. Rod dysplasia. Exp Eye Res 26:233, 1978b.

Aguirre GD, Bistner SI: Microphakia with lenticular luxation and subluxation in cats. Vet Med Small Anim Clin 68:498, 1973a.

Aguirre GD, Bistner SI: Posterior lenticonus in the dog. Cornell Vet 63:455, 1973b.

Aguirre GD, Farber D, Lolley R, et al: Rod-cone dysplasia in Irish setters: A defect in cyclic GMP metabolism in visual cells. Science 201:1133, 1978.

Aguirre GD, Rubin LF: Ophthalmitis secondary to congenitally open eyelids in a dog. J Am Vet Med Assoc 156:70, 1970.

Aguirre GD, Rubin LF: The early diagnosis of rod dysplasia in the Norwegian elkhound. J Am Vet Med Assoc 159:429, 1971.

Aguirre GD, Rubin LF: Pathology of hemeralopia in the Alaskan malamute dog. Invest Ophthalmol Vis Sci 13:231, 1974.

Aguirre GD, Rubin LF: Rod-cone dysplasia (progressive retinal atrophy) in Irish setters. J Am Vet Med Assoc 166:157, 1975.

Aguirre GD, Rubin LF, Bistner SI: Development of the canine eye. Am J Vet Res 33:2399, 1972.

Andersen AC, Shultz FT: Inherited (congenital) cataract in the dog. Am J Pathol 34:965, 1958.

Ashton N, Barnett KC, Sachs DD: Retinal dysplasia in the Sealyham terrier. J Pathol Bacteriol 96:269, 1968.

Barclay SM, Riis RC: Retinal detachment and reattachment associated with ethylene glycol intoxication in a cat. J Am Anim Hosp Assoc 15:719, 1979.

Barnett KC: Hereditary cataract in the dog. J Small Anim Pract 19:109, 1978.

Barnett KC: Hereditary cataract in the Welsh springer spaniel. J Small Anim Pract 21:621, 1980.

Barnett KC: Progressive retinal atrophy in the Abyssinian cat. J Small Anim Pract 23:763, 1982.

Barnett KC: Hereditary cataract in the miniature schnauzer. J Small Anim Pract 26:635, 1985a.

Barnett KC: The diagnosis and differential diagnosis of cataract in the dog. J Small Anim Pract 26:305, 1985b.

Barnett KC: Hereditary cataract in the German shepherd dog. J Small Anim Pract 27:387, 1986.

Barnett KC, Grimes TD: Unilateral persistence and hyperplasia of the primary vitreous in the dog. J Small Anim Pract 14:561, 1973.

Barrie KP, Lavach JD, Gelatt KN, et al: Diseases of the canine posterior segment. In Gelatt KN (ed): Textbook of Veterinary Ophthalmology. Philadelphia, WB Saunders, 1981, p 474.

Barrie KP, Peiffer RL, Gelatt KN, et al: Posterior lenticonus, microphthalmia, congenital cataracts, and retinal folds in an Old English sheepdog. J Am Anim Hosp Assoc 15:715, 1979.

Bedford PGC: Multifocal retinal dysplasia in the Rottweiler. Vet Rec 111:304, 1982.

Bellhorn RW, Barnett KC, Henkind P: Ocular colobomas in domestic cats. J Am Vet Med Assoc 159:1015, 1971.

Bellhorn RW, Bellhorn MB, Swarm RL, et al: Hereditary tapetal abnormality in the beagle. Ophthalmic Res 7:250, 1975.

Bergsjo T, Arnesen K, Heim P, et al: Congenital blindness with ocular developmental anomalies, including retinal dysplasia, in Doberman dogs. J Am Vet Med Assoc 184:1383, 1984.

Bertram T, Coignoul F, Cheville N: Ocular dysgenesis in Australian shepherd dogs. J Am Anim Hosp Assoc 20:177, 1984.

Blogg JR: The Eye in Veterinary Practice. Philadelphia, WB Saunders, 1980a, p 102.

Blogg JR: Diseases of the eyelids. In Blogg JR (ed): The Eye in Veterinary Practice: Extraocular Disease. Philadelphia, WB Saunders, 1980b, p 295.

Blogg JR: Diseases of the conjunctiva. In Blogg JR (ed): The Eye in Veterinary Practice: Extraocular Disease. Philadelphia, WB Saunders, 1980c, p 347.

Brightman AH, Ogilvie GK, Tompkins M: Ocular disease in FeLV-positive cats: 11 cases (1981–1986). J Am Vet Med Assoc 198:1049, 1991.

Brooks DE, Wolf ED, Merideth R: Ophthalmomyiasis interna in two cats. J Am Anim Hosp Assoc 20:157, 1984.

Carastro SM, Dugan SJ, Paul AJ: Intraocular dirofilariasis in dogs. Compend Contin Educ Pract Vet 14:209, 1992.

Carrig CB, MacMillan AD, Brundage S, et al: Retinal dysplasia associated with skeletal abnormalities in Labrador retrievers. J Am Vet Med Assoc 170:49, 1977.

Carrig CB, Sponenberg DP, Schmidt GM, et al: Inheritance of associated ocular and skeletal dysplasia in Labrador retrievers. J Am Vet Med Assoc 193:1269, 1988.

Carter JD: Combined operation for non-cicatricial entropion with districhiasis. J Am Anim Hosp Assoc 8:53, 1972.

Carter JD: Medial conjunctivoplasty for aberrant dermis of the Lhasa apso. J Am Anim Hosp Assoc 9:180, 1973.

Chambers ED, Slatter DH: Cryotherapy (N₂O) of canine districhiasis and trichiasis: An experimental and clinical report. Proc Am Coll Vet Ophthalmol, 1985, p 68.

Collier LL, Bryan GM, Prieur DJ: Ocular manifestations of the Chediak-Higashi syndrome in four species of animals. J Am Vet Med Assoc 175:587, 1979.

Corcoran K, Koch S, Peiffer RL: Glaucoma in the chow. Vet Comp Ophthalmol 4:193, 1994.

Cottrell BD, Barnett KC: Primary glaucoma in the Welsh springer spaniel. J Small Anim Pract 29:185, 1988.

Coulter DB, Martin CL, Alvarado TP: Waardenburg syndrome in cats. Calif Vet 34:11, 1980.

Creel DJ: Visual system anomaly associated with albinism in the cat. Nature 231:465, 1971.

Curtis R, Barnett KC: Progressive retinal atrophy in miniature longhaired Dachshund dogs. Br Vet J 149:71, 1993.

Dausch D, Wegner W, Michaelis W, et al: Eye changes in the merle syndrome in the dog. Graefes Arch Klin Exp Ophthalmol 206:135, 1978.

Davidson MG, Nasisse MP, English RV, et al: Feline anterior uveitis: A study of 53 cases. J Am Anim Hosp Assoc 27:77, 1991.

Dice PF: Primary corneal disease in the dog and cat. Vet Clin North Am Sm Anim Pract 10:339, 1980.

Dice PF: Corneal dystrophy in the Shetland sheepdog. Proc Am Coll Vet Ophthalmol 15:241, 1984.

Duddy JA, Powzaniuk WC, Rubin LF: Hyaloid artery patency in neonatal beagles. Am J Vet Res 44:2344, 1983.

Dugan SJ, Severin GA, Hungerford LL, et al: Clinical and histologic evaluation of the prolapsed third eyelid gland in dogs. J Am Vet Med Assoc 201:1861, 1992.

Dziezyc J, Brooks DE: Canine cataracts. Compend Contin Educ Pract Vet 5:81, 1983.

Dziezyc J, Millichamp NJ: Surgical correction of eyelid agenesis in a cat. J Am Anim Hosp Assoc 25:513, 1989.

Gaunt PS, Confer AW, Carter JD, et al: Intraocular strongyloidiasis in a dog. J Am Anim Hosp Assoc 18:120, 1982.

Gelatt KN: Congenital cataract associated with persistent hyaloid in a dog. Vet Med Small Anim Clin 68:511, 1973.

Gelatt KN: Feline ophthalmology. Compend Contin Educ Pract Vet 1:576, 1979a.

Gelatt KN: Inherited retinopathies in the dog. Compend Contin Educ Pract Vet 1:307, 1979b.

Gelatt KN: Lens and cataract formation in the dog. Compend Contin Educ Pract Vet 1:75, 1979c.

Gelatt KN, Powell NG, Huston K: Inheritance of microphthalmia with coloboma in the Australian shepherd dog. Am J Vet Res 42:1686, 1981.

Gelatt KN, Samuelson DA, Barrie KP, et al: Biometry and clinical characteristics of congenital cataracts and microphthalmia in the miniature schnauzer. J Am Vet Med Assoc 183:99, 1983a.

Gelatt KN, Samuelson DA, Bauer JE, et al: Inheritance of congenital cataracts and microphthalmia in the miniature schnauzer. Am J Vet Res 44:1130, 1983b.

Gelatt KN, Whitley RD, Lavach JD: Familial cataracts in the Chesapeake Bay retriever. J Am Vet Med Assoc 175:1176, 1979.

Gelatt KN, Whitley RD, Samuelson DA, et al: Ocular manifestations of viral diseases in small animals. Compend Contin Educ Pract Vet 7:968, 1985.

Glaze MB, Blanchard GL: Nutritional cataracts in a Samoyed litter. J Am Anim Hosp Assoc 19:951, 1983.

Grimes TD, Mullaney J: Persistent hyperplastic primary vitreous in a greyhound. Vet Rec 85:607, 1969.

Gwin RM, Gelatt KN: The canine lens. In Gelatt KN (ed): Textbook of Veterinary Ophthalmology. Philadelphia, Lea & Febiger, 1981a, p 438.

Gwin RM, Wyman M, Lim DJ, et al: Multiple ocular defects associated with partial albinism and deafness in the dog. J Am Anim Hosp Assoc 17:401, 1981b.

Halliwell WH: Surgical management of canine districhia. J Am Vet Med Assoc 150:874, 1967.

Haskins ME, Aguirre GD, Jezyk PF, et al: The pathology of the feline model of mucopolysaccharidosis. VI. Am J Pathol 101:657, 1980.

Haskins ME, Bingel SA, Northington JW, et al: Spinal cord compression and hindlimb paresis in cats with mucopolysaccharidosis. VI. J Am Vet Med Assoc 182:983, 1983.

Haskins ME, Jezyk PF, Desnick RJ, et al: Mucopolysaccharidosis in a domestic short-haired cat—A disease distinct from that seen in the Siamese cat. J Am Vet Med Assoc 175:384, 1979.

Hendy-Ibbs PM: Familial feline epibulbar dermoids. Vet Rec 116:13, 1985.

Heywood R, Wells GAH: A retinal dysplasia in the beagle dog. Vet Rec 87:178, 1970.

Irby NI: Hereditary cataracts in the British shorthair cat. Presented at the American College of Veterinary Ophthalmology Genetics Workshop, 1983.

Jezyk PF, Haskins ME, Newman LR: Alpha-mannosidosis in a Persian cat. J Am Vet Med Assoc 189:1483, 1986.

Johnson BW: Non-surgical correction of entropion in shar-pei puppies. Vet Med 83:482, 1988.

Johnson BW, Campbell KL: Dermatoses of the canine eyelid. Compend Contin Educ Pract Vet 11:385, 1989.

Johnson BW, Helper LC, Szajerski ME: Intraocular Cuterebra in a cat. J Am Vet Med Assoc 193:829, 1988.

Keep JM: Clinical aspects of progressive retinal atrophy in the Cardigan Welsh corgi. Aust Vet J 48:197, 1972.

Keller WF, Blanchard GL, Krehbiel JD: Congenital dysplasia in a canine eye. J Am Anim Hosp Assoc 8:29, 1972.

Kelly DF, Lewis DG: Rapidly progressive diffuse retinal degeneration in a kitten. J Small Anim Pract 26:317, 1985.

Kern TJ, Riis RC: Optic nerve hypoplasia in three miniature poodles. J Am Vet Med Assoc 178:49, 1981a.

Kern TJ, Riis RC: Persistent hyperplastic primary vitreous and microphthalmia in a dog. J Am Vet Med Assoc 178:1169, 1981b.

Koch SA: Cataracts in interrelated Old English sheepdogs. J Am Vet Med Assoc 160:299, 1972.

Koch SA: Congenital ophthalmic abnormalities in the Burmese cat. J Am Vet Med Assoc 174:90, 1979.

Kratz KE, Spear PD, Smith DC: Postcritical-period reversal of effects of monocular deprivation on striate cortex cells in the cat. J Neurophysiol 39:501, 1976.

Krehbiel JD, Sanger VL, Ravi A: Ophthalmic lesions in feline infectious peritonitis: Gross, microscopic and ultrastructural changes. Vet Pathol 11:443, 1974.

Langloss JM, Zimmerman LE, Krehbiel JD: Malignant intraocular teratoid medulloepithelioma in three dogs. Vet Pathol 13:343, 1976.

Lappin MR, Marks A, Greene CE, et al: Serologic prevalence of selected infectious diseases in cats with uveitis. J Am Vet Med Assoc 201:1005, 1992.

Laratta LJ, Riis RC, Kern TJ, et al: Multiple congenital ocular defects in the Akita dog. Cornell Vet 75:381, 1985.

Lavach JD, Murphy JM, Severin GA: Retinal dysplasia in the English springer spaniel. J Am Anim Hosp Assoc 14:192, 1978.

Lavach JD, Severin GA: Posterior lenticonus and lenticonus internum in a dog. J Am Anim Hosp Assoc 13:685, 1977.

Leon A, Curtis R, Barnett KC: Hereditary persistent hyperplastic primary vitreous in the Staffordshire bull terrier. J Am Anim Hosp Assoc 22:765, 1986.

Loew ER, Riis RC: Congenital nyctalopia in the Tibetan terrier. Proc Am Coll Vet Ophthalmol 14:83, 1983.

Lombard CW, Twitchell MJ: Tetralogy of Fallot, persistent left cranial vena cava and retinal detachment in a cat. J Am Anim Hosp Assoc 14:624, 1978.

MacMillan AD, Lipton DE: Heritability of multifocal retinal dysplasia in American cocker spaniels. J Am Vet Med Assoc 172:568, 1978.

MacMillan AD, Waring GO, Spangler WL, et al: Crystalline corneal opacities in the Siberian husky. J Am Vet Med Assoc 175:829, 1979.

Martin CL: Strabismus associated with extraocular muscle agenesis in a dog. J Am Anim Hosp Assoc 14:486, 1978.

Martin CL: Feline ophthalmology. Proc Am Anim Hosp Assoc 48:287, 1981.

Martin CL, Kaswan R: Distemper-associated keratoconjunctivitis sicca. J Am Anim Hosp Assoc 21:355, 1985.

Martin CL, Leipold HW: Aphakia and multiple ocular defects in Saint Bernard puppies. Vet Med Small Anim Clin 69:448, 1974.

Meyers VN, Jezyk PF, Aguirre GD, et al: Short-limbed dwarfism and ocular defects in the Samoyed dog. J Am Vet Med Assoc 9:975, 1983.

Miller WW, Albert RA: Canine entropion. Compend Contin Educ Pract Vet 10:431, 1988.

Millichamp NJ, Curtis R, Barnett KC: Progressive retinal atrophy in the Tibetan terrier. J Am Vet Med Assoc 192:769, 1988.

Moore CP, Whitley RD: Visual disturbance in the dog. II. Diseases of the retina and optic papilla. Compend Contin Educ Pract Vet 6:585, 1984.

Morgan RV: Systemic hypertension in four cats: Ocular and medical findings. J Am Anim Hosp Assoc 22:615, 1986.

Morgan RV, Duddy JM, McClurg K: Prolapse of the gland of the third eyelid in dogs: A retrospective study of 89 cases (1980–1990). J Am Anim Hosp Assoc 29:56, 1993.

Munger RJ, Carter JD: A further modification of the Kuhnt-Szymanowski procedure for correction of atonic ectropion in dogs. J Am Anim Hosp Assoc 20:651, 1984.

Murray JA, Blakemore WF, Barnett KC: Ocular lesions in cats with GM-1 gangliosidosis with visceral involvement. J Small Anim Pract 18:1, 1977.

Nafe LA, Carter JD: Canine optic neuritis. Compend Contin Educ Pract Vet 3:978, 1981.

Narfstrom K: Cataract in the West Highland white terrier. J Small Anim Pract 22:467, 1981.

Narfstrom K, Dubielzig R: Posterior lenticonus, cataracts and microphthalmia; congenital ocular defects in the Cavalier King Charles spaniel. J Small Anim Pract 25:669, 1984.

Nasisse MP, Guy JS: Feline ocular disease and the rhinotracheitis virus. Vet Med Report 1:155, 1989.

Nelson DL, MacMillan AD: Multifocal retinal dysplasia in field trial Labrador retrievers. J Am Anim Hosp Assoc 19:388, 1983.

Noden DM, de Lahunta A: The Embryology of Domestic Animals. Developmental Mechanisms and Malformations. Baltimore, Williams & Wilkins, 1985, p 116.

Olesen HP, Hensen OA, Norn MS: Congenital hereditary cataract in the cocker spaniel. J Small Anim Pract 15:741, 1974.

Palmer AC, Malinowski W, Barnett KC: Clinical signs including papilledema associated with brain tumours in twenty-one dogs. J Small Anim Pract 15:359, 1974.

Parshall CJK, Wyman M, Nitroy S, et al: Photoreceptor dysplasia: An inherited progressive retinal atrophy of miniature schnauzer dogs. Prog Vet Comp Ophthalmol 1:187, 1991.

Peiffer RL: Bilateral congenital aphakia and retinal detachment in a cat. J Am Anim Hosp Assoc 18:128, 1982a.

Peiffer RL: Inherited ocular diseases of the dog and cat. Compend Contin Educ Pract Vet 4:152, 1982b.

Peiffer RL, Belkin PV: Keratolenticular dysgenesis in a kitten. J Am Vet Med Assoc 182:1242, 1983.

Peiffer RL, Gelatt KN: Cataracts in the cat. Feline Pract 4:34, 1974.

Peiffer RL, Gelatt KN: Congenital cataracts in a Persian kitten. Vet Med Small Anim Clin 70:1334, 1975.

Peiffer RL, Gelatt KN, Gwin RM: Persistent primary vitreous and a pigmented cataract in a dog. J Am Anim Hosp Assoc 13:478, 1977.

Peiffer RL, Gelatt KN, Karpinski LG: Canine eyelids. In Gelatt KN (ed): Textbook of Veterinary

Ophthalmology. Philadelphia, Lea & Febiger, 1981, p 277.

Peterson-Jones SM, Zhu FX: Development and use of a polymerase chain reaction–based diagnostic test for the causal mutation of progressive retinal atrophy in Cardigan Welsh corgi. Am J Vet Res 61:844, 2000.

Rebhun WC: Persistent hyperplastic primary vitreous in a dog. J Am Vet Med Assoc 169:620, 1976.

Remillard RL, Pickett JP, Thatcher CD, et al: Comparison of kittens fed queen's milk with those fed mild replacers. Am J Vet Res 54:901, 1993.

Riis RC, Aguirre GD: The briard problem. Proc Am Coll Vet Ophthalmol 14:62, 1983.

Roberts SR, Bistner SI: Persistent pupillary membranes in basenji dogs. J Am Vet Med Assoc 153:523, 1968.

Roberts SR, Helper LC: Cataracts in Afghan hounds. J Am Vet Med Assoc 160:427, 1972.

Rubin LF: Heredity of retinal dysplasia in Bedlington terriers. J Am Vet Med Assoc 152:260, 1968.

Rubin LF: Hereditary microphakia and microphthalmia syndrome in the beagle. Proc Am Coll Vet Ophthalmol 2:50, 1971.

Rubin LF: Atlas of Veterinary Ophthalmoscopy. Philadelphia, Lea & Febiger, 1974a, p 236.

Rubin LF: Cataract in golden retrievers. J Am Vet Med Assoc 165:457, 1974b.

Rubin LF: Hereditary cataract in Himalayan cats. Feline Pract 16:14, 1986.

Rubin LF, Flowers RD: Inherited cataract in a family of standard poodles. J Am Vet Med Assoc 161:207, 1972.

Rubin LF, Lipton DE: Retinal degeneration in kittens. J Am Vet Med Assoc 162:467, 1973.

Rubin LF, Nelson EJ, Sharp CA: Collie eye anomaly in Australian shepherd dogs. Prog Vet Comp Ophthalmol 1:105, 1991.

Rubin LF, Saunders LZ: Intraocular larva migrans in dogs. Pathol Vet 2:566, 1965.

Scagliotti RH, MacMillan AD: Retinal degeneration in the borzoi. Proc Am Coll Vet Ophthalmol 8:67, 1977.

Schiavo DM, Field WE: The incidence of ocular defects in a closed colony of beagle dogs. Lab Anim Sci 24:51, 1974.

Schmidt GM, Ellersieck MR, Wheeler CA, et al: Inheritance of retinal dysplasia in the English springer spaniel. J Am Vet Med Assoc 174:1089, 1979.

Slatter DH: Fundamentals of Veterinary Ophthalmology, 2nd ed. Philadelphia, WB Saunders, 1990.

Slatter DH: Textbook of Small Animal Surgery. Philadelphia, WB Saunders, 1985, p 1509.

Stades FC: Persistent hyperplastic tunica vasculosa lentis and persistent hyperplastic primary vitreous in Doberman pinschers: Genetic aspects. J Am Anim Hosp Assoc 19:957, 1983a.

Stades FC: Persistent hyperplastic tunica vasculosa lentis and persistent hyperplastic primary vitreous in Doberman pinschers: Techniques and results of surgery. J Am Anim Hosp Assoc 19:393, 1983b.

Stades FC: Persistent hyperplastic tunica vasculosa lentis and persistent hyperplastic primary vitreous (PHTVL/PHPV) in 90 closely related Doberman pinschers: Clinical aspects. J Am Anim Hosp Assoc 16:739, 1980.

Stades FC: Hereditary retinal dysplasia (RD) in a family of Yorkshire terriers. Tijdschr Diergeneeskd 103:1087, 1978.

Szymanski C: The eye. In Holzworth J (ed): Diseases of the Cat. Philadelphia, WB Saunders, 1987, p 706.

Van Rensburg IBJ, Petrick SW, van der Lugt JJ, et al: Multiple inherited eye anomalies including persistent hyperplastic tunica vasculosa lentis in Bouvier des Flandres. Prog Vet Comp Ophthalmol 2:133, 1992.

Waring GO, MacMillan A, Reveles P: Inheritance of crystalline corneal dystrophy in Siberian huskies. J Am Anim Hosp Assoc 22:655, 1986.

Wen GY, Sturman JA, Wisniewski HM, et al: Chemical and ultrastructural changes in tapetum of beagles with a hereditary abnormality. Invest Ophthalmol Vis Sci 23:733, 1982.

West-Hyde L, Buyukmihci N: Photoreceptor degeneration in a family of cats. J Am Vet Med Assoc 181:243, 1982.

Wyman M, Donovan EF: Eye anomaly of the collie. J Am Vet Med Assoc 155:866, 1969.

Yakely WL: A study of heritability of cataracts in the American cocker spaniel. J Am Vet Med Assoc 172:814, 1978.

Yakely WL, Wyman M, Donovan EF, et al: Genetic transmission of an ocular fundus anomaly in collies. J Am Vet Med Assoc 152:457, 1968.

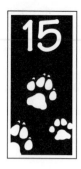

The Hematopoietic and Lymphoid Systems

Kenneth D. Clinkenbeard, Rick L. Cowell, James H. Meinkoth,
Lilli S. Decker, Mary K. Boudreaux, and Kenita S. Rogers

Hematology of Normal Dogs and Cats and Responses to Disease

Kenneth D. Clinkenbeard, Rick L. Cowell, James H. Meinkoth, and Lilli S. Decker

This chapter is intended to provide pertinent information about normal hematologic values and the evaluation of the hematologic changes seen in healthy and diseased puppies and kittens younger than 6 months. Some general principles of hematologic interpretation are described, reference values for complete blood counts (CBCs) are discussed, and hematologic changes associated with inherited disorders and diseases in puppies and kittens are reviewed. The chapter is not intended to be a comprehensive review of small animal hematology, and the reader is referred elsewhere for a more complete presentation of hematology as it applies to the adult dog and cat (Cowell and Tyler, 1991; Duncan et al, 1994; Jain, 1993; Latimer, 1995; Weiser, 1995).

NORMAL HEMATOLOGIC VALUES FOR PUPPIES AND KITTENS

Currently, there are no published sets of normal hematologic reference values for mixed-breed puppies or kittens younger than 6 months. What is available are reference value sets for closed research colonies composed of a few selected breeds. Tables 15–1 and 15–2 contain

reference value sets derived from these studies (Andersen and Gee, 1958; Anderson et al, 1971; Meyers-Wallen et al, 1984). Unfortunately, these value sets are of limited utility for veterinarians because the values may depend on the particular breed and are influenced by nutritional, environmental, and pathologic factors specific to the research colony. The values in these reference sets are sufficiently divergent that the validity of a consensus reference set derived from combining these data is questionable. Hematologic values for a puppy or kitten that are well below or above those for one of these reference value sets or for the adult reference range for the hematologic laboratory in which the testing was conducted should be suspected of being abnormal.

Although the research colony reference value sets do not provide precise value ranges applicable to most puppies and kittens seen in veterinary practice, analysis of these value sets does provide insight into trends in normal hematologic values for puppies and kittens younger than 6 months (see Tables 15–1 and 15–2).

At birth, the fetal red blood cells (RBCs) are larger than those of adults as measured by the mean corpuscular volume (MCV). Between birth and 2 to 3 months of age, these larger fetal RBCs are replaced with smaller adult

Table 15-1 Hematologic Values of Growing, Healthy Beagle Dogs

HEMATOLOGIC PARAMETER*	AGE (IN WEEKS)										
	BIRTH	1†	2†	3†	4†	6†	8†	12‡	16‡	20‡	24‡
RBC (× 10^6/µl)	4.7–5.6 (5.1)	3.6–5.9 (4.6)	3.4–4.4 (3.9)	3.5–4.3 (3.8)	3.6–4.9 (4.1)	4.3–5.1 (4.7)	4.5–5.9 (4.9)	6.34	6.38	6.93	7.41
Hemoglobin (g/dl)	14.0–17.0 (15.2)	10.4–17.5 (12.9)	9.0–11.0 (10.0)	8.6–11.6 (9.7)	8.5–10.3 (9.5)	8.5–11.3 (10.2)	10.3–12.5 (11.2)	14.3	15.0	16.0	16.7
PCV (%)	45.0–52.5 (47.5)	33.0–52.0 (40.5)	29.0–34.0 (31.8)	27.0–37.0 (31.7)	27.0–33.5 (29.9)	26.5–35.5 (32.5)	31.0–39.0 (34.8)	40.9	43.0	44.9	47.6
MCV (fl)	93.0	89.0	81.5	83.0	73.0	69.0	72.0	64.6	67.4	64.8	64.2
MCH (pg)	30.0	28.0	25.5	25.0	23.0	22.0	22.5	22.8	23.5	23.0	22.5
MCHC (%)	32.0	32.0	31.5	31.0	32.0	31.5	32.0	35.3	34.8	35.6	35.1
N-RBC/100 WBC	0–13 (2.3)	0–11 (4.0)	0–6 (2.0)	0–9 (1.6)	0–4 (1.2)	0–0 —	0–1 (0.2)				
Reticulocytes (%)	4.5–9.2 (6.5)	3.8–15.2 (6.9)	4.0–8.4 (6.7)	5.0–9.0 (6.9)	4.6–6.6 (5.8)	2.6–6.2 (4.5)	1.0–6.0 (3.6)				
Total WBC (×10^3/µl)	6.8–18.4 (12.0)	9.0–23.0 (14.1)	8.1–15.1 (11.7)	6.7–15.1 (11.2)	8.5–16.4 (12.9)	12.6–26.7 (16.3)	12.7–17.3 (15.0)	17.1	16.3	14.6	15.6
Band neutrophils	0–1.5 (0.23)	0–4.8 (0.50)	0–1.2 (0.21)	0–0.5 (0.09)	0–0.3 (0.06)	0–0.3 (0.05)	0–0.3 (0.08)	0.08	0.09	0.02	0.02
Segmented neutrophils	4.4–15.8 (8.6)	3.8–15.2 (7.4)	3.2–10.4 (5.2)	1.4–9.4 (5.1)	3.7–12.8 (7.2)	4.2–17.6 (9.0)	6.2–11.8 (8.5)	9.8	9.0	8.9	9.1
Lymphocytes	0.5–4.2 (1.9)	1.3–9.4 (4.3)	1.5–7.4 (3.8)	2.1–10.1 (5.0)	1.0–8.4 (4.5)	2.8–16.6 (5.7)	3.1–6.9 (5.0)	5.7	5.9	4.5	5.3
Monocytes	0.2–2.2 (0.9)	0.3–2.5 (1.1)	0.2–1.4 (0.7)	0.1–1.4 (0.7)	0.3–1.5 (0.8)	0.5–2.7 (1.1)	0.4–1.7 (1.0)	0.9	0.9	0.8	0.7
Eosinophils	0–1.3 (0.4)	0.2–2.8 (0.8)	0.08–1.8 (0.6)	0.07–0.9 (0.3)	0–0.7 (0.25)	0.1–1.9 (0.5)	0–1.2 (0.4)	0.4	0.4	0.3	0.5
Basophils	0.0	0–0.2 (0.01)	0.0	0.0	0–0.15 (0.01)	0.0	0.0				

*RBC = Red blood cells; PCV = packed cell volume expressed as percentage; MCV = mean corpuscular volume expressed in femtoliters; MCH = mean corpuscular hemoglobin expressed in picograms; MCHC = mean corpuscular hemoglobin concentration expressed as percentage; N-RBC/100 WBC = number of nucleated red blood cells per 100 white blood cells; total WBC = total number of white blood cells.

†Normal ranges and/or mean values from Earl FL, Melvegar BA, Wilson RL: The hemogram and bone marrow profile of normal neonatal and weanling beagle dogs. Lab Anim Sci 23:630, 1973.

‡Mean values from Anderson AC, Gee W: Normal blood values in the beagle. Vet Med 53:135, 1958.

Table 15-2 Hematologic Values of Growing, Healthy Cats

HEMATOLOGIC PARAMETER*	AGE (IN WEEKS)								
	0–2†	2–4†	4–6†	6–8†	8–9†	12–13†	16–17†	20‡	30‡
RBC ($\times 10^6$/µl)	5.29 ± 0.24	4.67 ± 0.10	5.89 ± 0.23	6.57 ± 0.26	6.95 ± 0.09	7.43 ± 0.23	8.14 ± 0.27	7.4 ± 0.7	8.0 ± 0.5
Hemoglobin (g/dl)	12.1 ± 0.6	8.7 ± 0.2	8.6 ± 0.3	9.1 ± 0.3	9.8 ± 0.2	10.1 ± 0.3	11.0 ± 0.4	10.7 ± 1.2	12.1 ± 1.8
PCV (%)	35.3 ± 1.7	26.5 ± 0.8	27.1 ± 0.8	29.8 ± 1.3	33.3 ± 0.7	33.1 ± 1.6	34.9 ± 1.1	33.4 ± 3.3	37.1 ± 3.4
MCV (fl)	67.4 ± 1.9	53.9 ± 1.2	45.6 ± 1.3	45.6 ± 1.0	47.8 ± 0.9	44.5 ± 1.8	43.1 ± 1.5	45.0 ± 5.2	46.0 ± 3.5
MCH (pg)	23.0 ± 0.6	18.8 ± 0.8	14.8 ± 0.6	13.9 ± 0.3	14.1 ± 0.2	13.7 ± 0.4	13.5 ± 0.4		
MCHC (%)	34.5 ± 0.8	33.0 ± 0.5	31.9 ± 0.6	30.9 ± 0.5	29.5 ± 0.4	31.3 ± 0.9	31.6 ± 0.8	32.0 ± 2.0	33.0 ± 3.3
Total WBC ($\times 10^3$/µl)	9.67 ± 0.57	15.31 ± 1.21	17.45 ± 1.37	18.07 ± 1.94	23.68 ± 1.89	23.20 ± 3.36	19.70 ± 1.12	15.9 ± 6.0	21.9 ± 6.7
Band neutrophils	0.06 ± 0.02	0.11 ± 0.04	0.20 ± 0.06	0.22 ± 0.08	0.12 ± 0.09	0.15 ± 0.07	0.16 ± 0.07		
Segmented neutrophils	5.96 ± 0.68	6.92 ± 0.77	9.57 ± 1.65	6.75 ± 1.03	11.00 ± 1.41	11.00 ± 1.77	9.74 ± 0.92	9.5 ± 1.27	15.5 ± 1.66
Lymphocytes	3.73 ± 0.52	6.56 ± 0.59	6.41 ± 0.77	9.59 ± 1.57	10.17 ± 1.71	10.46 ± 2.61	8.7 ± 1.06	6.2 ± 1.27	5.7 ± 1.5
Monocytes	0.01 ± 0.01	0.02 ± 0.02	0	0.01 ± 0.01	0.11 ± 0.06	0	0.02 ± 0.02		
Eosinophils	0.96 ± 0.43	1.40 ± 0.16	1.47 ± 0.25	1.08 ± 0.20	2.28 ± 0.31	1.55 ± 0.35	1.00 ± 0.19		
Basophils	0.02 ± 0.01	0	0	0.02 ± 0.02	0	0.03 ± 0.03	0		

*RBC = Red blood cells; PCV = packed cell volume expressed as percentage; MCV = mean corpuscular volume expressed in femtoliters; MCH = mean corpuscular hemoglobin expressed in picograms; MCHC = mean corpuscular hemoglobin concentration expressed as percentage; total WBC = total number of white blood cells.

†Normal ranges from Meyers-Wallen VN, Haskins ME, Patterson DF: Hematologic values in healthy neonatal, weanling, and juvenile kitens. Am J Vet Res 45:1322, 1984.

‡Normal ranges from Anderson L, Wilson R, Hay D: Haematological values in normal cats from four weeks to one year of age. Res Vet Sci 12:579, 1971.

RBCs, with the MCV decreasing to the adult normal range by 1 to 3 months of age. During this time of replacement of fetal RBCs with adult RBCs, the combined effect of replacement and dilution by increase in body size (and thus circulatory volume) results in a lower packed cell volume than the adult normal range. The iron content of maternal milk is low such that anemia by any mechanism in puppies and kittens may result in an iron deficiency anemia with low hemoglobin and microcytosis. In the normal puppy or kitten, packed cell volume begins to increase at 2 months of age and reaches the adult normal level sometime between 2 and 6 months of age. This replacement of fetal RBCs can also result in high RBC polychromasia and reticulocyte counts.

At birth, most puppies and kittens have normal serum or plasma albumin concentrations and decreased serum or plasma gamma globulin concentrations. The gamma globulins increase after birth (partly from assimilation of colostrum) and typically reach adult levels by 6 months of age. In one study of puppies, the ranges of total plasma protein concentrations were 5.0 to 6.5 g/dl at 8 weeks, 5.5 to 6.5 g/dl at 10 to 12 weeks, and 6.3 to 7.0 g/dl at 4 to 6 months of age (Jain, 1993).

Age-related changes in the white blood cell (WBC) and differential WBC counts are slight to moderate in magnitude such that the WBCs of puppies and kittens younger than 6 months remain within the reference value range for adults. For puppies, the WBC as well as neutrophil and lymphocyte counts are relatively high at birth, decline during the first month of life, increase by the second month, and then slowly decline over the life of the puppy. One study reported increased band neutrophils (>500 cells/μl) during the first 2 weeks of life (Earl et al, 1971). For kittens, WBC as well as neutrophil and lymphocyte counts at birth are within the adult reference range but increase above the adult reference range for kittens at 3 to 4 months of age. This leukocytosis, composed primarily of a mature neutrophilia and lymphocytosis, may be a physiologic leukocytosis resulting from excitement caused during blood sample collection.

EVALUATION OF THE ERYTHROGRAM

Those parameters needed for evaluating changes in the RBC circulating mass as it relates to disease are provided for the most part by the CBC. Anemia is the most common and diagnostically significant hematologic change. Anemias are never a primary disease; therefore, determining the cause of an anemia in puppies or kittens provides the veterinarian with a good first step in the diagnosis of the primary disease. The cause of the anemia can often be determined by classifying the anemia into a pathophysiologic classification of regenerative, iron deficiency, or nonregenerative anemia based on changes in the erythrogram.

Regenerative anemias are caused by either hemorrhage or hemolysis and are characterized by increased polychromatophilic RBCs and reticulocytes in circulation. After an acute episode of hemorrhage or hemolysis, increased polychromasia and reticulocytes may be detected as early as 2 days but require 5 to 7 days to reach maximal regenerative response. Reticulocytes are more reliable for evaluation of the regenerative response than is polychromasia. Reticulocytes can be more accurately quantified, whereas polychromasia is judged semiquantitatively and is affected by stain type and quality. Evaluation of polychromasia provides the veterinarian with a quick means of detecting a regenerative response when it is not timely or possible to conduct a reticulocyte count. Nucleated RBCs (N-RBCs) can be increased in regenerative anemias, but they are not a specific or selective indicator of regenerative response. This is because many processes not related to regenerative anemia increase N-RBCs, and the number of N-RBCs may not be increased in animals with regenerative anemias.

Polychromatophilic RBCs are detected on Wright's stained blood smears as blue-gray-tan, being less intensely stained than the more intensely stained orange-tan mature RBCs. Also, polychromatophilic RBCs are typically larger than mature RBCs and may have a slightly irregular folded shape. It is difficult to detect polychromasia with a Diff-Quik stain because all RBCs stain bluer than with Wright's type stains. The number of polychromatophilic RBCs needed to be considered an adequate regenerative response varies with the packed cell volume of the animal. The lower the packed cell volume, the greater the number of polychromatophilic RBCs needed to support an interpretation of regenerative anemia. The guidelines for evaluating the regenerative response in adult animals are likely sufficient for puppies and kittens older than 4 months (Table 15–3). A greater regenerative response should be observed in animals that are younger than 4 months.

Increased reticulocytes are the preferred

Table 15-3 Use of the Number of Polychromatophilic Red Blood Cells (RBCs) per Oil Immersion Field or the Subjective Polychromasia Score to Judge the Adequacy of a Regenerative Response

FOR AN ADEQUATE REGENERATIVE RESPONSE, THE NUMBER OF POLYCHROMATOPHILIC (PC) RBCs PER OIL IMMERSION FIELD (OIF) OR SUBJECTIVE POLYCHROMASIA SCORE (1 to 4+) SHOULD BE THIS VALUE OR GREATER

MAGNITUDE OF ANEMIA (PACKED CELL VOLUME [%])	DOGS		CATS	
	PC RBCs/OIF	Polychromasia	PC RBCs/OIF	Polychromasia
25–35	2–4	1–2+	1–2	1–2+
15–25	4–8	2–3+	3–5	2–3+
<15	>8	4+	>5	4+

Courtesy of the Clinical Pathology Section teaching files, Oklahoma State University, Stillwater.

means to evaluate the regenerative response in puppies and kittens. Reticulocytes are immature anucleate RBCs that still contain polyribosomes for hemoglobin synthesis. These polyribosomes are aggregated and stained by new methylene blue stain. Polyribosomes of reticulocytes stain as multiple fine blue aggregates, whereas the remainder of the RBC does not stain with the new methylene blue stain. Cats have two types of reticulocytes. Feline aggregate reticulocytes appear similar to canine reticulocytes, and feline punctate reticulocytes have individual fine blue clots rather than aggregates (Fig. 15–1). Feline aggregate reticulocytes are most reliable for evaluating moderate to severe anemias, but punctate reticulocytes can be useful for evaluating the regenerative response in mild anemias. Reticulocytes are quantified as a percentage of all RBCs. Like polychromasia, the more severe the anemia, the greater the percentage of reticulocytes required for consideration of the anemia to be regenerative. Animals younger than 4 months should have a greater reticulocyte response than that considered to be regenerative in adult dogs and cats.

Several approaches to evaluating reticulocyte response are used. To evaluate the regenerative response (Table 15–4), many veterinarians use a "rule of thumb" table based on the packed cell volume and reticulocyte count. Corrected reticulocyte percentage or absolute reticulocyte count can be used to evaluate the regenerative response in most cats and dogs, and reticulocyte

production index can also be used for most dogs (Table 15–5).

Once the anemia has been determined to be regenerative, then the total plasma (or serum) protein concentration is assessed to help determine whether the cause of the anemia is hemorrhage or hemolysis. The total plasma protein concentration is usually low in hemorrhage, whereas it is usually within the normal reference range or high in hemolysis. The magnitude of the decrease in total plasma protein concentration for hemorrhage depends on the severity of the hemorrhage; the greater extent and duration of the hemorrhage, the lower the total plasma protein concentration. The common causes of a hemorrhagic anemia in puppies and kittens include inherited or acquired coagulopathies, excessive hemorrhage after trauma or surgeries, and hematophagous parasitism.

If the cause of a hemorrhagic anemia is not corrected and continual blood loss occurs, the sequela of depletion of body iron stores produces an iron deficiency anemia. Initially, blood loss anemias are regenerative with a low total protein, but iron stores with increasing duration are diminished, and hemoglobin synthesis in immature RBCs declines (Table 15–6). The hallmark of iron deficiency anemia is microcytic hypochromic RBCs, which are detected by CBC parameters of low MCV and mean corpuscular hemoglobin concentration (MCHC). Microcytic hypochromic RBCs can also be detected by examination of RBC morphology on blood smears. Although the smaller size of these RBCs is difficult to detect on blood smears, the larger pale centers and thin halo of hemoglobin support hypochromia rather then normochromic RBCs, which have smaller pale centers and a wider rim of hemoglobin (Fig. 15–2).

In contrast to the regenerative hemorrhagic anemia, regenerative hemolytic anemias typically have normal or increased total protein because plasma is not lost with this type of anemia. Hemolytic anemias occur because of immune-mediated disease, oxidative injury and Heinz body formation, microangiopathy, and hemoparasites. There is no indication that puppies and kittens are especially prone to hemolytic anemias, but any one of these causes could result in hemolytic anemia. The most common cause of immune-mediated hemolytic anemia in newborn kittens is neonatal isoerythrolysis.

Red blood cell morphology is important in distinguishing the possible causes of the hemolytic anemias. As indicated in Table 15–7, various RBC morphologic changes can be used to identify the cause of the hemolytic anemia. In

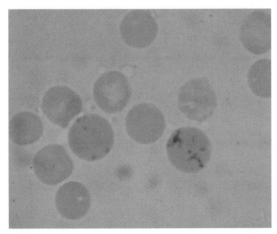

Figure 15–1. New methylene blue–stained blood smear from a kitten with hemolytic anemia demonstrating aggregate and punctate reticulocytes. (Courtesy of the Department of Veterinary Pathobiology teaching files, College of Veterinary Medicine, Oklahoma State University, Stillwater.)

Table 15–4 Rule of Thumb for Evaluating Regenerative Response Using an Uncorrected Reticulocyte Percentage

MAGNITUDE OF THE ANEMIA (PACKED CELL VOLUME [%])	FOR AN ADEQUATE REGENERATIVE RESPONSE, THE UNCORRECTED RETICULOCYTE PERCENTAGE SHOULD BE THIS VALUE OR GREATER	
	DOG	CAT*
25	5	2.5
10	10	5
5	20	10

*Aggregate reticulocytes.
Courtesy of the Clinical Pathology Section teaching files, Oklahoma State University, Stillwater.

Table 15–5 Use of Various Reticulocyte Parameters to Interpret the Adequacy of a Regenerative Anemia Response

PARAMETER	FOR A MINIMAL ADEQUATE REGENERATIVE RESPONSE, THE TEST RESULT SHOULD BE THIS VALUE	
	DOG	CAT*
Corrected reticulocyte (%)	>2	>0.4
Absolute reticulocyte count (/μl)	>80,000	>60,000
Reticulocyte production index	>1	Not applicable

*Aggregate reticulocytes.

Table 15–6 Hypothetical Development of Blood Loss Iron Deficiency Anemia and its Effect on Red Blood Cell Parameters

PARAMETERS	DURATION AND SEVERITY OF BLOOD LOSS		
	SHORT DURATION (DAYS) (MODERATE TO SEVERE LOSS)	INTERMEDIATE DURATION (DAYS TO WEEKS; MILD TO MODERATE LOSS)	LONG DURATION (WEEKS TO MONTHS; MILD TO MODERATE LOSS)
Packed cell volume	Mildly to moderately anemic	Moderately anemic	Moderately to severely anemic
MCV	Macrocytic	Normocytic	Microcytic
MCHC	Hypochromic	Hypochromic	Hypochromic
RBC morphology	Polychromatophilic RBCs	Polychromatophilic RBCs	Microcytic, hypochromic RBCs
Regenerative anemia response	Adequate	Inadequate	Inadequate or no regenerative response
Total plasma protein	Low	Low or low normal	Low or low normal

MCHC = mean corpuscular hemoglobin concentration; MCV = mean corpuscular volume; RBCs = red blood cells.

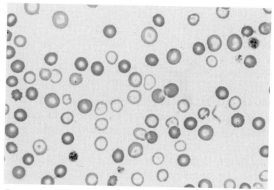

Figure 15–2. Wright-stained blood smear from a puppy with chronic blood loss anemia secondary to parasitism demonstrating hypochromic red blood cells. (Courtesy of the Department of Veterinary Pathobiology teaching files, College of Veterinary Medicine, Oklahoma State University, Stillwater.)

those cases in which the veterinarian suspects that hemolytic anemia is present (regenerative anemia with normal or high total protein), it is best to examine the blood smear for the RBC morphologic changes presented in Table 15–7.

Immune-mediated hemolytic anemia associated with immune reaction against antigens from infectious agents or drugs or from self-antigens on RBCs is diagnosed by spherocytosis (identifying the presence of more than one spherocyte per microscopic oil immersion field

in the blood smear of dogs and not cats), microagglutination, and/or a positive Coombs' test. Oxidative injury to RBCs by a variety of food, drug, and plant substances and disease-related factors causes denaturation of hemoglobin in RBCs and Heinz body formation. Splenic removal of RBCs containing Heinz bodies results in the hemolytic anemia. Diseases, such as feline infectious peritonitis, that cause fibrin deposition in or sclerosis of arterioles, capillaries, or venules may cause a microangiopathic anemia. Hitting the sclerosed vessel walls or fibrin strands damages the RBCs, and they are removed by the spleen precipitating the hemolytic anemia. The damaged RBCs are identified as blister cells, keratocytes, and schistocytes on blood smears.

Hemolytic anemia can result from a primary hemoparasitic infection and the resulting animal's immune response, or the hemolytic anemia may occur from recrudescence of a carrier state of the hemoparasite that is precipitated by some other disease process. For hemolytic anemias caused by primary hemoparasites, the anemia is usually regenerative, but in those cases in which the hemoparasite infection is secondary to another disease process, the hemolytic anemias are most often nonregenerative even though the initial cause of the anemia is hemolysis. Nonregenerative parasitic hemolytic anemias are uncommon in puppies and kittens

Table 15–7	**Various Red Blood Cell (RBC) Morphologic Features Useful for Diagnosis of Hemolytic Anemias**	
HEMOLYTIC PROCESS	**RBC MORPHOLOGIC FEATURE**	**DESCRIPTION**
Immune mediated	Microagglutination	Clumps of RBCs that are not dispersed when diluted at a 1:5 ratio in normal saline solution
	Spherocytosis	Small RBCs with no pale center (cannot be readily distinguished in cats from normocytes)
Heinz body	Heinz bodies	Single blocky structure in or protruding from RBCs Diff-Quik stain: nonstaining Wright's stain: normal hemoglobin or slightly whitish New methylene blue stain: blue
Microangiopathies	Blister cells	Eccentric holes in RBCs
	Keratocytes or helmet cells	Football or aviator helmet-shaped RBCs with strap-like structures extending from the earmuffs
	Schistocytes	RBC fragments
Hemoparasites	*Haemobartonella*	Dark-staining, small round or rod-shaped dots often on the periphery of RBCs
	Babesia	Large pyriform bodies often present as single, pairs or tetrads in RBCs
	Cytauxzoon	Small signet ring bodies usually singly in RBCs

because hemoparasite carrier states are uncommon at this age.

The least common cause of anemias in puppies and kittens is nonregenerative anemias. These anemias are caused by shortened RBC life spans, low erythropoietin activity, low iron availability, or cytokine suppression of bone marrow. They are usually associated with renal failure, endocrinopathies, and inflammatory, viral, or neoplastic diseases. The nonregenerative anemias that are secondary to an inflammatory or neoplastic disease are termed *anemia of chronic disease* or *anemia of inflammatory disease*. The nonregenerative anemias are diagnosed by the CBC parameters of MCV and MCHC being within the normal reference range and by poor reticulocyte response as well as an absence of polychromasia. Classically, these anemias develop over a period of weeks to months, but under unusual circumstances these anemias can develop in a few days. Although some chronic diseases do occur in young animals, such as congenital renal failure of small-breed dogs, a nonregenerative anemia may or may not be seen before 6 months of age.

EVALUATION OF THE LEUKOGRAM

Leukocyte morphology and changes in leukocyte circulating numbers are usually detected by the observation of particular patterns in the leukogram portion of the CBC. Such leukogram patterns may include physiologic leukocytosis, stress leukogram, regenerative and degenerative left shifts, and mature neutrophilia (Table 15–8). When one of these patterns is observed, it is often a reliable indicator of the disease process present in the puppy or kitten. In some cases, although the disease process exists, no changes in the leukogram may be seen because the leukocytes are just passing through the circulation to reach the tissue where they are functional. A random blood sampling of circulating leukocytes does not always adequately reflect what is occurring in the tissues. Therefore, the absence of a change in the leukogram does not rule out a particular physiologic or pathophysiologic process.

The physiologic leukocytosis and stress leukogram are caused primarily by physiologic processes and are of limited diagnostic importance. The veterinarian should nevertheless note these patterns so that these physiologic responses are not confused with the diagnostically important inflammatory-related leukogram patterns. The physiologic leukocytosis, consisting of a mature neutrophilia, lymphocytosis, and occasionally a monocytosis, is the most common leukogram pattern seen in puppies and kittens, especially in young kittens. The physiologic leukocytosis typically signifies an epinephrine response to the puppy's or kitten's anxiety about phlebotomy. Occasionally, the lymphocytosis seen with a physiologic leukocytosis can be confused with the lymphocytosis of lymphocytic leukemia, particularly if atypical lymphocytes are noted in the blood smear. Atypical lymphocytes are large lymphocytes with a larger nucleus and more abundant cytoplasm that can be derived from immune stimulation or neoplastic transformation. Atypical lymphocytes caused by immune stimulation are termed *reactive lymphocytes* and are more commonly noted in recently vaccinated puppies (Earl et al, 1971). In cases of lymphocytosis and presence of atypical lymphocytes, it is advisable to have a veterinary clinical pathologist examine the blood smear to determine whether the atypical lymphocytes are reactive or neoplastic in origin.

The stress leukogram pattern, consisting of a mature neutrophilia, lymphopenia, and occasionally a monocytosis and eosinopenia, is caused by the action of endogenous or exogenous corticosteroids. A stress leukogram typically results in a WBC count of not more than 30,000 cells/µl in puppies and not more than 35,000 cells/µl in kittens. Stress associated with an inflammatory disease may cause a stress leukogram that is coincident with a regenerative left shift in the neutrophils.

The inflammatory leukogram is important in that it may alert the veterinarian to the presence of a significant inflammatory process occurring somewhere in the animal's body. The inflammatory leukogram may also help the veterinarian to assess the quality of the inflammatory process that is occurring in the puppy or kitten. The regenerative left shift is the most common inflammatory leukogram and is elicited by various inflammatory causes in an animal with adequate bone marrow reserves of neutrophils. It can be initiated quickly and last for a few hours to several days. If the inflammatory process continues for a few weeks and the utilization of neutrophils in the inflamed tissue does not exceed the bone marrow production, then a mature neutrophilia may result. In general, the detection of a regenerative left shift or a mature neutrophilia suggests that the animal's bone marrow is responding appropriately to the inflammatory incident.

In certain situations, the virulence of an infectious agent may be so significant that the

Table 15–8	Leukogram Characteristics						
LEUKOCYTE PATTERN	PHYSIOLOGIC	STRESS	REGENERATIVE LEFT SHIFT	LEUKOPENIC DEGENERATIVE LEFT SHIFT	LEUKOCYTOTIC DEGENERATIVE LEFT SHIFT	MATURE NEUTROPHILIA
Cause	Anxiety Fear	Stress >1 h duration	Acute inflammation	Acute overwhelming inflammation	Prolonged overwhelming inflammation	Prolonged inflammation
Mechanism	Epinephrine	Corticosteroids	Inflammatory mediators	Inflammatory mediators	Inflammatory mediators	Inflammatory mediators
Leukogram features	Neutrophilia	Neutrophilia	Neutrophilia	Neutropenia	Neutrophilia or occasionally normal neutrophil count	Neutrophilia
	Lymphocytosis	Lymphopenia	Bands >500 cells/μl	Immature neutrophils >10% WBC	Immature neutrophils $\geq$ mature neutrophils	
	Occasional monocytosis	Occasional monocytosis Occasional eosinopenia				

tissue involvement is widespread or the ability of the animal's bone marrow to respond is so compromised that a leukopenia with a left shift results. This leukocyte pattern response is termed *leukopenic degenerative left shift* and may indicate an overwhelming challenge to the animal's general immune response. A leukopenic degenerative left shift can occur early or late in the development of disease process.

Another situation that can arise is a continued high demand for neutrophils in the tissue for a sufficient period of time that the bone marrow increases its granulopoiesis but not sufficient enough to avoid a left shift. This leukocyte pattern response is termed a *leukocytic degenerative left shift*. Both leukopenia and leukocytic degenerative left shifts alert the veterinarian to an urgency in identifying and treating the inciting cause of the disease process.

Inflammation often causes changes in neutrophil morphology known as *toxic changes* (Table 15–9). These morphologic changes are caused by defects in the maturation process of neutrophils in the bone marrow. The detection of toxic changes in the neutrophils in the blood smear, with the exception of Döhle bodies in cats, indicates the presence of a significant inflammatory response in the puppy or kitten. Detection of toxic changes in which there is no inflammatory leukogram pattern, such as regenerative or degenerative left shift, alerts the veterinarian to the presence of an inflammatory process in the animal. Toxic changes are more common with inflammatory responses secondary to bacterial infections, but nonbacterial causes such as viral infections, pancreatitis, renal failure, and neoplasia may result in toxic changes. In general, the more severe the toxic changes observed, the more likely that bacterial infection is involved. For example, observation of 4+ toxic granulation in neutrophils makes bacterial infection more likely than bacterial infection or other processes with 2+ Döhle bodies.

DISEASES OF PUPPIES AND KITTENS CAUSING CHANGES IN THE HEMOGRAM
Neonatal Isoerythrolysis

The clinical disease caused by maternal immune-mediated lysis of neonatal RBCs known as *neonatal isoerythrolysis* is uncommon in kittens and extremely rare in puppies. In kittens, neonatal isoerythrolysis can occur when RBC alloantigen type A kittens are born to type B primiparous or multiparous queens that have anti-A alloantibodies (Callan and Giger, 1994). These anti-A alloantibodies are agglutinating and hemolytic. After ingestion and assimilation of colostrum, kittens may demonstrate loss of the suckle reflex, lethargy progressing to depression, anemia, icterus, hemoglobinuria, and death by 48 to 60 hours of life (Gandolfi, 1988; Jonsson et al, 1990; Wilkerson et al, 1991).

Only a small fraction of litters with type A

Table 15–9	Neutrophil Toxic Changes			

FEATURES	CYTOPLASMIC TOXIC CHANGES			NUCLEAR TOXIC CHANGE
Type	Döhle bodies	Cytoplasmic basophilia and diffuse vacuolation	Toxic granulation	Giant nuclei
Morphologic appearance	1–4 1–2-μm slate blue bodies	Blue cytoplasm with very fine granular or foamy appearance	Numerous small blue to red rod-shaped granules	Band-form nuclei 2–3 times larger than normal neutrophils
Cause	Denatured endoplasmic reticulum	Retained RNA, lysosomal leakage	Failure of maturation of 1° neutrophil granules	Failure of nuclear division resulting in polyploidy
Diagnostic significance	Slight in dogs, none in cats	Usually associated with significant inflammatory processes	Usually associated with significant inflammatory processes	Usually associated with significant inflammatory processes

kittens born to type B queens develop neonatal isoerythrolysis, even though all type B queens possess anti-A alloantibodies. Acquisition of these alloantibodies does not require prior exposure of queens to type A alloantigens, but by an as yet uncharacterized mechanism type B queens begin to develop anti-A alloantibodies by 6 to 8 weeks of age with maximal titers around 3 months of age (Bücheler and Giger, 1993). The prevalence of type B alloantigens is related to breed and varies with geographical locale. The highest prevalence of type B alloantigen is in Exotic and British short-haired and Cornish and Devon Rex cats. Several of the reported cases of neonatal isoerythrolysis have occurred in Persian cats, although there are also reported cases in domestic short-haired and long-haired cats (Cain and Suzuki, 1985; Gandolfi, 1988).

Diagnosis is based on age, clinical signs, and pathologic lesions and can be further established by a slide hemagglutination test. A tentative diagnosis of neonatal isoerythrolysis should be considered for neonatal kittens that are initially vigorous, but between birth and 48 hours of age they exhibit weakness and hemoglobinuria. Slide hemagglutination can be done by mixing a drop of sera from the queen with a drop of EDTA-anticoagulated blood from an affected kitten. After gentle mixing and 5 minutes of incubation at room temperature, the slide is examined microscopically for hemagglutination recognized as clumped RBCs (Fig. 15–

3). Occasionally, hemolysis occurs rather than agglutination. Hemolysis should be considered as a positive endpoint. Hemagglutination will be positive for all type B queens with type A kittens, whether the kittens are affected by neonatal isoerythrolysis or not.

The potential for neonatal isoerythrolysis can be avoided by blood typing queens and sires before breeding. Breeding of type B queens with type A sires should be avoided. Although type A queens also possess anti-B alloantibodies, isoerythrolysis is not observed in litters containing type B kittens born to type A queens. This may result from the fact that the anti-B alloantibodies in type A queens are weak agglutinins and hemolysins in contrast to the strong hemagglutination and hemolytic activity of anti-A alloantibodies of type B queens.

Nutritional Iron Deficiency Anemia

Nutritional iron deficiency anemias are extremely rare in dogs and cats. Transient nutritional iron deficiency anemia can, however, be seen in kittens and rarely in puppies at 2 to 8 weeks of age. The effects of rapid growth, replacement of fetal RBCs, and low iron content of maternal milk may combine at weaning to cause iron deficiency anemia in some kittens. Iron deficiency anemia can be detected in these kittens by the presence of increased microcytes (Weiser and Kociba, 1983). These microcytes are not readily discernible on morphologic ex-

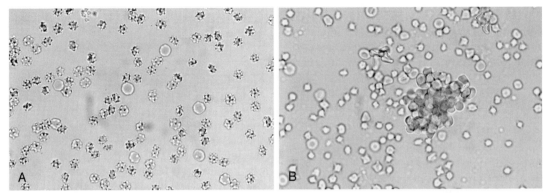

Figure 15–3. Wet preparation of blood diluted in normal saline solution from a normal kitten (**A**) and a kitten with feline leukemia virus infection (**B**) demonstrating microagglutinated red blood cells. (Courtesy of the Department of Veterinary Pathobiology teaching files, College of Veterinary Medicine, Oklahoma State University, Stillwater.)

amination of blood smears or by decreased MCV or MCHC but require detection by the percentage of RBCs with an MCV of less than 27 fl. Iron-deficient kittens did have statistically detectable lower serum iron and percentage of transferrin saturation than normal kittens, but again these changes were not dramatic enough to be practically useful for diagnosis in most veterinary practice situations. Red blood cell fragmentation detected on blood smears is an ancillary finding in iron deficiency anemia and is observed in approximately 50% of iron-deficient kittens. Kittens with packed cell volume of less than 20% at 2 to 3 weeks of age with the presence of RBC fragments should be considered as potentially iron deficient. Iron-dextran injections given at 2 to 3 weeks of age to kittens with these criteria resulted in the packed cell volume increasing to within the reference range by 5 weeks of age.

Chronic Blood Loss Anemias

Persistent blood loss from flea and tick infestations in puppies and kittens and from the hookworm *Ancylostoma caninum* infection in puppies can result in iron deficiency anemias. Of these causes, *Ancylostoma caninum* infection is common and can develop as early as 3 to 5 weeks of age (Miller, 1971). In heavy infections, not only will anemia be observed but also respiratory signs from migrating larvae may be seen. The anemia from *Ancylostoma caninum* infection can range from acute hemorrhagic anemia with some regenerative response to a true regenerative anemia to a classic microcytic, hypochromic iron deficiency anemia. The duration and severity of *Ancylostoma caninum* infection and of

blood loss and the age of the puppy are factors that will impact the characteristics of the anemia observed. The anemia can be identified as arising from blood loss by the low total plasma protein. *Ancylostoma caninum* infection can be identified by the observation of characteristic ova on fecal flotation.

Pelger-Huet Anomaly

Pelger-Huet anomaly is a rare inherited disorder of development in granulocytes that is characterized by hyposegmentation of the nuclei of neutrophils, basophils, and eosinophils (Feldman and Roman, 1976; Latimer et al, 1985). The nuclei of Pelger-Huet granulocytes appear hyposegmented, often resembling band neutrophils, metamyelocytes, or myelocytes, but with a coarse mature chromatin pattern. The anomaly is usually detected incidentally when a persistent left shift is found with a normal WBC count in an otherwise healthy animal (Latimer et al, 1985). Pelger-Huet anomaly has been seen in domestic short-haired cats (Weber et al, 1981) and in various dog breeds such as the Australian shepherd; Australian blue heeler; basenji; Boston terrier; black-and-tan, blue tick, and redbone coonhounds; cocker spaniel; English-American foxhound; German shepherd; Samoyed; and mongrel (Latimer et al, 1989b). The inheritance mode is assumed to be autosomal dominant (Bowles et al, 1979). Most cases are the heterozygous state with no abnormalities in neutrophil function, whereas the homozygous form may be pathologic with fetal death (Latimer et al, 1989b).

Mucopolysaccharidases

Mucopolysaccharidases are a group of inherited lysosomal storage disorders that rarely occur in dogs and cats. Lack of a specific enzyme's production or function results in accumulation of coarse metachromatic granules in most of the mature neutrophils (Fig. 15–4), in a few lymphocytes, and in some large cells resembling histiocytes (Jezyk et al, 1977). These granules, visible with Wright-Giemsa stain, are seen more easily when the blood smear is stained with toluidine blue. The numbers of neutrophils and lymphocytes and their functions are not altered in affected animals. Affected dogs or cats generally are not brought to the veterinarian because of their hematologic abnormalities but rather for the skeletal deformities, neurologic deficits of the central nervous system, and/or other signs attributed to enzyme deficiency in the catabolism of mucopolysaccharides.

Cholesteryl Ester Storage Disease

A cholesteryl ester storage disease (acid lipase/cholesteryl hydrolase deficiency) has been reported in two 11-month-old sibling Siamese kittens (Thrall et al, 1991). Clinical signs consisted of corneal clouding, vomiting and diarrhea, hepatomegaly, lymphadenopathy, and muscle wasting. Hematologic abnormalities included anemia and vacuolated lymphocytes in the peripheral blood and vacuolated sea-blue macrophages in bone marrow aspirates. Trans-

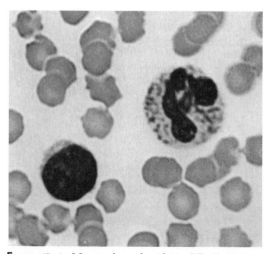

Figure 15–4. Mucopolysaccharidosis VI. Prominent cytoplasmic granules are present in most polymorphonuclear leukocytes in routine blood smears from cats with this disorder. (Wright-Giemsa stain; ×2000.) (From Haskins ME, Patterson DF: Inherited metabolic diseases. *In* Holzworth J [ed]: Diseases of the Cat: Medicine and Surgery, vol 1. Philadelphia, WB Saunders, 1987, p 812.)

mission is possibly as an autosomal recessive trait.

Hereditary Red Blood Cell Enzyme Deficiencies

Inherited deficiencies of the glycolytic enzymes, such as phosphofructokinase (PFK) and pyruvate kinase (PK), occur in dogs, and rarely in cats, resulting in regenerative anemias (Harvey, 1997). Clinical signs of these congenital conditions can be detected in puppies younger than 6 months. The anemia may be mild to marked. When the anemia is mild, the regenerative response may seem exaggerated or super-regenerative—although the severity of the anemia is mild, the degree of regenerative response as detected by polychromasia or reticulocytosis is much higher than that expected for that particular packed cell volume. Because these enzyme deficiencies are inherited, these conditions are most common in particular breeds of dogs.

Phosphofructokinase deficiency has been observed in English springer spaniels and American cocker spaniels. Persistent mild, super-regenerative anemia and periodic hemolytic crises characterize this condition. The hemolytic crises are often precipitated by hyperventilation-induced alkalemia, which causes the intravascular hemolysis of the alkaline-fragile PFK-deficient RBCs. The clinical signs during these crises of weakness, hemoglobinuria, pale and/or icteric mucous membranes, hepatosplenomegaly, and fever are referable to the intravascular hemolysis. Affected puppies can be identified by measurement of low PFK levels in the RBCs.

Pyruvate kinase deficiency has been reported in basenji, beagle, West Highland white terrier, Cairn terrier, American Eskimo dog, and Abyssinian cat. Puppies with PK deficiency develop mild super-regenerative to severe regenerative anemias. The clinical disease also involves musculoskeletal lesions and results in death at 3 to 4 years of age from bone marrow failure or hepatic insufficiency. Because affected puppies have decreased levels of the normal R-type PK isozyme but increased levels of a fetal-type M_2 PK isozyme in RBCs, the diagnosis is complex. Increased RBC PK activity along with increased accumulation of glycolytic intermediates and increased M_2 PK isozyme in RBCs as detected by enzyme stability, immunoreactivity, or electrophoresis supports a diagnosis of PK deficiency in puppies.

Dyserythropoiesis of English Springer Spaniels

A nonregenerative anemia associated with a polysystemic disorder occurs in English springer spaniel dogs from 3.5 months to 2 years of age (Holland et al, 1991). The dogs exhibit a moderate dyserythropoietic anemia, polymyopathy with megaesophagus, and varying degrees of cardiomyopathy. The dyserythropoiesis is characterized by abnormal erythroid cells with arrested or abnormal mitoses in the bone marrow and many nucleated red blood cells in the peripheral blood without appropriate reticulocytosis. Microcytes, spherocytes, schizocytes, and other poikilocytes are seen on peripheral blood smears.

Canine Cyclic Hematopoiesis

Canine cyclic hematopoiesis, formerly called *gray collie syndrome* or *canine cyclic neutropenia*, is an uncommon disorder that is inherited as a simple autosomal recessive trait in gray collies (Campbell, 1985). At 1 week of age, affected puppies are usually smaller and weaker than their littermates. All affected collies have a specific silver-gray to beige dilution of hair color and regular cyclic fluctuations of all cellular blood elements, including platelets. In affected puppies, the episodes occur at 11- to 12-day cycles, starting as early as the eighth day of life, with each cycle lasting an average of 3 days. Neutropenia is followed by a normal to slightly increased neutrophil count that lasts for 6 to 7 days. The neutrophil cycle typically corresponds to episodes of infection, which may or may not be associated with illness before 2 months of age. After weaning, episodes of malaise, anorexia, fever, painful joints, severe bilateral keratitis, and respiratory and enteric infections frequently occur 1 to 2 days after the episodes of neutropenia. Most affected dogs develop increasing dependency on antimicrobial therapy and die within 6 months of age from moderate to severe secondary infections (Yang, 1978). Amyloidosis is a common sequela in animals that survive 3 months or longer.

Feline Chediak-Higashi Syndrome

Chediak-Higashi syndrome is an inherited, autosomal recessive disorder that occurs mostly in Persian cats with blue-smoke haircoat (Kramer et al, 1977; Renshaw et al, 1974). The syndrome is associated with an increased susceptibility to upper respiratory infections and septicemia; the production of abnormally large primary granules in neutrophils (Fig. 15–5), basophils, and eosinophils; enlarged lysosomal granules in lymphocytes and many other cell types (liver and kidney); and the formation of enlarged melanin granules (Guilford, 1987). Affected cats, because of their defective melanin pigmentation, have lighter colored haircoats, light-colored irises, and red fundic light reflections and are photophobic. Cataracts tend to form at an early age. In addition, affected cats have a tendency to bleed after minor surgery and to form hematomas at venipuncture sites. Coagulation times and platelet counts are usually normal, but platelet function may be abnormal (Guilford, 1987). Diagnosis of Chediak-Higashi syndrome in affected Persian cats is made by examination of blood smears for the presence of enlarged granules in neutrophils and by finding enlarged melanin granules in the hair shafts. Allogenic bone marrow transplantation is successful in correcting the neutrophil migration defect and platelet storage pool deficiency (Colgan et al, 1991). Otherwise, treatment for the syndrome is entirely symptomatic care.

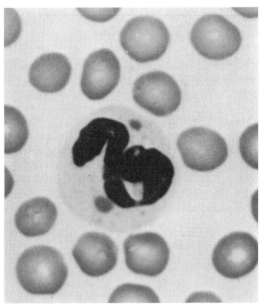

Figure 15–5. Chediak-Higashi syndrome. Large cytoplasmic granules in a neutrophil of a cat affected with this disorder. (Wright-Giemsa stain; original magnification, ×1900.) (From Prasse KW, Mahaffey EA: Hematology of normal cats and characteristic responses to disease. *In* Holzworth J [ed]: Diseases of the Cat: Medicine and Surgery, vol 1. Philadelphia, WB Saunders, 1987, p 748; courtesy of Dr. John W. Kramer.)

Lead Poisoning

Lead poisoning can occur at any age, but the propensity of puppies, in particular, to chew on or ingest foreign objects makes them more likely to develop lead poisoning. In affected puppies or kittens, the characteristic hematologic changes associated with lead poisoning are only observed in animals exhibiting either the gastrointestinal or neurologic signs. The hematologic changes observed are increased N-RBCs, basophilic stippled RBCs, and polychromasia. These changes typically occur in an animal with a packed cell volume within the reference range or only slightly anemic.

The numbers of N-RBCs and basophilic stippled RBCs present can range from 0 to more than 200 N-RBCs/100 WBCs or 0 to more than 40 basophilic stippled RBCs/10,000 RBCs. The presence of N-RBCs in blood smears is not specific to lead poisoning. The observation of more than 40 basophilic stippled RBCs/10,000 RBCs has been proposed as being pathognomonic for lead poisoning. Because basophilic stippling can result from intense regenerative responses in anemic dogs and cats, however, caution should be used to assess the nature and severity of the anemia before accepting the increased basophilic stippling as support for a diagnosis of lead poisoning (Zook et al, 1970). Typically, no or only mild anemia is present in lead poisoning.

A tentative diagnosis of lead poisoning should be considered for puppies or kittens exhibiting acute gastrointestinal or neurologic signs with no or only a slight anemia but with increased polychromasia, N-RBCs, and/or basophilic stippled RBCs. A definitive diagnosis of lead poisoning can be sought by evaluating serum and urine lead levels.

Zinc-Induced Hemolytic Anemia

The propensity of puppies to ingest foreign objects and the change from primarily copper to primarily zinc content of U.S. pennies minted after 1982 are likely the reasons for increased zinc-induced hemolytic anemia in puppies (Robinette, 1990). Signs include vomiting, diarrhea, depression, anemia, hemoglobinemia, and hemoglobinuria. Radiographic examination of the stomach often reveals radioopaque objects compatible with U.S. pennies. Zinc-containing pet carrier screw nuts or plumbing nuts as well as zinc-containing ointments have been involved in some cases (Ackerman et al, 1990). Rapid dissolution of metallic zinc items under the action of gastric secretions results in high plasma, tissue, and urine zinc levels.

The anemia observed is typically regenerative with increased reticulocytes, polychromasia, and a normal serum or plasma total protein concentration, indicating that it is a hemolytic anemia. The mechanism of zinc-induced hemolysis is unknown, and a variety of RBC morphologic changes have been observed in some cases, including Heinz bodies, N-RBCs, spherocytes, and basophilic stippling (Latimer et al, 1989a; Luttgen et al, 1990; Meurs et al, 1991). Other laboratory findings are a regenerative left shift, hyperbilirubinemia, and azotemia. In some cases, zinc-containing foreign objects in the stomach may dissolve so rapidly that no radioopaque objects are observed on radiography, and none are recovered on endoscopy or gastrotomy. Diagnosis can be confirmed by elevated serum, tissue, or urine zinc levels (Ackerman et al, 1990; Luttgen et al, 1990; Robinette, 1990).

Babesiosis

Babesiosis, a tick-borne hematozoon disease, affects dogs and cats of all ages and results in a progressive anemia as the primary physical finding during apparent disease. Three species of causative organisms are associated with canine babesiosis: *Babesia canis*, *Babesia gibsoni*, and *Babesia vogeli*. Puppies 4 months of age or younger are quite susceptible to these *Babesia* species and frequently acquire a more severe infection than do adult dogs. *Babesia canis* and *Babesia vogeli* are of similar size, 2.4 × 5.0 and 4.0 × 5.0 μm, respectively, and are usually seen as paired piriform trophozoites within red blood cells. *Babesia gibsoni* is smaller (1.0 × 3.2 μm), pleomorphic, and usually found as singular, annular bodies in red blood cells. Under natural conditions, ticks are the principal vectors for *Babesia* species. Feline babesiosis primarily affects cats younger than 2 years of age. Four species are known to infect domestic and wild cats: *Babesia cati*, *Babesia felis*, *Babesia herpailuri*, and *Babesia pantherae*. These *Babesia* species occur either singly or as paired piriform bodies within red blood cells and are similar in size to *Babesia gibsoni*, approximately 1.0 × 2.5 to 1.3 × 3.4 μm.

Babesia species in the young dog or cat induce a parasitemia that causes both intravascular and extravascular hemolysis. Early in the disease, babesiosis is characterized predominantly by intravascular hemolysis, resulting in a regenerative anemia without suppression of erythropoiesis. The hemolytic anemia usually corresponds to increased parasitemia, especially during the first month of the infection. Nucleated red blood cells are frequently numerous in late infections. The packed cell volume may be less than 10%, and the hemoglobin concentration is often less than 3.9 g/dl in terminal stages of the disease. Other laboratory findings may include thrombocytopenia, hyperbilirubinemia, bilirubinuria, hemoglobinuria, cellular and granular casts in the urine sediment, and azotemia. Metabolic acidosis and disseminated intravascular coagulation may develop as complications of infection. Some dogs have spherocytes and a positive result of a direct Coombs' test. Definitive diagnosis requires identification of the *Babesia* organisms in red blood cells of a Wright-stained or Giemsa-stained peripheral blood smear. Unlike canine babesiosis, which is characterized by a normocytic, normochromic anemia, a macrocytic, hypochromic anemia is often found in feline babesiosis and is most likely related to a lower grade hemolytic anemia. A mild anemia generally persists in the infected, asymptomatic carriers of canine babesiosis, and parasitemia often is undetectable because few organisms are present in the peripheral blood at any one time. When babesiosis is suspected but the organism cannot be demonstrated, the

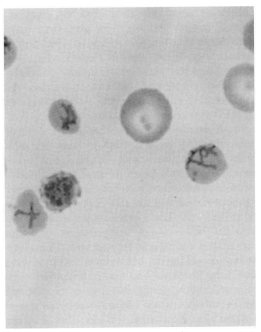

Figure 15–7. Four red blood cells parasitized by *Haemobartonella canis* organisms from an infected dog. (Wright-Giemsa stain; ×1500.) (From Harvey JW: Haemobartonellosis. *In* Greene CE [ed]: Clinical Microbiology and Infectious Diseases of the Dog and Cat. Philadelphia, WB Saunders, 1984, p 578.)

indirect fluorescent antibody test for *Babesia canis* and *Babesia gibsoni* is a reliable means of detecting patent or occult parasitemia in dogs. Antibody titers greater than 1:40 are considered seropositive for either *Babesia canis* or *Babesia gibsoni*. Babesiosis in the dog commonly occurs along with other erythroparasites, such as *Ehrlichia canis* and *Haemobartonella canis*. Treatment for babesiosis in the young dog or cat is similar to that for the adult and is described elsewhere.

Haemobartonellosis

Haemobartonellosis occurs fairly commonly in dogs and cats of all ages throughout the world but is mostly a disease of the domestic cat. *Haemobartonella felis* infects domestic cats, whereas domestic dogs are infected with *Haemobartonella canis*. *Haemobartonella felis* is highly pleomorphic and often appears as cocci that can be arranged singly or in short chains (Fig. 15–6). Ring and rod forms may also occur. *Haemobartonella canis* appears as cocci or short rods that occur singly or in short chains (Fig. 15–7). *Haemobartonella* organisms are about 0.5 μm in diameter and, unlike other erythroparasites, attach themselves in depressions or deep in-

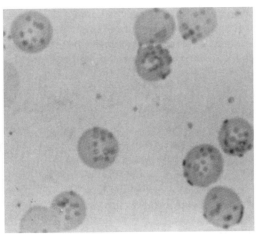

Figure 15–6. *Haemobartonella felis* organisms parasitizing red blood cells from an infected cat. Note that some free organisms displaced during blood smear preparation are present. (Wright-Giemsa stain; ×1600.) (From Harvey JW: Haemobartonellosis. *In* Greene CE [ed]: Clinical Microbiology and Infectious Diseases of the Dog and Cat. Philadelphia, WB Saunders, 1984, p 577.)

foldings on the surface of the red blood cell and cause distortion of the red blood cell to which they attach. The organisms are easily dislodged from the surface of the red blood cell, as can occur with refrigerated or anticoagulated blood; therefore, fresh, thin-prepared, well-stained blood smears are best for the definitive identification of *Haemobartonella* organisms.

With haemobartonellosis, evidence of a regenerative anemia is present by the time dogs or cats are presented with symptoms of an apparent illness. Red blood cells are usually macrocytic, with an increased MCV, and frequently hypochromic, with a reduced MCHC. The magnitude of the regenerative response observed in blood samples depends on the duration of the anemia. If the packed cell volume decreases rapidly, the MCV may be normal with little polychromasia and few reticulocytes present until the bone marrow begins to respond. Results of the direct Coombs' test commonly become positive 1 to 2 weeks after detected parasitemia in the infected cat and remain positive during the early stages of the disease whether or not parasitemia is present. Cats that are infected, asymptomatic carriers of *Haemobartonella* organisms generally have low-grade parasitemia. Their packed cell volume tends to fluctuate over time and may be normal or slightly to moderately decreased. Slight polychromasia and reticulocytosis and increased MCV are present at times. *Haemobartonella* infection has been associated with feline leukemia virus and feline immunodeficiency infections. The preferred diagnostic procedure to detect occult *Haemobartonella felis* infection is the polymerase chain reaction (PCR), which also evaluates response to medical treatment and clearance of the organisms. The PCR will be positive before the onset of clinical signs of infection and visible organisms and is positive before detectable seroconversion. The PCR will maintain positivity until all organisms are cleared from the infected cat. Treatment of haemobartonellosis in young dogs and cats is similar to that in the adult.

Cytauxzoonosis

Cytauxzoonosis is a hematozoon disease of the domestic cat and is caused by the organism *Cytauxzoon felis*. At the time *Cytauxzoon*-infected cats present with apparent illness, the red blood cell counts average 1% to 4% parasitized red cells, and evidence of moderate regenerative anemia is usually present. Hemoglobinuria and

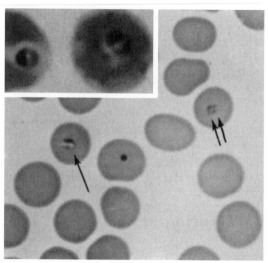

Figure 15–8. Red blood cells parasitized by *Cytauxzoon* piroplasms. Ring form (single arrow) and dividing form (double arrows). Inset, Enlarged view of ring forms in parasitized red blood cells. Compare their appearance with that of a Howell-Jolly body. (Giemsa-Triton stain; ×1000.) (From Kier AB: Cytauxzoonosis. *In* Greene CE [ed]: Clinical Microbiology and Infectious Diseases of the Dog and Cat. Philadelphia, WB Saunders, 1984, p 793.)

bilirubinuria are only rarely observed. Diagnosis of cytauxzoonosis is made by demonstrating the organisms in Wright-stained or Giemsa-stained thin blood smears (Fig. 15–8). *Cytauxzoon* organisms appear as rounded "signet rings" or oval "safety pin" bodies. In general, the treatment of cytauxzoonosis in young cats yields poor results; supportive therapy with fluids and broad-spectrum antimicrobial agents may prolong the course of illness but does not effect a cure.

Feline Panleukopenia

Cats younger than 1 year have the highest incidence of feline panleukopenia. Leukopenia ranging from 100 to 2000 cells/μl is the most common hematologic change. This leukopenia is composed of an absolute neutropenia without an increase in band neutrophils and often a lymphopenia (Jain, 1986). Although feline panleukopenia can cause a bloody diarrhea, typically no anemia is observed (Carpenter, 1971). It is likely that a mild to moderate acute blood loss anemia is present but is masked by an accompanying hemoconcentration secondary to dehydration. The total plasma protein concentration is often within the reference range for the age of the kitten affected or slightly to moderately increased. During the convalescent and recovery phase of the infection, the leukogram may change to a degenerative left shift and occasionally to a regenerative left shift.

Canine Parvovirus Infection

The highest incidence of canine parvovirus infection is in puppies between 6 and 20 weeks of age. At presentation, only a few puppies may exhibit leukopenia, but a moderate to marked leukopenia is detected in most puppies by serial WBC counts on subsequent days (Jacobs et al, 1980). This leukopenia often ranges from 500 to 6000 cells/µl and is composed of a neutropenia and lymphopenia. The severity of the leukopenia may parallel the severity of the clinical signs. A mild anemia and panhypoproteinemia can be observed at 2 to 5 days after presentation. Convalescence can be associated with a rebound leukocytosis.

Canine Distemper

The incidence of canine distemper is most common in puppies from 2 months to 2 years of age. The hematologic changes observed with canine distemper are extremely variable and range from slight anemia to polycythemia and from leukopenia to leukocytosis (Jain, 1986). The anemias are mild, and packed cell volume is 23% to 37% and may actually represent packed cell volume values within the reference range for some ages of puppies. The polycythemias are attributed to hemoconcentration secondary to dehydration. Lymphopenia is a common feature of the leukogram. This lymphopenia is attributed to viral-induced lymphoid atrophy or necrosis. The leukograms observed in puppies with canine distemper can be leukopenias composed of a lymphopenia with or without a neutropenia, leukocyte counts within the reference range with a lymphopenia or a leukocytosis composed of a lymphopenia, regenerative left shift or mature neutrophilia, and/or monocytosis. The variability of the leukogram may reflect the varied clinical course of canine distemper involving both viral and secondary bacterial infections.

Viral inclusion composed of the distemper viral nucleocapsid can rarely be observed in RBCs, neutrophils, or lymphocytes. These distemper inclusions may be seen more commonly during the viremic stage of the disease, although an association with hardening of the footpads has also been reported (Jain, 1986). The inclusion bodies are small, but variable sized, round to irregularly shaped, red to blue in Romanosky-type stain of RBCs and in the cytoplasm of neutrophils and lymphocytes (Fig. 15–9).

Canine Ehrlichiosis

In canine ehrlichiosis, morulae of *Ehrlichia* species are detected in the cytoplasm of various leukocytes of Wright-stained or Giemsa-stained peripheral blood smears (Fig. 15–10), buffy coat smears, or bone marrow aspirates (Fig. 15–11). The morulae stain bluish purple and are usually found transiently and in low numbers early in *Ehrlichia* infections.

Canine Hepatozoonosis

Gametocytes of *Hepatozoon* species may be found in neutrophils and monocytes of Wright-stained or Giemsa-stained peripheral blood or buffy coat smears (Fig. 15–12). The organisms appear as ice-blue, oval intracytoplasmic inclusions measuring approximately 5×10 µm. If blood smears are not made shortly after blood collection, the gametocytes appear to leave the host cells, and a nonstaining capsule is all that remains. When a dog has a detectable parasitemia, only 1 to 2 cells/1000 leukocytes are usually infected. Infection with *Hepatozoon* species is often inapparent but may cause severe disease that is characterized by anorexia, leth-

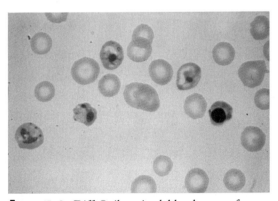

Figure 15–9. Diff-Quik–stained blood smear from a puppy with canine distemper demonstrating inclusions in red blood cells. A nucleated red blood cell is also present. (Courtesy of the Department of Veterinary Pathobiology teaching files, College of Veterinary Medicine, Oklahoma State University, Stillwater.)

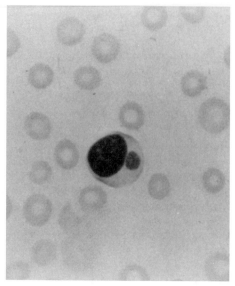

Figure 15–10. Intracytoplasmic morula in a leukocyte from a dog infected with *Ehrlichia canis*. (Giemsa stain; ×1000.) (Courtesy of Dr. S.D. Gaunt, Louisiana State University, Baton Rouge.)

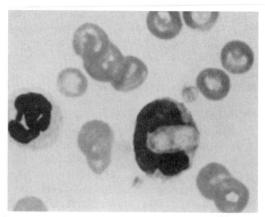

Figure 15–12. Gametocyte of *Hepatozoon* species in a neutrophil from a peripheral blood smear. (Giemsa stain; ×1200.) (From Craig TM: Hepatozoonosis. *In* Greene CE [ed]: Clinical Microbiology and Infectious Diseases of the Dog and Cat. Philadelphia, WB Saunders, 1984, p 776.)

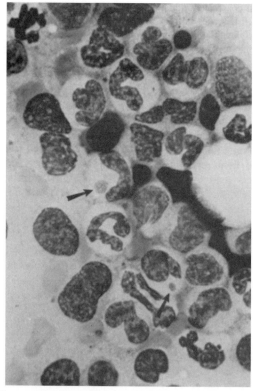

Figure 15–11. Intracytoplasmic morulae in two neutrophils (arrows) in a bone marrow biopsy sample from a dog infected with *Ehrlichia canis*. (Wright-Giemsa stain; ×1000.) (Courtesy of Dr. T.N. Hribernik, Ft. Walton, FL.)

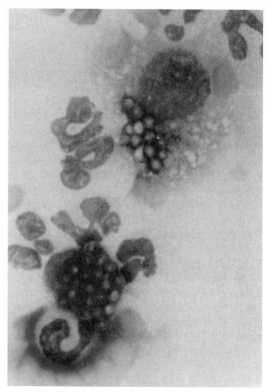

Figure 15–13. Intracellular organisms of *Histoplasma capsulatum* from a peripheral blood smear. (Wright's stain; ×1000.) (From Barsanti JA: Histoplasmosis. *In* Greene CE [ed]: Clinical Microbiology and Infectious Diseases of the Dog and Cat. Philadelphia, WB Saunders, 1984, p 693; courtesy of Dr. Ken Latimer.)

argy, fever, muscle pain, stiffness, periosteal new bone formation, and marked leukocytosis with or without a left shift. Transmission of the parasite occurs via ingestion of infected *Rhipicephalus sanguineus* ticks. Canine hepatozoonosis appears to have a limited distribution in the United States and occurs mostly in the states along the Gulf Coast.

Histoplasmosis

Histoplasma capsulatum yeast is identified in the cytoplasm of neutrophils and monocytes on Wright-stained or Giemsa-stained peripheral blood smears (Fig. 15–13), buffy coat smears, and bone marrow aspirates in disseminated cases. The organisms appear as 2- to 4-μm oval basophilic inclusions surrounded by an unstained halo.

Leishmaniasis

Leishmania species are seen in the cytoplasm of infected monocytes on peripheral blood smears and bone marrow aspirates (Fig. 15–14). Amastigotes appear in the cytoplasm of the monocyte as round bodies with a dark blue kinetoplast and nucleus.

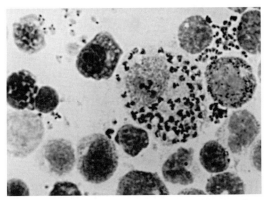

Figure 15–14. *Leishmania* amastigotes in the cytoplasm of a bone marrow macrophage of a dog with visceral leishmaniasis. (Wright-Giemsa stain; ×1000.)

Birman Cat Neutrophil Granulation Anomaly

An autosomal recessive anomaly that is characterized by fine eosinophilic intracytoplasmic granules in neutrophils occurs in highly inbred Birman cats (Hirsch and Cunningham, 1984). The granules are not seen in other granulocytes. This anomaly must be differentiated from toxic granulation, which is usually associated with a left shift, and from mucopolysaccharidosis type VI, which usually is associated with facial dysmorphia.

Disorders of Hemostasis

Mary K. Boudreaux

NORMAL HEMOSTASIS

Normal hemostasis depends on the complex interaction of plasma coagulation, antithrombotic and fibrinolytic proteins, platelets, and the blood vasculature. After injury of the vessel wall, vasoconstriction retards extravascular blood loss and slows local blood flow, enhancing the adherence of platelets to exposed subendothelial surfaces and the activation of the coagulation process. The adherence of platelets at sites of vascular injury is an important early event in hemostasis and is mediated by a plasma protein known as von Willebrand's factor. After adhesion, additional platelets are recruited in response to components released from platelet granules, including adenosine 5'-diphosphate and serotonin. Platelets also synthesize thromboxane A_2 and platelet-activating factor, which are potent platelet-aggregating agonists and, in the case of thromboxane A_2, enhance vasoconstriction.

Exposure of subendothelial surfaces and/or the generation of tissue factors also leads to the sequential activation of a series of coagulation proteins (Fig. 15–15). These proteins, a series of enzymes and cofactors, ultimately convert prothrombin to thrombin. Thrombin cleaves fibrinogen into fibrin monomers and activates factor XIII, which serves to crosslink and stabilize the resulting fibrin network. The activity of

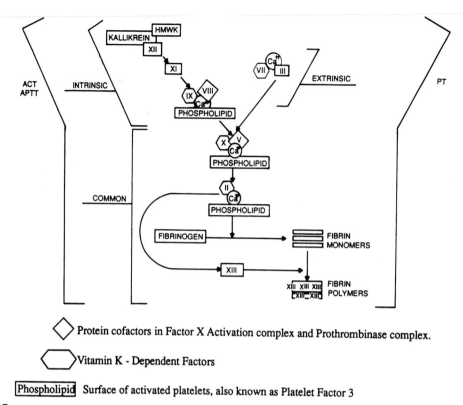

Protein cofactors in Factor X Activation complex and Prothrombinase complex.

Vitamin K - Dependent Factors

Phospholipid Surface of activated platelets, also known as Platelet Factor 3

Figure 15–15. A series of enzymes and cofactors ultimately convert prothrombin to thrombin. Thrombin cleaves fibrinogen into fibrin and activates factor XIII, resulting in the formation of a stable fibrin network. ACT = activated coagulation time; APTT = activated partial thromboplastin time; HMWK = high molecular weight kininogen; PT = prothrombin time.

many of the coagulation factors depends not only on calcium but also on the phospholipid provided by the surface of activated platelets. Binding of coagulation proteins to a common surface in close proximity enhances the efficiency of serial activation of the coagulation factors in a fairly discrete area. Thrombin formed in excess binds to thrombomodulin on endothelial cells distal to the injury site. Thrombin bound to thrombomodulin activates protein C, which, in concert with protein S, inactivates factors Va and VIIIa. This serves to limit fibrin formation to local areas of injury. Simultaneous to the activation of the coagulation cascade, plasminogen is converted to plasmin, the agent of fibrinolysis, not only by coagulation contact factors such as kallikrein, but also by tissue plasminogen activator. The latter activation requires fibrin, thus limiting the production of plasmin to the site of thrombus formation. The localization of plasmin is important because the enzyme is fairly nonspecific in its activity and will destroy not only fibrin but also fibrinogen, factor V, and factor VIII.

In general, after vascular injury, platelets and the vasculature serve to temporarily stem blood flow, whereas the coagulation proteins provide a more permanent repair. The antithrombotic system aids in the containment of the thrombus locally, and the fibrinolytic system slowly destroys the fibrin network as healing ensues. Qualitative and quantitative platelet defects are usually manifested by superficial ecchymotic or petechial bleeding, especially from mucous membranes, whereas coagulation protein abnormalities are characterized by delayed deep-tissue hemorrhage and hematoma formation.

COAGULOPATHIES

Disorders of hemostasis may be due to congenital or acquired defects in coagulation proteins, platelets, and/or the vasculature. Congenital coagulopathies are usually first recognized between birth and 6 months of age. Defects in coagulation at this time are exacerbated by a normally immature hemostatic mechanism (Buchanan, 1978) related to a young, developing liver, the site of synthesis of most coagulation proteins. Puppies and kittens with major coagulopathies due to deficiencies in factors vital for hemostasis are often stillborn or die of massive hemorrhage shortly after birth. Major coagulopathies include the existence of less than 1% of normal activity of factors VIII, IX, II, and I. Animals with less severe coagulopathies (factor activities between 1% and 5% of normal levels) usually survive the neonatal period but may encounter hemostatic difficulties between 1 and 6 months of age. Before they reach 6 months of age, puppies and kittens are subjected to a number of routine procedures, including vaccination, deworming, tail docking and dewclaw removal, ear cropping, neutering, and declawing. In addition, normal physiologic processes such as the shedding of deciduous teeth and the onset of estrus also occur, events not tolerated well by individuals with a compromised hemostatic response. Animals with factor activities between 5% and 10% usually do not bleed spontaneously. The coagulopathy is usually only apparent after trauma or surgery. Small dogs and cats with congenital coagulopathies, even with factor activities less than 5% of normal levels, are more likely to have minimal or no spontaneous hemorrhage than are large dogs with similarly diminished factor activity. Small dogs and cats with congenital coagulopathies that are not subjected to trauma or surgery may be several years old before their coagulation defect is recognized.

Acquired coagulopathies are more common than congenital coagulopathies and can occur at any age. Because congenital coagulopathies are usually first apparent before 6 months of age, however, the origin of a bleeding diathesis at this young age may be difficult to discern at initial examination. Also, minor congenital hemostatic defects may not become apparent unless superimposed with an acquired coagulopathy. A thorough history and evaluation of coagulation screening tests and a platelet count will be helpful in determining the reason for a bleeding problem. Proper blood collection procedures and considerations are provided in Table 15–10.

COAGULATION SCREENING TESTS

Activated Coagulation Time

The activated coagulation time (ACT) is a useful screen for evaluation of the intrinsic and common pathways. Whole blood (2 ml) is added to a tube containing diatomaceous earth as a contact activator, and the tube is gently agitated at specific intervals while timing until clot formation. A 37° C heating block is recommended for consistent results (Middleton and Watson, 1978). If a heating block is not available, a Styrofoam cup and 37° C tap water is preferable to performing the assay at room temperature. The ACT test relies on platelet phospholipids to support the reaction; therefore, platelet counts of less than 10,000 cells per μl may result in a prolonged ACT. Published reference ranges should not be used for this assay. Ideally, a reference range should be established for the veterinary facility based on times obtained by repeatedly performing the test on animals known to be normal (different ranges for each species and possibly separate ranges for puppies and kittens younger than 2 months should be established).

Activated Partial Thromboplastin Time

The activated partial thromboplastin time (APTT) assay is an indicator of the function of coagulation factors in the intrinsic and common pathways. Phospholipids as a substitute for platelets, calcium, and a negatively charged surface activator such as kaolin are added to citrated plasma at 37° C, and the time to clot formation is recorded. The test is a useful screen for the function of a number of clotting factors; however, specific factor activities must usually be less than 30% for a prolonged APTT to occur, and the detection of a prolonged APTT is not always clinically significant. Deficiencies of factor XII and kallikrein will prolong the APTT without an associated hemorrhagic diathesis. A prolonged APTT in conjunction with overt bleeding and a normal prothrombin time (see following section) warrants the evaluation of specific coagulation factors. This requires the careful collection of citrated blood (1 part 3.8% trisodium citrate to 9 parts blood) and isolation and immediate freezing of plasma for factor analysis by a specialized hemostasis laboratory. Because young animals may normally have decreased factor activity compared with adults, age-matched controls are important for evaluating not only the APTT but also specific factor activities (Dodds et al, 1975). Young animals may normally have a slight prolongation in the APTT (1 to 3 seconds) compared with adults; however, they should not have markedly prolonged APTTs (greater than 5 seconds) or severe deficiencies in individual factors (less than 10% of normal activity levels). Usu-

Table 15–10	Sample Collection for Coagulation Testing

1. The sample should be collected with minimal excitement of the animal, as excitement can be associated with elevated platelet counts, enhanced platelet activity, and elevated factor VIII levels.
2. Faulty venipuncture technique is the most common cause of abnormal coagulation tests, particularly the APTT. Tissue fluids and hemolysis rapidly activate clotting. Ideally, the sample should be obtained with minimal probing for the vessel and minimal venous stasis.
3. Blood samples for coagulation procedures should never be collected through intravenous catheters that have been used for heparin therapy.
4. It is important that the surface of any collection, holding, or transfer containers be consistent, that is, all plastic or all siliconized, to avoid activation of factor XII and to prevent spontaneous platelet clumping.
5. The preferred anticoagulant is 3.8% trisodium citrate. The ratio of anticoagulant to blood is 1:9. Any deviation from this ratio can limit calcium availability in the test systems and cause erratic results. Ethylenediaminetetraacetic acid (EDTA) is not an acceptable anticoagulant for coagulation testing. EDTA is a much more avid binder of calcium than citrate and will chelate calcium added to the sample during testing.
6. The sample should be centrifuged and the plasma removed within 30 min of blood collection.
7. The plasma should be stored in an ice bath and capped to prevent changes in pH. If these precautions are followed, the sample should be stable for 4 h.
8. If it is necessary to freeze the sample and mail it to an outside laboratory, centrifuge the blood sample at a high speed (2200 $\times$ g) for 15 min and remove the plasma with a plastic pipette. Freeze the plasma rapidly to prevent formation of ice crystals. Slow freezing or thawing of samples induces cryoprecipitation of coagulation factors, particularly factor VIII, and can be a major source of erratic results in the APTT. The sample should subsequently be stored or transported at $-20°C$ or lower. Packing the specimen in a large amount of dry ice (10 to 20 lb) in a Styrofoam container is necessary to maintain this temperature. Similar processing of blood from a normal individual of the same species is recommended to rule out artifacts induced during sample collection and transportation.

APTT = Activated partial thromboplastin time.

ally by 6 months of age, factor activity levels of puppies and kittens are equivalent to those of adults.

Prothrombin Time

An indicator of the functional activity of factors in the extrinsic and common pathways, the prothrombin time (PT) assay requires citrated plasma, a source of tissue factor, and calcium. The PT is a sensitive indicator of warfarin toxicity. Because factor VII is the vitamin K–dependent factor with the shortest half-life, the PT may be prolonged within 24 hours after warfarin ingestion, before the occurrence of a significant alteration in the APTT or the appearance of clinical signs. As with the APTT, age-matched controls are important, and specific factor activity must usually be less than 30% for a prolongation in the PT to occur. Because factor VII deficiency is usually not accompanied by hemorrhage, a bleeding diathesis of longer than 24 hours' duration is not likely to be characterized solely by a prolonged PT.

Thrombin Time

The thrombin time (TT) assay is a direct measurement of functional fibrinogen and entails the addition of thrombin to citrated plasma and the timing of clot formation. The rate of clot formation is directly proportional to the concentration of functional fibrinogen and is especially useful in the diagnosis and/or evaluation of individuals with disseminated intravascular coagulation (DIC). Although the test will also detect individuals with congenital hypofibrinogenemia or dysfibrinogenemia, these conditions are rare.

Fibrinogen/Fibrin Degradation Products

The assay of fibrinogen/fibrin degradation products (FDPs) detects the presence of elevated levels of circulating fibrinogen or fibrin degradation products by the use of specific antibodies coupled to latex beads. The sample requires serum taken from blood collected into a tube containing thrombin and a trypsin inhibitor (provided with the Thrombo-Wellcotest for FDP determination, Burroughs Wellcome). The test is useful for evaluation of animals with known or suspected DIC. The FDP assay results may also be elevated for animals with indwelling catheters, in severe warfarin toxicity, or for animals with abdominal or thoracic hemorrhage.

Antithrombin III

Antithrombin III (ATIII) is a circulating protein inhibitor of several coagulation factors, including factors XII, XI, X, IX, and thrombin (II). The activity of ATIII is greatly enhanced by heparin. Antithrombin III is an α_2-globulin, synthesized by the liver, with a molecular weight of 62,000 daltons. Decreases in ATIII can occur secondary to hepatic failure, as a result of protein-losing conditions, such as protein-losing enteropathy or glomerulopathy, or secondary to consumption as a result of DIC. Individuals with ATIII concentrations of less than 70% are at risk for the development of thrombosis. Because ATIII is often depleted in DIC, the assay is useful in the evaluation or diagnosis of this syndrome. The test was not, however, useful for cats with DIC after experimental infection with feline infectious peritonitis virus (Boudreaux et al, 1988a,b). The test requires citrated plasma, and age-matched controls are recommended.

COAGULATION PROTEIN DISORDERS

Coagulation protein abnormalities may be either congenital or acquired. Acquired coagulopathies can be complicated by thrombocytopenia and/or vascular disorders and may progress to the development of DIC if untreated. Congenital coagulopathies (Table 15–11) are less common and if severe often require a specialized, isolated environment for successful management.

CONGENITAL COAGULATION AND VASCULAR DISORDERS

Prekallikrein Deficiency

Prekallikrein deficiency is a rare disorder in domestic animals and has only been described in a poodle (Chinn et al, 1986), a family of miniature horses (Turrentine et al, 1986), and a family of Belgian horses (Geor et al, 1990). The disorder is not usually associated with clinical bleeding and is often diagnosed fortuitously during the performance of routine coagulation screening tests. Affected animals have a prolonged APTT and ACT and a normal PT. The poodle with prekallikrein deficiency was 14 years old before the diagnosis was made, and the miniature horses also did not have clinical bleeding. One of the Belgian horses did hemorrhage excessively after castration; however, this

is the only report of a possible bleeding diathesis associated with prekallikrein deficiency.

Factor XII

Factor XII deficiency or Hageman's disease is not associated with a bleeding diathesis (Bennett, 1984). Diagnosis of factor XII deficiency is often made fortuitously during the conduction of routine screening procedures and is characterized by a prolonged APTT and ACT. The disorder has been described in cats (Kier et al, 1980), as well as in a German short-haired pointer, a standard poodle (Dodds, 1984a), and a family of miniature poodles (Randolph et al, 1986). The coexistence of factor XII deficiency with von Willebrand's disease (Randolph et al, 1986) or factor IX deficiency (Dillon and Boudreaux, 1988) did not seem to exacerbate bleeding. Although factor XII deficiency is not associated with apparent bleeding, affected individuals may be predisposed to infection and/or thrombosis. This may be related to the central role of factor XII in the activation of the complement cascade and the fibrinolytic pathway (Kane, 1984). Possible enhanced thrombosis and/or infection associated with factor XII deficiency has only been described in humans. This may be related to the relatively short life span of domestic animals compared with humans. Factor XII is normally lacking in the plasma of birds, marine mammals, and reptiles (Dodds, 1981).

Factor XI Deficiency

Individuals with severe factor XI deficiency characteristically have a minor bleeding diathesis that becomes major following trauma or surgery (Dodds and Kull, 1971). The disease is relatively rare and has only been described in the springer spaniel, Great Pyrenees, Weimaraner, and Kerry blue terrier (Dodds, 1984a). The occurrence of a circulating factor XI inhibitor, resulting in epistaxis, has been described in an adult cat (Feldman et al, 1983). The mode of inheritance is autosomal; it is not clear whether the gene is dominant or recessive. Affected individuals with factor XI levels less than 30% to 40% will usually have a prolonged APTT and ACT. Bleeding episodes can be curtailed by the intravenous infusion of fresh or fresh-frozen autologous plasma at 6 to 10 ml/kg of body weight. Factor XI deficiency has also been recognized in holstein cattle (Dodds, 1981; Kociba et al, 1969).

Table 15–11 Congenital Coagulation Protein Disorders				
FACTOR	INCIDENCE	CLINICAL SIGNIFICANCE	SCREENING TESTS	TREATMENT
XII	Cats, standard poodle, German short-haired pointer	None	APTT, ACT	None
XI	English springer spaniel, Great Pyrenees, Weimaraner, Kerry blue terrier	Moderate to severe	APTT, ACT	Fresh or fresh-frozen plasma
X	American cocker spaniel	Severe in newborns and puppies	ACT, APTT, PT	Fresh or fresh-frozen plasma
IX	Numerous dog breeds, British short-haired cat, Siamese-cross cat	Moderate to severe (may be mild to moderate in small dogs and in cats)	ACT, APTT	Fresh or fresh-frozen plasma; supernatant fluid from cryoprecipitate
VIII	Numerous dog breeds, cats	Same as for factor IX	ACT, APTT	Fresh or fresh-frozen plasma; cryoprecipitate
VII	Beagle, miniature schnauzer, Alaskan malamute, boxer, bulldog	None to mild	PT	Fresh or fresh-frozen plasma
II	English cocker spaniel	Moderate	ACT, APTT, PT	Fresh or fresh-frozen plasma
I	Saint Bernard, vizsla, Russian wolfhound	Mild to severe	ACT, APTT, PT, TT	Fresh or fresh-frozen plasma, cryoprecipitate

ACT = Activated coagulation time; APTT = activated partial thromboplastin time; PT = prothrombin time; TT = thrombin time.

Factor X Deficiency

Factor X deficiency is a rare hemorrhagic disorder that to date has only been described in a family of American cocker spaniels (Dodds, 1973). The inheritance pattern is autosomal dominant with variable penetrance. Individuals homozygous for the gene are usually stillborn or die within the first weeks of life with massive pulmonary and/or abdominal hemorrhage. Heterozygotes have intermediate levels of factor X and have a mild to severe bleeding tendency. Individuals with factor X levels less than 30% usually have a prolonged PT, APTT, and ACT. Treatment to control bleeding requires the intravenous infusion of fresh or fresh-frozen autologous plasma.

Factor IX Deficiency

Factor IX deficiency, or hemophilia B, is a sex-linked hemorrhagic disorder identical in presentation to that of factor VIII deficiency (hemophilia A). Although not as common as factor VIII deficiency, factor IX deficiency has been described in one mixed-breed dog (Littlewood et al, 1986) and nine purebred dogs (Campbell et al, 1983; Peterson and Dodds, 1979; Sherding and DiBartola, 1980; Verlander et al., 1984). In addition, the defect has been recognized in one family of British short-haired cats (Dodds, 1981) and one family of Siamese-cross cats (Dillon and Boudreaux, 1988). In the latter group of cats, danazol proved to be ineffective in increasing factor IX activity (Boudreaux and Dillon, 1988). In 1989, the author acquired a factor IX–deficient (3% factor IX activity) domestic medium-haired cat donated from a local small animal clinic. The veterinarian, a recent graduate, had an unforgettable experience when she declawed and castrated the young, undiagnosed hemophiliac. She was able to save the cat with repeated blood transfusions over a several-week period. The cat is now an adult and in a household with 3 other cats. The only evidence of a hemostatic defect is the periodic occurrence of lameness associated with joint hemorrhage. These bleeds have been self-limiting; transfusions have not been required.

In cases of severe factor IX deficiency (less

than 1%), puppies or kittens may die at or immediately after birth. Excessive bleeding from the umbilical cord or tail and feet at the time of tail docking and dewclaw removal is a common sign. Hemarthrosis, gingival bleeding during tooth eruption, and spontaneous hematoma formation are other typical manifestations. Individuals with factor IX levels between 5% and 10% may not be recognized as being hemophiliacs unless challenged with trauma or surgery. Small dogs and cats also often go unrecognized as having a bleeding disorder despite the presence of very low levels of factor IX, presumably due to their light weight and usually protected environments. Affected individuals will have a prolonged ACT and APTT. Carriers of hemophilia B usually have factor IX levels between 40% and 60% and cannot be detected with routine coagulation screening tests. Identification of a carrier state in animals less than 6 months of age by factor activity evaluation should be done with caution because young animals may normally have a lower activity than adults. As with factor VIII deficiency, the disorder primarily affects males except in closely inbred families where females may be affected as well. Transfusion of fresh or fresh-frozen homologous plasma at 6 to 10 ml/kg every 12 hours is the recommended treatment for acute bleeding episodes. Although external hemorrhage is fairly easy to discern, affected individuals often bleed internally into either the thorax or abdomen, between fascial planes separating muscle groups, or into the brain. These bleeding episodes are often not recognized until a crisis exists. Unchecked hemorrhage can result in muscle necrosis, paralysis, seizures, and/or hypovolemic shock.

Factor VIII Deficiency

Factor VIII deficiency, or hemophilia A, is one of the most common inherited hemostatic defects in dogs and cats (Dodds, 1984a). The defect has also been recognized in Arabians, standardbreds, quarter horses, and thoroughbreds (Dodds, 1975b; Henninger, 1988; Littlewood and Bevan, 1991). Due to the X-linked nature of the disorder, males are usually affected, whereas females are asymptomatic carriers. The birth of affected female progeny requires the mating of an affected male to a carrier female, a possibility in closely inbred families. The other possibility is the spontaneous development of hemophilia A as a result of a gene mutation. This may have been the cause of hemophilia in an adult female

cocker spaniel–poodle cross examined at Tufts University (Murtaugh and Dodds, 1988).

Puppies with factor VIII deficiency usually experience prolonged bleeding from the umbilicus at birth, from the gingiva during tooth eruption, and after routine surgical procedures such as tail docking and ear cropping. Spontaneous hematoma formation, hemarthrosis, and hemorrhagic body cavity effusions are also common manifestations. Individuals having a less than 5% factor VIII activity level usually experience the most severe bleeding diathesis. Factor VIII levels between 5% and 10% may not be associated with spontaneous hemorrhage; the hemostatic defect in puppies thus affected is often not recognized before a traumatic or surgical event. A recurrent shifting leg lameness may be the only manifestation observed (Johnstone and Norris, 1984). Factor VIII deficiency in cats can be associated with spontaneous hematoma formation, but, presumably due to their light weight and agility, affected cats often do not experience prolonged hemorrhage except after trauma or surgery (Cotter et al, 1978). A similar presentation may also be observed in small-breed dogs.

Factor VIII deficiency is characterized by a prolonged APTT and ACT. Factor VIII activity levels are often less than 10%, whereas von Willebrand factor levels are normal or higher than normal (Dodds, 1984a). Carriers of hemophilia A have intermediate levels of factor VIII (40% to 60%), but identification of carriers should be done with caution for animals younger than 6 months. Carriers usually have a normal APTT and ACT. Treatment for hemophilia A requires repeated transfusions of fresh whole blood, plasma, or frozen plasma concentrates at 6 to 10 ml/kg of body weight two to three times a day until bleeding is under control. Plasma transfusions are preferred due to the possible sensitization of the animal to red blood cell antigens.

Factor VII Deficiency

Factor VII deficiency has been recognized in beagles, miniature schnauzers, Alaskan malamutes, boxers, and bulldogs (Dodds, 1984a). The disorder is usually not accompanied by detectable bleeding, although affected individuals may experience bruising or prolonged bleeding after surgery. Postpartum hemorrhage has also been described as a potential complication (Spurling et al, 1974). Factor VII deficiency is usually discovered fortuitously during screening tests for blood clotting ability. The disorder is characterized by a prolonged PT. The inheritance pattern is autosomal with incomplete dominance.

Factor II Deficiency

Disorders of prothrombin or factor II are extremely rare and have only been described in the English cocker spaniel (Hill et al, 1982) and boxer breeds (Dodds, 1979). In humans and in the boxer the defect has been characterized as having an autosomal recessive inheritance pattern. The disorder in the boxer was one of dysprothrombinemia; immunologic levels of the prothrombin molecule were normal. The existence of an abnormal prothrombin level or an actual prothrombin deficiency was not determined in the cocker spaniel. Signs in affected puppies included epistaxis and gingival bleeding. In adults, bleeding episodes became milder, and individuals experienced easy bruising and/or dermatitis. Coagulation studies in untreated puppies were characterized by a prolonged ACT, APTT, and PT. The TT was normal. Transfusion of fresh whole blood successfully arrested bleeding episodes for up to 3 days. Fresh or fresh-frozen plasma transfusions, however, are preferred if the animal does not require red blood cells as well.

Factor I (Fibrinogen) Deficiency

Congenital afibrinogenemia has not been described in dogs or cats, but dysfibrinogenemia has been recognized in one inbred family of Russian wolfhounds (Dodds, 1984a). Coagulation screening test results included a prolonged ACT, APTT, PT, and TT. Fibrinogen could be detected by quantitative but not by qualitative methods. Affected animals experienced mild bleeding manifested by lameness and epistaxis; challenge with surgery or trauma resulted in life-threatening bleeding. Hypofibrinogenemia has been reported in the Saint Bernard and vizsla. Bleeding was severe, and coagulation screening test results were similar to those of dysfibrinogenemia; however, a quantitative reduction in fibrinogen was determined (Dodds, 1978). Congenital afibrinogenemia has been reported in one family of Saanen dairy goats (Dodds, 1984a). Treatment to arrest protracted bleeding includes the intravenous infusion of fresh or fresh-frozen plasma or plasma cryoprecipitate.

Vitamin K–Dependent Multifactor Coagulopathy

A congenital coagulopathy has been described in Devon Rex cats (Maddison et al, 1990) that is characterized by hematoma formation and hemorrhage into the conjunctiva, joints, and thoracic and abdominal cavities. Affected cats have prolonged PT and APTT and diminished levels of factors II, VII, IX, and X. Hemorrhage can be controlled with vitamin K_1 treatment. Factor deficiencies seem to be due to a defective γ-glutamylcarboxylase that has a decreased affinity for both vitamin K hydroquinone and propeptide (Soute et al, 1992). The inheritance pattern appears to be autosomal.

Cutaneous Asthenia (Ehlers-Danlos Syndrome)

Cutaneous asthenia is an uncommon, congenital, inherited connective tissue disorder characterized by loose, hyperextensible, fragile skin (Muller et al, 1983). The defect has been recognized in both dogs and cats, as well as in humans, mink, cows, sheep, and horses. The underlying defect is in the synthesis and/or maturation of type I collagen, and, as a result of lack of vascular support, affected animals often experience subcutaneous hematomas (Poulsen et al, 1985). A platelet function defect may also be present in this disease (George et al, 1984). There is no treatment.

ACQUIRED COAGULATION AND VASCULAR DISORDERS

Coumarin/Indanedione Toxicity

Rodenticide-induced coagulopathies are fairly common in the dog and cat. Clinical signs can vary and may include lethargy, respiratory distress, lameness, petechial and ecchymotic hemorrhages, epistaxis, and hemoptysis (Schulman et al, 1986). Occasionally, sudden death occurs without prior signs of illness. Anticoagulant rodenticides interfere with the vitamin K–dependent carboxylation of factors II, VII, IX, and X. The epoxide-reductase enzyme necessary for the recycling of vitamin K is inhibited, resulting in depletion of body stores of vitamin K. As a result, only nonfunctional precursors of the vitamin K–dependent factors are synthesized (Davis, 1982). Coumarin compounds, including warfarin and coumafuryl, have a half-life of up to 55 hours. In contrast, indanedione compounds (pindone, valone, diphacinone, and chlorophacinone) have a half-life as long as 15 to 20 days (Mount and Feldman, 1983). In addition, the indanedione compounds may interfere with exocrine pancreatic function, resulting in reduced intestinal absorption of vitamin K (Mount and Feldman, 1983). Brodifacoum and bromadiolone seem to have half-lives intermediate between those described for warfarin and indanedione compounds.

Coagulation screening tests for uncomplicated rodenticide toxicity are usually characterized by a prolonged ACT, APTT, and PT with a normal TT. Because factor VII has the shortest half-life of the vitamin K–dependent factors, it is conceivable that with early detection only the PT will be prolonged. Bleeding will likely not, however, be present at this time, and there will be a history of rodenticide ingestion within the past 24 hours. Untreated or high-dose rodenticide toxicity can also be associated with thrombocytopenia and/or DIC. Because of the marked difference in the duration of action of coumarin versus indanedione compounds, it is helpful to determine the source of toxicity before instituting treatment.

The recommended treatment for coumarin toxicity is 0.25 to 2.5 mg of vitamin K_1 per kg for 4 to 6 days. In contrast, treatment for indanedione toxicity may require doses of vitamin K_1 as high as 5 mg/kg for 3 to 6 weeks. High-dose vitamin K_1 therapy should, however, be administered with caution because vitamin K_1 was reported to induce Heinz body anemia in a dog when administered at 4 mg/kg for 5 days (Fernandez et al, 1984). In life-threatening situations, initiation of therapy by subcutaneous or intramuscular injection, followed by oral dosing, may be required. Intravenous injection is not recommended, nor is therapy with vitamin K_3.

Rocky Mountain Spotted Fever

Rickettsia rickettsii, the causative agent of Rocky Mountain spotted fever (RMSF), is an obligate intracellular parasite transmitted principally by the vector ticks *Dermacentor variabilis* and *Dermacentor andersoni*. The organism invades vascular endothelial cells leading to cell necrosis, increased vascular permeability, and perivascular hemorrhage and edema (Greene and Phillip, 1984). The developing vasculitis is accompanied by thrombocytopenia and variable activation of the coagulation mechanism (Davidson et al, 1990). Early signs may include petechial and ecchymotic hemorrhages of the skin and mucous membranes, retinal hemorrhage, epistaxis,

melena, and hematuria. Severely affected individuals may develop DIC. The most useful test for diagnosing RMSF is the microimmunofluorescence test. Although cross-reactions do develop between other rickettsial organisms, the titer is usually highest for the specific rickettsia causing the infection. Paired acute and convalescent serum samples (10 to 14 days apart) are recommended for testing.

Tetracycline, chloramphenicol, or enrofloxacin is the recommended therapy. Chloramphenicol should be administered with caution to young dogs and cats, however, to avoid toxicity related to reduced drug metabolism by an immature liver. Intravenous fluid therapy should also be used with caution due to the presence of enhanced vascular permeability. Although RMSF has been recognized extensively in the dog, its significance for the cat is unknown.

Canine Herpesvirus Infection

Although its incidence is sporadic, herpesvirus infection can result in the rapid death of puppies usually between the ages of 7 and 21 days. The disease is characterized by multiple hemorrhages throughout numerous tissues, including the liver, kidney, brain, gastrointestinal tract, and lung, as a consequence of a virally induced necrotizing vasculitis (Carmichael, 1977). Puppies usually die within 24 hours; treatment is often unsuccessful.

Liver Disease

The liver is the major site of synthesis for most of the coagulation, fibrinolytic, and antithrombotic proteins. The liver is also responsible for clearance of activated factors and end and intermediate products of fibrinolysis (Mammen, 1992). Because coagulation factors have a relatively short half-life (4 hours to 2 days), hepatic disease may result in a fairly rapid change in factor activity. Hepatic degeneration, inflammation, cirrhosis, or neoplasia may result in decreases in factor activity, particularly factors XI, IX, X, VII, and II and proteins C and S. Decreases in factor activity may or may not be sufficient to cause increases in coagulation screening tests because factor activity generally must be less than 30% to affect these tests. In two studies performed in dogs, however, the PT and/or APTT was abnormal in 50% to 66% of dogs with liver disease (Badylak and Van Fleet, 1981; Badylak et al, 1983). Although screening tests such as the PT and APTT may be fairly sensitive in detecting coagulation factor abnormalities associated with liver disease, they are not specific and cannot be used to predict the type of liver pathology present. Fibrinogen and von Willebrand's factor levels may actually be increased with liver disease. This may be related to the nature of fibrinogen (acute phase reactant) and the extrahepatic synthesis of von Willebrand's factor.

Disseminated Intravascular Coagulation

Disseminated intravascular coagulation is a pathologic process involving overwhelming activation and consumption of coagulation proteins and platelets often accompanied by enhanced fibrinolysis (Fruchtman and Aledort, 1986; Kane, 1984). The syndrome may occur secondarily to a variety of events, including viral, bacterial, protozoal, or rickettsial infections, parasite migration, heat stroke, burns, shock, or trauma. In newborn humans the most common triggering events for the induction of DIC are hypothermia, hypoxia, shock, and sepsis. Important contributing factors include the immaturity of the newborn's clotting mechanism and reduced or inadequate protective functions such as reduced ATIII and protein C activities (Greffe et al, 1989) and impaired immune-phagocytic clearance mechanisms (Buchanan, 1978). Gastrointestinal disease often results in hemostatic abnormalities in horses (Johnstone and Crane, 1986; Morris et al, 1988). This includes disease secondary to colitis, torsion/obstruction, impaction, or *Ehrlichia risticii* (Potomac horse fever; equine ehrlichial colitis).

Laboratory abnormalities usually include increased fibrinogen concentrations and a prolonged APTT. The FDP concentrations may or may not be increased. Recently, protein C and plasminogen were found to be decreased in horses with intestinal ischemia and endotoxemia (Welles et al, 1991). In the future, protein C and plasminogen may be useful predictors for the outcome of equine colic. The occurrence of laminitis in horses with gastrointestinal disease may be secondary to activation of hemostasis resulting in microvascular thrombosis and digital ischemia.

Dogs with vascular tumors (hemangiomas and hemangiosarcomas) may develop localized or disseminated consumptive coagulopathy. Cutaneous vascular tumors should be excised as early as possible. Hemostatic parameters should be evaluated before surgery (Hammer et al, 1991; Hargis and Feldman, 1991). Although DIC is not a primary event, if left unchecked it will often result in the death of the animal due to thrombosis and/or hemorrhage within vital organs. A key to the control of DIC is identification and elimination of the underlying cause. Acute DIC is characterized by prolongation of the ACT, APTT, PT, and TT, elevated FDP levels (greater than 40 µg/ml), a reduction in ATIII levels, and thrombocytopenia. Chronic DIC is often more difficult to recognize; compensation by the liver and bone marrow in coagulation factor and platelet production, respectively, may result in normalization or even shortening of many of the coagulation screening test times. Horses commonly demonstrate a chronic DIC type of pattern. Horses with DIC are rarely hypofibrinogenemic and are almost always hyperfibrinogenemic. This is probably related to the ability of the equine liver to rapidly synthesize this acute phase reactant protein in response to inflammation.

Treatment for DIC should be centered on the identification and treatment of the underlying cause. Supportive therapy including intravenous fluids to maintain fluid volume and organ perfusion is vital. Heparin therapy is controversial and often must be accompanied by plasma transfusions to obtain effective ATIII activity.

PLATELET SCREENING TESTS
Platelet Count

Acquired thrombocytopenia is the most common cause of platelet-related bleeding disorders. There are many causes of acquired thrombocytopenia, including vaccines, rickettsial agents, viruses, and drugs. Accurate platelet counts are important in the monitoring of thrombocytopenic animals to determine if treatment has been successful. Platelet counts are usually determined in a veterinary facility with the use of the Unopet system, a hemocytometer, and a microscope. In some veterinary facilities and most clinical pathology laboratories, platelet counts are performed with automated instruments. Many of these instruments will also determine the mean platelet volume (MPV). The MPV is an indication of the size of the circulating platelet population. A high MPV in the face of thrombocytopenia generally means that megakaryocytes are attempting to respond to the low platelet number by releasing larger platelets into the circulation; this is a favorable sign. A low MPV in the face of thrombocytopenia may indicate that there are insufficient numbers of megakaryocytes present or that they are failing to respond. The sample of choice for the determination of platelet number is a blood sample collected into ethylenediaminetetraacetic acid (EDTA).

Platelet counts can be performed on citrated whole blood before the centrifugation of the sample to remove plasma for coagulation testing. Samples collected for platelet counts should not be sent through the mail; platelet counts should be performed on samples within 2 to 4 hours of collection. Normal platelet counts are usually greater than 150,000 cells per μl, although there are species differences. Prediction of whether an animal will bleed excessively cannot be made based on circulating platelet number. Some individuals with platelet numbers as low as 10,000 per μl will not spontaneously bleed, whereas others with platelet numbers as high as 100,000 per μl will have hemorrhagic tendencies. Variables such as platelet size and function, and vascular integrity, may all contribute to the variability observed clinically. Platelet number can be estimated by evaluating a blood smear; however, this technique is not recommended if the animal is suspected of having thrombocytopenia. Smear evaluation yields too crude an estimate of platelet number for critical assessment of response to treatment.

Bleeding Time

The bleeding time is generally considered to be an indicator of primary hemostasis or platelet status. This procedure has much more applicability to humans, but many techniques have been attempted and described in animals. The existence of hairy, thick skin and relative lack of a consistent surface to perform bleeding times on are but two of the obstacles veterinarians face. The buccal mucosa bleeding time (Jergens et al, 1987; Parker et al, 1988) has been described in dogs and cats and appears to be a fairly reliable indicator of primary hemostasis.

In this technique, the bleeding time is performed on the buccal mucosa using a spring-loaded cassette that delivers a precise depth and length of cut. The technique avoids the hair and thick skin normally encountered when attempting to perform a bleeding time. The technique does, however, usually require that the animal be inactive. Use of the bleeding time to evaluate primary hemostasis generally should be reserved for those animals in which platelet number is known to be adequate but platelet function is questioned. The technique would be especially useful for Doberman pinschers just before ear cropping.

Clot Retraction

The clot retraction test is a test of platelet function that can be performed in a clinical setting (Table 15–12). As with the bleeding time, this technique should be reserved for animals known to have normal platelet numbers but questionable platelet function. Also, the clot retraction test should not be performed in animals known to be receiving medication that will inhibit platelet function. The clot retraction test is a test of platelet function that relies on the normal interaction between thrombin, platelet receptors, and fibrinogen. Because it is a fairly specific test of platelet function, not all animals with a platelet function defect will have an abnormal clot retraction test result. Basset hounds with canine thrombopathia have platelets that will interact with thrombin and express fibrinogen receptors; therefore, the clot retraction test in these animals is normal. Otterhounds with thrombasthenic thrombopathia have platelets that either lack or have reduced amounts of the receptor needed for normal interaction with fibrinogen. These animals have abnormal clot retraction. Gray collies with cyclic hematopoiesis also have reduced clot retraction due to decreased reactivity of platelets to thrombin (Lothrop et al, 1991). Animals with von Willebrand's disease have normal clot retraction because their in vivo adhesion defect is extrinsic to the platelet, and platelets of these individuals respond normally to thrombin.

Platelet Aggregation

Platelet evaluation using a platelet aggregometer is presently the definitive means for

Table 15–12	Clot Retraction Test*

1. Draw 0.5 ml of blood directly into a plastic syringe containing 4.5 ml of cold saline solution. Mix gently.
2. Dispense 2 ml of the above mixture into each of two glass tubes containing 0.1 ml of 10 units/ml thrombin (1 unit final).
3. Cap and mix the tubes. Place the tubes in a refrigerator for 30 min.
4. Transfer the tubes to a 37° C water bath.
5. Record the degree of clot retraction at 1 and 2 hours as 1+ to 4+.

*Always test a normal control simultaneously. Always perform the test in duplicate. Technique obtained from Comparative Hemostasis Laboratory, Wadsworth Center for Laboratories and Research, New York State Department of Health, Albany, New York 12201.

evaluating platelet function. The technique is highly specialized and not readily available. Platelet function testing requires the collection of 10 to 20 ml of citrated, whole blood and the isolation of platelet-rich plasma. Because testing must be completed within 4 hours of collection, the animal being tested must be on or near the premises; samples cannot be sent through the mail. Although human laboratories are more likely to be equipped for the performance of platelet function testing, use of one of these laboratories is not recommended unless the lab is well-versed in the isolation and testing of platelets in the particular species of interest.

PLATELET DISORDERS

Platelet disorders can be generally divided into four categories (Table 15–13), congenital and acquired thrombocytopenias and congenital and acquired functional platelet disorders. Congenital thrombocytopenia has not been described in animals. Congenital abnormalities in platelet function are further categorized as defects in adhesion, aggregation, and/or secretion. These defects may be either intrinsic or extrinsic to the

Table 15–13	Qualitative and Quantitative Platelet Disorders

Functional Disorders of Platelets
 Congenital (intrinsic)
  Chediak-Higashi syndrome (cats, cattle, mink, mice)
  Canine thrombopathia (basset hounds)
  Glanzmann's thrombasthenia (otterhounds, Great Pyrenees)
  Cutaneous asthenia? (many dog breeds, cats)
  Spitz thrombopathia
  Cyclic hematopoiesis (gray collies)
 Congenital (extrinsic)
  von Willebrand's disease
 Acquired
  Feline leukemia virus
  Ehrlichia platys?
  Ehrlichia canis?
  Drug induced
Thrombocytopenia
 Acquired
  Ehrlichia platys
  Ehrlichia canis
  Feline leukemia virus
  Drug induced
  Vaccine induced
  Rocky Mountain spotted fever
  Canine herpesvirus
  Disseminated intravascular coagulation

platelet. The prevalence of intrinsic congenital platelet function disorders in animals is not known, mainly due to the scarcity of specialized laboratories equipped to evaluate platelet function in nonhuman species. The common practice by professional breeders of mating closely related individuals to maintain selected desirable traits also increases the risk of producing congenital defects. Intrinsic platelet function defects may be difficult to recognize but should be suspected in young nonmedicated animals experiencing mucosal or superficial bleeding in the presence of normal coagulation screening tests, normal levels of von Willebrand's factor, and a normal platelet count. Although documentation is scarce, newborn puppies are believed to have platelet numbers comparable with those of adults (Earl et al, 1973). Platelet functionality in newborn dogs and cats is not known but is reported to be normal in human infants (Blifeld et al, 1986). Acquired platelet function disorders are also often characterized by thrombocytopenia.

Congenital Intrinsic Platelet Function Disorders

CHEDIAK-HIGASHI SYNDROME

Chediak-Higashi syndrome is an autosomal recessive genetic disorder characterized by abnormal leukocyte, melanocyte, and platelet granulation (Meyers et al, 1982). Platelets of affected individuals lack discernible dense granules and are deficient or reduced in storage pools of adenine nucleotides, serotonin, and divalent cations. Studies of platelet ultrastructure indicate that Chediak-Higashi syndrome platelets do not form tight aggregates in response to adenosine diphosphate in vitro. The disease has been identified in a line of Persian cats; all of the affected animals exhibited a "blue smoke" hair color and pale irises with the development of bilateral nuclear cataracts in several individuals (Collier et al, 1979; Kramer et al, 1977; Prieur et al, 1979). Affected cats experienced prolonged bleeding at incision sites and the development of hematomas after venipuncture. Chediak-Higashi syndrome has also been diagnosed in mink, cattle, and mice.

CANINE THROMBOPATHIA

Canine thrombopathia is a hereditary intrinsic platelet disorder that has only been described in basset hounds (Johnstone and Lotz, 1979). Affected individuals exhibit signs typical of quantitative or qualitative platelet defects, that is, epistaxis, gingival bleeding, and petechiation. The mode of inheritance for the defect is unknown, but evaluation of affected families suggests an autosomal dominant inheritance with variable penetrance (Catalfamo et al, 1986; Dodds and Catalfamo, personal communication, 1986). The platelet defect is characterized by abnormal fibrinogen receptor exposure and impaired dense granule release. The underlying dysfunction is related to defective stimulus–response–coupled platelet activation. Thrombopathic platelets have been shown to have elevated basal levels of cyclic adenosine monophosphate (Boudreaux et al, 1985). The presence of impaired phosphodiesterase activity in intact cell studies but normal phosphodiesterase activity in disrupted cell preparations implies that the defect is one of regulatory control (Boudreaux et al, 1986a,b). Signs referable to platelet dysfunction in nonthrombocytopenic basset hounds with normal levels of von Willebrand's factor are suggestive of canine thrombopathia. Unfortunately, a reliable diagnosis of the disease requires that the affected individual be presented at specialized facilities equipped for the evaluation of platelet function; the clot retraction test in this disorder is normal.

GLANZMANN'S THROMBASTHENIA

Glanzmann's thrombasthenia (GT) is an intrinsic platelet function defect resulting from reduced to absent amounts of the glycoprotein complex IIb-IIIa on the surface of platelets. This receptor, also known as the integrin $\alpha_{IIb}\beta_3$, is necessary for normal platelet aggregation. Type I GT is characterized by severe reduction to absence of the glycoprotein complex. Type II GT is characterized by moderate to mild reduction in the complex. Two breeds of dogs have been identified as having members with type I GT, otterhounds and Great Pyrenees. The otterhound defect, previously described as *thrombasthenic thrombopathia*, had originally been described as having features of both Bernard Soulier's disease (a platelet defect involving glycoprotein complex Ib-IX) and GT (Raymond and Dodds, 1979). More recent studies failed to demonstrate a combined defect (Boudreaux and Catalfamo, in press). In affected Great Pyrenees and otterhounds, platelets fail to aggregate in response to adenosine diphosphate, collagen, platelet-aggregating factor (PAF), or thrombin, and clot retraction is markedly impaired.

Young dogs with type I GT usually demonstrate excessive mucosal bleeding during teething. Some affected puppies may also have chronic epistaxis (Boudreaux et al, 1996). Spontaneous bleeding usually subsides when animals become young adults; however, excessive hemorrhage will still occur with routine surgical procedures or trauma. Young animals with chronic mucosal-type bleeding are highly susceptible to the development of iron deficiency anemia and should be monitored at least monthly for iron status. Oral iron is often not sufficient to maintain iron levels; iron injections are recommended to maintain iron levels in young growing animals with chronic hemorrhage. Recent genetic studies have determined that although the otterhound defect is distinct from the Great Pyrenees defect, both involve the gene encoding for glycoprotein IIb (Boudreaux and Catalfamo, in press; Lipscomb et al, in press).

SPITZ THROMBOPATHIA

An intrinsic platelet disorder has been described in two spitz dogs that presented at the Auburn University Small Animal Clinic (Boudreaux et al, 1994). Both were female dogs and were presented at separate times (approximately 18 months apart) with histories of chronic epistaxis and gingival bleeding. One of the dogs had a shifting leg lameness. Both dogs were anemic from chronic blood loss at the time of presentation. The platelets of the dogs did not aggregate in response to adenosine disposphate, collagen, or PAF. The platelets did aggregate in response to thrombin, but there was a lag phase. The clot retraction test was normal. The functional platelet disorder is very similar to the one described in basset hounds (canine thrombopathia).

CYCLIC HEMATOPOIESIS

Cyclic hematopoiesis is an autosomal recessive disorder described in gray collies and characterized by cyclic fluctuations in the number of circulating neutrophils, reticulocytes, and platelets (Cheville, 1975; DiGiacomo et al, 1983). The basis for the disease is a bone marrow stem cell defect resulting in neutropenic episodes occurring approximately every 12 days. Mortality rates are high; most puppies die before 6 months of age due to fulminating infection. Platelet number usually does not decline below the normal range and fluctuates between 300,000 and 700,000 cells per μl. Platelet reactivity to collagen, PAF, tissue plasminogen activator, and possibly thrombin is defective. Platelet granule storage pools of serotonin and adenine nucleotides are markedly reduced. Clot retraction and platelet adhesiveness are impaired (Lothrop et al, 1991).

Congenital Extrinsic Platelet Function Disorders: von Willebrand's Disease

Von Willebrand's disease, due to defective or deficient von Willebrand's factor, is the most common inherited bleeding disorder of dogs (Dodds, 1984b). Two inheritance patterns exist; one is autosomal recessive, and the other is autosomal with an incompletely dominant expression (Dodds, 1975a). One study seemed to indicate that the inheritance pattern for von Willebrand's disease in Doberman pinschers is autosomal recessive (Moser et al, 1996). Signs include mucosal bleeding primarily manifested by gingival bleeding, epistaxis, and hematuria. Stillbirths, neonatal deaths, and prolonged bleeding at tail docking, ear cropping, and dewclaw removal are other common manifestations. Von Willebrand's factor circulates as a complex with factor VIII coagulant, the protein deficient in hemophilia A. Factor VIII coagulant activity may also be reduced in severe forms of von Willebrand's disease. In most cases of von Willebrand's disease, however, all coagulation screening tests are normal. Because von Willebrand's factor is important in mediating the adhesion of platelets to subendothelial surfaces, the presentation mimics an intrinsic platelet function defect or thrombocytopenia. Because platelets are normal in this syndrome, however, von Willebrand's disease is considered an extrinsic platelet function disorder.

Puppies experiencing a bleeding diathesis in the absence of abnormal coagulation screening tests or thrombocytopenia should be tested for von Willebrand's disease. At present, most assays are quantitative and involve electroimmunodiffusion techniques (Benson et al, 1983); however, a qualitative assay has also been developed (Johnson et al, 1985), as has an enzyme-linked immunosorbent assay (ELISA) technique (Benson et al, 1991). Citrated plasma samples to be analyzed for von Willebrand's factor should be frozen immediately and sent frozen in plastic tubes to a veterinary diagnostic laboratory within 2 weeks of collection. Puppies should not have been vaccinated or received medication within 2 weeks of sampling. Affected puppies may only experience bleeding problems after vaccination or surgical procedures. The administration of drugs known or suspected to alter platelet function should be avoided.

Hemorrhagic crises can be arrested by the transfusion of autologous fresh whole blood or plasma at 6 to 10 ml/kg. Plasma is preferred, especially if crossmatching cannot be performed, because these dogs may require repeated transfusions. Desmopressin acetate (DDAVP), a synthetic analogue of vasopressin, has been administered intravenously in humans to raise the concentration of circulating von Willebrand's factor (Warrier and Lusher, 1983). A maximal response (twofold or greater rise in factor level) is usually reached within 1 to 2 hours after a dosage of 0.3 μg/kg body weight. Unfortunately, equivalent responses have not been seen in normal healthy dogs or in Doberman pinschers with von Willebrand's disease even at dosages as high as 3 μg/kg body weight (Giger and Dodds, 1989). Despite the lack of observable elevation in von Willebrand's factor antigen, the bleeding times of dogs with von Willebrand's disease did shorten to the normal range 2 hours after administration of DDAVP. Possibly, DDAVP may be useful for some dogs as a transient relief to a bleeding episode. DDAVP has also been administered to canine plasma donors within 2 hours of the collection of blood to enhance the efficacy of the plasma transfusion. Von Willebrand's disease is rare in the cat (French et al, 1987) and horse (Brooks et al, 1991), with only one case being described for each of these species.

Acquired Platelet Function Disorders
FELINE LEUKEMIA VIRUS INFECTION

Viral replication and accumulation within the cytoplasm of megakaryocytes results in the infection of circulating platelets (Beck et al, 1986). Feline leukemia virus–associated thrombocytopenia may be due to aplasia or atrophy of bone marrow stem cells, immune-mediated clearance of infected cells, or extravascular sequestration within lymphoid tissue. Thrombocytopenia, thrombocytosis, and/or impairment of platelet function may accompany feline leukemia virus–induced myeloproliferative disease (Boyce et al, 1986). Hemorrhage occurring in the face of a normal or elevated platelet count and a normal coagulation profile is an indication of impaired platelet function. Abnormal platelet function has been demonstrated in numerous cases of myeloproliferative disease in humans (Schafer, 1984) and in a dog with radiation-induced megakaryoblastic leukemia (Cain et al, 1986).

DRUG-INDUCED DISORDERS

Drugs can impair platelet function by inhibiting receptor binding of agonists, by inhibiting transduction of messages received at the platelet surface, or by inhibiting the execution of the platelet response (Table 15–14), including aggregation, secretion, or the generation of thromboxane A_2 (Cowan, 1982). Drug-induced impairment of platelet function may not be clinically significant unless coupled with another underlying platelet function defect such as von Willebrand's disease.

Acquired Thrombocytopenia

EHRLICHIA PLATYS INFECTION

Ehrlichia platys is the causative agent of canine infectious cyclic thrombocytopenia (Harvey et al, 1978). The disease is characterized by thrombocytopenic episodes occurring at 1- to

Table 15–14	Drugs Mediating Qualitative and Quantitative Platelet Disorders

I. Impairment of platelet function
  A. Receptor blockade or alteration in membrane charge or permeability
    1. Furosemide
    2. Phentolamine
    3. Chlorpromazine
    4. Lidocaine
    5. Penicillin, carbenicillin
  B. Impairment of signal transduction
    1. Papaverine
    2. Dipyridamole
    3. Caffeine
    4. Theophylline
  C. Impairment of execution
    1. Aspirin
    2. Phenylbutazone
    3. Indomethacin
    4. Pentobarbital
    5. Sulfinpyrazone
    6. Ticlopidine
    7. Acetaminophen
II. Thrombocytopenia
  A. Marrow suppression
    1. Chloramphenicol
    2. Phenylbutazone
    3. Diphenylhydantoin
    4. Sulfonamides
    5. Estrogens
  B. Platelet consumption or destruction
    1. Ristocetin
    2. Acetaminophen
    3. Aspirin
    4. Diphenylhydantoin
    5. Levamisole
    6. Methicillin, penicillin
    7. Sulfisoxazole

2-week intervals after cycles of enhanced parasitemia in acutely affected individuals. Single to multiple round or oval basophilic inclusions may be observed in infected platelets immediately before periods of thrombocytopenia; however, the percentage of infected platelets declines with each succeeding wave of parasitemia. Chronic infections may not be cyclic and may present as slowly resolving thrombocytopenias.

Ehrlichia platys infection alone has not been reported to be associated with overt bleeding; however, concomitant infection with other disorders may exacerbate an already impaired hemostatic mechanism. Diagnosis of *Ehrlichia platys*, as with *Ehrlichia canis*, is most reliably made by an indirect fluorescent antibody test (French and Harvey, 1983). Paired serum samples 10 days to 2 weeks apart are ideal. The antibody test for *Ehrlichia platys* does not cross-react with that for *Ehrlichia canis*; however, there is a high incidence of concomitant infection. Although the mode of transmission has not been determined, the tick is a likely vector. Tetracycline is the recommended therapy.

EHRLICHIA CANIS INFECTION

The occurrence of hemorrhage manifested by hematoma formation or prolonged bleeding from venipuncture or surgical incision sites, epistaxis, gingival bleeding, retinal hemorrhages, melena, petechiae, or ecchymoses is common in canine ehrlichiosis (Greene and Harvey, 1984). Affected individuals may or may not demonstrate thrombocytopenia. Abnormal platelet function and vasculitis have been proposed as the cause of bleeding in individuals with normal platelet counts because in most cases the PT and APTT are normal. As a consequence, the severity of bleeding does not always correspond to circulating platelet number. Thrombocytopenia is associated with decreased platelet survival, enhanced platelet consumption being mediated by immune, inflammatory, or coagulatory mechanisms (Lovering et al, 1980; Pierce et al, 1977; Smith et al, 1975). Impaired platelet function may be due to an acquired platelet membrane defect associated with marked elevations in serum globulin concentrations as seen in some cases of multiple myeloma (Kuehn and Gaunt, 1985).

DRUG-INDUCED THROMBOCYTOPENIA

Drugs can induce thrombocytopenia in humans and animals by enhancing peripheral platelet destruction or by suppressing marrow production. Increased platelet consumption can be related to a direct toxic effect of the drug or to an immune-mediated destruction. Drug-induced immune thrombocytopenia may occur due to binding of the drug to the platelet surface with subsequent antibody production to the drug-platelet complex or as a result of nonspecific absorption of immune complexes on the platelet membrane. Many drugs are suspected or have been demonstrated to induce thrombocytopenia (see Table 15–14). Drug-induced immune thrombocytopenia is often idiosyncratic, making prediction of a reaction to a drug impossible. Removal of the inducing drug usually results in a rapid return to normal platelet numbers. Rarely, drugs can induce an autoimmune phenomenon, and thrombocytopenia persists even after discontinuation of the drug. Drug-induced marrow suppression usually occurs at the stem cell level, resulting in a pancytopenia and hypocellular bone marrow.

VACCINE-INDUCED THROMBOCYTOPENIA

Attenuated-live adenovirus and *Paramyxovirus* vaccines have been reported to induce thrombocytopenia in some individuals (Jones, 1984). The mechanism is unknown but is likely an immune-mediated event associated either with antibody production against viral antigens adhered to the platelet membrane or with the nonspecific binding of antibody-virus complexes to the surface of platelets. The phenomenon occurs within 3 to 10 days after a challenge administration of vaccine and is therefore most likely to occur in young animals receiving routine booster injections. Vaccine-induced thrombocytopenias are usually transitory and may not be recognized unless superimposed on another platelet or coagulation defect. Routine surgical procedures such as tail docking and ear cropping should be avoided for 2 weeks after a repeat vaccination.

IDIOPATHIC THROMBOCYTOPENIC PURPURA

Idiopathic thrombocytopenic purpura (ITP) is a thrombocytopenic condition that is probably immune mediated. It has been described in horses and dogs (Byars and Greene, 1982; Larson et al, 1983) and is characterized by blood platelet concentrations of less than 100,000 cells per μl in the absence of other hematologic abnormalities. Megakaryocytes may be increased or absent in these animals, depending on the target of the immune response. Treatment for ITP in humans has included corticosteroids, danazol, splenectomy, and ascorbate (Brox et al, 1988). Danazol has been an effective treatment for corticosteroid-resistant immune-mediated thrombocytopenias in dogs (Bloom et al, 1989; Holloway et al, 1990). Splenectomy has been suggested as being useful in the management of dogs with relapsing immune-mediated thrombocytopenia (Jans et al, 1990).

The Lymphoid System

Kenita S. Rogers

THE LYMPH NODES

In dogs, the primordial structure of the largest lymph nodes is present at 35 to 38 days of gestation, and lymphocytic colonization of the nodes is prominent at 52 to 53 days of gestation (Rogers et al, 1993b). At birth, puppies and kittens have readily recognizable lymph nodes with a loose reticular structure, low lymphocyte density, and limited organization into cortex and medulla that rapidly proliferates into cortical nodules and medullary cords. Lymph nodes and lymphatic vessels vary in location and number, but their primary function is to participate in immunologic reactions by filtering lymph and recirculating the lymphocytes (Couto et al, 1995). Antigens that gain access to particular body tissues are ultimately found in lymphatic vessels that drain these tissues, making it logical that elements of the immune system are strategically positioned along lymphatic vessels. Although lymph node architecture is relatively uniform throughout the body, nodes near portals of entry of external antigens (mandibular and mesenteric lymph node areas) are often more reactive than nodes in other locations.

Lymph Node Disorders

As a major site of immunologic recognition, lymph nodes are expected to respond to various local and systemic inflammatory, infectious, and neoplastic stimuli. Lymphadenopathy may be characterized by enlargement of lymph nodes that are normally palpable, the presence of nodes that are not usually apparent on examination, or nodes that are simply altered in texture on palpation. Lymph nodes that are typically palpable in dogs and cats are the mandibular, superficial cervical, superficial inguinal, and popliteal lymph nodes. More than one lymph node may be palpable at each anatomic location. The tonsils may be visualized in the oral cavity, and buccal or facial lymph nodes may be found in some normal healthy puppies. Pathology is indicated if the axillary, accessory axillary, cervical, femoral, or retropharyngeal lymph nodes are palpable. Sublumbar and mesenteric lymph nodes must be enlarged to be detected on rectal or abdominal palpation (Rogers et al, 1993a).

Puppies and kittens are presented with many new antigenic stimuli early in life, and increased lymph node size is an expected part of the immunologic response. Indeed, lymphadenopathy is often noted after routine vaccination. As the animal ages, lymph node size often decreases. Two basic mechanisms result in lymphadenopathy. First, and most commonly, there can be increased number and size of lymphatic follicles with proliferation of lymphocytes and reticuloendothelial elements (immune stimulation). Disease processes causing reactive changes in lymph nodes are listed in Table 15–15. Second, infiltration of cells that are not normally found in the lymph node (neoplasia) could produce lymphadenopathy. Fortunately, neoplasia is a rare cause of nodal enlargement in puppies and kittens.

Evaluation of lymphadenopathy should include a detailed history and physical examination. Distribution of the adenopathy is important in determining the type of underlying disease process. If one lymph node or regional group of lymph nodes is involved, the sites drained by these lymph nodes should be carefully examined for evidence of inflammation, infection, or neoplasia. If lymph node involvement is more widespread, primary lymphoid neoplasia or diseases causing systemic antigenic stimulation should be considered.

Useful diagnostic tests include aspiration cytology, biopsy for histologic evaluation, bacterial culture, laboratory testing including serology, survey radiographs, and ultrasonography. Aspiration cytology can be a particularly useful and cost-effective screening test when evaluating animals with lymphadenopathy. The largest lymph node is usually not ideal for the aspiration procedure because it may have a necrotic center and areas of hemorrhage. Mandibular lymph nodes are also not ideal because they typically have reactive changes associated with regional drainage from the oral cavity. Cytology may provide a definitive diagnosis when microorganisms (i.e., bacteria or fungi) are identified and in the rare circumstance of large cell lymphoma. It can also provide a supportive picture of reactive changes that can occur secondary to local or systemic antigenic stimulation with increased numbers of inflammatory cells, including plasma cells, neutrophils, eosinophils, and macrophages.

Several specific disorders affecting lymph nodes in puppies and kittens deserve particular attention. Canine juvenile cellulitis (commonly known as *puppy strangles*) is a granulomatous and pustular disorder of the face, pinnae, and mandibular lymph nodes of puppies (Scott et al, 1995). Typical affected puppies are between 3 and 16 weeks of age; one or several in a litter may have the condition. Clinical signs include an acutely swollen face with papules and pustules progressing to ulceration and striking mandibular lymphadenopathy. The puppies may also exhibit lethargy, anorexia, pyrexia, and joint pain. Cytologic examination reveals pyogranulomatous inflammation with no microorganisms identified or cultured. Daily treatment with corticosteroids is indicated until the disease is inactive. If there is clinical evidence of secondary bacterial infection, bactericidal antimicrobial agents should be administered simultaneously.

Reactive lymphoid hyperplasia in young cats can present as a transient generalized lymphadenopathy that can develop in the initial viremic stage of many viral infections, including feline leukemia virus and feline immunodeficiency virus. However, in a retrospective study of 132 feline lymph node biopsy specimens, many cases of lymphadenopathy (82) were not associated with a specific cause and were designated as idiopathic (Moore et al, 1986). Fourteen cats in this study had lymph node hyperplasia with unique histologic features including severely distorted nodal architecture, making differentiation from lymphoma difficult. The cats were young (5 to 24 months old), and lymph nodes were judged to be two to three times normal

Table 15–15 Diseases Associated with Lymphadenopathy

Causes of Reactive Hyperplasia	
Infectious	Aspergillosis
Bacterial	Zygomycosis
Staphylococcus species	Rickettsial
Streptococcus species	Ehrlichiosis
Pasteurella species	Rocky Mountain spotted fever
Corynebacterium species	Salmon poisoning
Bartonella species	Protozoal
Brucellosis	Toxoplasmosis
Salmonellosis	Hepatozoonosis
Actinomyces species	Leishmaniasis
Nocardia species	Algal
Mycobacterial infection	Prototothecosis
Septicemia	Noninfectious
Viral	Postvaccination
Feline leukemia virus	Allergic skin disease
Feline immunodeficiency	Immune-mediated disorders
virus	Eosinophilic granuloma complex
Feline infectious peritonitis	Dermatopathic lymphadenopathy
Canine distemper	Localized inflammation
Infectious canine hepatitis	Idiopathic lymphadenopathy of
Parasitic	young cats
Demodicosis	Tumor-related reactive hyperplasia
Sarcoptes	Extramedullary hematopoiesis
Flea infestation	**Primary Lymphoid Neoplasia (rare)**
Tick infestation	Lymphoma
Fungal	Leukemias
Histoplasmosis	Systemic mast cell disease
Blastomycosis	**Metastatic Neoplasia (rare)**
Cryptococcosis	Mast cell tumor
Coccidioidomycosis	Transmissible venereal tumor
Sporotrichosis	Malignant melanoma
	Carcinomas

size. Six of nine cats tested for feline leukemia virus were positive. Prominent generalized peripheral lymphadenopathy was also identified in six cats with biopsy specimens that had histologic features compatible with lymphoma (Mooney et al, 1987). One cat was euthanized, but in the remaining five cats the lymph nodes regressed in size without therapy within 1 to 17 weeks. These studies emphasize the importance of careful interpretation of lymph node biopsy results, particularly for young cats. Infections in young cats with one of the *Bartonella* species may also contribute to a palpable lymphadenopathy, and can be reported by the veterinary pathologist as reactive lymphoid hyperplasia.

Lymphoma is rare in dogs and cats younger than 12 months (Shell et al, 1989; Rogers et al, 1989; Mooney et al, 1989; Jeglum et al, 1987). In one study, the hematopoietic system, brain, and skin were the most frequently affected sites for neoplasia in immature dogs younger than 6 months (Keller et al, 1992). The age-specific

incidence for lymphoma for dogs younger than 1 year old was estimated to be 1.5/100,000 dogs per year (Dorn et al, 1970). The multicentric form is the most common form of canine lymphoma, making chemotherapy the optimal therapy. Remission rates and survival times vary with the chemotherapy protocol used.

When neoplasia is diagnosed in young cats, hematopoietic neoplasms and lymphoma predominate (Greenlee et al, 1994). Cats with lymphoma should be tested for feline leukemia virus and feline imunodeficiency virus, as both viruses may be associated with an increased incidence of lymphoproliferative disease. In very young animals, anterior mediastinal and multicentric are the most frequent forms and are often associated with positive retrovirus status. The stage of disease is significantly related to response to chemotherapy, with less advanced stages being more likely to achieve a complete response (Mooney et al, 1989). The stage of disease and feline leukemia virus status are both significantly related to survival time, even though feline leukemia virus status does not affect response to therapy (Mooney et al, 1989; Cotter, 1983). Combination chemotherapy is recommended for multifocal lymphoma, but radiation can be effective for the limited number of cases with localized disease (Elmslie et al, 1991).

Lymphedema

Congenital lymphedema usually becomes evident at a young age, often at birth (Fossum and Miller, 1992). Primary lymphedema is caused by an abnormality or disease of the lymph conduction elements of the lymph vessels or nodes. Lymphedema usually has an insidious onset, is initially pitting in nature, painless, and typically begins in the distal part of the limb and progresses proximally (Fossum et al, 1992). Lameness and pain are uncommon unless there is massive enlargement or cellulitis. The primary differential diagnosis is an abnormality of the venous system such as venous stasis or arteriovenous fistula. If the edema is bilateral, systemic causes of edema including hypoproteinemia and heart failure must be ruled out.

THE THYMUS

The thymus is a pale, lobulated organ occupying a portion of the cranial mediastinum. Organ size can vary considerably, with its relative size being greatest in the newborn and its absolute size greatest at puberty. Gradual and continuing thymic involution accelerates after puberty and often coincides with the loss of deciduous teeth. The thymus atrophies, and its cortex is gradually replaced with loose connective tissue and fat. Remnants of the organ do, however, persist until old age (Tizard, 1995; Banks, 1993). In the young animal, the thymus can frequently be identified on ventrodorsal or dorsoventral thoracic radiographs as it lies in the cranioventral mediastinal reflection. It is not easily seen on lateral views as it may silhouette with and obscure the cranial margin of the heart (Thrall, 1994).

In mammals, the thymus is a primary lymphoid organ that is essential for development of T lymphocytes (Banks, 1993). Lymphocytes differentiating in the thymus leave and populate secondary lymphoid organs (lymph nodes, spleen, and bone marrow) and other aggregates of scattered lymphoid nodules with T cells. Continual circulation of T cells through the spleen and lymph nodes is important in immune recognition and stimulation. The role of the thymus in immunity is demonstrated by neonatal thymectomy that leads to an impaired ability to mount a delayed hypersensitivity response. The ability to produce an antibody-mediated response is also impaired because antibody production requires T-cell assistance (Banks, 1993).

Developmental disorders of the thymus have been reported in both dogs and cats. The organ grossly appears rudimentary; the decreased size may be from reduced numbers of lymphocytes, decreased epithelial framework, or both. The thymus may be involved in cases of wasting syndrome in puppies and kittens that cannot be attributed to a specific etiology (Roth, 1987). Other than viral-induced disease, thymic hypoplasia is rare, and presenting clinical signs are likely to be related to immunosuppression (Modiano and Helfand, 1997). Recognized congenital abnormalities include an X-linked, severe combined immunodeficiency in a colony of basset hounds established from a single affected female, growth hormone deficiency resulting in immunodeficient dwarfism in a family of Weimaraners, a syndrome of thymic atrophy in Mexican hairless dogs, acrodermatitis with immunodeficiency in bull terriers, and thymic aplasia associated with a syndrome of hairlessness in Birman cats (Modiano and Helfand, 1997; Searcy, 1995).

Infectious agents, toxins, neoplasia, or malnutrition may cause injury to the thymus resulting in variable degrees of immunodeficiency. Infection with feline leukemia virus, feline immunodeficiency virus, feline infectious peritonitis, canine distemper virus, canine parvovirus, and feline panleukopenia can be associated with thymic and lymph node atrophy at necropsy (Searcy, 1995). Canine distemper virus, canine parvovirus, and feline panleukopenia are lympholytic and result in thymic necrosis. Feline leukemia virus induces thymocyte apoptosis (a programmed cell death), but thymic hypoplasia does not always occur with feline immunodeficiency virus. Thymic function may be impaired in young animals with severe protein malnutrition resulting in diminished immunoglobulin synthesis, and zinc deficiency in pups has also been shown to result in severe atrophy of the thymus (Roth, 1987; Searcy, 1995). Thymic involution is part of the normal process of aging and may be accelerated by any toxic insult.

Thymic neoplasia is usually identified as lymphoma or thymoma. Lymphoma has a higher incidence in cats than dogs and is often associated with feline leukemia virus in this age group.

Benign cysts of the ventral mediastinum are uncommon congenital defects and can arise from diverse cell lines including thymic (Bauer and Woodfield, 1995). Puppies and kittens are typically asymptomatic, and the cysts are incidental findings on thoracic radiographs. After aspiration, benign cysts should be radiographically diminished in size. A mediastinal cystic lymphangioma associated with progressive dyspnea was diagnosed and successfully surgically resected in an 8-week-old puppy (Remedios et al, 1990).

An uncommon syndrome of spontaneous thymic hemorrhage has been reported in the canine, often as a cause of death (Klopfer et al, 1985; Linde-Sipman et al, 1987; Coolman et al, 1994). Although it is unlikely to be a specific pathogenic entity, spontaneous hemorrhage appears to be confined to the age of thymic involution, as most dogs are younger than 1 year. Some investigators feel that the syndrome may be related to specific histologic changes associated with thymic involution (Klopfer et al, 1985). During involution, blood vessels within the stroma of the thymus lose their tissue support, dilate, and become thin walled. In one study, some form of trauma was often noted in the immediate history (Linde-Sipman et al, 1987). Thirteen of 20 dogs had a history that involved a major or minor trauma such as being hit by a car or having the head suddenly pulled back by the owner when running at the end of a leash. The authors speculated that trauma resulting in sudden overstretching of the relaxed neck could be followed by rupture of small vessels in loose tissues like thymus. At necropsy, diffuse thymic hemorrhage, cranial hemomediastinum, and hemothorax are seen. Treatment of spontaneous thymic hemorrhage is immediate blood replacement therapy and other supportive care. Surgical removal of the thymus is seldom needed.

THE SPLEEN

The normal spleen may be palpable in most puppies and infrequently in kittens as a flat structure oriented dorsoventrally in the left anterior abdominal quadrant (Couto et al, 1995). The spleen is one of the major hematopoietic organs during fetal development, although this activity diminishes before or shortly after birth. Although normal adult canine and feline spleens have no hematopoietic activity, the ability to initiate extramedullary hematopoiesis is retained. The spleen, which is the largest mass of lymphatic tissue in the body, has multiple

Table 15–16	Diseases Associated with Splenomegaly

Inflammatory
  Infectious
    Bacterial (sepsis, pyometra, peritonitis, endocarditis, brucellosis)
    Fungal (histoplasmosis, blastomycosis, sporotrichosis)
    Rickettsial (ehrlichiosis, haemobartonellosis)
    Viral (feline infectious peritonitis, infectious canine hepatitis)
    Protozoal (toxoplasmosis, leishmaniasis)
  Noninfectious
    Hemolytic disorders
    Eosinophilic gastroenteritis
    Hypereosinophilic syndrome
  Other
    Splenic torsion
    Penetrating abdominal wounds
    Migrating foreign body
Noninflammatory
  Congestive
    Splenic torsion
    Pharmacologic (tranquilizers, anticonvulsants)
    Portal hypertension (right-sided heart failure, intrahepatic obstruction)
  Infiltrative
    Extramedullary hematopoiesis
    Neoplasia (lymphoma, leukemias, mastocytosis)
  Other
    Hematoma
    Splenic rupture secondary to trauma

functions including blood cell formation, hemoglobin and iron metabolism, red blood cell destruction, blood filtration, blood storage, phagocytosis, and immune response (Banks, 1993).

The spleen has a unique vascular structure through which blood circulates in close contact with macrophages, allowing for ample biologic filtration of cells and particles (Couto et al, 1995). Just as lymph nodes filter lymph, the spleen filters blood (Tizard, 1995). It is an organ of great immunologic significance because it is a major site for production of antibodies and effector T cells. Formation and storage of red blood cells and antigen trapping occur in the red pulp, whereas the immune response occurs in the white pulp. The spleen helps clear poorly opsonized bacteria and remains a critical line of defense against blood-borne bacteria (Couto et al, 1995). Sepsis after splenectomy and hyposplenism, however, appears to be rare in the puppy and kitten. Postoperative sepsis is more likely to occur in animals that are already immunosuppressed. An intact spleen does provide protection from parasitemia in animals with hemoparasitic infections.

The spleen is a target for many pathologic processes because it is located between the portal and systemic circulation (Neer, 1996). The spleen may be a primary disease site, but it can also be affected secondarily by systemic disease and may act as a sentinel organ for an underlying disease process. Diseases that may be associated with splenomegaly in puppies and kittens are listed in Table 15–16. Diagnostic evaluation for the specific splenic disorder may include the history, physical examination, hematology, serology, imaging (radiography, ultrasonography), aspiration cytology, and biopsy and would be done in a similar manner for the adult dog and cat.

References and Supplemental Reading

HEMATOLOGY OF NORMAL DOGS AND CATS AND RESPONSES TO DISEASE

Ackerman N, Spencer CP, Sundlof SF, et al: Zinc toxicosis in a dog secondary to ingestion of pennies. Vet Radiol 31:155, 1990.

Andersen AC, Gee W: Normal blood values in the beagle. Vet Med 53:135, 1958.

Anderson L, Wilson R, Hay D: Haematological values in normal cats from four weeks to one year of age. Res Vet Sci 12:579, 1971.

Bowles CA, Alsaker RD, Wolfe TL: Studies of the Pelger-Huet anomaly in foxhounds. Am J Pathol 96:237, 1979.

Bücheler J, Giger U: Alloantibodies against A and B blood types in cats. Vet Immunol Immunopathol 38:283, 1993.

Cain GR, Suzuki Y: Presumptive neonatal isoerythrolysis in cats. J Am Vet Med Assoc 187:46, 1985.

Callan MB, Giger U: Transfusion medicine. In August JR (ed): Consultations in Feline Internal Medicine, 2nd ed. Philadelphia, WB Saunders, 1994, p 525.

Campbell KL: Canine cyclic hematopoiesis. Compend Contin Educ Pract Vet 7:57, 1985.

Carpenter JL: Feline panleukopenia: Clinical signs and differential diagnosis. J Am Vet Med Assoc 158:857, 1971.

Colgan SP, Hull-Thrall MA, Gasper PW, et al: Restoration of neutrophil and platelet function in feline Chediak-Higashi syndrome by bone marrow transplantation. Bone Marrow Tranplant 7:365, 1991.

Cowell RL, Tyler RD: Diagnosis of anemia. In August JR (ed): Consultations in Feline Internal Medicine, 1st ed. Philadelphia, WB Saunders, 1991, p 335.

Duncan JR, Prasse KW, Mahaffey EA: Veterinary Laboratory Medicine, 3rd ed. Ames, Iowa State University Press, 1994, p 3.

Earl FL, Melveger E, Wilson RL: The hemogram and bone marrow profile of normal neonatal and weaning beagle dogs. Lab Anim Sci 23:690, 1971.

Feldman BF, Roman AV: The Pelger-Huet anomaly of granulocytic leukocytes in the dog. Canine Pract 3(5):22, 1976.

Gandolfi RC: Feline neonatal isoerythrolysis: A case report. Calif Vet 42:9, 1988.

Guilford WG: Primary immunodeficiency diseases of dogs and cats. Compend Contin Educ Pract Vet 9:641, 1987.

Harvey JW: The erythrocyte: Physiology, metabolism, and biochemical disorders. In Kaneko JJ, Harvey JW, Bruss ML (eds): Clinical Biochemistry of Domestic Animals, 5th ed. New York, Academic Press, 1997, p 157.

Hirsch VM, Cunningham TA: Hereditary anomaly of neutrophil granulation in Birman cats. Am J Vet Res 45:2170, 1984.

Holland CT, Canfield PJ, Watson AD, et al: Dyserythropoiesis, polymyopathy, and cardiac disease in three related English springer spaniels. J Vet Intern Med 5:151, 1991.

Jacobs RM, Weiser MG, Hall RL, et al: Clinicopathologic features of canine parvovirus enteritis. J Am Anim Hosp Assoc 16:809, 1980.

Jain NC: Schalm's Veterinary Hematology. Philadelphia, Lea & Febiger, 1986, p 1046.

Jain NC: Essentials of Veterinary Hematology. Philadelphia, Lea & Febiger, 1993, p 1.

Jezyk, PF, Haskins ME, Patterson DF, et al: Mucopolysaccharidosis in a cat with arylsulfatase B deficiency: A model of Maroteaux-Lamy syndrome. Science 198:834, 1977.

Jonsson NN, Pullen C, Watson ADJ: Neonatal isoerythrolysis in Himalayan kittens. Austral Vet J 67:416, 1990.

Kramer JW, Davis WC, Prieur DJ: The Chediak-Higashi syndrome of cat. Lab Invest 36:554, 1977.

Latimer KS: Leukocytes in health and disease. In Ettinger SJ, Feldman EC (eds): Textbook of Veterinary Internal Medicine, 4th ed. Philadelphia, WB Saunders, 1995, p 1892.

Latimer KS, Jain AV, Inglesby HB, et al: Zinc-induced hemolytic anemia caused by ingestion of pennies by a pup. J Am Vet Med Assoc 195:77, 1989a.

Latimer KS, Kircher IM, Lindl PA, et al: Leukocyte function in Pelger-Huet anomaly of dogs. J Leukocyte Biol 45:301, 1989b.

Latimer KS, Rakich PM, Thompson DF: Pelger-Huet anomaly in cats. Vet Pathol 22:370, 1985.

DISORDERS OF HEMOSTASIS

Badylak SF, Dodds WJ, Van Fleet JF: Plasma coagulation factor abnormalities in dogs with naturally occurring hepatic disease. Am J Vet Res 44(12):2336, 1983.

Badylak SF, Van Fleet JF: Alterations of prothrombin

time and activated thromboplastin time in dogs with hepatic disease. Am J Vet Res 42(12):2053, 1981.

Beck ER, Harris CK, Macy DW: Feline leukemia virus: Infection and treatment. Compend Contin Educ Pract Vet 8(8):567, 1986.

Bennett JS: Blood coagulation and coagulation tests. Med Clin North Am 68(3):557, 1984.

Benson RE, Catalfamo JL, Brooks M, et al: A sensitive immunoassay for von Willebrand factor. J Immunol 12(3):371, 1991.

Benson RE, Jones DW, Dodds WJ: Efficiency and precision of electroimmunoassay for canine factor VIII–related antigen. Am J Vet Res 44(3):399, 1983.

Blifeld C, Courtney JT, Gross JR: Assessment of neonatal platelet function using a viscoelastic technique. Ann Clin Lab Sci 16(5):373, 1986.

Bloom JC, Meunier LD, Thiem PA, et al: Use of danazol for treatment of corticosteroid-resistant immune-mediated thrombocytopenia in a dog. J Am Vet Med Assoc 194(1):76, 1989.

Boudreaux MK, Caralfamo JL: The molecular basis for Glanzmann's thrombasthenia in otterhounds. Am J Vet Res, in press.

Boudreaux MK, Catalfamo JL, Dodds WJ: Elevated cyclic AMP levels in canine thrombopathia. Thromb Haemost 54:278, 1985 (abstract).

Boudreaux MK, Crager C, Dillon AR, et al: Identification of an intrinsic platelet function defect in spitz dogs. J Vet Intern Med 8(2):93, 1994.

Boudreaux MK, Dillon AR: The effect of danazol treatment on factor IX deficiency in cats. Vet Clin Pathol 17(4):84, 1988.

Boudreaux MK, Dodds WJ, Slauson DO, et al: Evidence for regulatory control of canine platelet phosphodiesterase. Blochem Biophys Res Commun 140(2):589, 1986a.

Boudreaux MK, Dodds WJ, Slauson DO, et al: Impaired cAMP metabolism associated with abnormal function of thrombopathic platelets. Biochem Biophys Res Commun 140(2):595, 1986b.

Boudreaux MK, Kvam K, Dillon AR, et al: Type I Glanzmann's thrombasthenia in a Great Pyrenees dog. Vet Pathol 33:503, 1996.

Boudreaux MK, Weiss RC, Cox N, et al: Evaluation of antithrombin III activity as a co-indicator of DIC in cats experimentally infected with feline infectious peritonitis virus. Am J Vet Res 50(11):1910, 1988a.

Boudreaux MK, Weiss RC, Cox N, et al: Evaluation of antithrombin III activity in cats with FIP virus–induced DIC. Am Soc Vet Clin Pathol Conf Proc, 1988b, p 10 (abstract).

Boyce JT, Kociba GJ, Jacobs RM, et al: Feline leukemia virus–induced thrombocytopenia and macrothrombocytosis in cats. Vet Pathol 23:16, 1986.

Brooks M, Leith GS, Allen AK, et al: Bleeding disorder (von Willebrand disease) in a quarter horse. J Am Vet Med Assoc 198(1):114, 1991.

Brox AG, Howson-Jan K, Fauser AA: Treatment of idiopathic thrombocytopenic purpura with ascorbate. Br J Haematol 70:341, 1988.

Buchanan GR: Neonatal coagulation: Normal physiology and pathophysiology. Clin Haematol 7:85, 1978.

Byars TD, Greene CE: Idiopathic thrombocytopenic purpura in the horse. J Am Vet Med Assoc 180(12): 1422, 1982.

Cain GR, Feldman BF, Kawakami TG, et al: Platelet dysplasia associated with megakaryoblastic leukemia in a dog. J Am Vet Med Assoc 188(5):529, 1986.

Campbell KL, Greene CE, Dodds WJ: Factor IX deficiency (hemophilia B) in a Scottish terrier. J Am Vet Med Assoc 182(2):170, 1983.

Carmichael LE: Canine herpesvirus infection in puppies. In Kirk RW (ed): Current Veterinary Therapy VI. Philadelphia, WB Saunders, 1977, p 1296.

Catalfamo JL, Raymond SL, White JG, et al: Defective platelet-fibrinogen interaction in hereditary canine thrombopathia. Blood 67(6):1568, 1986.

Cheville NF: The gray collie syndrome (cyclic neutropenia). J Am Anim Hosp Assoc 11:350, 1975.

Chinn DR, Dodds WJ, Selcer BA: Prekallikrein deficiency in a dog. J Am Vet Med Assoc 188(1):69, 1986.

Collier LL, Bryan GM, Prieur DJ: Ocular manifestations of the Chediak-Higashi syndrome in four species of animals. J Am Vet Med Assoc 175(6):587, 1979.

Corapi WV, Elliott RD, French TW, et al: Thrombocytopenia and hemorrhages in veal calves infected with bovine viral diarrhea virus. J Am Vet Med Assoc 196(4):590, 1990.

Cotter SM, Brenner RM, Dodds WJ: Hemophilia A in three unrelated cats. J Am Vet Med Assoc 172(2):166, 1978.

Cowan DH: Acquired Disorders of Platelet Function. Hemostasis and Thrombosis Basic Principles and Clinical Practice. Philadelphia, JB Lippincott, 1982, p 516.

Davidson MG, Breitschwerdt EB, Walker DH, et al: Vascular permeability and coagulation during Rickettsia rickettsii infection in dogs. Am J Vet Res 51(1):165, 1990.

Davis LE: Vitamin K and its therapeutic importance. J Am Vet Med Assoc 180(11):1354, 1982.

DiGiacomo RF, Hammond WP, Kunz LL, et al: Clinical and pathologic features of cyclic hematopoiesis in grey collie dogs. Am J Pathol 111(2):224, 1983.

Dillon AR, Boudreaux MK: Combined factors IX and XII deficiencies in a family of cats. J Am Vet Med Assoc 193(7):833, 1988.

Dodds WJ: Canine factor X (Stuart-Prower factor) deficiency. J Lab Clin Med 82(4):560, 1973.

Dodds WJ: Further studies of canine von Willebrand's disease. Blood 45(2):221, 1975a.

Dodds WJ: Inherited hemorrhagic disorders. J Am Anim Hosp Assoc 11:366, 1975b.

Dodds WJ: Inherited bleeding disorders. Canine Pract 5(6):49, 1978.

Dodds WJ: Prothrombin (factor II) deficiencies. In Dodds WJ (ed): Spontaneous Animal Models of

Human Disease. New York, Academic Press, 1979, p 267.

Dodds WJ: Second International Registry of Animal Models of Thrombosis and Hemorrhagic Diseases. ILAR News 24(4):R1, 1981.

Dodds WJ: Bleeding diseases of small animals. Vet Ref Lab Newslett 8(2), 1984a.

Dodds WJ: Von Willebrand's disease in dogs. Mod Vet Pract 65(9):681, 1984b.

Dodds WJ, Kull JE: Canine factor XI (plasma thromboplastin antecedent) deficiency. J Lab Clin Med 78(5):746, 1971.

Dodds WJ, Moynihan AC, Benson RE, et al: The value of age- and sex-matched controls for coagulation studies. Br J Haematol 29:305, 1975.

Earl FL, Melveger BE, Wilson RL: The hemogram and bone marrow profile of normal neonatal and weanling beagle dogs. Lab Anim Sci 23(5):690, 1973.

Feldman BF, Soares CJ, Kitchell BE, et al: Hemorrhage in a cat caused by inhibition of factor XI (plasma thromboplastin antecedent). J Am Vet Med Assoc 182(6):589, 1983.

Fernandez FR, Teachout DJ, Christopher MM: Vitamin K–induced Heinz body formation in dogs. J Am Anim Hosp Assoc 20:711, 1984.

French TW, Fox LE, Randolph JF, et al: A bleeding disorder (von Willebrand's disease) in a Himalayan cat. J Am Vet Med Assoc 190(4):437, 1987.

French TW, Harvey JW: Serologic diagnosis of infectious cyclic thrombocytopenia in dogs using an indirect fluorescent antibody test. Am J Vet Res 44(12):2407, 1983.

Fruchtman S, Aledort LM: Disseminated intravascular coagulation. J Am Coll Cardiol 8(6):159B, 1986.

Geor RJ, Jackson ML, Lewis KD, et al: Prekallikrein deficiency in a family of Belgian horses. J Am Vet Med Assoc 197(6):741, 1990.

George JN, Nurden MD, Phillips DR: Molecular defects in interactions of platelets with the vessel wall. N Engl J Med 311(17):1084, 1984.

Giger U, Dodds JW: Effect of desmopressin in normal dogs and dogs with von Willebrand's disease. Vet Clin Pathol 18(2):39, 1989.

Greene CE, Harvey JW: Canine ehrlichiosis. In Greene CE (ed): Clinical Microbiology and Infectious Diseases of the Dog and Cat. Philadelphia, WB Saunders, 1984, p 545.

Greene CE, Philip RN: Rocky Mountain spotted fever. In Greene CE (ed): Clinical Microbiology and Infectious Diseases of the Dog and Cat. Philadelphia, WB Saunders, 1984, p 562.

Greffe BS, Marlar RA, Manco-Johnson MJ: Neonatal protein C: Molecular composition and distribution in normal term infants. Thromb Res 56(1):91, 1989.

Hackett T, Kelton JG, Powers P: Drug-induced platelet destruction. Semin Thromb Hemost 8(2):116, 1982.

Hammer AS, Couto CG, Swardson C, et al: Hemostatic abnormalities in dogs with hemangiosarcoma. J Vet Intern Med 5(1):11, 1991.

Hargis AM, Feldman BF: Evaluation of hemostatic defects secondary to vascular tumors in dogs: 11 cases (1983–1988). J Am Vet Med Assoc 198(5):891, 1991.

Harvey JW, Simpson CF, Gaskin JM: Cyclic thrombocytopenia induced by a rickettsia-like agent in dogs. J Infect Dis 137:182, 1978.

Henninger RW: Hemophilia A in two related quarter horse colts. J Am Vet Med Assoc 193(1):91, 1988.

Hill BL, Zenoble RD, Dodds WJ: Prothrombin deficiency in a cocker spaniel. J Am Vet Med Assoc 181(3):262, 1982.

Holloway SA, Meyer DJ, Mannella C: Prednisolone and danazol for treatment of immune-mediated anemia, thrombocytopenia, and ineffective erythroid regeneration in a dog. J Am Vet Med Assoc 197(8):1045, 1990.

Jans HE, Armstrong PJ, Price GS: Therapy of immune mediated thrombocytopenia. A retrospective study of 15 dogs. J Vet Intern Med 4(1):4, 1990.

Jergens AE, Turrentine MA, Kraus KH, et al: Buccal mucosa bleeding times of healthy dogs and of dogs in various pathologic states, including thrombocytopenia, uremia, and von Willebrand's disease. Am J Vet Res 48(9):1337, 1987.

Johnson GS, Turrentine MA, Tomlinson JL: Detection of von Willebrand's disease in dogs with a rapid qualitative test based on venom-coagglutinin–induced platelet agglutination. Vet Clin Pathol 14(2):11, 1985.

Johnstone IB, Crane S: Hemostatic abnormalities in equine colic. Am J Vet Res 47(2):356, 1986.

Johnstone IB, Lotz F: An inherited platelet function defect in basset hounds. Can Vet J 20:211, 1979.

Johnstone IB, Norris AM: A moderately severe expression of classical hemophilia in a family of German shepherd dogs. Can Vet J 25:191, 1984.

Jones BEV: Platelet aggregation in dogs after live-virus vaccination. Acta Vet Scand 25:504, 1984.

Kane KK: Fibrinolysis—A review. Ann Clin Lab Sci 14(6):443, 1984.

Kier AB, Bresnahan JF, White FJ, Wagner JE: The inheritance pattern of factor XII (Hageman) deficiency in domestic cats. Can J Comp Med 44:309, 1980.

Kociba GJ, Ratnoff OD, Loeb WF, et al: Bovine plasma thromboplastin antecedent (factor XI) deficiency. J Lab Clin Med 74:37, 1969.

Kramer JW, Davis WC, Prieur DJ: The Chediak-Higashi syndrome of cats. Lab Invest 36(5):554, 1977.

Kuehn NF, Gaunt SD: Clinical and hematologic findings in canine ehrlichiosis. J Am Vet Med Assoc 186(4):355, 1985.

Larson VL, Perman V, Stevens JB: Idiopathic thrombocytopenic purpura in two horses. J Am Vet Med Assoc 183(3):328, 1983.

Lipscomb DL, Bourne C, Boudreaux MK: Two genetic defects in alpha IIb are associated with type I Glanzmann's thrombasthenia in a Great Pyrenees dog: A 14-base insertion in exon 13 and a splicing defect of intron 13. Vet Pathol, accepted for publication.

Littlewood JD, Bevan SA: Haemophilia A (classic haemophilia, factor VIII deficiency) in a thoroughbred colt foal. Equine Vet J 23(1):70, 1991.

Littlewood JD, Matic SE, Smith N: Factor IX deficiency (haemophilia B, Christmas disease) in a crossbred dog. Vet Rec 118:400, 1986.

Lothrop CD, Candler RV, Pratt HL, et al: Characterization of platelet function in cyclic hematopoietic dogs. Exp Hematol 19:916, 1991.

Lovering SL, Pierce KR, Adams LG: Serum complement and blood platelet adhesiveness in acute canine ehrlichiosis. Am J Vet Res 41(8):1266, 1980.

Maddison JE, Watson ADJ, Eade IG, et al: Vitamin K–dependent multifactor coagulopathy in Devon Rex cats. J Am Vet Med Assoc 197(11):1495, 1990.

Mammen EF: Coagulation abnormalities in liver disease. Hematol Oncol Clin North Am 6(6):1247, 1992.

Meyers KM, Hopkins G, Holmsen H, et al: Ultrastructure of resting and activated storage pool deficient platelets from animals with the Chediak-Higashi syndrome. Am J Pathol 106(3):364, 1982.

Middleton DJ, Watson ADJ: Activated coagulation times of whole blood in normal dogs and dogs with coagulopathies. J Small Anim Pract 19:417, 1978.

Morris DD, Messick J, Whitlock RH, et al: Effect of equine ehrlichial colitis on the hemostatic system in ponies. Am J Vet Res 49(7):1030, 1988.

Moser J, Meyers KM, Russon RH: Inheritance of von Willebrand factor deficiency in Doberman pinschers. J Am Vet Med Assoc 209(6):1103, 1996.

Mount ME, Feldman BF: Mechanism of diphacinone rodenticide toxicosis in the dog and its therapeutic implications. Am J Vet Res 44(11):2009, 1983.

Muller GH, Kirk RW, Scott DW: Congenital and Hereditary Defects. Cutaneous Asthenia. Small Animal Dermatology, 3rd ed. Philadelphia, WB Saunders, 1983, p 561.

Murtaugh RJ, Dodds WJ: Hemophilia A in a female dog. J Am Vet Med Assoc 193(3):351, 1988.

Parker MT, Collier LL, Kier AB, et al: Oral mucosa bleeding times of normal cats and cats with Chediak-Higashi syndrome or Hageman trait (factor XII deficiency). Vet Clin Pathol 17(1):9, 1988.

Peterson ME, Dodds WJ: Factor IX deficiency in an Alaskan malamute. J Am Vet Med Assoc 174(12):1326, 1979.

Pierce KR, Marrs GE, Hightower D: Acute canine ehrlichiosis: Platelet survival and factor 3 assay. Am J Vet Res 38(11):1821, 1977.

Poulsen PH, Thomsen MK, Kristensen F: Cutaneous asthenia in the dog. A report of two cases. Nord Vet Med 37:291, 1985.

Prieur DJ, Collier LL, Bryan GM, et al: The diagnosis of feline Chediak-Higashi syndrome. Feline Pract 9(5):26, 1979.

Randolph JF, Center SA, Dodds WJ: Factor XII deficiency and von Willebrand's disease in a family of miniature poodle dogs. Cornell Vet 76:3, 1986.

Raymond SL, Dodds WJ: Platelet membrane glyco-

proteins in normal dogs and dogs with hemostatic defects. J Lab Clin Med 93(4):607, 1979.

Schafer AI: Bleeding and thrombosis in the myeloproliferative disorders. Blood 64(1):1, 1984.

Schulman A, Lusk R, Lippincott CL, et al: Diphacinone-induced coagulopathy in the dog. J Am Vet Med Assoc 188(4):402, 1986.

Sherding RG, DiBartola SP: Hemophilia B (factor IX deficiency) in an Old English sheepdog. J Am Vet Med Assoc 176(2):141, 1980.

Smith RD, Ristic M, Huxsoll DL, et al: Platelet kinetics in canine ehrlichiosis: Evidence for increased platelet destruction as the cause of thrombocytopenia. Infect Immun 11(6):1216, 1975.

Soute BAM, Ulrich MMW, Watson ADJ, et al: Congenital deficiency of all vitamin K–dependent blood coagulation factors due to a defective vitamin K–dependent carboxylase in Devon Rex cats. Thromb Haemost 68(5):521, 1992.

Spurling NW, Peacock R, Pilling T: The clinical aspects of factor-VII deficiency including some case histories. J Small Anim Pract 15:229, 1974.

Turrentine MA, Sculley PW, Green EM, et al: Prekallikrein deficiency in a family of miniature horses. Am J Vet Res 47(11):2464, 1986.

Verlander JW, Gorman NT, Dodds WJ: Factor IX deficiency (hemophilia B) in a litter of Labrador retrievers. J Am Vet Med Assoc 185(1):83, 1984.

Warrier AL, Lusher JM: A useful alternative to blood components in moderate hemophilia A and von Willebrand's disease. J Pediatr 102:175, 1983.

Welles EG, Prasse KW, Moore JN: Use of newly developed assays for protein C and plasminogen in horses with signs of colic. Am J Vet Res 52(2):345, 1991.

THE LYMPHOID SYSTEM

Banks WJ: Lymphatic system and immunity. In Banks WJ (ed): Applied Veterinary Histology, 3rd ed. St. Louis, Mosby Yearbook, 1993, p 277.

Bauer T, Woodfield JA: Mediastinal, pleural, and extrapleural diseases. In Ettinger SJ, Feldman EC (eds): Textbook of Veterinary Internal Medicine, 4th ed. Philadelphia, WB Saunders, 1995, p 812.

Coolman BR, Brewer WG, D'Andrea GH, et al: Severe idiopathic thymic hemorrhage in two littermate dogs. J Am Vet Med Assoc 205:1152, 1994.

Cotter SM: Treatment of lymphoma and leukemia with cyclophosphamide, vincristine, and prednisone: II. Treatment of cats. J Am Anim Hosp Assoc 19:166, 1983.

Couto CG, Hammer AS: Diseases of the lymph nodes and spleen. In Ettinger SJ, Feldman EC (eds): Textbook of Veterinary Internal Medicine, 4th ed. Philadelphia, WB Saunders, 1995, p 1930.

Dorn CR, Taylor DON, Schneider R: The epidemiology of canine leukemia and lymphoma. Bibl Haematol 36:403, 1970.

Elmslie R, Ogilvie G, Gillette E, et al: Radiotherapy with and without chemotherapy for localized lymphoma in 10 cats. Vet Radiol 32:277, 1991.

Fossum TW, King LA, Miller MW, et al: Lymphedema: Clinical signs, diagnosis, and treatment. J Vet Intern Med 6:312, 1992.

Fossum TW, Miller MW: Lymphedema: etiopathogenesis. J Vet Intern Med 6:283, 1992.

Greenlee PG, Patnaik AK, Tappe J: Prevalence and incidence of neoplasms by site and cell type. *In* August JR (ed): Consultations in Feline Medicine, 2nd ed. Philadelphia, WB Saunders, 1994, p 535.

Jeglum KA, Whereat A, Young K: Chemotherapy of lymphoma in 75 cats. J Am Vet Med Assoc 190:174, 1987.

Keller ET, Madewell BR: Locations and types of neoplasms in immature dogs: 69 cases (1964–1989). J Am Vet Med Assoc 200:1530, 1992.

Klopfer U, Perl S, Yakobson B, et al: Spontaneous fatal hemorrhage in the involuting thymus in dogs. J Am Anim Hosp Assoc 21:261, 1985.

Linde-Sipman JS, Dijk JE: Hematomas in the thymus of dogs. Vet Pathol 24:59, 1987.

Modiano JF, Helfand SC: Diseases of the thymus. *In* Morgan RV (ed): Handbook of Small Animal Practice. Philadelphia, WB Saunders, 1997, p 805.

Mooney SC, Hayes AA, MacEwen EG, et al: Treatment and prognostic factors in lymphoma in cats: 103 cases (1977–1981). J Am Vet Med Assoc 194:696, 1989.

Mooney SC, Patnaik AK, Hayes AA, et al: Generalized lymphadenopathy resembling lymphoma in cats: Six cases (1972–1976). J Am Vet Med Assoc 190:897, 1987.

Moore FM, Emerson WE, Cotter SM, et al: Distinctive peripheral lymph node hyperplasia of young cats. Vet Pathol 23:386, 1986.

Neer TM: Clinical approach to splenomegaly in dogs and cats. Compend Contin Educ Pract Vet 18:35, 1996.

Remedios A, Bauer M, McMurphy R, et al: Mediastinal cystic lymphangioma in a dog. J Am Anim Hosp Assoc 26:161, 1990.

Rogers KS, Barton CL, Landis M: Canine and feline lymph nodes. Part II. Diagnostic evaluation of lymphadenopathy. Compend Contin Educ Pract Vet 15:1493, 1993a.

Rogers KS, Janovitz EB, Fooshee SK, et al: Lymphosarcoma with disseminated skeletal involvement in a pup. J Am Vet Med Assoc 195:1242, 1989.

Rogers KS, Landis M, Barton CL: Canine and feline lymph nodes. Part I. Anatomy and function. Compend Contin Educ Pract Vet 15:397, 1993b.

Roth JA: Possible association of thymus dysfunction with fading syndromes in puppies and kittens. Vet Clin North Am 17:603, 1987.

Scott DW, Miller WH, Griffin CE: Miscellaneous skin diseases. *In* Scott DW, Miller WH, Griffin CE (eds): Small Animal Dermatology, 5th ed. Philadelphia, WB Saunders, 1995, p 902.

Searcy GP: Hemopoietic system. *In* Carlton WW, McGavin MD (eds): Thomson's Special Veterinary Pathology, 2nd ed. St. Louis, Mosby, 1995, p 285.

Shell L, Davenport DJ, Barber DL, et al: Generalized skeletal involvement of a hematopoietic tumor in a dog. J Am Vet Med Assoc 194:1077, 1989.

Thrall DE: The mediastinum. *In* Thrall DE (ed): Textbook of Veterinary Diagnostic Radiology, 2nd ed. Philadelphia, WB Saunders, 1994, p 277.

Tizard IR: The lymphoid organs. *In* Tizard IR (ed): Immunology: An Introduction, 4th ed. Philadelphia, Saunders College Publishing, 1995, p 108.

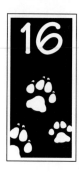

16

Endocrine and Metabolic Systems

Deborah S. Greco and C. B. Chastain

The Endocrine System

Deborah S. Greco

Endocrine and metabolic disorders affecting puppies and kittens from birth until 6 months of age may manifest as clinical problems related to growth or to polydipsia and polyuria or as episodic weakness. Most commonly, endocrine and metabolic disorders affect growth, and puppies are often presented to the veterinarian for assessment of delayed or aberrant growth. Other endocrine disorders of small animals, such as juvenile-onset diabetes insipidus or diabetes mellitus, affect water metabolism, resulting in excessive thirst and urination or in difficulty in house-breaking. Finally, the third manner in which endocrine and metabolic diseases may present is that of episodic weakness. Disorders that fall into this category include juvenile-onset hypoadrenocorticism and various inborn errors of metabolism that may result in hypoglycemia or hyperammonemia.

ENDOCRINE DISEASES THAT AFFECT STATURAL GROWTH

Many pediatric endocrine disorders, including hypothyroidism and growth hormone deficiency, are manifested as abnormalities of statural growth. Growth charts for kittens and puppies are shown in Figures 16–1 and 16–2, and skeletal development as determined by the radiographic appearance of ossification centers is shown in Table 16–1. Causes of inadequate

growth can be divided into two broad categories: intrinsic defects of growing tissues (skeletal dysplasias, chromosomal abnormalities, dysmorphic dwarfism) and abnormalities in the environment of growing tissues (nutritional, metabolic, environmental, and endocrine).

Intrinsic defects of growing tissues include most of the genetic and chromosomal abnormalities that result in growth failure. Genetic disorders may be suspected on the basis of clustering of disease in certain breeds or lines of dogs and cats (i.e., chondrodystrophy of Alaskan malamutes). Diagnosis may require pursuing pedigree analysis, genetic testing, or both.

Abnormalities of the environment of growing tissues are the most common and easily identified disorders. A thorough dietary history will reveal inadequate quantity and/or quality of feeding. Metabolic disorders, such as congenital portosystemic shunting, exocrine pancreatic insufficiency, congenital heart disease, and chronic renal failure, may be identified by characteristic clinical signs and laboratory data. Endocrine causes of growth retardation include juvenile hypothyroidism, juvenile type I diabetes mellitus, juvenile hyperadrenocorticism, and hypopituitarism.

Endocrine growth abnormalities can be divided into two groups based on the type of dwarfism present. A proportionate dwarf exhibits small stature but precisely the same di-

344

CANINE GROWTH CHART

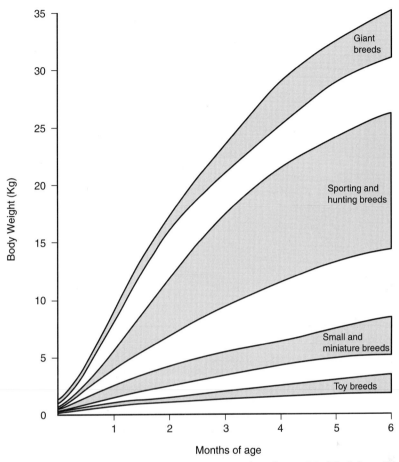

Figure 16–1. Canine growth chart from birth to 6 months of age. (Modified from Kirk RW, Bistner SI [eds]: Handbook of Veterinary Procedures and Emergency Treatment, 4th ed. Philadelphia, WB Saunders, 1985, p 885.)

mensions as the adult animal; proportionate dwarfism is characteristic of isolated growth hormone deficiency. In contrast, a disproportionate dwarf has a normal-sized head and trunk with short legs; disproportionate dwarfism is characteristic of hypothyroid dwarfism. Other endocrine causes of abnormal growth (i.e., diabetes mellitus) result in subnormal stature (not true dwarfism) and a proportionate, emaciated animal.

Pituitary Dwarfism

The pituitary gland is composed of the adenohypophysis (pars distalis or anterior lobe), the neurohypophysis (pars nervosa or posterior lobe), the pars intermedia (intermediate lobe),

and the pars tuberalis. The adenohypophysis is formed from an area of the roof of the embryonic oral ectoderm called Rathke's pouch, which extends upward to meet the neurohypophysis, which extends downward from the floor of the third ventricle. The adenohypophysis is composed of the pars distalis and the pars intermedia. The major hormones produced by the anterior pituitary include growth hormone (GH) or somatotropin, prolactin, thyroid-stimulating hormone (TSH), follicle-stimulating hormone (FSH), luteinizing hormone (LH), and adrenocorticotropin (ACTH). Growth hormone is produced by acidophilic somatotropes as a single-chain protein that contains two disulfide bonds. It is uniquely species specific in its activity. As shown in Figure 16–3, GH mediates its

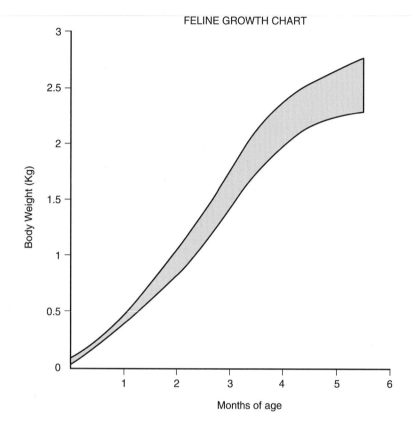

Figure 16–2. Feline growth chart from birth to 6 months of age. (Modified from Kirk RW, Bistner SI [eds]: Handbook of Veterinary Procedures and Emergency Treatment, 4th ed. Philadelphia, WB Saunders, 1985, p 888.)

Table 16-1 Age at Appearance of Ossification Centers and of Bony Fusion in Puppies and Kittens

| | AGE AT APPEARANCE | | | |
| | Ossification Center (Weeks) | | Fusion (Months) | |
ANATOMIC SITE	Puppies*	Kittens†	Puppies*	Kittens†
Proximal epiphysis of humerus	1–2	2–3	10–13	2
Proximal epiphysis (head) of femur	2	2–3	7–11	6
Proximal epiphysis of radius	3–5	3–4	6–11	7
Tuber calcis of calcaneus	6	8–9	3–8	6
Epiphysis of accessory carpal bone	7	3–4	4	7
Tuber scapulae of scapula	7	12–13	4–7	7
Olecranon of ulna	8	7–8	6–10	5
Trochanter major of femur	8	4–5	6–10	6
Tibial tuberosity	8	10–11	6–12‡	6
Proximal epiphysis of fibula	9	10–11	8–12	6
Tuber ischii of pelvis	12	12–13	8–10	6

*Condensed from Ticer JW: General principles. *In* Ticer JW (ed): Radiographic Techniques in Veterinary Practice, 2nd ed. Philadelphia, WB Saunders, 1984, p 107.

†From Horvath A: Rontgenanatomische Untersuchungen zur postnatalen Entwicklung des Hintergliedmassenskeletts der Hauskatze *(Felis catus):* Rongenanatomische Untersuchungen zur postnatalen Entwicklung des Vordergliedmassenskeletts der Hauskatze *(Felis catus).* Dissertation from Ludwig-Maximilians-Universität München, 1983, pp 59–70.

‡To shaft.

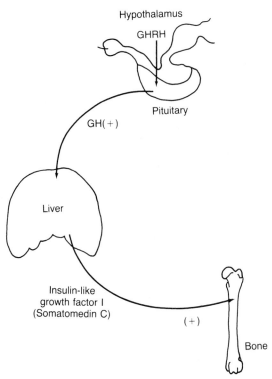

Figure 16–3. Growth hormone (GH) mediates its effects on growth plates of bones through induction of insulin-like growth factor I. GHRH = Growth hormone–releasing hormone.

effects on bone growth through induction of somatomedins (insulin-like growth factor 1 [IGF-1]).

Pituitary dwarfism results from destruction of the pituitary gland via an anomalous process. It may be associated with decreased production of pituitary hormones, including TSH, ACTH, LH, FSH, and GH.

Pituitary dwarfism is most common in German shepherd dogs aged 2 to 6 months (Fig. 16–4). Other affected breeds include carnelian bear dogs, spitz, toy pinschers, and Weimaraners. The disease is inherited as a simple autosomal recessive trait in German shepherd dogs and occurs as a result of cystic Rathke's pouch. The first observable clinical signs of pituitary dwarfism are slow growth noticed in first 2 to 3 months of life and mental retardation usually manifested as difficulty in house-training. Physical examination findings may include proportionate dwarfism, retained puppy haircoat, hypotonic skin, trunkal alopecia, cutaneous hyperpigmentation, infantile genitalia, and delayed dental eruption (Campbell, 1988).

Clinicopathologic features include eosino-philia, lymphocytosis, mild normocyctic normochromic anemia, hypophosphatemia, and occasionally hypoglycemia resulting from secondary adrenal insufficiency. Differential diagnoses include other causes of stunted growth such as hypothyroid dwarfism, portosystemic shunt, diabetes mellitus, hyperadrenocorticism, malnutrition, and parasitism. The characteristic signalment and clinical signs may allow a presumptive diagnosis, but pituitary dwarfism should be confirmed by measuring serum growth hormone concentrations or serum somatomedin C (IGF-1). Canine and feline GH assays are not currently available in the United States; however, serum IGF-1 or somatomedin C assays are available in some endocrine laboratories. The advantage of serum IGF-1 measurement over GH measurement is that it is not species specific. Normal serum IGF-1 concentrations, in German shepherd puppies, are 345 ± 50 ng/ml; this is much higher than the normal concentrations in adult dogs. The mean IGF-1 concentrations for pituitary dwarf German shepherd dogs are 11 ± 2 ng/ml (Campbell, 1988). There is usually a subnormal response to exogenous TSH and ACTH stimulation tests; furthermore, endogenous TSH and ACTH are decreased in affected dogs as a result of panhypopituitarism.

Growth hormone preparations (somatotropins) are expensive and may be difficult to obtain. If available, recommended therapy includes GH (bovine, porcine, or human) at a dosage of 0.1 U/kg subcutaneously three times weekly for 4 to 6 weeks (Campbell, 1988). Growth hormone treatment can be repeated if clinical signs recur. Overtreatment with GH preparations should be avoided, as somatotropin is an extremely diabetogenic hormone. Thyroid hormone supplementation (22 to 44 µg/kg per day, orally) may reverse many of the dermatologic and skeletal consequences of TSH deficiency. This may be a treatment option for owners who cannot afford somatotropin therapy. Prognosis for affected pituitary dwarfs is poor. Eventually, neurologic sequelae of the expanding cystic Rathke's pouch, such as seizures or ataxia, will become apparent. Most dogs do not live more than 3 to 4 years after diagnosis even with appropriate hormone supplementation.

Congenital Hypothyroidism

Congenital hypothyroidism, which occurs in approximately 1 in 4000 births, is a relatively common endocrine disorder of human infants (LaFranchi, 1979). In contrast, reports of con-

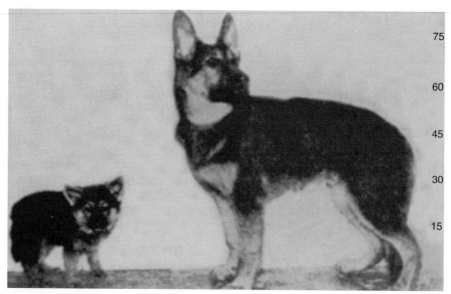

75

60

45

30

15

Figure 16–4. Pituitary dwarfism in a 5.5-month-old German shepherd dog (left) compared with its normal littermate (right). (From Andresen E, Willeberg P: Pituitary dwarfism in German shepherd dogs: Additional evidence of simple autosomal recessive inheritance. Nord Vet Med 23:481, 1976.)

genital hypothyroidism in dogs and cats are relatively few (Greco et al, 1985; Feldman and Nelson, 1987; Chastain et al, 1983; Medleau et al, 1985; Robinson et al, 1988; Jones et al, 1992). Only 3.6% of the cases of canine hypothyroidism occur in dogs younger than 1 year of age. In contrast, most of the cases of feline hypothyroidism have been reported in kittens as congenital hypothyroidism. Congenital hypothyroidism may be caused by aplasia or hypoplasia of the thyroid gland, thyroid ectopia, dyshormonogenesis, maternal goitrogen ingestion, maternal radioactive iodine treatment, iodine deficiency (endemic goiter), autoimmune thyroiditis, hypopituitarism, isolated thyrotropin deficiency, hypothalamic disease, or isolated thyrotropin-releasing hormone (TRH) deficiency (Feldman and Nelson, 1987).

Because thyroid hormone secretion is essential for normal postnatal development of the nervous and skeletal systems, congenital hypothyroidism is characterized by disproportionate dwarfism, central and peripheral nervous system abnormalities, and mental deficiency. In addition, many of the signs of adult-onset hypothyroidism, such as lethargy, inappetence, constipation, dermatopathy, and hypothermia, may be observed (Greco et al, 1985).

Congenital hypothyroidism, regardless of cause, results in characteristic historical and physical examination features. Both dogs and infants have a history of large birth weight (in

babies this is the result of prolonged gestation), which is followed by aberrant and delayed growth (Feldman and Nelson, 1987; Kenny et al, 1975). In puppies, the first signs or abnormal growth occur as early as 3 weeks after birth, and abnormal body proportions are evident by 8 weeks of age. This is similar to the pattern in human infants, who are normal at birth but, if undiagnosed, exhibit characteristic signs by 6 to 8 weeks of age (LaFranchi, 1979). Historical findings in hypothyroid puppies, such as lethargy, mental dullness, weak nursing, delayed dental eruption, and abdominal distension, are also observed in hypothyroid children (LaFranchi, 1979).

Physical features of hypothyroid dwarfism in children include hypotonia, umbilical hernia, skin mottling, large anterior and posterior fontanelles, macroglossia, hoarse cry, distended abdomen, dry skin, jaundice, pallor, slow deep tendon reflex, delayed dental eruption, and hypothermia (LaFranchi, 1979; Fisher, 1980). In the dogs with congenital hypothyroidism, hypotonia, macroglossia, distended abdomen, dry skin, delayed dental eruption, and hypothermia have been described (Fig. 16–5). In addition, because dogs develop more rapidly and become weight bearing sooner than human infants, gait abnormalities and disproportionate dwarfism are prominent features of canine congenital hypothyroidism. Midface hypoplasia, broad nose, and a large protruding tongue are some of the

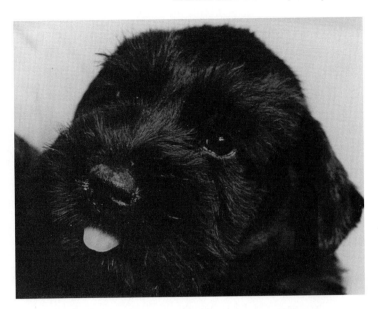

Figure 16–5. Photograph of a 16-week-old hypothyroid giant schnauzer puppy. Note macroglossia.

sequelae of untreated hypothyroidism in humans (Loevy et al, 1987; Isreal et al, 1983). Similar facial features, such as broad maxillas and macroglossia, were observed in affected puppies and kittens. In humans, delayed eruption of permanent teeth is observed in untreated congenitally hypothyroid individuals (Loevy et al, 1987); delayed dental eruption is characteristic of hypothyroid puppies treated after 4 months of age. In humans and in dogs, both macroglossia and effusions of the body cavities are the result of myxedematous fluid accumulation (Sawin, 1985). Hypothyroid animals often exhibit haircoat abnormalities, including retention of the puppy haircoat and thinning of the haircoat. Congenitally hypothyroid rats exhibit alterations in hair shaft morphology as a result of thyroid hormone deficiency during development (Essman, 1984).

Thyroid hormone is crucial for proper postnatal development of the nervous system. As a result, a significant number of properly treated and all untreated hypothyroid infants exhibit poor coordination and speech impediments later in life (Noguchi and Sugisaki, 1984; Moschini, 1986). Delayed treatment often results in low perceptual-motor, visual-spatial, and language scores in children with congenital hypothyroidism (Rovet et al, 1987). If treatment is delayed beyond 4 to 6 months in human babies, intelligence is irreversibly affected and mental retardation may ensue (LaFranchi, 1979). Mental retardation is also likely to occur in hypothyroid puppies; however, no objective evidence of delayed or abberant intelligence is available to assess affected puppies. Because the

bulk of cerebellar development occurs postnatally, Purkinje cell growth is also significantly affected by congenital hypothyroidism (Rovet et al, 1987). In humans and puppies, if treatment is delayed, signs of cerebellar dysfunction, such as ataxia, are observed.

Skeletal abnormalities such as delayed maturation and epiphyseal dysgenesis are the hallmark of congenital hypothyroidism (Fig. 16–6). Delayed epiphyseal maturation is observed in the vertebral bodies and long bones of affected puppies and kittens. Epiphyseal dysgenesis, which is characterized by a ragged epiphysis with scattered foci of calcification, is observed in both humans and dogs with untreated congenital hypothyroidism. Normal epiphyseal development proceeds from a single center; however, in hypothyroidism, thyroid deficiency leads to the development of multiple epiphyseal centers, each with its own calcification progression (Wilkins, 1941). Disorderly epiphyseal calcification leads to secondary arthropathies in children suffering from untreated congenital hypothyroidism (Johansen, 1985).

Clinicopathologic features of congenital hypothyroidism include hypercholesterolemia, hypercalcemia, and mild anemia. Hypercholesterolemia develops in both congenital and adult-onset hypothyroidism because of decreased hepatic metabolism and decreased fecal excretion of cholesterol. Hypercalcemia secondary to congenital hypothyroidism is the result of decreased renal clearance and increased gastrointestinal absorption of calcium (Tau et al, 1986). Decreased thyroid hormone stimulation of erythropoietic precursors results in a mild normocytic, nor-

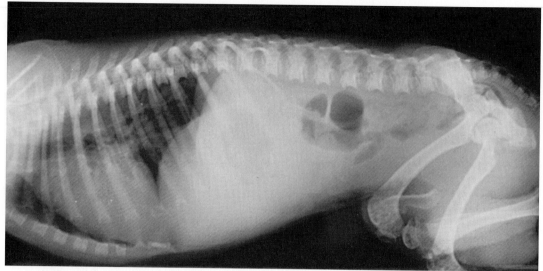

Figure 16–6. Lateral radiograph of a 16-week-old hypothyroid puppy showing epiphyseal dysgenesis and delayed epiphyseal maturation of the spine and long bones.

mochromic anemia in some animals suffering from hypothyroidism (Cline and Berlin, 1963).

It has been well established that thyroxine is essential for the proper transcription, translation, and secretion of GH by pituitary somatotrophs (Wood et al, 1987). In humans (and most likely in dogs), circulating GH concentrations are very high during the first few days after birth but rapidly decrease during the subsequent few weeks to levels just slightly above those in adults (Feldman and Nelson, 1987). In a previously reported case of congenital hypothyroidism, the dog exhibited a blunted GH response to xylazine but had a normal GH response to provocative stimulation after treatment of the hypothyroid state (Medleau et al, 1985).

Diagnosis of congenital hypothyroidism is based on clinical signs, supporting clinicopathology, and thyroid function testing. It is vital to remember that normal puppies aged 5 to 6 weeks have serum total thyroxine (TT_4) concentrations two to three times higher than normal adult dogs. Therefore, a serum TT_4 of 2.0 μg/dl, which is normal for an adult dog, would be low for a 6-week-old puppy and indicative of thyroid dysfunction. Serum free thyroxine (FT_4) would also be expected to be higher in neonatal dogs. Indeed, a recent report of TT_4, FT_4, total triiodothyronine (TT_3), free triiodothyronine (FT_3), and reverse T3 (rT_3) in puppies from birth to 12 weeks confirmed the suspicion that TT_4 and FT_4 are high in neonates (Casal et al, 1994). At birth, TT_4 was within the normal range, but by 1 week of age and until 5 weeks of age the serum TT_4 was two to three times the normal adult range. Surprisingly, TT_3 and FT_3 were much lower in these neonatal puppies, suggesting an inability of neonatal animals to convert T_4 to T_3 peripherally. The advent of the endogenous canine TSH assay should allow discrimination of primary congenital hypothyroidism from secondary hypothyroidism (TSH deficiency). Puppies with primary hypothyroidism (thyroid dysgenesis, dyshormonogenesis, and so forth) would be expected to have elevated endogenous TSH concentrations, whereas puppies with TSH deficiency should have subnormal endogenous TSH concentrations. Specific studies on endogenous TSH in neonatal canines have yet to be performed.

Treatment of congenital hypothyroid dwarfism in puppies consists of levothyroxine supplementation (22 to 44 μg/kg per day, orally) with name brand medication (Soloxine). Prognosis for treatment is excellent if thyroid supplementaion occurs before 6 months of age; after that time, neurologic and skeletal damage may become irreversible. In kittens, thyroid hormone supplementation should be started at 0.05 to 0.1 mg per kitten once daily. As in adult dogs and cats, TT_4 concentrations should at least be in the high normal range 6 hours after oral administration. Supplementation of puppies and kittens may require an even greater degree of elevation of TT_4 after supplementation to stimulate normal growth and development.

DISORDERS THAT RESULT IN POLYDIPSIA AND POLYURIA

Juvenile endocrine disorders may not affect growth primarily, but may manifest as disorders of water metabolism. Diseases that fall into this category include diabetes insipidus (DI), diabetes mellitus, hyperadrenocorticism, and primary hyperparathyroidism. All of these diseases result in primary polyuria, although by different mechanisms. For example, diabetes mellitus causes primary polyuria by osmotic diuresis; DI causes polyuria via problems with antidiuretic hormone (ADH) either as a result of vasopressin deficiency (central DI) or because of a congenital lack of ADH receptors (nephrogenic DI). Hyperadrenocorticism and hyperparathyroidism cause polyuria because of secondary nephrogenic DI; cortisol and calcium can interfere with the action of the ADH receptors in the kidney, resulting in polyuria.

Diabetes Insipidus: Antidiuretic Hormone

The neurohypophysis is composed of axons that originate within the supraoptic and paraventricular nuclei of the hypothalamus. The main activity of vasopressin, which is produced by the neurohypophysis, is the enhancement of water retention by the kidney. As a consequence, the hormone is often called *antidiuretic hormone*. Vasopressin is the most important hormone for the control of water balance. Control of vasopressin secretion is a result of changes in plasma osmolality. An increase in osmolality stimulates cells in the hypothalamus to synthesize and release vasopressin. Vasopressin acts on receptors in the collecting ducts of the kidney, causing an increase in urine osmolality and conservation of body fluid.

Juvenile Diabetes Insipidus

Diabetes insipidus is a disorder of water metabolism characterized by polyuria, urine of low specific gravity or osmolality, and polydipsia (Bruyette, 1991). It is caused by defective secretion of ADH (central DI [CDI]) or by the inability of the renal tubule to respond to ADH (nephrogenic DI) (Fig. 16–7). Deficiency of vasopressin can be partial or complete. Central diabetes insipidus (CDI) is characterized by an absolute or relative lack of circulating ADH and is classified as primary (idiopathic and congenital) or secondary. Congenital CDI has been reported in male toy poodles (Greene et al, 1979).

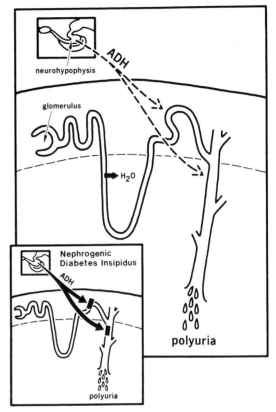

Figure 16–7. Hypothalamic diabetes insipidus. Nephrogenic diabetes insipidus is shown in inset. ADH = Antidiuretic hormone. (From Chastain CB, Ganjam VK: Clinical Endocrinology of Companion Animals. Philadelphia, Lea & Febiger, 1986, p 100.)

Secondary CDI usually results from congenital neurologic anomalies, head trauma, parasites, or neoplasia. Congenital CDI has been reported in a female kitten with cystic aplasia of the neurohypophysis (Winterbotham and Mason, 1983) and in dogs with craniopharyngiomas (Hawkins et al, 1986; Neer and Reavis, 1983). Finally, CDI was reported as a result of visceral larva migrans in a young hound puppy (Lieberman et al, 1979).

Central DI may appear at any age, in any breed, and in either gender; however, young adults (6 months of age) are most commonly affected. The major clinical signs of DI are profound polyuria and polydipsia (more than 100 ml/kg per day; normal, 40 to 70 ml/kg per day), nocturia, and incontinence usually of several months' duration. The severity of the clinical signs varies because DI may result from a partial or a complete defect in ADH secretion or action. Another less consistent sign is weight loss because these animals are constantly dehydrated.

Routine complete blood count and serum biochemical and electrolyte profiles are usually normal in animals with DI. Plasma osmolality will often be high (>310 mOsm/L) in central or nephrogenic DI as a result of *dehydration.* Animals with primary polydipsia will often exhibit low plasma osmolality (<290 mOsm/L) as a result of *overhydration.* When abnormalities such as slightly increased hematocrit or hypernatremia are present on initial evaluation, they are usually secondary to dehydration from water restriction by the pet owner. In DI, the urinalysis is unremarkable except for the finding of a persistently dilute urine (urine specific gravity 1.004 to 1.012) (Nichols, 1989).

Diagnostic tests to confirm and differentiate central DI, nephrogenic DI, and psychogenic polydipsia include the modified water deprivation test or response to ADH supplementation (Krause, 1987; Nichols, 1992) (Table 16–2). The modified water deprivation test is designed to determine whether endogenous ADH is released in response to dehydration and whether the kidneys can respond to ADH. The more common causes of polyuria and polydipsia should be ruled out before this procedure. Failure to recognize renal failure before water deprivation may lead to an incorrect or inconclusive diagnosis or cause significant patient morbidity.

Some owners may be unable to afford any mediation and may opt for no treatment other than unlimited access to water. Other owners will want to supplement puppies and kittens suffering from CDI with hormone replacement. Because most cases of congenital DI are central in origin, desmopressin (DDAVP) administration is recommended. Administration of DDAVP (Ferring), a synthetic arginine ADH, results in complete resolution of polydipsia and polyuira caused by vasopressin deficiency. Although there is considerable variability in the pharmacokinetics of DDAVP, many animals can be managed by once or twice daily administration of DDAVP in the conjunctival sac (Nichols,

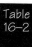

Table 16–2 **Procedures for the Modified Water Deprivation Test and the Antidiuretic Hormone Supplementation Test**

MODIFIED WATER DEPRIVATION TEST

1. The animal is confined to a cage with no food or water and is weighed at 1- to 2-h intervals after the urinary bladder is emptied and an initial body weight is obtained.
2. When more than 5% of body weight has been lost, the urinary bladder should be completely emptied and the urine checked for specific gravity and osmolality.
3. A urine specific gravity of more than 1.025 or a urine osmolality of more than 900 mOsm/L is generally considered an adequate response to water deprivation.
4. Failure to concentrate urine to this degree in the absence of renal disease indicates either central or nephrogenic diabetes insipidus and/or medullary washout.
5. Immediately after water deprivation, if the animal fails to concentrate urine adequately after losing 5% or more of its body weight, an ADH response test is performed.
6. A synthetic form of ADH (desmopressin acetate [DDAVP]) may be given subcutaneously or intravenously, or 20 μg of DDAVP (approximately 4 drops of the 100 μg/ml intranasal preparation) can be administered as intranasal or conjunctival drops.
7. Urine concentrating ability is then monitored every 2 h for 6–10 h.
8. Increases in urine specific gravity of more than 1.025 or a urine osmolality of more than 900 mOsm/L after administration of aqueous vasopressin or DDAVP is suggestive of central diabetes insipidus.
9. An inability to concentrate urine after ADH administration indicates nephrogenic diabetic insipidus or severe medullary washout.

Frequent patient monitoring is essential because severe dehydration, possible neurologic complications, and even death could ensue.

DDAVP THERAPEUTIC TRIAL

1. The owner should measure the animal's 24-h water intake 2–3 days before the therapeutic trial with DDAVP is initiated, allowing free-choice water intake.
2. The intranasal preparation of DDAVP is administered in the conjunctival sac (1 to 4 drops every 12 h) for 3–5 d.
3. A dramatic reduction in water intake (>50%) during the first few treatment days would strongly suggest an ADH deficiency.
4. When the polyuria is due to other causes, the decrease is seldom more than 30%.

ADH = antidiuretic hormone.

1992). Cost of DDAVP can be considerable; however, purchase of the product without the nasal administration apparatus results in improved affordability.

Adjuvant therapy of CDI includes the use of diuretics and sulfonylureas. Chlorpropamide is a first-generation sulfonylurea that stimulates secretion of ADH (for patients with partial DI) and sensitizes the renal tubules to ADH by increasing cyclic adenosine monophosphate within renal tubular cells. The recommended dosage is 10 to 40 mg/kg per day, and common side effects include hypoglycemia (frequent feedings are needed), nausea, and skin eruptions (Nichols, 1989). Both nephrogenic and central DI patients may benefit from thiazide diuretics. Thiazide diuretics cause extracellular fluid volume contraction, increased proximal tubular sodium/water resorption, and hence decreased water delivery (reducing urine volume) by inhibition of sodium resorption in the ascending loop of Henle (Nichols, 1989). The initial starting dose of chlorothiazide is 20 to 40 mg/kg orally twice daily.

Juvenile Diabetes Mellitus

Diabetes mellitus is a common endocrinopathy of adult dogs and cats, but less than 1.5% of diabetic dogs have juvenile-onset diabetes and rarely is the disease observed in kittens. All reported cases of juvenile diabetes mellitus have been type I or insulin-dependent diabetes mellitus. Juvenile-onset diabetes mellitus has been described in the keeshond, West Highland terrier, Alaskan malamute, Old English sheepdog, Doberman pinscher, schipperke, German shepherd, Labrador retriever, Finnish spitz, Manchester terrier, English springer spaniel, whippet, chow, miniature pinscher, standard poodle, miniature schnauzer, and mongrel (Anderson et al, 1986; Kramer and Evermann, 1982; Lettow et al, 1983). A genetic basis for diabetes mellitus is suspected in the keeshond and golden retriever. In humans, an association between juvenile diabetes and viral disease is suspected; similarly, viral disease (canine distemper) has been implicated in the pathogenesis of canine juvenile diabetes mellitus. Viral infections often present as diabetes mellitus.

Diabetic puppies and kittens present with the classic clinical signs of polyuria and polydipsia. Dramatic and rapid weight loss in an animal with a good or even ravenous appetite will often alert the owner to seek veterinary advice. Polyphagia is a common historical finding in diabetic kittens and puppies. Occasional inappetence may, however, be explained by the presence of ketoacidosis. In puppies and kittens, progressive polyuria, polydipsia, and weight loss develop relatively rapidly, usually over a period of several days or weeks. Another common presenting complaint of diabetes mellitus in puppies is that of acute onset of blindness caused by cataract formation. Diabetic cataracts can develop rapidly, and the owner may notice that the puppy is suddenly bumping into furniture and other obstacles. Physical examination findings of nonketotic diabetes mellitus in kittens and puppies are typically nonspecific. The most common physical examination findings are dehydration, muscle wasting or thin body condition, and failure to thrive. Emaciated diabetic juveniles often have concurrent underlying disorders, such as exocrine pancreatic insufficiency.

A diagnosis of diabetes mellitus should be based on the presence of clinical signs compatible with diabetes mellitus and evidence of fasting hyperglycemia and glycosuria. The presence of only clinical signs may be misleading. In puppies, exocrine pancreatic insufficiency may present with signs similar to to those of diabetes mellitus (i.e., polyphagia and weight loss) but with the additional signs of severe diarrhea or steatorrhea resulting from impaired fat digestion.

Treatment of type I diabetes mellitus requires insulin therapy. Human recombinant insulin (neutral protamine Hagedorn [NPH] or Lente) is the most available insulin preparation and is perfectly acceptable as insulin therapy for all puppies and kittens; NPH insulin is more rapidly absorbed and may be more appropriate for young animals.

Initial insulin therapy for the uncomplicated diabetic should be designed to mimic physiologic insulin concentrations without induction of hypoglycemia. This is extremely difficult to achieve in a young, growing animal. Initial insulin therapy should be conservative, followed by incremental increases in insulin dosage based on resolution of clinical signs, urine glucose monitoring, and serial blood glucose curves. Aggressive insulin therapy using NPH insulin two to three times daily combined with multiple feedings should allow the puppy or kitten to grow during the critical period between 2 and 6 months of age. For puppies, the starting insulin dose is 0.4 to 0.5 U/kg of NPH insulin two to three times daily. For kittens, the initial insulin dosage ranges from 0.2 to 0.4 U/kg of NPH insulin two to three times daily. The timing of the insulin injections should be coincidental with feeding. The author recommends feeding the animal and injecting the insulin at the same time. If the puppy does not eat, the insulin dosage can be reduced (usually by one half) or skipped entirely and the animal evaluated by the veterinarian to determine the cause of the anorexia.

Nutritionally balanced diets with protein of high biologic values should be fed. The quantity of food should be calculated using standard age and breed feeding charts, and energy needs should be recalculated every 2 weeks during periods of rapid growth (ages 1 to 6 months). Puppies and kittens should be fed at least twice daily and preferably three to four times daily; if more frequent feedings are given, supplemental injections of regular insulin may also be administered with the meals. Physical activity, water consumption, and urine output should be maintained with in normal limits.

Management of concurrent exocrine pancreatic insufficiency may be particularly problematic. The veterinarian should be alerted to the possibility of exocrine pancreatic insufficiency by the persistence of clinical signs such as diarrhea or steatorrhea, weight loss, or lack of weight gain in a growing puppy or by hypoglycemic episodes after administration of low doses of insulin. Replacement therapy with exocrine pancreatic enzyme preparations is indicated. Insulin dosage should be increased after supplementation to compensate for the increased caloric intake.

In general, the owner should be instructed to monitor the insulin effect and gross regulation of hyperglycemia by noting changes in appetite, attitude, body condition, polydipsia, polyuria, and urine glucose and ketone levels. Ideally, glucosuria (<250 to 500 mg/dl) without ketonuria should be detected. Consistently high urine glucose readings coupled with uncontrolled clinical signs, such as polyuria and polydipsia, indicate that the insulin dose may be inadequate. Conversely, consistently negative readings on urine glucose may indicate that insulin dosages are either adequate or excessive. A serial glucose curve is required to differentiate between adequate insulin therapy and excessive therapy that could result in hypoglycemic shock. The insulin dose should be adjusted no more frequently than every 3 to 4 days. Adjustments should be made in 0.5- to 3-unit increments, depending on the size of the animal and the initial insulin dosage. The reader is referred to Table 16–3 for a summary of recommended insulin and feeding regimens.

Diabetic Ketoacidosis

With insulin deficiency, the *hormone-sensitive lipase* system, which is normally suppressed by

Table 16–3 Treatment Outline for Juvenile Diabetes Mellitus

1. Diet
   a. Energy requirements for growth
   b. High-quality protein
   c. Feeding frequency: Three to four times daily
2. Exercise
   a. Regularly scheduled, consistent
3. Insulin therapy
   a. Initial dose (0.5–1 U/kg, SC)
   b. NPH insulin (human recombinant)
   c. Frequency: Two to three times daily
   d. May administer in combination with regular insulin or as NPH 70/30
4. Monitoring therapy in puppies
   a. Assess body weight every 2 wk
   b. Assess glucose curve every 2 wk
   c. Monitor urine glucose and ketones twice weekly
   d. Adjust dose based on new weight and glucose curve
5. Concurrent exocrine pancreatic insufficiency
   a. Supplement with pancreatic enzymes (1 tsp/feeding)
   b. Conservative insulin dosage (0.5 U/kg, bid)

bid = twice daily; NPH = neutral protamine Hagedorn; SC = subcutaneously.

insulin, becomes activated. As a consequence of this increased lipase activity, adipose tissue is broken down at an accelerated rate into nonesterified fatty acids. The unrestrained lipolytic activity of hormone-sensitive lipase results in the clinical sign of weight loss in a previously obese or overweight animal. Hepatic assimilation of these fatty acids, which depends on the rate of lipolysis, also proceeds at an accelerated rate. Nonesterified fatty acids are released in the bloodstream and delivered to the liver for repackaging as triglycerides. With insulin deficiency, lipid metabolism in the liver becomes deranged, and nonesterified fatty acids are converted to acetyl coenzyme A, which accumulates in the liver, ultimately being converted into acetoacetyl coenzyme A and then to acetoacetic acid. Finally, the liver starts to generate large amounts of ketones.

As insulin deficiency culminates in diabetic ketoacidosis (DKA), in which the accumulation of ketones and lactic acid in the blood and loss of electrolytes and water in the urine results in profound dehydration, hypovolemia, metabolic acidosis, and shock. Ketonuria and osmotic diuresis caused by glycosuria causes sodium and potassium loss in the urine, thus exacerbating hypovolemia and dehydration. Nausea, anorexia, and vomiting caused by stimulation of the chemoreceptor trigger zone via ketonemia contribute to the dehydration caused by osmotic diuresis. Dehydration and shock lead to prerenal azotemia and a decline in glomerular filtration rate. Stress hormones, such as cortisol and epinephrine, contribute to the hyperglycemia in a vicious cycle. Eventually severe dehydration may result in hyperviscosity, thromboembolism, severe metabolic acidosis, renal failure, and death.

The most dramatic clinical signs and physical examination findings occur in animals with acute DKA. The most common historical findings in DKA are anorexia, weakness, depression, and vomiting. Animals suffering from severe DKA often present in shock. Physical examination findings may include depression, tachypnea, dehydration, weakness, vomiting, and, occasionally, a strong acetone odor on the breath. Dehydration may be severe in puppies and kittens with DKA. Kussmaul's breathing (slow, deep respirations) has been described in animals with severe DKA. Gastrointestinal signs such as vomiting, abdominal distension, and abdominal pain should be differentiated from pancreatitis (which can occur currently with DKA), peritonitis, and other causes of acute abdomen. Clinicopathologic features of DKA include severe metabolic acidosis, hyperglycemia, hypercholesterolemia, azotemia, hyperosmolality, stress leukogram, hyponatremia, hypochloremia, hyperkalemia, hyperphosphatemia, hyperbilirubinemia, and increased liver enzymes.

Treatment of DKA includes the following steps, in order of importance: (1) fluid therapy initially using shock doses of 0.9% saline solution, (2) insulin therapy (low-dose intramuscular or intravenous), (3) electrolyte supplementation (potassium chloride and/or potassium phosphate), and (4) reversal of metabolic acidosis.

Fluid therapy should consist of 0.9% saline solution supplemented with potassium when insulin therapy is initiated. Normal saline is the fluid of choice initially, and, when the blood glucose decreases to below 250 mg/dl, fluid therapy is changed to 5% or 2.5% dextrose in water and 0.45% saline solution when the blood glucose falls below 250 mg/dl. A large central venous catheter should be used to administer fluid therapy because puppies with DKA are severely dehydrated and require rapid fluid administration. Insulin therapy should be initiated as soon as possible, and the author prefers intravenous insulin therapy as described elsewhere (Macintire, 1995). Regular insulin is mixed in a 250-ml saline bag at a dosage of 2.2 units of regular insulin/kg of body weight for dogs and 1.1 U/kg for cats. Approximately 50 ml of fluid and insulin is allowed to run through the intravenous drip set and is discarded because insulin binds to the plastic tubing.

The diluted regular insulin is administered initially at a rate of 10 ml/h via an infusion pump and decreased according to the drop in serum glucose. As serum glucose decreases, the insulin fluid rate is decreased from 10 to 7 to 5 ml/h and finally discontinued as blood glucose approaches the normal range (100 mg/dl). When blood glucose decreases below 250 mg/dl, the fluid is changed to 2.5% dextrose and 0.45% saline solution. When the blood glucose falls below 150 mg/dl, the fluids are changed to 5% dextrose and 0.45% saline solution. With this method, blood glucose decreases to below 250 mg/dl by approximately 10 hours in dogs and about 16 hours in cats. Insulin is administered through a separate catheter than the fluids to allow for more flexible insulin administration. Once euglycemia has been acheived, the puppy is maintained on subcutaneous regular insulin (0.1 U/kg subcutaneously every 3 to 4 hours) until it starts to eat and/or the ketosis has resolved. Another protocol is to use low-dose intramuscular insulin at an initial dosage of 0.2 U/kg followed by hourly intramuscular injections of 0.1 U/kg until the blood glucose concentration is below 250 mg/dl. After the blood glucose drops to less than 250 mg/dl, regular insulin is administered subcutaneously every 6 to 8 hours.

Electrolyte, specifically potassium, balance may be difficult to manage during a ketoacidotic crisis. Potassium should be supplemented as soon as insulin therapy is initiated. Although serum potassium may be normal or elevated in DKA, the animal actually suffers from total body depletion of potassium. Furthermore, correction of the metabolic acidosis tends to drive potassium into cells in exchange for hydrogen ions. Insulin facilitates this exchange, and the net effect is a dramatic decrease in serum potassium that must be attenuated with appropriate potassium supplementation in fluids. According to general guidelines, 40 to 80 mEq/L is appropriate supplementation. Monitoring serum potassium level frequently during the course of treatment of DKA is essential to avoid undersupplementation or oversupplementation of potassium and other electrolytes. Serum and tissue phosphorus may also be depleted during a ketoacidotic crisis, and a portion of the potassium supplementation should consist of potassium phosphate (0.01 to 0.03 ml phosphate/kg per hour), particularly for small dogs and cats, which are most susceptible to hemolysis caused by hypophosphatemia.

Finally, serum pH should be monitored after administration of fluids, insulin, and potassium. Often, the first three steps will result in normalization of serum acid-base status; however, bicarbonate therapy may be necessary for some patients. Caution with bicarbonate therapy is recommended as metabolic alkalosis may be difficult to reverse. General guidelines for bicarbonate therapy are to calculate the base deficit (body weight [kg] × 0.1 × 24 − HCO$_3$ [mEq/L]) to obtain the number of milliliters of intravenous sodium bicarbonate to administer.

In some cases, juvenile diabetics may be in transition from complicated diabetes and ketoacidosis to maintenance therapy. The decision to change from regular insulin to intermediate-acting or long-acting insulin should be made on the basis of resolution of ketosis and clinical signs. In these cases, the initial dose of regular insulin may be used as a guide for maintenance dosages of intermediate-acting or long-acting insulin. Often, the transition from hospital to home maintenance therapy can be made by using a low dose (1 to 2 U) of regular insulin combined with the intermediate-acting maintenance insulin at the recommended dosages.

Juvenile Hyperadrenocorticism

The control of secretion of glucocorticoids by the zona fasciculata and zona reticularis is mediated by the tropic hormone ACTH. A negative feedback system exists, whereby glucocorticoids inhibit the release of hypothalamic corticotropin-releasing hormone (CRH), which in turn results in decreased ACTH secretion by the pituitary. The glucocorticoids, produced by the zona fasciculata and zona reticularis, are important in the regulation of all aspects of metabolism, either directly or through an interaction with other hormones. The major form of glucocorticoid is cortisol. The mechanism of action of adrenal hormones involves penetration of the cell membrane and interaction in the cytoplasm with specific cytosolic receptors. This complex is transferred to the nucleus with a resultant transcription of certain genes and the synthesis of specific proteins that effect the biologic action of the adrenal hormones.

Juvenile-onset hyperadrenocorticism (Cushing's syndrome) may be caused by pituitary lesions resulting in excessive ACTH production, by adrenal hyperplasia, or, more commonly, by administration of corticosteroids to a growing

animal (iatrogenic). Spontaneous juvenile hyperadrenocorticisim has been identified in four dogs less than 1 year of age; however, juvenile-onset hyperadrenocorticism has not been described in kittens. Dogs with juvenile-onset hyperadrenocorticism usually suffer from stunted growth because of the effects of glucocorticoid excess on epiphyseal growth centers. The most common clinical signs associated with canine juvenile hyperadrenocorticism are growth retardation, polydipsia, polyuria, polyphagia, abdominal enlargement or "pot belly," panting, obesity, and muscle weakness. Dermatologic manifestations of canine hyperadrenocorticism include alopecia, thin skin, phlebectasias, comedones, bruising, cutaneous hyperpigmentation, calcinosis cutis, pyoderma, dermal atrophy, seborrhea, and secondary demodicosis.

Serum chemistry abnormalities associated with hypercortisolemia in puppies include increased serum activities of alkaline phosphatase (ALP) and alanine transferase (ALT), hypercholesterolemia, hyperglycemia, and decreased blood urea nitrogen. The hemogram is often characterized by evidence of erythroid regeneration (nucleated red blood cells and a classic "stress leukogram"). Basophilia is occasionally observed. Puppies may have evidence of urinary tract infection without pyuria. Urine specific gravity is usually decreased and may be hyposthenuric.

Screening tests for hyperadrenocorticism, such as the low-dose dexamethasone suppression (LDDS) test and the ACTH stimulation test, work on the principle of suppression or stimulation of the pituitary-adrenal axis. In the case of the LDDS, dexamethasone is administered at a low dosage to cause negative feedback to the pituitary gland. In a normal animal, this negative feedback results in a decrease in endogenous ACTH secretion and a resultant decrease in circulating cortisol concentrations. Dexamethasone is the only synthetic corticosteroid that does not cross-react with the cortisol assay. The ACTH stimulation test is used to determine the extent of adrenal hyperplasia or atrophy. Adrenal glands that are hyperplastic will show an exaggerated response to exogenous ACTH; conversely, puppies with iatrogenic hyperadrenocorticism will show a subnormal response to exogenous ACTH.

Treatment of endogenous juvenile hyperadrenocorticism of pituitary or adrenal origin is similar to that for adult-onset hyperadrenocorticism (i.e., mitotane, ketoconazole). Iatrogenic hyperadrenocorticism should be treated by gradual withdrawal of glucocorticoids to allow pituitary secretion of ACTH to become normal.

Juvenile Hyperparathyroidism

The main endocrine organ involved in the control of calcium and phosphate metabolism is the parathyroid gland. The synthesis of parathyroid hormone (PTH) is similar to other protein hormones. Prepro-PTH is synthesized in the rough endoplasmic reticulum and then cleaved to form pro-PTH. A 6 amino acid pro-portion is removed, resulting in the formation of PTH, which is secreted by the process of exocytosis. Parathyroid hormone is rapidly metabolized by the liver and kidneys and has a relatively short half-life of 5 to 10 minutes in blood.

Hypercalcemia has a variety of etiologies, including hypercalcemia of malignancy, hyperparathyroidism, fungal disease, osteoporosis, hypoadrenocorticism, chronic renal disease, hypervitaminosis D, and primary hyperplasia of the parathyroid glands (Feldman and Nelson, 1996). The initial signs of hypercalcemia are polydipsia and polyuria resulting from impaired response of distal renal tubules to ADH. Listlessness, depression, and muscle weakness result from depressed excitability of neuromuscular tissue. Mild gastrointestinal signs of hypercalcemia include inappetence, vomiting, and constipation. Persistent mild elevations in serum calcium (12 to 14 mg/dl) can cause uroliths and signs of urinary tract disease such as hematuria and stranguria. On the other hand, severe hypercalcemia (>14 mg/dl) can progress rapidly to acute renal failure when the calcium-phosphate product (Ca [mg/dl] $\times$ PO$_4$ [mg/dl]) exceeds 60 to 80 because of mineralization of renal tissues.

In young animals, the primary differential diagnosis for hypercalcemia is renal failure. This is the most difficult differential to exclude because other causes of hypercalcemia may result in renal damage because of soft tissue mineralization of the kidneys. Therefore, an animal with hypercalcemia, azotemia, and hyperphosphatemia could suffer from primary hyperparathyroidism, primary renal failure with secondary renal hyperparathyroidism, or vitamin D intoxication. Furthermore, patients with hypercalcemia secondary to renal disease may also exhibit elevations in intact PTH. Diagnosis of primary hyperparathyroidism is based on the findings of hypercalcemia (preferably ionized), hypophosphatemia (unless azotemic), high normal to elevated serum PTH concentrations, and a mass in the cervical region that may be small and go undetected. Intact PTH, using a sandwich assay

validated for use in the dog and cat, should be measured. It should be emphasized that a normal PTH concentration in the face of elevated total and/or ionized calcium is *inappropriate* for the calcium level and would be considered diagnostic for primary hyperparathyroidism.

German shepherd puppies may suffer from primary hyperplasia of the parathyroid glands. This condition is inherited as an autosomal recessive trait. Clinical findings include stunted growth, polyuria, polydipsia, and muscular weakness (Chastain, 1990). Laboratory findings consist of hypophosphatemia associated with increased fractional clearance of phosphorus, elevated plasma PTH concentrations, and hypercalcemia. Radiographs may reveal decreased bone density.

DISORDERS THAT RESULT IN WEAKNESS, COLLAPSE, OR ENCEPHALOPATHY

The adrenal cortex produces two major types of steroid hormones. The mineralocorticoids, produced by the zona glomerulosa, play an important role in electrolyte balance and in the regulation of blood pressure. The major mineralocorticoid is aldosterone.

Mineralocorticoids are produced in the outer zone (zona glomerulosa) of the adrenal cortex. Electrolyte balance and blood pressure homeostasis are the main physiologic effects of mineralocorticoids. These actions are carried out at the level of the distal tubules in the kidney. The effect of the mineralocorticoids is to promote sodium retention and potassium and hydrogen secretion. In the case of mineralocorticoids, the main controlling factors are produced in the target organ, the kidney. Cells in the juxtaglomerular apparatus of the kidney produce an enzyme, *renin*, in response to decreases in blood pressure. This enzyme acts on angiotensinogen, which results in the production of angiotensin I. Angiotensin I is further hydrolyzed to angiotensin II by angiotensin-converting enzyme. Angiotensin II stimulates the zona glomerulosa to produce mineralocorticoids and increases peripheral resistance of the blood vascular system by causing vasoconstriction of smooth muscle of the blood vessels. Another major regulatory factor in the control of mineralocorticoid secretion is blood potassium concentration. An increase in potassium concentration stimulates the zona glomerulosa to secrete mineralocorticoids, whereas a decline in potassium has the opposite effect.

Primary hypoadrenocorticism is most commonly diagnosed in young dogs and may have an immune-mediated etiology; however, congenital adrenal hypoplasia has been described in an 8-week-old puppy (Ruben et al, 1985). Secondary hypoadrenocorticism resulting from ACTH deficiency is relatively common in puppies suffering from pituitary deficiencies.

Historical findings compatible with hypoadrenocorticism include intermittent vomiting, diarrhea, weight loss, lethargy, anorexia, and weakness. These symptoms often resolve with fluid therapy and/or corticosteroid treatment. Physical examination of animals in an acute hypoadrenal crisis reveals weak pulse, bradycardia, prolonged capillary refill time, severe mental depression, and profound muscle weakness. Clinical features of hypoadrenocorticism that should heighten the index of suspicion include a normal or slow heart rate in the face of circulatory shock and the "waxing and waning" course of disease before collapse.

Electrolyte abnormalities consisting of severe hyponatremia and hypochloremia associated with hyperkalemia are the hallmarks of hypoadrenocorticism. Although a serum Na:K ratio of less than 27:1 is considered suggestive of hypoadrenocorticism, it is not pathognomonic. Gastrointestinal disease, acute renal failure, and postrenal azotemia may also cause a low sodium to potassium ratio. Furthermore, some patients with hypoadrenocorticism, in particular those with glucocorticoid deficiency only, will not show classic electrolyte imbalances. Azotemia and hyperphosphatemia also attend primary hypoadrenocorticism, making it difficult to differentiate from acute renal failure. Azotemia may be prerenal as a result of dehydration, and hypovolemia or increased blood urea nitrogen may be due to gastrointestinal hemorrhage. Hematologic abnormalities consist of eosinophilia and lymphocytosis or normal eosinophil and lymphocyte counts in the face of severe metabolic stress. The anemia of hypoadrenocorticism has classically been attributed to lack of glucocorticoid effects on the bone marrow. Recent studies suggest, however, that hemorrhagic gastroenteritis contributes significantly to the anemia. Although hypoglycemia is more common with secondary or atypical hypoadrenocorticism, it is rarely seen with typical hypoadrenocorticism.

Urine specific gravity is frequently low and is attributed to medullary washout (inadequate medullary gradient due to sodium depletion) and decreased medullary blood flow. Dilute urine in the face of azotemia and hyperkalemia may easily be mistaken for acute renal failure.

Hormonal assays are required to confirm the presence or absence of adrenal disease and to differentiate between hypoadrenocorticism and renal failure.

Diagnosis of primary hypoadrenocorticism is based on clinical signs, classic electrolyte imbalances, and confirmation with an ACTH response test. The baseline cortisol sample should be collected with the initial blood work, and synthetic ACTH (Cortrosyn, 0.25 mg) should be administered intravenously during the initial fluid therapy. A 1-hour, post-ACTH sample may then be drawn and glucocorticoids administered after the 1-hour sample is taken. Intramuscular injection of ACTH (gel or synthetic) may not be absorbed in animals in circulatory shock; therefore, intravenous administration of synthetic ACTH is preferred. If glucocorticoids must be administered before cortisol is measured, dexamethasone sodium phosphate is preferred because dexamethasone will not interfere with the cortisol assay. Endogenous plasma ACTH may be measured to determine if the hypoadrenocorticism is primary or secondary. This specimen must be collected in an EDTA tube, spun within 1 hour of sampling, and stored in plastic *before corticosteroids are administered*.

Dogs and cats with primary hypoadrenocorticism will exhibit a subnormal response to ACTH administration. The baseline cortisol concentration is usually low or undetectable, and the post-ACTH cortisol concentration is also low or undetectable. Endogenous plasma ACTH concentrations are dramatically increased in animals with primary hypoadrenocorticism as a result of loss of negative feedback to the pituitary caused by decreased serum cortisol concentrations. In the case of secondary hypoadrenocorticism, which is caused by a pituitary deficiency of ACTH, the endogenous ACTH concentrations are typically decreased (<20 pg/ml). The response to exogenous ACTH is diminished but not as dramatically as for primary hypoadrenocorticism. Baseline cortisol and post-ACTH cortisol concentrations may be in the normal range.

Treatment of the addisonian crisis consists of four parts: (1) fluid therapy and electrolyte stabilization, (2) glucocorticoid replacement therapy, (3) treatment of gastrointestinal hemorrhage, and (4) mineralocorticoid replacement therapy. Normal saline solution is the drug of choice for hypoadrenal crises; in fact, shock doses of normal saline alone are enough to reverse the circulatory shock caused by the loss of sodium and chloride in the kidney resulting from aldosterone deficiency. Treatment of hyperkalemia can be achieved with fluid therapy alone. Normal saline solution without potassium supplementation is the fluid of choice. If hyperkalemia is life threatening, intravenous administration of calcium chloride or calcium gluconate may be used to counteract the effects of potassium on the heart. Alternately, insulin and glucose and/or sodium bicarbonate can be administered. However, bicarbonate may take up to 24 hours to be fully effective in lowering serum potassium by which time the potassium would have been diluted by appropriate fluid therapy.

Glucocorticoid and mineralocorticoid therapy must be initiated after diagnostic tests for hypoadrenocorticism have been performed. Glucocorticoid therapy, using ultrashort-acting corticosteroids such as dexamethasone sodium phosphate and prednisolone sodium succinate,

is indicated. Dexamethasone may be preferred for animals that require immediate glucocorticoid administration as it will not interfere with the cortisol assay; in addition, a single dose of short-acting corticosteroid will not suppress the hypothalamic pituitary adrenal axis.

Long-term therapy of primary hypoadrenocorticism involves the use of mineralocorticoid supplementation as oral fludrocortisone (0.1 mg/10 lb orally every 24 hours) or injectable deoxycorticosterone pivalate (1 mg/lb every 25 days). Electrolytes should be monitored once weekly until the puppy is stable on replacement therapy and then twice yearly thereafter. All puppies with secondary hypoadrenocorticism and those supplemented with deoxycorticosterone pivalate require a low dose of glucocorticoid (0.2 mg/kg orally every 24 hours). About 50% of addisonians supplemented with fludrocortisone require glucocorticoid supplementation. Prognosis with treatment is excellent.

The Metabolic System

C. B. Chastain

Metabolic disorders occurring between birth and 6 months of age are usually congenital or nutritional. Congenital causes are often genetic in origin and should be considered so until proved otherwise. However, puppies and kittens can develop most of the acquired metabolic disorders that are more common in adults.

Inbreeding practices are used by most breeders of purebred dogs and cats. The risk of inherited endocrine and metabolic disorders is thereby increased. In humans from civilized countries who rarely inbreed, the collective incidence of inborn errors of metabolism is 1 in 500 in the United States (Cederbaum, 1986). It is reasonable to assume that the incidence of such disorders will be more frequent in purebred dogs and cats than in the general human population.

INBORN ERRORS OF METABOLISM

Errors of metabolism are enzyme deficiencies caused by gene abnormalities. Any metabolic

pathway can be affected. Thus, any organ and tissue can be involved. Garrod described the first recognized error of metabolism in humans, alkaptonuria, in 1902 (Thompson and Thompson, 1991). Several hundred errors of metabolism have since been described in humans. Collectively, 1 occurs in every 500 live human births. Some have been recognized in puppies and kittens (Table 16–4). A few are benign, and others are serious.

The gene defects are usually autosomal recessive or sex-linked recessive. Heterozygote carriers may be identified by tracing pedigrees. Definitive diagnosis of apparently affected animals usually requires enzyme assays of organs or tissue involved.

Two basic types of enzyme deficiency exist. One type of enzyme deficiency results in an accumulation of small-molecular-weight, water-soluble metabolic intermediates. The second type are lysosomal enzyme deficiencies that impair the degradation of complex carbohydrates.

Common features of the errors of metabolism are mental and physical developmental retardation, a failure to thrive, vomiting, orga-

Table 16–4 A Partial List of Inborn Errors of Metabolism

FAMILIAL DEFECT	ENZYME OR END-PRODUCT DEFICIENCY	CLINICAL FEATURES
Substrate: Amino Acids		
Albinism	Tyrosinase	Lack of pigmentation
Alkaptonuria	Homogentisate oxidase	Arthritis, pigmented cartilage, dark urine
Phenylketonuria	Phenylalanine hydroxylase	Seizures, behavioral problems
Homocystinuria	Cystathionine synthetase	Seizures, osteoporosis, thrombosis
Maple syrup urine disease	Branched-chain ketoacid dehydrogenase	Vomiting, seizures, hypoglycemia, hypertonia, burnt sugar urine odor
Urea cycle (citrullinemia)*	Argininosuccinic acid synthetase	Vomiting, seizures, mental retardation
Substrate: Carbohydrates		
Fructose intolerance	Fructose-1-phosphate aldolase	Hypoglycemia, vomiting, hepatosplenomegaly
Galactosemia	Galactose-1-phosphate uridyltransferase	Liver failure, hepatomegaly, cataracts, vomiting, mental retardation
Lactose intolerance†	Lactase	Colic, diarrhea
Glycogen storage disorders**	Glucose-6-phosphatase	Hypoglycemia, hepatomegaly, lactic acidosis, hyperlipidemia, xanthomas, thromboasthenia
	Amylo-1,6-glucosidase‡	Hypoglycemia, hepatosplenomegaly, myopathy
	Hepatic phosphorylase	Hypoglycemia, hepatomegaly
	Phosphorylase kinase	Hypoglycemia, hepatomegaly
Glycogen synthetase deficiency	Glycogen synthetase	Hypoglycemia, hepatomegaly
Substrate: Lipids		
Hyperchylomicronemia§	Lipoprotein lipase	Pancreatitis, eruptive xanthomas, neuropathy, hepatosplenomegaly
Hypercholesterolemia	Defective synthesis of low-density lipoprotein receptors	Atherosclerosis, tendon xanthoma
Dysbetalipoproteinemia¶	Defective synthesis of apolipoprotein E-III	Seizures, pancreatitis, atherosclerosis, plantar xanthoma
Hypertriglyceridemia	?	Glucose intolerance, insulin resistance
Hyperlipoproteinemia	?	Pancreatitis, eruptive xanthomas, hepatosplenomegaly, sensory neuropathy, glucose intolerance

*Reported in dogs (Strombeck et al, 1975).
†Reported in cats (Drochner and Muller-Schlosser, 1980).
‡Reported in German shepherd dogs (Ceh et al, 1976; Rafiquazzaman et al, 1976).
§Reported in cats and dogs (Baum et al, 1969; Jones et al, 1983, 1986; Olin et al, 1976; Rogers et al, 1975).
¶Reported in dogs (miniature schnauzers) (Rogers et al, 1975).
**Reported in dogs (Brix et al, 1995).

nomegaly, peculiar body odors, and ocular or cutaneous abnormalities. Laboratory findings may include ketonuria, inappropriate aminoaciduria, and reducing substances in the urine. Blood analyses may reveal pancytopenia, acidosis, hypoglycemia, or ketonemia. A review of the family history often reveals inbreeding or similarly affected relatives. Some possible inborn errors of metabolism is listed in Table 16–4.

At present, the most commonly recognized sign of disordered metabolism in puppies is hypoglycemia. Hypoglycemia is very rarely recognized in kittens.

HYPOGLYCEMIA IN PUPPIES
Maintenance of Blood Glucose Levels

Blood glucose levels are normally kept in a relatively narrow range by a complex mechanism involving hormones, hepatic enzymes, and glucose substrate availability (Atkins, 1983; Turnwald and Troy, 1983). Under usual metabolic conditions, the brain is wholly dependent on plasma glucose as a source of energy. As the glucose drops after the end of the absorptive phase of digestion, pancreatic A (or α) cells are directly stimulated to release glucagon. Glucagon is the key hormone that mobilizes glucose

from hepatic stores, a process called *glycogenolysis*. If the stimulus for hepatic glucose production is prolonged, gluconeogenesis occurs. Gluconeogenesis is the transformation of glucose substrates into glucose by the liver (Fig. 16–8). During early fasting, blood glucose is maintained principally (75%) by glycogenolysis and 25% by gluconeogenesis. As fasting continues, gluconeogenesis is increasingly responsible for maintaining blood glucose levels.

If a sudden drop in blood glucose deprives the brain of enough glucose to meet its metabolic needs, an autonomic response is triggered to mobilize glycogen and fat. Released catecholamines, particularly epinephrine, are additional stimuli of the direct effects of hypoglycemia on the pancreatic A cells for glucagon secretion. Epinephrine also mobilizes glycogen from muscle, while free fatty acids and glycerol are released from fat depots. Fasted adult dogs release more glycerol per kilogram than do fasted humans (de Bruijne et al, 1981).

Acute deprivation of glucose to the brain also causes the release of ACTH and GH. Adrenocorticotropin causes cortisol secretion from the adrenal cortex. Cortisol facilitates lipolysis and mobilization of amino acids from muscle to be converted to glucose by the liver. Growth hormone activates lipolysis and antagonizes the ac-

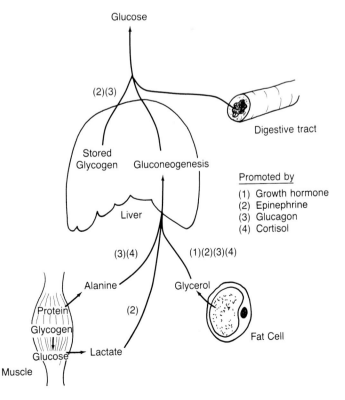

Figure 16–8. Sources of plasma glucose.

tion of insulin. Plasma insulin levels are normally suppressed by low blood glucose levels. Lowered plasma insulin levels facilitate the mobilization of glycogen, fat, and amino acids; increases enzymes necessary for conversion of energy stores to glucose; and inhibits muscle use of remaining blood glucose. A reduction in fasting plasma insulin levels has been demonstrated in adult dogs (de Bruijne et al, 1981). Plasma glucagon levels were not increased, but, with the reduction of plasma insulin levels, the effects of glucagon become dominant during fasting in adult dogs.

Substrates for glucose production are lactate and pyruvate, amino acids (alanine, glycine, serine, and threonine [particularly alanine]), and glycerol. The only storage form of carbohydrate is glycogen, which is present in all tissue, but most is stored in the liver and skeletal muscle. Glycogen is a highly branched polymer of glucose residues. During fasting, glycogen is mobilized from the liver by glucagon. Exhaustive physical exertion causes epinephrine release, which causes hepatic glycogenolysis and mobilization of glycogen from skeletal muscle for use during exercise or hypoxia. Glycogenolysis requires glycogenolytic hormones (glucagon or

epinephrine), glycogenolytic enzymes, and normal stores of hepatic and muscle glycogen.

If fasting is prolonged or physical exertion continues for more than a few hours postprandially, glycogen stores become insufficient and glucose is generated from gluconeogenesis. Lactate and pyruvate are end products of glucose used by peripheral tissue. Alanine is mobilized from skeletal muscle. Glycerol is released from fat depots. Gluconeogenesis requires the presence of gluconeogenic hormones, especially cortisol and glucagon, and, to a lesser extent, GH and thyroid hormone; the presence of a normal liver with the necessary gluconeogenic enzymes; and normal skeletal muscle and hepatic tissue. With prolonged fasting, gluconeogenesis occurs in the kidneys as well as the liver.

Glycogen is formed in the liver, beginning with the entry of glucose (Fig. 16–9). Glucose is converted to glucose-6-phosphate, which is then converted to glucose-1-phosphate. The hepatic enzyme glycogen synthetase links glucose-1-phosphate in chains, and a branching enzyme forms links between the chains of glucose-1-phosphate.

Hepatic glycogen breakdown begins with the enzyme hepatic phosphorylase, which splits

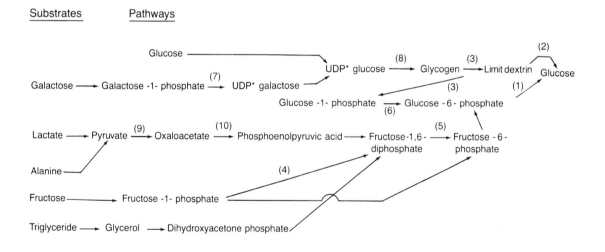

Important Enzymes involved in glycogen synthesis, glycogenolysis, and gluconeogenesis

(1) Glucose - 6 - phosphatase	(6) Phosphoglucomutase
(2) Amylo -1,6- glucosidase	(7) Galactose -1- phosphate uridyltransferase
(3) Phosphorylase	(8) Glycogen synthetase
(4) Fructose -1- phosphate aldolase	(9) Pyruvate carboxylase
(5) Fructose -1,6 - diphosphatase	(10) Phosphoenolpyruvate carboxykinase

*UDP=Uridine diphosphate

Figure 16–9. Pathways for glycogen synthesis, glycogenolysis, and gluconeogenesis.

some of the links in the glucose-1-phosphate chains, creating "limit dextrin." At this point, another enzyme, 4α-glucanotransferase, exposes the branch points so that the debrancher enzyme amylo-1,6-glucosidase can split the branch points, liberating free glucose. Less than 10% of stored glycogen is liberated to glucose by the debrancher enzyme. Phosphorylase can further convert "limit dextrin" to glucose-1-phosphate, which is converted to glucose-6-phosphate by phosphoglucomutase. Glucose-6-phosphate liberates glucose by the action of glucose-6-phosphatase.

Gluconeogenesis requires four key enzymes: (1) glucose-6-phosphatase, (2) fructose-1,6-diphosphatase, (3) pyruvate carboxylase, and (4) phosphoenolpyruvate carboxykinase. Deficiency of glucose-6-phosphatase causes profound hypoglycemia during fasting because it is required in the final step for the release of glucose from either glycogenolysis or gluconeogenesis. Without glucose-6-phosphatase, no glucose is generated from glycogen or glucose substrates except for a small amount produced by the debrancher enzyme's action on "limit dextrin." Fructose-1,6-diphosphatase deficiency in humans is associated with hypoglycemia during prolonged fasting or with infections. Pyruvate carboxylase or phosphoenolpyruvate carboxykinase deficiency can also cause hypoglycemia.

CAUSE

The most common causes of hypoglycemia in puppies are transient hypoglycemia in newborns and recurrent fasting substrate-limited hypoglycemia (transient juvenile hypoglycemia). Other causes of persistent or recurrent hypoglycemia similar to substrate-limited hypoglycemia in puppies are listed in Table 16–5. Cases of insulinomas and extrapancreatic tumor hypoglycemia have not been reported in puppies and are unlikely to occur.

Transient hypoglycemia of newborn puppies is probably the most common cause of hypoglycemia during the nursing period and is associated with inadequate glycogen or protein substrate stores or immature liver enzyme function. Predisposing factors include premature birth of a litter, birth at term of a runt, debilitation of the bitch at parturition, or diabetes in the bitch.

Substrate-limited hypoglycemia is probably the most common cause of hypoglycemia in puppies that survive past weaning. It is caused by a failure to adapt to fasting during the postweaning period. There are insufficient glycogen stores or glucose substrate, especially alanine from skeletal muscle (Strombeck et al, 1978). Concurrent infections, vaccinations, strenuous physical exertion, gastrointestinal disturbances, hypothermia, poor nutrition, and prolonged fasting are predisposing factors. Prolonged fast-

Table 16–5 Possible Causes of Hypoglycemia in Puppies	
FASTING	**POSTPRANDIAL**
Substrate-limited hypoglycemia	Hyperinsulinism
Neonatal (transient) hypoglycemia	Leucine hypersensitivity
Substrate-limited hypoglycemia*	Deficiency of contrainsulin hormones
Carnitine deficiency*	Glucagon deficiency
Deficiency of contrainsulin hormones	Hepatic enzyme deficiency
Glucagon deficiency	Galactosemia
Cortisol/adrenocorticotropin deficiency*	Fructose intolerance
Growth hormone deficiency	
Thyroid hormone deficiency*	
Catecholamine deficiency	
Hepatic disease	
Hepatitis	
Portosystemic shunts*	
Hepatic enzyme deficiency	
Glycogen storage diseases*	
Glycogen synthetase deficiency	
Maple syrup urine disease	
Gluconeogenic enzyme deficiency	
Bacteremia*	
Drug-induced hypoglycemia*	

*Reported in dogs (Atkins, 1984a,b; Chastain et al, 1983; Keene, 1986; Leifer and Peterson, 1984; Strombeck et al, 1978; Turnwald and Troy, 1983, 1984).

ing can be the result of the owner failing to feed three to four times per day, as is necessary for postweaning puppies, illness, or prolonged sleep (van Toor et al, 1991). Maple syrup urine disease, a rare reason for glucose substrate insufficiency in humans and a possible cause of hypoglycemia in puppies and kittens, causes a block in the oxidative decarboxylation of branched-chain amino acids (Sperling, 1994).

Other causes of fasting hypoglycemia and more common causes of persistent hypoglycemia include hepatic vascular anomalies (portosystemic shunts) or other severe hepatic diseases. If more than 70% of the normal functioning hepatic mass is impaired, inadequate hepatic glycogen stores and hepatic enzyme insufficiencies occur. Approximately one-third of the puppies with portosystemic shunts develop hypoglycemia (Atkins, 1984a). Deficiencies of gluconeogenic hormones, such as cortisol, GH, and T_4, are rare in puppies. Others, such as glucagon and epinephrine deficiencies, have not been reported in dogs. Deficiency of gluconeogenic enzymes (fructose-1,6-diphosphatase, phosphoenolpyruvate carboxykinase, or pyruvate carboxylase) can cause hypoglycemia. Deficiency of glycogen synthetase prevents the formation of hepatic glycogen, which can cause fasting hypoglycemia. Multiple hormone or enzyme deficiencies or additional predisposing factors as mentioned for ketotic hypoglycemia are, however, generally necessary to cause hypoglycemia. Single gluconeogenic hormone or enzyme deficiencies without deficiency of substrates rarely cause hypoglycemia.

Bacteremia is a multifactorial cause of hypoglycemia. Increased glucose utilization, decreased glycogen stores, inhibition of gluconeogenesis, and hypotension are contributing factors to the occurrence of hypoglycemia associated with bacteremia (Breitschwerdt et al, 1981). In a survey of canine surgical patients with sepsis, 27% were found to be hypoglycemic (Hardie et al, 1986). Iatrogenic excess of insulin or drugs that cause the secretion of insulin, that increase sensitivity to insulin, or that inhibit glycogenolysis can cause hypoglycemia. Drugs that can cause hypoglycemia include sulfonylureas, salicylates, ethanol, and ethylene glycol.

Glycogen storage diseases are inherited deficiencies of glycogenolytic enzymes normally present in the liver or skeletal muscle. Twelve glycogen storage diseases are known to occur in humans. Only four are associated with hypoglycemia. These enzyme deficiencies are glucose-6-phosphatase (type I), amylo-1,6-glucosidase (type III), hepatic phosphorylase (type VI), and phosphorylase kinase (type IX). Glucose-6-phosphatase deficiency, von Gierke's disease, which causes a serious hypoglycemia, has been suspected for many years in toy breed puppies (Bardens, 1966; Bardens et al, 1961) and documented in a litter of Maltese puppies (Brix et al, 1995). Amylo-1,6-glucosidase deficiency (Cori's disease or "limit dextrinosis"), a cause of moderate hypoglycemia after a long fast, has been confirmed in some female German shepherd dogs. Signs begin at around 2 months of age (Ceh et al, 1976; Rafiquzzaman et al, 1976).

Hypoglycemia in puppies initiated by ingestion of a meal could be caused by glucagon deficiency, fructose intolerance, galactosemia, or leucine hypersensitivity. Glucagon secretion precedes the postprandial secretion of insulin and antagonizes insulin's hypoglycemia effects. Glucagon deficiency results in inadequate opposition to postprandial insulin effects on blood glucose values (Kolle et al, 1978). Fructose intolerance, a deficiency of fructose-1-phosphate aldolase, can lead to hypoglycemia because of the resulting accumulation of fructose-1-phosphate, which inhibits some of the gluconeogenic enzymes. Fructose is present in fruits and vegetables, particularly potatoes. Galactosemia is a deficiency of the enzyme galactose-1-phosphate uridyl transferase. Deficiency of this enzyme prevents utilization of galactose, a major constituent of milk. The resultant accumulation of galactose-1-phosphate inhibits the conversion of glucose-1-phosphate into glucose-6-phosphate. Leucine hypersensitivity provokes hyperinsulinemia after the ingestion of leucine and other amino acids in milk, among other sources.

INCIDENCE

Hypoglycemia is the most commonly recognized disorder of metabolism in puppies. Recognition is based on seizures and other dramatic clinical signs that can be induced by hypoglycemia. Blood glucose levels or the recovery in response to the administration of glucose can be easily ascertained to verify the diagnosis.

Puppies are at greater risk to develop hypoglycemia than are adult dogs because puppies have a smaller liver and skeletal muscle mass and a larger brain size in proportion to the remainder of the body. Relative to adult dogs, puppies are deficient in glucose substrates and glycogen stores. Very young puppies cannot tolerate fasting more than a few hours. Orphaned nursing puppies must be fed at least every 6 hours.

A common occurrence in practice is for a puppy that has not been fed that day to be presented for vaccination and deworming. During the struggling of the trip, examination, vaccination, or deworming, the puppy becomes disoriented and weak, may collapse, or may even have a seizure due to hypoglycemia. Recovery occurs with rest, feeding, or administration of 10% to 25% dextrose by intravenous injection. Recurrence is rare if the frequency of feeding is increased.

CLINICAL FEATURES

Hypoglycemia should be the first cause to be ruled out in a puppy presenting with seizures. Signs of hypoglycemia are due to deficient glucose supply to the brain (neuroglucopenia) or to increased epinephrine secretion induced by falling blood glucose levels. Presenting signs of neuroglucopenia are any or all of the following: seizures, hypothermia, depression, amaurosis, confusion, a change in behavior, polyphagia, and syncope (Atkins, 1984b; Sperling, 1986). Signs of epinephrine release are seen in puppies more than 1 week old and include increased pulse rate and blood pressure, restlessness, increased respiratory rate, muscular weakness, and incoordination.

Glucose is virtually the only energy source normally used by the brain. Hypoglycemia restricts oxygen uptake by brain cells. The brain contains a very limited supply of glycogen. When the body is at rest, the human brain consumes two thirds of the liver's output of glucose (Turnwald and Troy, 1984). Different areas of the central nervous system vary in their susceptibility to hypoglycemia. The most susceptible area is the cerebral cortex, particularly the occipital lobes. The diencephalon is intermediate in its sensitivity to low levels of blood glucose. If hypoglycemia is severe and prolonged, permanent neural damage can result.

The degree of hypoglycemia does not always correlate with clinical signs of neural dysfunction. The brain is able to adapt to low glucose levels, particularly in periods of rest. The rate of fall of blood glucose and the degree of neural adaptation are important factors governing the clinical signs produced. Persistent hypoglycemia of 20 to 60 mg/dl in a resting animal usually does not cause clinical signs of neural dysfunction in puppies.

Hepatomegaly is a prominent finding in puppies with hypoglycemia caused by a glycogen storage disease (Brix et al, 1995). Fructose-1,6-diphosphatase deficiency or galactosemia would probably cause hepatomegaly in affected puppies as it does in children. In contrast, portosystemic hepatic venous anomalies are associated with small liver size.

Deficiencies of adenohypophyseal hormones associated with hypoglycemia are usually multiple, resulting in impaired general physical growth and mental development. Congenital hypothyroidism is characterized by strabismus, a protruding swollen tongue, poor development of the haircoat, and in some cases goiter. Bacteremias should be suspected in puppies or kittens with hypoglycemia associated with petechial or ecchymotic hemorrhage, pyrexia, or embolic phenomenon.

LABORATORY FINDINGS

Blood glucose levels of less than 30 mg/dl in neonates and 40 mg/dl in puppies 2 weeks to 6 months of age should be considered significant if accompanied by clinical signs typical of hypoglycemia or if persistent when spurious causes have been ruled out (Atkins, 1984b). Spurious hypoglycemia can occur if blood samples are improperly handled. Plasma or serum should be separated from blood cells within 30 minutes and then refrigerated until measurements are possible. Whole blood should be analyzed as soon as possible, if whole-blood measurements are intended. If whole blood remains at room temperature, blood cells will consume glucose at about 10 mg/dl per hour, depending on cell counts and ambient temperature (Turnwald and Troy, 1983). Whole-blood glucose concentration is diluted by blood cells. Whole-blood glucose levels are approximately 15% lower than plasma or serum levels.

Ketones are generated by hepatic conversion of free fatty acids, which are liberated when serum insulin is persistently low and relative serum glucagon levels are high. More ketones are generated in fasting humans than in fasting dogs (de Bruijne et al, 1981). In fasting adult dogs, ketones are not detected until after 2 to 3 days of fasting, but puppies and kittens develop ketonemia and ketonuria more rapidly. Ketones are then used as an alternate source of energy for the central nervous system when blood glucose levels are low. If ketones are not present in the urine, transient hypoglycemia, an excess of insulin, or a deficiency of glucagon should be suspected. Insulin excess can be caused by overadministration of treatment for juvenile diabetes mellitus or by leucine hypersensitivity in humans.

Carnitine deficiency has been discovered in

boxers, a Samoyed, and a Doberman pinscher with cardiomyopathy (Keene, 1986). Carnitine is a lysine derivative that greatly stimulates fat oxidation. Hypoglycemia can occur with carnitine deficiency or deficiency of its transferase enzyme acyl-carnitine transferase because they are essential for the transport of free fatty acids into mitochondria, where free fatty acids produce energy for gluconeogenesis. Free fatty acids also provide energy for ketogenesis, so carnitine deficiency causes recurrent fasting hypoglycemia without ketonemia or ketonuria due to insufficient adenosine triphosphate to maintain gluconeogenesis.

DIAGNOSIS

To identify the cause of hypoglycemia in a puppy, it should first be determined if the hypoglycemia is transient or persistent (or recurrent). Almost all neonatal hypoglycemias occur during fasting. The puppy's general physical condition, diet, history of any recent drug administration, and frequency of feeding should be determined. Minimum laboratory evaluation should include blood glucose and urine ketone determinations.

Transient Hypoglycemia

Transient hypoglycemia usually occurs in 6- to 12-week-old, small-breed puppies during a period of fasting and stress. Substrate-limited hypoglycemia is the presumed cause if the puppy is in a fasting state, the liver size is normal, and urine ketones are present. Urine ketones may not occur if fasting is of less than 3 days' duration.

Further confirmation is rarely necessary or economically warranted. This requires assays for plasma insulin, ketones, alanine, cortisol, GH, T_4, and glucagon during either symptomatic episodes of hypoglycemia or fasting. Results consistent with substrate-limited ketotic hypoglycemia are normal to high plasma cortisol, GH, T_4 and glucagon levels, and high plasma ketone level.

Persistent or Recurrent Hypoglycemia

Persistent or recurrent hypoglycemia in a puppy indicates the need for further laboratory evaluations to prevent permanent brain damage or death. If drug-induced causes and bacteremia can be excluded, particular attention should be directed to determining the size and function of the liver to rule out severe hepatic disease or vascular anomalies. An abnormally small liver suggests a congenital portosystemic venous shunt or hepatic fibrosis. Puppies with an enlarged liver should be evaluated for deficiencies of enzymes required for gluconeogenesis or glycogenolysis. Puppies with persistent or recurrent hypoglycemia, a normal-sized liver, and apparently normal hepatic function should be suspected of having substrate-limited hypoglycemia, hyperinsulinemia, or a deficiency of hormone-mediated gluconeogenesis.

After a carefully supervised 24-hour fast, baseline blood glucose and urine ketone samples should be obtained. Additional plasma should be frozen for possible insulin, cortisol, GH, T_4, glucagon, lactate, free fatty acid, ketones, alanine, lactate, and uric acid determinations at a later date, if indicated. After collection of baseline samples, 30 µg/kg glucagon should be administered intramuscularly and plasma again collected after 30 minutes. The glucagon tolerance test should also be performed again 3 hours after feeding or after 20% glucose per os. Urine should be tested for glucose with glucose oxidase test strips (Chemstrip bG, Boehringer Mannheim Corporation, Germany) and for reducing sugars (galactose or fructose) (Clinitest Tablets, Miles Inc., Elkhart, IN). If blood glucose levels increase more than 40 mg/dl above baseline levels after glucagon administration, hyperinsulinemia or glucagon deficiency should be suspected, and stored baseline plasma should be assayed for insulin and glucagon. Small to no increase in blood glucose indicates possible glycogen storage disease or gluconeogenic hormone deficiency. If signs or other laboratory findings are suggestive of hypoadrenocorticism, pituitary disease, or hypothyroidism, baseline plasma cortisol, GH, or T_4, respectively, should be assayed.

When gluconeogenic enzyme deficiency or glycogen storage disease is suspected, a liver biopsy should be performed. Hepatic lipidosis associated with hypoglycemia is compatible with a deficiency of a gluconeogenic enzyme or glycogen synthetase. Glycogen storage diseases are characterized by excess glycogen accumulation in the liver. Glycogen storage disease III (GSD III) leads to formation of glycogen with abnormally short outer branches. Definitive diagnosis of any of these enzyme deficiencies can be confirmed if 1 g of frozen liver is assayed at a special reference laboratory. A deficiency of amylo-1,6-glucosidase (GSD III) may be detectable in leukocytes of affected puppies (Ceh et al, 1976).

Urine that tests positive for reducing substances, but not for glucose, with glucose oxidase test strips may indicate galactosemia or fructose intolerance. Differential features of the causes of hypoglycemia in puppies are summarized in Table 16–6.

Management of Hypoglycemia

Puppies with clinical signs suggestive of hypoglycemia should be screened for blood glucose levels with a glucose oxidase–hydrogen peroxidase paper test strip (Chemstrip bG, Bio-Dynamics, Indianapolis, IN). A needle should be placed intravenously, if possible, with a tubing line to 5% to 10% dextrose solution. If intravenous administration is not possible, the solution should be given orally by gavage tube. Fifty percent dextrose causes severe phlebitis. From 2 to 4 ml/kg body weight should be infused over 30 to 60 seconds. When hypoglycemia has been confirmed and treatment has corrected the signs, the infusion should be continued at a slow drip rate. Affected puppies should be kept in an environment with an ambient temperature of 29.4° to 32.2° C (85° to 90° F) with a humidity of 85% to 90% Feeding should then be attempted and the puppy slowly weaned off the intravenous infusion.

Transient hypoglycemia and recurrent substrate-limited hypoglycemia can be successfully managed by frequent daily feedings of high-carbohydrate, high-protein, and/or high-fat foods. In addition to monitoring for signs of hypoglycemia, urine should be checked for ketones. The disappearance of ketonuria signals adequate therapy. Puppies gradually mature out of substrate limitations. Carnitine deficiency is treated with dietary supplementation with levocarnitine (Carnitor, Sigma-Tau Pharmaceuticals, Inc., Gaithersburg, MD).

Deficiencies of cortisol or thyroid hormone can be easily replaced with oral supplements. Deficiency of GH can be corrected, when GH is available, by subcutaneous injections. There is no satisfactory treatment for glucagon or catecholamine deficiencies.

Hepatic diseases may or may not be correctable, depending on the cause. Portosystemic venous shunts can often be surgically corrected.

Hepatic enzyme deficiencies cannot be replaced. Glycogen storage disease I and gluconeogenic enzyme deficiencies are treated with frequent feedings of glucose during the day to supplement normal feedings and uncooked cornstarch in the evenings. Glycogen synthetase deficiency and GSD III are treated in the same manner as glycogen storage disease I, but protein can be given in large quantities to animals with GSD III or glycogen synthetase deficiency because there is an intact gluconeogenic pathway. There is no satisfactory treatment for hepatic phosphorylase or phosphorylase kinase deficiencies. Maple syrup urine disease can sometimes be adequately treated with large doses of the vitamin coenzyme thiamine (B_1) (Sperling, 1986). Intake of branched-chain amino acids should also be controlled.

Bacteremias are treated by the appropriate antimicrobial agents and elimination of the cause. Drug-induced hypoglycemia is corrected

Table 16–6	Differential Features of Selected Causes of Hypoglycemia in Puppies								
				BLOOD GLUCOSE RESPONSE TO GLUCAGON		FOLLOWING 24-h FAST			
CONDITION	HYPOGLYCEMIA	URINE KETONES	HEPATOMEGALY	Fed	Fasted	Glucose	Insulin	Alanine	Lactate
Hyperinsulinemia	F, P	−	−	+	+	↓	↑	N	N
Substrate-limited hypoglycemia	F	+	−	+	±	↓	↓	↓	N
Hypopituitarism	F (mild)	+	−	+	±	↓	↓	↓	N
Hypoadrenocorticism	F (mild)	+	−	+	±	↓	↓	↓	N
Glucose-6-phosphatase deficiency	Persistent	+	+	−	−	↓	↓	↑	↑
Amylo-1,6-glucosidase deficiency	F	+	+	+	−	↓	↓	↓	N

F = fasting; N = no change; P = postprandial; + = present; − = absent; ± = may be present; ↑ = increased; ↓ = decreased.

by eliminating the drug usage or adjusting the dosage or frequency so that the risk of recurrence of hypoglycemia is reduced.

Leucine hypersensitivity, galactosemia, and fructose intolerance are managed by avoiding dietary sources of leucine, galactose, and fructose, respectively. Principal sources of leucine and galactose for puppies are milk and milk products. Fructose is in its highest concentrations in fruits and potatoes.

References and Suggested Reading

The Endocrine System

Anderson PG, Braund KG, Dillon AR, et al: Polyneuropathy and hormone profiles in a chow puppy with hypoplasia of the islets of Langerhans. Vet Pathol 23:528, 1986.

Bruyette DS: Polyuria and polydipsia. In August JR (ed): Consultations in Feline Internal Medicine. Philadelphia, WB Saunders, 1991, p 227.

Burns MG, Kelly AB, Hornof WJ, et al: Pulmonary artery thrombosis in three dogs with hyperadrenocorticism. J Am Vet Med Assoc 178:388, 1981.

Campbell KL: Growth hormone–related disorders in dogs. Compend Contin Educ Pract Vet 10:477, 1988.

Casal ML, Zerbe CA, Jezyk PF, et al: Thyroid profiles in healthy puppies from birth to 12 weeks of age. Proc Am Coll Vet Intern Med, San Francisco, 1994, p 989.

Cederbaum SD: Introduction to inborn errors of metabolism. In Lavin N (ed): Manual of Endocrinology and Metabolism. Boston, Little Brown & Co, 1986, p 527.

Chastain CB: Endocrine and metabolic systems. In Hoskins JD (ed): Veterinary Pediatrics: Dogs and Cats from Birth to Six Months, 2nd ed. Philadelphia, WB Saunders, 1995, p 377.

Chastain CB, Franklin RT, Granham VK, et al: Evaluation of the hypothalamic pituitary-adrenal axis in clinically stressed dogs. J Am Anim Hosp Assoc 22:435, 1986.

Chastain CB, McNeil SV, Graham CL, et al: Congenital hypothyroidism in a dog due to an iodide organification defect. Am J Vet Res 44:1257, 1983.

Chew DJ, Meuten DJ: Disorders of calcium and phosphorus metabolism. Vet Clin North Am Small Anim Pract 12:411, 1982.

Cline MJ, Berlin NI: Erythropoiesis and red cell survivial in the hypothyroid dog. Am J Physiol 204:415, 1963.

Contreras LN, Hane S, Tyrrell JB: Urinary cortisol in the assessment of pituitary-adrenal function: Utility of 24-hour and spot determinations. J Clin Endocrinol Metab 65:965, 1986.

Dibartola SP: Disorders of sodium and water: Hypernatremia and hyponatremia. In Dibartola SP (ed): Fluid Therapy in Small Animal Practice. Philadelphia, WB Saunders, 1992, p 57.

Dorner JL, Hoffman WE, Long GB: Corticosteroid induction of an isoenzyme of alkaline phosphatase in the dog. Am J Vet Res 35:1457, 1974.

Essman EJ: Alterations in hair shaft morphology in the cretin rat. Biol Clin Lab 14:657, 1984.

Feldman BF, Feldman EC: Routine laboratory abnormalities in endocrine disease. Vet Clin North Am Small Anim Pract 7:433, 1977.

Feldman EC: Comparison of ACTH response and dexamethasone suppression as screening tests in canine hyperadrenocorticism. J Am Vet Med Assoc 182:505, 1983a.

Feldman EC: Distinguishing dogs with functioning adrenocortical tumors from dogs with pituitary-dependent hyperadrenocorticism. J Am Vet Med Assoc 183:195, 1983b.

Feldman EC, Mark RE: Urine cortisol:creatinine ratio as a screening test for hyperadrenocorticism in the dog. J Am Vet Med Assoc 200:1637, 1992.

Feldman EC, Nelson RW: Hypothyroidism. In Feldman EC, Nelson RW (eds): Canine and Feline Endocrinology and Reproduction. Philadelphia, WB Saunders, 1987, p 55.

Feldman EC, Nelson RW: Hypercalcemia and primary hyperparathyroidism. In Feldman EC, Nelson RW (eds): Canine and Feline Endocrinology and Reproduction. Philadelphia, WB Saunders, 1996, p 497.

Fisher DA: Medical management of suspected cases of congenital hypothyroidism. In Burrow GN (ed): Neonatal Thyroid Screening. New York, Raven Press, 1980, p 237.

Greco DS, Peterson ME, Cho DY: Juvenile-onset hypothyroidism in a dog. J Am Vet Med Assoc 187:948, 1985.

Greene CE, Wong PE, Finco DR: Diagnosis and treatment of diabetes insipidus in two dogs using two synthetic analogs of antidiuretic hormone. J Am Anim Hosp Assoc 15:371, 1979.

Hawkins KL, Diters RW, McGrath JT: Craniopharyngioma in a dog. J Comp Pathol 95:469, 1986.

Isreal H, Johnson GF, Fierro-Benitez R: Craniofacial malformation among endemic cretins in Ecuador. J Craniofac Genet Dev Biol 3:3, 1983.

Johansen NA: Endocrine arthropathies. Clin Rheum Dis 11:297, 1985.

Jones BR, Gruffydd-Jones TJ, Sparkes AH, et al: Preliminary studies on congenital hypothyroidsm in a family of Abyssinian cats. Vet Rec 131:145, 1992.

Kaplan AJ, Peterson ME, Kemppainen RJ: Effects of nonadrenal disease on the results of diagnostic tests for hyperadrenocorticism in dogs. J Vet Intern Med 8:161, 1994 (abstract).

Kemppainen RJ, Clark TP, Peterson ME: Aprotinin preserves immunoreactive adrenocorticotropin in canine plasma. J Vet Intern Med 8:163, 1984 (abstract).

Kenny FM, Klein AH, Augustin AV, et al: Sporadic cretinism. In Fisher DA, Gurrow GN (eds): Perinatal Thyroid Physiology and Disease. New York, Raven Press, 1975, p 73.

Kidney BA, Jackson ML: Diagnostic value of alkaline phosphatase isoenzyme separation by affinity electrophoresis in the dog. Can J Vet Res 52:106, 1988.

Kornegay JN: Hypocalcemia in dogs. Compend Contin Educ Pract Vet 4:103, 1982.

Kramer JW, Evermann JF: Early-onset genetic and familial diabetes mellitus in dogs. Proc Kal Kan Symp 6:59, 1982.

Krause KH: The use of desmopressin in diagnosis and treatment of diabetes insipidus in cats. Compend Contin Educ Pract Vet 9:752, 1987.

LaFranchi SH: Hypothyroidism. Pediatr Clin North Am 26:33, 1979.

Lettow VE, Opitz M, Brieger H, et al: Juveniler Diabetes mellitus bei einem Hund. Kleintier Praxis 28:119, 1983.

Lieberman LL, Kircher CH, Lein DH: Polyuria and polydipsia associated with pituitary visceral larva migrans in a dog. J Am Anim Hosp Assoc 15:237, 1979.

Loevy HT, Aduss H, Rosenthal IM: Tooth eruption and craniofacial development in congenital hypothyroidism: Report of a case. J Am Dent Assoc 115:429, 1987.

Macintire DK: Emergency therapy of diabetic crises: Insulin overdose, diabetic ketoacidosis, and hyperosmolar coma. Vet Clin North Am (Small Anim Pract) 25:139, 1995.

Mark RE, Feldman EC: Comparison of two low-dose dexamethasone suppression protocols as screening and discrimination tests in dogs with hyperadrenocorticism. J Am Vet Med Assoc 197:1603, 1990.

Mark RE, Feldman EC, Wilson SM: Diagnosis of hyperadrenocorticism in dogs. Compend Contin Educ Pract Vet 16:311, 1994.

Medleau L, Eigenmann JE, Saunders HM, et al: Congenital hypothyroidism in a dog. J Am Anim Hosp Assoc 21:341, 1985.

Milne KI, Hayes HM: Epidemiologic features of canine hypothyroidism. Cornell Vet 71:3, 1981.

Moschini L, Costa P, Marinelli E, et al: Longitudinal assessment of children with congenital hypothyroidism detected by neonatal screening. Helv Paediatr Acta 41:415, 1986.

Neer TM, Reavis DU: Craniopharyngioma and associated central diabetes insipidus and hypothyroidism in a dog. J Am Vet Med Assoc 182:519, 1983.

Nichols CE: Endocrine and metabolic causes of polyuria and polydipsia. In Kirk RW, Bonagura JD (eds): Current Veterinary Therapy XI. Philadelphia, WB Saunders, 1992, p 293.

Nichols R: Diabetes insipidus. In Kirk RW (ed): Current Veterinary Therapy X. Philadelphia, WB Saunders, 1989, p 973.

Noguchi T, Sugisaki T: Hypomyelination in the cerebrum of the congenitally hypothyroid mouse (hyt). J Neurochem 42:891, 1984.

Owens JM, Drucker WD: Hyperadrenocorticism in the dog: Canine Cushing's syndrome. Vet Clin North Am Small Anim Pract 7:583, 1977.

Parfitt AM, Kleerekoper M: Clinical disorders of calcium, phosphorus, and magnesium metabolism. In Maxwell M, Kleeman CR (eds): Clinical Disorders of Fluid and Electrolyte Metabolism. New York, McGraw-Hill Book Co, 1980, p 1026.

Peterson M: Hyperadrenocorticism. Vet Clin North Am Small Anim Pract 14:731, 1984.

Peterson ME: Hypoparathyroidism and other causes of hypocalcemia in cats. In Kirk RW, Bonagura JA (eds): Current Veterinary Therapy XI. Philadelphia, WB Saunders, 1992, p 376.

Peterson ME, Ferguson DC: Thyroid diseases. In Ettinger SJ (ed): Textbook of Veterinary Internal Medicine: Diseases of the Dog and Cat, 3rd ed. Philadelphia, W.B. Saunders, 1989, p 1632.

Peterson ME, Gilbertson SR, Drucker WD: Plasma ortisol response to exogenous ACTH in 22 dogs with hyperadrenocorticism caused by adrenocortical neoplasia. J Am Vet Med Assoc 180:542, 1982.

Reimers TJ: Radioimmunoassays and diagnostic tests for thyroid and adrenal disorders. Compend Contin Educ Pract Vet 4:65, 1982.

Rijnberk A: Iodine Metabolism and Thyroid Disease in the Dog. PhD thesis. University of Utrecht, the Netherlands, 1971.

Rijnberk A, van Wees A, Mol JA: Assessment of two tests for the diagnosis of canine hyperadrenocorticism. Vet Rec 122:178, 1988.

Robinson WF, Shaw SE, Stanley B, et al: Congenital hypothyroidism in Scottish deerhound puppies. Aust Vet J 65:386, 1988.

Rovet J, Ehrlich R, Sorbara D: Intellectual outcome in children with fetal hypothyroidism. J Pediatr 10:700, 1987.

Ruben JM, Walker MJ, Lonstaffe JA: Addison's disease in a puppy. Vet Rec 116:91, 1985.

Sawin CT: Hypothyroidism. Med Clin North Am 69:989, 1985.

Schalm OW, Jain NC, Carroll EJ: Veterinary Hematology, 3rd ed. Philadelphia, Lea & Febiger, 1975, p. 89.

Schick MP: Calcinosis cutis secondary to percutaneous penetration of calcium chloride in dogs. J Am Vet Med Assoc 191:207, 1987.

Smiley LE, Peterson ME: Evaluation of a urine cortisol:creatinine ratio as a screening test for hyperadrenocorticism in dogs. J Vet Intern Med 7:163, 1993.

Tau C, Garagedian M, Farriaux JP, et al: Hypercalcemia in infants with congenital hypothyroidism and its relation to vitamin D and thyroid hormones. J Pediatr 109:808, 1986.

White SD, Ceragioli KL, Bullock LP, et al: Cutaneous markers of canine hyperadrenocorticism. Compend Contin Educ Pract Vet 4:446, 1989.

Wilkins L: Epiphyseal dysgenesis associated with hypothyroidism. Am J Dis Child 61:13, 1941.

Wilson SM, Feldman EC: Diagnostic value of the steroid-induced isoenzyme of alkaline phosphatase in the dog. J Am Anim Hosp Assoc 28:245, 1992.

Wood DF, Franklyn JA, Docherty K: The effect of thyroid hormones on growth hormone gene expression in vivo in rats. J Endocrinol 112:459, 1987.

The Metabolic System

Atkins CE: Disorders of glucose homeostasis in neonatal and juvenile dogs: Hyperglycemia. Compend Contin Educ Pract Vet 5:851, 1983.

Atkins CE: Disorders of glucose homeostasis in neonatal and juvenile dogs: Hypoglycemia. Part I. Compend Contin Educ Pract Vet 6:197, 1984a.

Atkins CE: Disorders of glucose homeostasis in neonatal and juvenile dogs: Hypoglycemia. Part II. Compend Contin Educ Pract Vet 6:358, 1984b.

Bardens JW: Glycogen storage disease in puppies. Vet Med Small Anim Clin 61:1174, 1966.

Bardens JW, Bardens GW, Bardens B: Clinical observations on a von Gierke-like syndrome in puppies. Allied Vet 32:4, 1961.

Baum D, Schweld AK, Porte D, et al: Congenital lipoprotein lipase deficiency and hyperlipemia in the young puppy. Proc Soc Exp Biol Med 131:183, 1969.

Breitschwerdt EB, Loar AS, Hribernik TN, et al: Hypoglycemia in four dogs with sepsis. J Am Vet Med Assoc 178:1072, 1981.

Brix AE, Howerth EW, McConkie-Rosell A, et al: Glycogen storage disease type Ia in two littermate Maltese puppies. Vet Pathol 32:460, 1995.

Cederbaum SD: Introduction to inborn errors of metabolism. In Lavin N (ed): Manual of Endocrinology and Metabolism. Boston, Little, Brown and Co, 1986, p 527.

Ceh L, Hauge JG, Svenkerud R, et al: Glycogenosis type III in the dog. Acta Vet Scand 17:210, 1976.

Chastain CB, McNeel SV, Graham CL, et al: Congenital hypothyroidism in a dog due to an iodide organification defect. Am J Vet Res 44:1257, 1983.

de Bruijne JJ, Altszuler N, Hampshire J, et al: Fat mobilization and plasma hormone levels in fasted dogs. Metabolism 10:199, 1981.

Drochner W, Muller-Schlosser S: Digestibility and tolerance of various sugars in cats. In Anderson RS (ed): Nutrition of the Dog and Cat. New York, Pergamon Press, 1980, p 101.

Hardie EM, Rawlings CA, Calvert CA: Severe sepsis in selected small animal surgical patients. J Am Anim Hosp Assoc 22:33, 1986.

Jones BR, Johnstone AC, Cahill JI, et al: Peripheral neuropathy in cats with inherited primary hyperchylomicronaemia. Vet Rec 119:268, 1986.

Jones BR, Wallace A, Harding DRK, et al: Occurrence of idiopathic, familial hyperchylomicronaemia in a cat. Vet Rec 112:543, 1983.

Keene B: Canine heart problem. In Companion Animal News. Englewood, CO, Morris Animal Foundation, Dec 1986, p 4.

Kolle LA, Monnens LA, Cejka V, et al: Persistent neonatal hypoglycemia due to glucagon deficiency. Arch Dis Child 53:422, 1978.

Leifer CE, Peterson ME: Hypoglycemia. Vet Clin North Am Small Anim Pract 1:873, 1984.

Olin DD, Rogers WA, MacMillan AD: Lipid-laden aqueous humor associated with anterior uveitis and concurrent hyperlipemia in two dogs. J Am Vet Med Assoc 168:861, 1976.

Rafiquzzaman M, Svenkerud R, Strande A, et al: Glycogenosis in the dog. Acta Vet Scand 17:196, 1976.

Rogers WA, Donovan EF, Kociba GJ: Idiopathic hyperlipoproteinemia in dogs. J Am Vet Med Assoc 166:1087, 1975.

Sperling MA: Hypoglycemia in infants and children. In Lavin N (ed): Manual of Endocrinology and Metabolism. Boston, Little, Brown and Co, 1994, p 443.

Strombeck DR, Meyer DJ, Freedland RA: Hyperammonemia due to a urea cycle enzyme deficiency in two dogs. J Am Vet Med Assoc 166:1109, 1975.

Strombeck DR, Rogers QR, Freedland R, et al: Fasting hypoglycemia in a pup. J Am Vet Med Assoc 173:299, 1978.

Thompson JS, Thompson MW: Human biochemical genetics. In Thomspon JS, Thompson MW (eds): Genetics in Medicine, 4th ed. Philadelphia, WB Saunders, 1991, p 79.

Turnwald GH, Troy GC: Hypoglycemia. Part I. Carbohydrate metabolism and laboratory evaluation. Compend Contin Educ Pract Vet 5:932, 1983.

Turnwald GH, Troy GC: Hypoglycemia. Part II. Clinical aspects. Compend Contin Educ Pract Vet 6:115, 1984.

van Toor AJ, van der Linde-Sipman JS, van den Ingh TSGAM, et al: Experimental induction of fasting hypoglycaemia and fatty liver syndrome in three Yorkshire terrier pups. Vet Q 13:16, 1991.

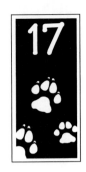

The Urinary System

John M. Kruger, Carl A. Osborne, Jody P. Lulich, David P. Polzin, and Scott D. Fitzgerald

Urinary tract disorders of puppies and kittens may result from heritable (genetic) or acquired disease processes affecting differentiation and growth of the developing urinary tract or from similar processes that eventually affect the structure or function of the mature urinary system. Successful management of urinary tract disorders depends on familiarity with the structure and functions of the kidneys, ureters, urinary bladder, and urethra.

DEVELOPMENTAL PHYSIOLOGY

Although the embryonic kidneys produce urine, maintenance of fetal homeostasis is primarily the responsibility of the placenta. Varying quantities of urine formed by the fetal kidneys pass from the developing urinary bladder through the urachus to the placenta, where unwanted waste products are absorbed by the maternal circulation and subsequently excreted in the mother's urine (Noden and deLahunta, 1985). Fetal urine also passes through the urethra into the amniotic cavity, where urine forms a major constituent of amniotic fluid. The latter part of gestation is characterized by rapid increases in nephron number and size and by maturation of glomerular and renal tubular functions (Guiguard, 1982; Maizels, 1992). Prenatal development of glomerular filtration and renal blood flow appears to parallel increases in fetal kidney size. Parturition is accompanied by dramatic increases in glomerular filtration rate (GFR) mediated largely by hemodynamic changes (increased cardiac output, increased systemic arterial blood pressure, and decreased renal vascular resistance) and by changes in intrinsic morphologic and functional characteristics of glomeruli (increased glomerular permeability and increased filtration surface area) (Guiguard, 1982). Inulin clearance studies in puppies have demonstrated that GFR increases sevenfold over the first month of life (Heller and Capek, 1965) (Fig. 17–1). Similarly, renal blood flow (RBF) increases nearly fourfold during the same time period (Heller and Capek, 1965; Horster and Valtin, 1971). Both GFR and RBF continue to increase after 4 weeks of age, reaching adult values approximately 10 weeks after birth (Horster and Valtin, 1971). Similarly, endogenous creatinine clearance studies suggest that GFR in kittens increases rapidly after birth, reaching adult values by 9 weeks of age (Hoskins et al, 1991).

The rate of maturation of intrinsic renal mechanisms regulating GFR, RBF, and distal delivery of water and solutes appears to vary in puppies (Fettman and Allen, 1991; Guiguard, 1982). Limited studies suggest that puppies are able to adequately increase proximal tubular resorption of at least water, sodium, and glucose in response to elevations in GFR (glomerulotubular balance) (Arant et al, 1974; Kleinman, 1975). Autoregulation of RBF and GFR in neonatal puppies appears to be relatively inefficient in response to rapid changes in systemic arterial blood pressures (Kleinmann and Lubbe, 1972). Maturity of renal tubular functions varies considerably with age. Newborn puppies have a limited ability to concentrate or dilute urine in response to changes in extracellular fluid volume (Fettman and Allen, 1991). The urine/plasma osmolality ratio (U/P Osm) in puppies rose from 2.0 at 2 weeks of age to 7.0 at 11

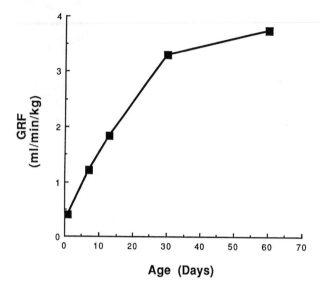

Figure 17–1. Mean inulin clearance values in 1- to 60-day-old puppies. GFR = Glomerular filtration rate. (Adapted from Heller J, Capek K: Changes in body water compartments and inulin and PAH clearance in the dog during postnatal development. Physiol Bohemoslov 14:433, 1965.)

weeks of age; normal U/P Osm values for adult dogs range from 3.3 to 8.4 (Hardy and Osborne, 1979; Horster and Valtin, 1971). The U/P Osm values in kittens rose from 4.6 at 4 to 6 weeks of age to 8.9 at 13 to 19 weeks of age (Crawford, 1990). Sodium balance appears to be relatively stable in newborn puppies. Whole kidney fractional resorption of sodium was constant in 2- to 77-day-old puppies and similar to values in mature dogs (less than 0.7%) (DiBartola et al, 1980; Horster and Valtin, 1971). Puppies younger than 3 weeks of age appear to have an impaired ability to excrete excess sodium compared with adult dogs. Puppies were able to excrete only 10% of an isotonic saline load within 2 hours of administration, whereas adult dogs were able to excrete up to 500% (Kleinman, 1975).

Significant differences in acid-base balance exist between puppies/kittens and adults. In vitro studies of kidney slices revealed that neonatal puppies, but not kittens, have an impaired ability to increase renal ammoniagenesis in response to an acid environment compared with adults (Robinson, 1954). Puppies challenged with ammonium chloride or sulfate developed more severe acidosis and were less able to increase renal ammoniagenesis, secrete protons, and acidify urine compared with adult dogs (Cort and McLance, 1954). Renal tubular resorption of amino acids is incomplete in 5-day-old puppies (Bovée et al, 1984). By 3 weeks of age, most amino acids are resorbed in puppies, and by 7 weeks of age adult patterns of amino acid resorption are evident. Incomplete tubular resorption of glucose is commonly observed in puppies. Glucosuria was detected in 50% of urinalyses obtained from 5-day-old puppies; glucosuria was not detected in puppies 21 days of age or older (Bovée et al, 1984). Although renal transport mechanisms for glucose appear to be relatively mature in puppies, transient glucosuria may be related to a greater proportion of immature nephrons and increased splay in puppies younger than 14 days of age (Arant et al, 1974).

The immaturity of glomerular and renal tubular function has significant clinical implications with regard to therapeutic management of puppies and kittens. Puppies and kittens are predisposed to rapid dehydration as a result of their higher water requirements and their decreased ability to maximally concentrate urine and resist osmotic diuresis (Fettman and Allen, 1991). Conversely, they are inherently more susceptible to fluid volume and solute overload (Kleinman, 1975). Although this paradox poses unique therapeutic challenges, use of conservative rates of fluid administration and careful monitoring during the course of fluid therapy may prove beneficial in managing immature animals. Puppies and kittens may be more susceptible to drug toxicity because of their limited capacity to eliminate those drugs and drug metabolites dependent on renal excretory mechanisms (Boothe and Tannert, 1992).

CONGENITAL AND HEREDITARY DISORDERS OF THE KIDNEY
Structural Anomalies of the Kidney
RENAL AGENESIS

Renal agenesis is the complete absence of one or both kidneys. Bilateral renal agenesis is fatal and is a cause of early death in puppies and kittens (Maxie and Prescott, 1991). Unilateral renal agenesis is more frequently observed in puppies and kittens than is bilateral agenesis (Lulich et al, 1987; Maxie and Prescott, 1991). Unilateral renal agenesis may affect either kidney and is usually accompanied by ipsilateral ureteral agenesis. The etiopathogenesis of renal agenesis in dogs and cats is uncertain. A familial predisposition for renal agenesis in beagles, Shetland sheepdogs, and Doberman pinschers supports a genetic basis for the anomaly (Table 17–1) (Brownie et al, 1988; Chew et al, 1982a; Vymetal, 1965). Unilateral renal agenesis may remain clinically silent, provided the contralateral kidney undergoes sufficient compensatory change to maintain normal hemostasis. Clinical findings may include an inability to palpate both kidneys or to detect a kidney by ultrasonography or contrast urography. Because of close associations in the development of the urogenital system, findings of abnormal or absent vas deferens, epididymal tails, or uterine horns at the time of castration or ovariohysterectomy should arouse suspicion of concurrent unilateral renal agenesis. Because unilateral renal agenesis is compatible with normal life, specific therapy is not indicated unless reduced renal function exists.

RENAL HYPOPLASIA

Hypoplastic kidneys appear as miniature replicas of normal kidneys composed of reduced numbers of histologically normal nephrons (Maxie and Prescott, 1991). Renal hypoplasia occurs sporadically in puppies and kittens (Lulich et al, 1987). Embryonic pathogenic mechanisms resulting in renal hypoplasia may involve inadequate metanephric blastema, insufficient branching of the ureteric bud, reduced nephron induction, or failure of postnatal renal tubular growth (Welling and Grantham, 1991). Clinical signs, therapy, and prognosis depend on the extent of involvement; unilateral disease may be clinically silent, whereas severe bilateral disease is typically associated with renal failure.

RENAL DYSPLASIA AND APLASIA

Renal dysplasia refers to disorganized parenchymal development characterized by segmental or focal areas of immature or anomalous structures in an otherwise normal kidney (Picut and Lewis, 1987c). Renal aplasia represents a more severe generalized form of dysplasia that affects the entire kidney. Renal dysplasia has been observed in male and female puppies, but rarely in kittens (see Table 17–1) (Lulich et al, 1987). Renal dysplasia is a familial disorder in the Lhasa apso, Shih Tzu, soft-coated wheaten terrier, and standard poodle (see Table 17–1) (DiBartola et al, 1983; Eriksen and Grondalen, 1984; Hoppe et al, 1990). In addition a hereditary basis is strongly suspected in keeshonds, chow chows, and miniature schnauzers (see Table 17–1) (Brown et al, 1990; Klopfer et al, 1975; Morton et al, 1990). Renal dysplasia has been associated with in utero inoculation of kitten fetuses with panleukopenia virus and in puppies with canine herpesvirus (Kilham et al, 1967; Percy et al, 1967).

Puppies with renal dysplasia may appear clinically normal for extended periods before development of signs of chronic renal failure (CRF). The rate at which renal dysplasia progresses to overt renal failure depends on the severity of initial renal lesions and factors resulting in progressive loss of renal functional mass (Table 17–2). Age of onset of clinical signs is variable, ranging from 4 weeks to more than 5 years; however, most cases of CRF are recognized in puppies younger than 2 years (O'Brien et al, 1982). Early signs of CRF are often subtle and may include lethargy, selective appetite, poor haircoat, variable weight loss, nocturia, and mild to moderate polyuria and polydipsia (Polzin and Osborne, 1995b). Severe dysplasias are associated with signs of advanced CRF and uremia (anorexia, depression, vomiting, diarrhea, dehydration, halitosis, oral ulceration, pale mucous membranes, and severe weight loss). Abdominal palpation may reveal small, irregularly shaped kidneys. Symmetric enlargement of the maxilla and mandible, bone pain, soft pliable mandibles ("rubber jaw"), and pathologic fractures are occasionally observed in young dogs with renal dysplasia and are indicative of severe renal osteodystrophy.

Laboratory findings with renal dysplasia reflect changes associated with CRF and typically include azotemia, hyperphosphatemia, metabolic acidosis, and normocytic normochromic nonregenerative anemia (Polzin and Osborne, 1995b). Serum calcium concentrations may be decreased, normal, or increased. Typically, serum calcium concentrations are normal to decreased in animals with CRF; however, some puppies develop hypercalcemia (DiBartola et al, 1983). Urinalysis usually reveals an inappropriately low urine specific gravity, an inactive urine sediment, and occasional mild to moderate proteinuria. A diagnosis of renal dysplasia is based on breed and clinical and laboratory findings

Table 17-1 Congenital Renal Diseases of Dogs and Cats

BREED PREDILECTION	DISORDER	INHERITANCE	SEX PREDILECTION	TYPICAL AGE AT DIAGNOSIS	SIGNS AND SYMPTOMS
Abyssinian cat	Amyloidosis	Unknown	None	1–5 y	Proteinuria, CRF
Basenji	Fanconi-like syndrome	Unknown	None	1–7 y	PU, glucosuria, ARF
Basset hound	Cystinuria	Unknown	M	Incidental	Cystine crystalluria, uroliths
Beagle	Unilateral agenesis	Unknown	None	Incidental	Asymptomatic
	Polycystic kidneys	Auto recessive	None	<2 y	Renomegaly, CRF
	Amyloidosis	Unknown	None	5–11 y	Proteinuria, CRF
	Glomerulopathy	Unknown	None	<9 y	Proteinuria, CRF
Bedlington terrier	Dysplasia	Unknown	None	<2 y	CRF
Bernese mountain dog	Glomerulopathy	Auto recessive	F > M	2–7 y	Proteinuria, CRF, NS
Bulldog	Cystinuria	Unknown	M	Incidental	Cystine crystalluria, uroliths
	Hyperuricuria	Unknown	M	Incidental	Urate crystalluria, uroliths
Bull terrier	Glomerulopathy	Auto dominant	None	1–8 y	Proteinuria, CRF
	Polycystic kidneys	Auto dominant	None	<2 y	Renomegaly, CRF
Cairn terrier	Polycystic kidneys	Auto recessive	None	<1 y	Renomegaly, CRF
Chow	Dysplasia	Unknown	None	<2 y	CRF
Cocker spaniel	Glomerulopathy*	Unknown	None	<2 y	Proteinuria, CRF
Dachshund	Cystinuria	Unknown	M	Incidental	Cystine crystalluria, uroliths
	Xanthinuria	Unknown	None	Incidental	Xanthine crystalluria, uroliths
Dalmatian	Hyperuricuria	Auto recessive	None	Incidental	Urate crystalluria, uroliths
	Glomerulopathy	Unknown	None	<5 y	Proteinuria, CRF
Doberman pinscher	Unilateral agenesis	Unknown	None	Incidental	Asymptomatic
	Glomerulopathy	Unknown	None	<6 y	Proteinuria, CRF, NS
Domestic long-haired cat	Polycystic kidneys	Unknown	None	<11 y	Renomegaly, CRF
Domestic short-haired cat	Hyperoxaluria	Unknown	None	<1 y	ARF
English cocker spaniel	Glomerulopathy	Auto recessive	None	<2 y	Proteinuria, CRF
English foxhound	Amyloidosis	Unknown	None	<9 y	Proteinuria, CRF
German shepherd	Cystadenocarcinomas	Auto dominant*	None	5–11 y	Renomegaly, hematuria, CRF
Irish terrier	Cystinuria	Auto recessive	M	Incidental	Cystine crystalluria, uroliths
Keeshond	Dysplasia	Unknown	None	<1 y	CRF
Lhasa apso	Dysplasia	Unknown	None	<5 y	CRF
Miniature schnauzer	Dysplasia	Unknown	None	<3 y	CRF

Breed	Disorder	Inheritance	Sex predisposition	Age	Clinical findings
Newfoundland	Cystinuria	Auto recessive	None	Incidental	Cystine crystalluria, uroliths
Norwegian elkhound	Tubulointerstitial nephropathy	Unknown	None	<5 y	CRF
	Primary glucosuria	Unknown	NR	NR	Glucosuria
Oriental short-haired cat	Amyloidosis	Unknown	None	<5 y	CRF
Persian cat	Polycystic kidneys	Auto dominant	None	<10 y	Renomegaly, CRF
Rottweiler	Glomerulopathy	Unknown	None	<1 y	Proteinuria, CRF
Samoyed	Glomerulopathy	X-linked dominant	M > F	<1 y	Proteinuria, CRF
Shar-pei	Amyloidosis	Unknown	None	1–6 y	Proteinuria, CRF NS
Shetland sheepdog	Unilateral agenesis	Unknown	None	Incidental	Asymptomatic
Shih Tzu	Dysplasia	Auto recessive	None	<9 y	CRF
Siamese	Amyloidosis	Unknown	None	<5 y	CRF
Soft-coated wheaten terrier	Dysplasia	Auto recessive	None	<3 y	CRF
	Glomerulopathy	Unknown	None	2–11 y	Proteinuria, CRF, NS
Standard poodle	Dysplasia	Unknown	None	<1 y	CRF
Tibetan spaniel	Hyperoxaluria	Unknown	None	<1 y	ARF
Welsh corgi	Telangiectasia	Unknown	None	2–8 y	Hematuria, renal pain
West Highland white terrier	Polycystic kidneys	Auto recessive*	None	<1 y	Renomegaly, CRF
None†	Ectopia/fusion	Unknown	None	Incidental	Asymptomatic
	Nephroblastoma	Unknown	None	<11 y	Renomegaly, hematuria
	Nephrogenic diabetes insipidus	Unknown	None	<2 y	PU

ARF = acute renal failure; auto = autosomal; CRF = chronic renal failure; F = female; M = male; NR = not reported; NS = nephrotic syndrome; PU = polyuria.

*Suspected.

†No specific breed association has been identified.

375

Table 17–2	Conditions That May Exacerbate Clinical Signs of Uremia or Promote Progressive Renal Damage

Prerenal conditions
 Intravascular volume depletion
  Dehydration
  Hemorrhage
 Diminished "effective" arterial blood volume
  Peripheral vasoconstriction
  Reduced cardiac output
  Hypoalbuminemia
 Primary renal hemodynamic alterations
  Prostaglandin synthetase inhibition (e.g.,
   administration of nonsteroidal
   antiinflammatory drugs)
  Hypercalcemia
Urinary obstruction
 a. Uroliths
 b. Blood clots
 c. Strictures
 d. Neoplasms
Urinary tract infection
Systemic hypertension
Concurrent nonrenal diseases

(Table 17–3). A definitive diagnosis of renal dysplasia depends on identification of primary dysplastic lesions by microscopic evaluation of renal tissues obtained by biopsy or necropsy. Primary lesions suggestive of renal dysplasia include (1) fetal or immature glomeruli and/or tubules, (2) persistent mesenchyme, (3) persistent metanephric ducts, (4) atypical tubular epithelium, and (5) dysontogenic metaplasia (Picut and Lewis, 1987c).

Renal dysplasia is an irreversible and often progressive disorder for which there is no specific therapy. Clinical and pathologic consequences of renal failure may, however, be minimized by supportive and symptomatic therapies designed to correct fluid, electrolytes, acid-base, endocrine, and nutritional imbalances. Therapeutic strategies for the management of CRF include the following: (1) ameliorate clinical signs of uremia; (2) correct fluid, electrolyte, and acid-base abnormalities; (3) minimize endocrine and hematologic disturbances; (4) provide adequate nutritional support; (5) modify progression of renal dysfunction; and (6) avoid conditions that exacerbate or promote progressive renal dysfunction (Table 17–4; see also Table 17–2) (Polzin and Osborne, 1995a). Recommendations regarding therapy should be individualized for each puppy (see Tables 17–3 and 17–4).

Because CRF associated with renal dysplasia is often progressive, serial clinical and laboratory evaluations are helpful for effective long-term management. Because moderate protein restriction is of benefit to uremic dogs and cats and may have potential long-term benefits with respect to renal hemodynamics, proteinuria, renal growth, and phosphate retention, it is logical to recommend feeding reduced-protein diets (Polzin and Osborne, 1995a). Optimal daily protein requirements for puppies and kittens with CRF are not known. Therefore, serial determinations of serum albumin concentration and body weight should be performed to monitor for malnutrition and hypoalbuminemia.

Hyperphosphatemia is a major factor promoting development of renal secondary hyperparathyroidism and progressive decline of renal function in dogs and cats with CRF (Polzin and Osborne, 1995b). A goal of medical therapy is to normalize serum phosphorus concentrations (Polzin and Osborne, 1995a). In early stages of CRF, hyperphosphatemia may be controlled by dietary phosphorus restriction alone. In advanced CRF, control of serum phosphorus concentrations may require administration of oral intestinal phosphate-binding agents. Serum phosphorus concentrations should be monitored regularly to evaluate therapeutic efficacy of dietary phosphate restriction and intestinal phosphate binders.

GLOMERULOPATHIES

Congenital renal diseases affecting predominantly the glomerulus have been described in young Bernese mountain dogs, English cocker spaniels, Samoyeds, Doberman pinschers, bull terriers, cocker spaniels, and Rottweilers (see Table 17–1) (Cook et al, 1993; Picut and Lewis, 1987a; Reusch et al, 1994). Proteinuria is the hallmark of glomerular disease. Although severe proteinuria may be associated with the nephrotic syndrome (i.e., proteinuria, hypoalbuminemia, hypercholesterolemia, and edema), most puppies and kittens with congenital glomerulopathies develop signs of advanced CRF. As functional and morphologic abnormalities of the glomeruli induce secondary changes in renal tubules, interstitium, and blood vessels, clinical manifestations of generalized renal dysfunction and renal failure supervene (Polzin and Osborne, 1995b).

Samoyed hereditary glomerulopathy is a genetic disorder of Samoyeds resulting from inheritance of an abnormal X-linked dominant gene (Jansen et al, 1986). The inherited defect results in

Table 17-3	Problem-Specific Database for Renal Failure in Immature Dogs and Cats

I. Medical history
   A. Note age, sex, and breed
   B. Note duration of signs
   C. Note potential exposure to nephrotoxins, infectious agents, or drugs
   D. Note previous illness, injury, surgery, or anesthetic episode
   E. Note concurrent illness in siblings
II. Physical examination
   A. Determine hydration status
   B. Examine oral cavity for ulcerations, loose or missing teeth, enlargement of maxillary tissues, and pallor of mucous membranes
   C. Palpate kidneys for number and changes in size, shape, position, consistency, and pain
   D. Palpate urinary bladder for size, shape, consistency, and position
   E. Palpate urethra per rectum
III. Complete urinalysis
IV. Quantitative urine culture (preferably collected by cystocentesis)
V. Complete blood count
VI. Serum biochemistries
   A. Urea nitrogen and creatinine concentration
   B. Sodium, potassium, and chloride concentrations
   C. Calcium and phosphorus concentrations
   D. Bicarbonate or total carbon dioxide concentrations
   E. Total protein and albumin concentrations
VII. Survey abdominal radiographs
   A. Kidneys—size, shape, location, number
   B. Uroliths—location, number, character
   C. Masses
   D. Urinary bladders—size, shape, location
VIII. Fundic examination
IX. Consider
   A. Renal ultrasonography
   B. Excretory urography
   C. Blood pressure determination
   D. Serum parathormone and ionized calcium concentrations
   E. Renal biopsy

alteration of type IV collagen molecules that are major components of the glomerular capillary basement membrane (Valli et al, 1991). Hereditary glomerulopathy of Samoyeds affects both male and female dogs; however, males are affected more frequently (Bloedow, 1981). Affected male dogs develop persistent proteinuria and, occasionally, microscopic hematuria as early as 2 to 4 months of age. Most affected male dogs develop signs of CRF and uremia; death due to end-stage CRF occurs between 8 and 16 months of age. Affected female dogs have milder clinical signs and are less likely to progress to overt renal failure (Jansen et al, 1984). Affected females may have mild proteinuria that persists for several years before clinical signs of CRF develop in middle or older age. In affected males, kidneys are reduced in size. Microscopic lesions are characterized by primary membranoproliferative glomerulonephritis progressing to glomerulosclerosis. Ultra-

structurally, multilaminar splitting of the lamina densa of glomerular capillary basement membranes is evident as early as 1 month of age and often precedes development of microscopic abnormalities (Jansen et al, 1984).

Bull terrier hereditary nephritis is a genetic disorder of bull terriers characterized by ultrastructural abnormalities of the glomerular capillary basement membrane similar to those observed in Samoyed hereditary glomerulopathy (Hood et al, 1990). Unlike the disorder in Samoyeds, hereditary nephritis of bull terriers appears to be inherited as an autosomal dominant gene (Hood et al, 1990). In addition, both male and female bull terriers appear to be affected with equal frequency and have similar clinical features (Robinson et al, 1989). Affected terriers usually die from CRF between 10 months and 9 years of age. Kidneys are usually small with finely irregular cortical surfaces. Lesions observed by microscopy include reduced numbers

Table 17–4	Medical Management of Chronic Renal Failure
PROBLEM	**THERAPEUTIC OPTIONS**
Dehydration	Parenteral fluids
	Free access to water
	Avoid stress
Uremia/vomiting	Dietary protein restriction
	Correct fluid, electrolyte, acid-base abnormalities
	H$_2$-receptor blockade
	Antiemetics (centrally acting)
Anorexia	Correct fluid, electrolyte, acid-base abnormalities
	Enhance palatability of diets
	H$_2$-receptor blockade
	Control vomiting
	Consider appetite stimulant
Hyperphosphatemia	Dietary phosphate restriction
	Intestinal phosphate binders
Metabolic acidosis	Alkalinizing therapy
Anemia	Recombinant erythropoietin
	Anabolic steroids
Systemic hypertension	Sodium restriction
	Antihypertensive drug therapy
Renal osteodystrophy	Dietary phosphate restriction
	Intestinal phosphate binders
	Calcitriol therapy
	Calcium supplementation
Drug reactions/overdose	Reduce dosages
	Avoid nephrotoxic drugs
Urinary tract infection	Appropriate antimicrobial therapy
	Monitor for pyuria, bacteriuria

of glomeruli, glomerular tuft atrophy, tubular dilation, corticomedullary fibrosis, mineralization of Bowman's capsule and renal tubules, and variable interstitial mononuclear cell infiltration. Extensive thickening and splitting of the basement membranes of glomerular capillaries, Bowman's capsule, and renal tubules are observed by electronic microscopy.

Doberman pinscher familial glomerulonephritis has been described in related Doberman pinschers (Chew et al, 1982a). Clinical signs of CRF are first observed between 6 weeks and 8 years of age. No sex predilection is apparent; however, males appear to be affected earlier (average age 20 months) than females (average age 31 months) (Chew et al, 1982a). Urinalyses typically reveal persistent marked proteinuria and variable glucosuria. Most, but not all, animals affected with familial glomerulonephritis develop clinical signs and laboratory abnormalities consistent with CRF. Dogs with advanced disease often die or are euthanized between 6 months and 9 years of age. Five of 20 female Dobermans with hereditary nephritis had concurrent unilateral renal and ureteral aplasia

(Wilcock and Patterson, 1979). Kidneys are usually normal or slightly small in size and have an irregularly pitted surface (Wilcock and Patterson, 1979). Microscopic lesions are suggestive of a primary membranoproliferative glomerulonephritis and accompanied by variable degrees of tubulointerstitial disease (Chew et al, 1982a). Renal lesions include glomerular sclerosis, cystic glomerular atrophy, atrophy and dilatation of renal tubules, interstitial mononuclear cell infiltration, fibrosis, and mineralization and hyperplasia of collecting duct epithelium. Glomerular ultrastructural lesions are characterized by multifocal irregular thickening of the glomerular basement membrane or diffuse thickening of the glomerular basement membrane zone (Picut and Lewis, 1987b). The pathogenic mechanisms involved in Doberman familial nephritis and mode of inheritance are unknown. Variability in clinical course and rate of progression may be indicative of different degrees of gene expression or, conversely, factors that potentiate heritable renal defects. Immunofluorescent studies have identified immunoglobulins and complement in glomeruli of some affected dogs. These findings appear, however, to be inconsistent features of Doberman familial glomerulonephritis.

Familial nephropathy of English cocker spaniels was first described as bilateral renal cortical hyperplasia (Krook, 1957). Subsequent investigations, however, suggest that familial nephropathy of English cocker spaniels may be considered a primary glomerulopathy (Robinson et al, 1985). The disorder appears to be transmitted as an autosomal recessive trait (Robinson et al, 1985). Clinical signs of CRF and uremia typically develop between 6 months to 2 years of age. There appears to be no sex predilection. Urinalyses consistently reveal moderate to severe proteinuria and occasional glucosuria and hematuria. Kidneys are usually normal to small in size with a mild to moderate decrease in cortical thickness (Lees et al, 1997; Robinson et al, 1985). Microscopic findings in more advanced cases include mesangial thickening, glomerular and periglomerular fibrosis, glomerular obsolescence, diffuse interstitial fibrosis, mild to moderate interstitial mononuclear cell infiltrates, tubular dilation, and mineralization of tubular basement membranes. Ultrastructural lesions are characterized by extensive thickening, multilaminar splitting, and fragmentation of the glomerular basement membrane (Lees et al, 1997).

Rottweiler atrophic glomerulopathy was described in four related Rottweilers and appears to be distinct from other canine hereditary glomerulopathies (Cook et al, 1993). Affected dogs develop clinical signs of CRF and uremia between 6 months and 1 year of age. Both male and female dogs are affected. Urinalysis typically reveals isosthenuria and moderate to severe proteinuria. Kidneys are usually moderately enlarged. Microscopic lesions are characterized by severe, diffuse global, atrophic membranous glomerulopathy with secondary degenerative changes. The familial nature of this disorder is suggestive of a genetic disorder; however, confirmation of this hypothesis requires further investigation.

A diagnosis of familial glomerulopathy is based on breed, age of onset of clinical signs, and laboratory abnormalities. Despite the presence of moderate to severe proteinuria, hypoalbuminemia and clinical signs consistent with the nephrotic syndrome are uncommonly observed in puppies with familial glomerular disease. A definitive diagnosis is based on microscopic evaluation of renal tissues obtained by biopsy or necropsy. The irreversible nature of familial glomerulopathies precludes specific therapy;

however, supportive or symptomatic therapy may improve the quality of life and minimize progression of renal dysfunction. Results of studies in young Samoyed dogs with hereditary nephritis suggest that dietary modification may be of benefit to puppies with some types of familial glomerulopathy (Valli et al, 1991). Affected puppies are to be fed a modified diet restricted in protein (14.8% dry matter basis), phosphorus (0.028% dry matter basis), and sodium (0.23% dry matter basis). Although dietary modification did not prevent development of terminal renal failure, it did appear to diminish the severity of glomerular lesions in affected males and carrier females and prolongs survival in affected male dogs.

TUBULOINTERSTITIAL NEPHROPATHIES

A noninflammatory tubulointerstitial nephropathy has been identified in related Norwegian elkhounds (Finco, 1976). This nephropathy affects both male and female dogs and is characterized by renal failure that varies in severity and rate of progression. The pathologic mechanisms responsible for familial renal disease in Norwegian elkhounds are unknown. Results of histologic, electron microscopic, and immunofluorescent studies do not provide evidence of glomerular, vascular, or immune-mediated renal disease (Finco et al, 1977). Based on a strong familial tendency, genetic factors are suspected; however, the mode of inheritance is unknown. Azotemia may be detected in affected puppies as early as 3 months of age; however, some affected dogs may remain nonazotemic for extended periods (Finco, 1976; Finco et al, 1977). In severely affected dogs, clinical signs and laboratory abnormalities are consistent with CRF and uremia. Urinalyses typically reveal impaired concentrating ability and occasional glucosuria and proteinuria. Microscopic renal lesions are not observed in affected puppies younger than 25 days (Finco et al, 1977). In advanced disease, kidneys are small, white, and firm, with thin cortices and radial streaks of fibrous connective tissue. Periglomerular fibrosis and parietal epithelial cell hyperplasia and hypertrophy were consistent early morphologic lesions observed by microscopy. As the disease progresses, severe corticomedullary interstitial fibrosis becomes evident. Although no specific treatment will reverse the nephropathy, puppies with advanced disease may benefit from supportive and symptomatic therapy.

POLYCYSTIC RENAL DISEASE

Polycystic renal disease has been described in several breeds of puppies and kittens (see Table 17–1). Polycystic renal disease is characterized by formation of multiple, variable-sized cysts throughout the renal medulla and cortex (Maxie and Prescott, 1991). Affected kidneys are enlarged and lobulated and contain multiple fluid-filled epithelial lined cysts ranging in size from 0.5 mm to several centimeters in diameter. Etiopathologic mechanisms resulting in renal cyst formation are unknown. A strong familial tendency in bull terriers, West Highland white terriers, Cairn terriers, beagles, Persian cats, and domestic long-haired cats suggests a genetic basis for polycystic disease in these species (see Table 17–1) (Burrows et al, 1994; Crowell et al, 1979; Eaton et al, 1997; Fox, 1964; McAloose et al, 1998; McKenna and Carpenter, 1980). Polycystic renal disease in West Highland white terriers, Cairn terriers, and domestic long-haired cats is often associated with concurrent formation of hepatic biliary cysts (Crowell et al, 1979; McAloose et al, 1998; McKenna and Carpenter, 1980). Polycystic renal disease may cause progressive irreversible renal failure as a result of cyst enlargement and compression of adjacent renal parenchyma. Animals often develop abdominal enlargement, renomegaly, and clinical signs and laboratory abnormalities consistent with CRF and uremia. Radiography, ultrasonography, and/or exploratory celiotomy and renal biopsy may help differentiate polycystic renal disease from other causes of abdominal mass lesions (i.e., renal ectopia, nonrenal neoplasms, foreign bodies, and pregnancy; Table 17–5). Symptomatic and supportive therapy may be of benefit to animals with renal failure.

AMYLOIDOSIS

Renal amyloidosis is characterized by extracellular deposition of amyloid in glomerular capillary walls, glomerular mesangium, and medullary interstitium (Maxie and Prescott, 1991). Renal amyloidosis is usually observed in older unrelated dogs; however, familial renal amyloidosis occurs in young related Abyssinian, Oriental short-haired, and Siamese cats and in beagle and Chinese shar-pei dogs (Bowles and Mosier, 1992; Chew et al, 1982b; DiBartola et al, 1990; Zuber, 1993). The condition is usually recognized at 1 to 6 years of age at which time clinical signs and laboratory abnormalities consistent with CRF and uremia develop. Affected Chinese shar-pei dogs may have a history of

Table 17–5	Problem-Specific Database for Abdominal Distention in Immature Dogs and Cats

I. Medical history
  A. Note age, sex, and breed
  B. Note duration and/or changes in degree of abdominal distention
  C. Note changes in micturition and/or defecation
II. Physical examination
  A. Auscultate heart and lungs for evidence of heart murmurs, pulmonary edema, or pleural effusions
  B. Identify peritoneal fluid
  C. Characterize position, size, shape, consistency, and attachments of abdominal masses
  D. Palpate liver, spleen, kidneys, urinary bladder, intestinal tract, and genital tract for changes in size, shape, position, and consistency
  E. Identify and localize abdominal pain
III. Laboratory evaluation
  A. Complete urinalysis
  B. Serum chemistry profile
  C. Complete blood count
IV. Survey abdominal radiography
V. Abdominal ultrasonography
VI. Consider
  A. Biopsy—aspiration, punch, or surgical
  B. Localizing contrast radiographic or ultrasonographic procedures
  C. Exploratory celiotomy

intermittent pyrexia and/or swelling of the tibiotarsal joints (so-called "swollen hock disease"). Unlike older animals with nonfamilial renal amyloidosis, severe proteinuria is an inconsistent clinical feature of familial renal amyloidosis in Abyssinian cats and Chinese shar-pei dogs. This disparity most likely reflects differences in the intrarenal location of amyloid deposits. The medullary interstitium is the primary site of amyloid deposition in these breeds. Diagnosis of familial renal amyloidosis is based on breed, clinical signs and laboratory findings consistent with CRF, and demonstration of renal amyloid deposits by microscopy. No therapy is capable of slowing or eliminating renal amyloid deposition. Because renal amyloidosis often results in progressive nephron destruction and deterioration of renal function, symptomatic and supportive therapy may be of benefit.

RENAL ECTOPIA AND FUSION

Renal ectopia (with or without fusion) describes congenital malposition of one or both kidneys

(Kaufmann et al, 1987; Lulich et al, 1987). *Renal ectopia* occurs when the mature kidney fails to reach its normal location or orientation within the abdomen (Welling and Grantham, 1991). *Renal fusion* represents the congenital union of normally lateralized kidneys. Fused kidneys may assume a variety of shapes; *horseshoe kidneys* are symmetrically fused along the medial border of either pole, resulting in a shape resembling that of a horseshoe. Not all cases of renal ectopia involve fusion. The etiopathogenesis of renal ectopia and the relationship of fusion to ectopic kidneys are not understood. Because renal ectopia and fusion do not directly result in damage to renal parenchyma, affected dogs and cats may appear clinically normal. Radiography, ultrasonography, or exploratory celiotomy may be of value in differentiating renal ectopia from other abdominal masses (see Table 17–5).

DUPLEX AND SUPERNUMERARY KIDNEYS

The presence of one or more accessory kidneys (supernumerary kidneys) or the presence of an enlarged kidney with two distinct pelves and ureters (duplex kidneys) appear to be uncommon in puppies and has not been reported in kittens (Odendaal, 1992; O'Handley et al, 1979). Most renal and ureteral duplications are asymptomatic; however, if pyelonephritis selectively affects a supernumerary kidney or a portion of the duplex kidney, surgical resection of the diseased moiety is recommended.

PRIMARY RENAL NEOPLASMS

Primary tumors of the kidneys are usually considered disorders of older animals; however, several renal malignancies, including nephroblastoma, lymphoma, carcinoma, and undifferentiated sarcoma, have been described in puppies and kittens (Caywood et al, 1980a). Nephroblastomas (embryonal nephroma, Wilms' tumor, congenital mixed tumor) occur in puppies younger than 6 months. Nephroblastomas are believed to be congenital tumors arising from the pluripotent metanephric blastema. Nephroblastomas vary markedly in size and usually affect a single kidney; bilateral involvement is rare (Caywood et al, 1980a). Invasion and compression of adjacent renal parenchyma progressively destroy the affected kidney. Tumors may penetrate the renal capsule and invade local tissue or metastasize to lungs, liver, mesentery, lymph nodes, and bone. Clinical signs associated with nephroblastomas vary with location, size, and duration of the neoplasm.

Nephroblastomas typically are recognized because of signs of persistent or intermittent hematuria and/or abdominal distention associated with a palpable mass. A diagnosis of primary renal neoplasia is based on physical examination and radiographic and ultrasonic findings (see Table 17–5). Definitive diagnosis requires microscopic identification of neoplastic cells in tissue samples obtained by biopsy or at the time of necropsy. Therapy has rarely been attempted for dogs with nephroblastoma, presumably due to widespread metastatic disease at the time of diagnosis. Nephrectomy and ureterectomy are recommended for animals with unilateral disease, adequate renal function in the contralateral kidney, and absence of identifiable metastatic disease (Caywood et al, 1980a). The therapeutic efficacy of adjunctive radiation or chemotherapy in dogs with primary renal neoplasia is unknown. A dog with unilateral nephroblastoma and distant metastases, however, survived over 15 months after treatment with combination therapy utilizing unilateral nephrectomy, local radiation, and periodic administration of actinomycin D (Caywood et al, 1980b).

Functional Anomalies of the Kidney
FANCONI'S SYNDROME

Generalized renal tubular dysfunction associated with impaired renal tubular resorption of amino acids, glucose, phosphate, sodium, potassium, and uric acid had been described in basenjis, Norwegian elkhounds, schnauzers, and Shetland sheepdogs (see Table 17–1) (Brown, 1989). Fanconi's syndrome in the basenji dog is familial and is strongly suggestive of a hereditary defect; however, the mode of inheritance is unknown (Easley and Breitschwerdt, 1976). Gentamicin-induced acquired Fanconi's syndrome has been reported in a dog (Brown et al, 1986). The syndrome has not been reported in cats. Clinical signs develop between 1 and 7 years of age in most affected dogs and depend on the severity of renal tubular dysfunction and concomitant renal failure (Bovée et al, 1979). Urinalyses typically reveal glucosuria, mild proteinuria, and urine specific gravity values of 1.005 to 1.018. Results of serum biochemistries and hemograms are usually normal. Some affected dogs may rapidly develop severe renal failure. Diagnosis of Fanconi's syndrome is based on breed, clinical signs of polyuria and polydipsia, and laboratory abnormalities of low urine specific gravity, normoglycemic glucosuria, aminoaciduria, nonanion gap metabolic acidosis, and hypokalemia (Brown, 1989). Treatment should be individualized for each dog and depends on specific cause, severity of serum biochemical abnormalities, and presence of overt renal failure.

PRIMARY RENAL GLUCOSURIA

Primary renal glucosuria is an isolated hereditary defect in proximal renal tubular resorption of glucose resulting in persistent glucosuria without concurrent hyperglycemia. Primary renal glucosuria has been reported in Scottish terriers, Norwegian elkhounds, and mixed-breed dogs (see Table 17–1) (Bovée, 1984). Primary renal glucosuria in Norwegian elkhounds appears to be familial; however, the mode of inheritance is unknown. Dogs with primary renal glucosuria are clinically asymptomatic. Laboratory findings include low urine specific gravity and persistent glucosuria in the absence of hyperglycemia. Primary renal glucosuria must be differentiated from other causes of glucosuria (i.e., diabetes mellitus, administration of dextrose-containing fluids, familial nephropathies, Fanconi's syndrome, acute tubular necrosis, and transient glucosuria due to physiologic stress hyperglycemia).

CYSTINURIA

Excessive urinary excretion of the amino acid cystine results from a heritable defect in renal tubular transport of cystine and other dibasic amino acids. Cystinuria has been observed in over 60 breeds of dogs and occasionally in cats (Case et al, 1992; DiBartola et al, 1991; Osborne et al, 1996). The disorder predominantly affects male dogs, and analyses of pedigrees of

Newfoundlands and Irish and Scottish terriers suggest a recessive mode of inheritance (Casal et al, 1995; Tsan et al, 1972). Cystinuric puppies and kittens have no detectable abnormalities associated with amino acid loss with the exception of formation of cystine uroliths. Although cystinuria represents a risk factor for development of urolithiasis, cystine uroliths are uncommon in puppies and kittens (see Tables 17–15 and 17–16, later). Observation of cystine crystals in urine sediment is expected with this disorder (Fig. 17–2).

HYPERURICURIA

Hyperuricuria in Dalmatian dogs is transmitted by a recessive nonsex-linked mode of inheritance (Keeler, 1940). Etiopathogenic factors responsible for hyperuricuria involve impaired hepatic conversion of uric acid to allantoin by the enzyme uricase and enhanced renal tubular secretion of uric acid (Giesecke and Tiemeyer, 1984). Although hyperuricuria predisposes affected dogs to urolithiasis, urate uroliths are uncommon in Dalmatian puppies (see Table 17–15, later). A high prevalence of ammonium urate uroliths has been observed in puppies with portal vascular anomalies (Marretta et al, 1981). Hyperuricuria may be detected by identification of characteristic uric acid, sodium, or ammonium urate (ammonium biurate) crystals in urine sediment.

XANTHINURIA

Congenital xanthinuria is an uncommon metabolic disorder of puppies and kittens characterized by a deficiency of xanthine oxidase, the hepatic enzyme that catalyzes the oxidation of hypoxanthine to xanthine and xanthine to uric

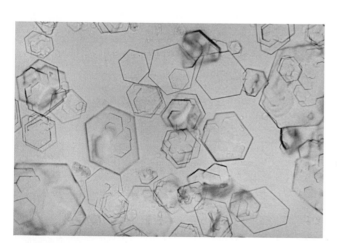

Figure 17–2. Photomicrograph of cystine crystals formed in urine collected from a 22-month-old male Newfoundland dog. (Unstained; ×100.) (From Osborne CA, Clinton CW, Bamman LK, et al: Prevalence of canine uroliths, Minnesota Urolith Center. Vet Clin North Am Small Anim Pract 16:58, 1986.)

acid. As a consequence, abnormal quantities of xanthine are excreted in the urine as a major end product of purine metabolism. Because xanthine is the least soluble urine purine metabolite, xanthinuria represents a risk factor for xanthine urolithiasis. Congenital xanthinuria and xanthine urolithiasis have been observed in dachshunds and mixed-breed cats (Kucera et al, 1997; Osborne et al, 1996; White et al, 1997). Because xanthine crystalluria cannot be reliably distinguished from urate crystalluria by routine microscopic urine sediment examination, a diagnosis of xanthinuria is based on detection of xanthine in uroliths analyzed by infrared spectroscopy or x-ray diffraction. Formation of xanthine uroliths in xanthinuric dogs and cats may be minimized by consumption of low-purine diets, alkalization of urine, and eradication or control of urinary tract infections.

PRIMARY HYPEROXALURIA

Primary hyperoxaluria is an inborn error of metabolism resulting in excessive oxalate production and increased urinary oxalate excretion. Hereditary primary hyperoxaluria has been recognized in domestic short-haired cats and Tibetan spaniels (see Table 17–1) (Jansen and Arnesen, 1990; McKerrel et al, 1989). The predominant clinical manifestation of primary hyperoxaluria in puppies and kittens is acute renal failure caused by deposition of calcium oxalate crystals in renal tubules. Affected puppies and kittens usually develop clinical signs of acute renal failure and uremia between 7 weeks and 1 year of age. Renal lesions observed by microscopy include interstitial fibrosis and dilated necrotic proximal tubules containing rosettes of birefringent calcium oxalate crystals. Specific therapy for management of primary hyperoxaluria has not been identified.

NEPHROGENIC DIABETES INSIPIDUS

Congenital nephrogenic diabetes insipidus has been described in puppies and is characterized by severe polyuria and polydipsia (5 to 10 times normal urine volume), nocturia, and poor growth (Breitschwerdt et al, 1981). Urine specific gravity values typically range from 1.002 to 1.004. Diagnosis of congenital nephrogenic diabetes insipidus is based on a history of persistent polyuria and polydipsia, hyposthenuric urine, and lack of response to water deprivation, partial water deprivation, hypotonic saline infusion, and antidiuretic hormone administration. Therapy for congenital nephrogenic diabetes

insipidus is limited to strategies designed to reduce the severity of the polyuria and polydipsia. Use of salt-restricted diets and the diuretic chlorothiazide have been reported to reduce the magnitude of polyuria by 20% to 65% in puppies with congenital nephrogenic diabetes insipidus (Breitschwerdt et al, 1981).

CONGENITAL AND HEREDITARY ANOMALIES OF THE URETERS

Ureteral Agenesis

Ureteral agenesis is the congenital absence of one or both ureters due to incomplete ureteral bud formation. Unilateral ureteral agenesis is the most common form observed in dogs and cats and is usually accompanied by ipsilateral renal aplasia (Lulich et al, 1987; Murti, 1965).

Ureteral Duplication

Ureteral duplication is a congenital disorder involving complete or partial duplication of one ureter. This disorder has been associated with a duplexed kidney and a supernumerary kidney in dogs; ureteral duplication has not been observed in cats (Odendaal, 1992; O'Handley et al, 1979).

Ureteral Valves

Congenital ureteral valves are persistent transverse folds of vestigial mucosa and smooth muscle fibers forming annular, semiannular, or diaphragmatic lesions in the ureter (Bauer et al, 1992). Semiannular ureteral valves have been described in a 6-month-old female collie with unilateral ureterectasis, hydronephrosis, and urinary incontinence (Pollock and Schoen, 1971). The etiopathogenesis of urinary incontinence associated with ureteral valves in this case is uncertain.

Ectopic Ureters

Ureteral ectopia is a congenital anomaly in which one or both ureters terminate abnormally in the urinary bladder. *Intramural ectopic ureters* contact and enter the bladder wall normally but continue submucosally through the trigone and terminate distally in the urethra or vagina (Fig. 17–3) (Osborne et al, 1995a). Intramural ectopic ureters may also form ureteral troughs, develop double ureteral openings, or fail to develop a distal orifice. *Extramural ectopic ureters* totally bypass the bladder before terminating in the urethra, vagina, or uterus (see Fig. 17–3). Fe-

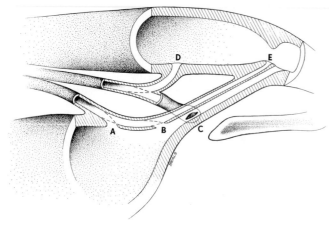

Figure 17–3. Schematic illustration of canine ectopic ureters showing **A**, normal position of the ureter; **B**, intramural ectopic ureter terminating in the proximal urethra; **C**, extramural ectopic ureter terminating in the proximal urethra; **D**, extramural ectopic ureter terminating in the vagina; and **E**, intramural ectopic ureter terminating in the vagina.

male puppies and kittens are affected more often than males (Hayes, 1984; Holt and Gibbs, 1992; Holt and Moore, 1995; Lulich et al, 1987). Most ectopic ureters in female dogs are unilateral (Holt and Moore, 1995). In male dogs, unilateral and bilateral ureteral ectopia appear to occur with similar frequencies. The urethra is the most common site of ectopic ureters in female dogs. In males, the prostatic urethra is the most common site of termination. Because of the close relationship between the metanephric duct system and development of the urogenital organs, ectopic ureters may be associated with other concurrent anomalies such as renal ectopia, renal hypoplasia, renal aplasia, ureteroceles, urachal remnants, urinary bladder, agenesis or hypoplasia, urethral agenesis or ectopia, phimosis, and persistent hyman (Holt and Moore, 1995; Pearson and Gibbs, 1971).

Although most cases occur in mixed-breed dogs, an increased frequency of ectopic ureters has been found in Siberian huskies, Labrador retrievers, Newfoundlands, English bulldogs, West Highland white terriers, fox terriers, golden retrievers, Skye terriers, Welsh corgis, and miniature and toy poodles (Hayes, 1984; Holt and Moore, 1995). Familial or breed predilections have not been identified in cats with ectopic ureters. Clinical signs of urethral ectopia vary, being dependent on the site of termination of the abnormal ureter and other urogenital abnormalities. Urinary incontinence is the predominant clinical sign. Ureteral ectopia is often recognized shortly after weaning, and its severity may vary from continuous involuntary dribbling to intermittent incontinence associated with rest, excitement, or changes in body position (Osborne et al, 1995a). Discoloration of the periurethral hair and urine scald dermatitis may also be observed.

Although urinary incontinence in immature animals is highly suggestive of ectopic ureters, other causes of incontinence should be considered (Tables 17–6 and 17–7). Excretory urography combined with retrograde contrast urethrography or vaginography appears to provide the most comprehensive means of establishing a de-

Table 17–6	**Causes of Urinary Incontinence in Immature Dogs and Cats**

Neurogenic
  Spinal dysraphism
  Spinal trauma
  Dysautonomia
  Others
Non-neurogenic
  Anatomic anomalies
    Ureteral ectopic
    Ureterocele
    Ureteral ectasia
    Ureteral valves
    Urinary bladder agenesis/hypoplasia
    Urinary bladder duplication
    Exstrophy
    Ectopic uterine horns
    Colorurocystic fistula
    Patent urachus
    Urethral agenesis
    Urethral hypoplasia
    Pseudohermaphroditism/intersex
    Epispadias/hypospadias
  Obstructive (paradoxical) incontinence
    Urolithiasis
    Ureterocele
    Urethral stricture
    Neoplasia
    Periurethral mass lesion
  Urge incontinence
Inappropriate (submissive) micturition

Table 17–7	Problem-Specific Database for Urinary Incontinence in Immature Dogs and Cats

I. Medical history
  A. Note age, sex, and breed
  B. Note owner's definition of incontinence
  C. Note age of onset and duration of incontinence
II. Physical examination
  A. Observe micturition
  B. Evaluate bladder size before and after micturition
  C. Verify incontinence
  D. Vaginal examination
  E. Neurologic examination
III. Quantitative urine culture
IV. Serum biochemistry (serum urea nitrogen and creatinine = minimum)
V. Consider
  A. Survey abdominal radiographs
  B. Excretory urography
  C. Contrast urethrography or vaginography
  D. Endoscopy (vaginoscopy, urethroscopy, cystoscopy)

finitive diagnosis (Osborne et al, 1995a). In addition, vaginoscopy, urethroscopy, and cystoscopy may allow direct visualization of an ectopic ureteral orifice (Osborne et al, 1985b). Urinary incontinence associated with ectopic ureters is helped only with surgery. Surgical strategies employed for correction of ectopic ureters include transection and reimplantation of the ureter, creation of a neostoma in situ, or complete removal of the kidney and its ureter. Dogs with postoperative incontinence due to urethral insufficiency may benefit from pharmacologic management with α-adrenergic agonists such as phenylpropanolamine.

Ureterocele

A ureterocele is a congenital cystic dilation of the terminal submucosal segment of the intravesicular ureter. *Orthotopic (simple) ureteroceles* are located at the trigone of the urinary bladder with the ureteral orifice in normal position. Ureteroceles accompanying ectopic ureters are classified as *ectopic ureteroceles*. Ureteroceles may be unilateral or bilateral and are typically ectopic (McLoughlin et al, 1989). Most ureteroceles have been observed in female puppies. Ureteroceles have not been reported in kittens. Puppies with orthotopic ureteroceles may be asymptomatic or may develop signs of lower urinary tract disease (i.e., dysuria, stranguria, pollakiuria, and hematuria). Puppies with ectopic ureteroceles typically develop urinary incontinence. A diagnosis of ureterocele is based on excretory urography, ultrasonography, and/or exploratory celiotomy and cystotomy. Treatment of ureteroceles is directed at alleviating clinical signs by ureterocelectomy or ureteronephrectomy and eliminating and/or preventing urinary tract infections.

Vesicoureteral Reflux

Vesicoureteral reflux is retrograde flow of urine from the bladder into the ureters and renal pelves. *Primary vesicoureteral reflux* denotes intrinsic maldevelopment of the ureterovesical junction; the term *secondary vesicoureteral reflux* implies an acquired disorder of the ureterovesical junction. Primary vesicoureteral reflux occurs in 79% of healthy puppies 2 to 4 months of age and in 47% of healthy puppies 4 to 6 months of age (Christie, 1973). As puppies mature, the frequency of primary vesicoureteral reflux decreases and is observed in less than 10% of adults. The cause of primary vesicoureteral reflux is unknown; however, it is believed to be related to delayed maturation of the vesicoureteral junction. Vesicoureteral reflux may also occur secondarily to urinary tract infection, congenital anomalies of the bladder and urethra (ureteral ectopia, ureteral duplication, and urinary bladder diverticula), urethral obstruction, and neurogenic bladder diseases (Klausner and Feeney, 1983). A diagnosis of vesicoureteral reflux is based on contrast radiography, preferably voiding or maximum distention retrograde contrast cystourethrography.

CONGENITAL AND HEREDITARY ANOMALIES OF THE URINARY BLADDER

Agenesis and Hypoplasia

Complete agenesis of the urinary bladder is extremely rare and has been reported in a 4-month-old mixed-breed female dog with a life-long history of urinary incontinence (Pearson et al, 1965). Hypoplasia of the urinary bladder has been typically associated with bilateral and, occasionally, unilateral ectopic ureters (Holt and Gibbs, 1992). Small urinary bladder capacity may contribute to postoperative urinary incontinence occasionally observed after surgical correction of ectopic ureters. Bladder capacity may, however, increase substantially over a period of several months after correction of ureteral ectopia.

Exstrophy

The term *exstrophy* encompasses a number of congenital anomalies characterized by ventral midline defects in the ventral abdominal wall, urinary bladder, intestines, and external genitalia. Life-long urinary incontinence, ascending urinary tract infection, and pyelonephritis are the predominant clinical features of exstrophy of the urinary bladder and ventral abdominal wall (Hobson and Ader, 1979). Correction of exstrophy requires reconstructive surgery, and success depends on the severity of the defect and the presence of other urinary tract abnormalities.

Anomalies of the Urachus

The urachus is a fetal conduit that allows urine to pass from the developing urinary bladder to the placenta (Noden and deLahunta, 1985). The urachus usually undergoes complete atrophy and is nonfunctional at birth. If the urachus fails to undergo complete atrophy, macroscopic or microscopic remnants may remain and result in persistent urachal patency or in formation of urachal cysts or diverticula (Osborne et al, 1987). A *persistent* (or *patent*) *urachus* exists when the entire urachal canal remains functionally patent between the bladder and the umbilicus (Fig. 17–4). A persistent urachus is associated with inappropriate loss of urine through the umbilicus and is often accompanied by omphalitis, ventral dermatitis, and a urinary tract infection. Rarely, a persistent urachus may terminate in the abdomen cavity, resulting in uroabdomen. *Urachal cysts* may develop if secreting urachal epithelium persists in isolated segments of a persistent urachus (see Fig. 17–4). *Vesicourachal diverticula* occur when that portion of urachus located at the bladder vertex fails to close (see Fig. 17–4). Microscopic urachal remnants persisting in the urinary bladder vertex after birth are usually clinically silent; however, macroscopic diverticula may develop at the bladder vertex of cats (and possibly dogs) with microscopic urachal remnants following the onset of concurrent but unrelated acquired diseases of the lower urinary tract (i.e., bacterial cystitis, urolithiasis, crystalline-matrix urethral plugs, and idiopathic disease) (Lulich et al, 1989; Osborne et al, 1989). Vesicourachal diverticula are best identified by positive-contrast or double-contrast cystography or by excretory urography. Survey abdominal radiographs and pneumocystography are inconsistent in identifying diverticula. Surgical management may be indicated for any of the urachal anomalies. Many macroscopic diverticula of cats (and possibly dogs) are, however, self-limiting after amelioration of clinical signs of lower urinary tract disease.

Duplication

Complete or partial duplication of the urinary bladder, with or without concomitant duplication of the urethra, is a rare congenital disorder of dogs (Hoskins et al, 1982; Longhofer et al, 1991). Similar anomalies have not been reported in cats. Clinical signs usually develop early in life and include dysuria, urinary incontinence, and abdominal distention. Anomalies involving duplication of the urinary bladder are amenable to surgical correction; however, prognosis is guarded and depends on the degree of

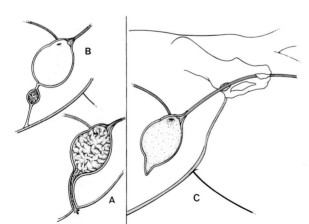

Figure 17–4. Congenital urachal anomalies. **A,** Persistent urachus. **A,** Persistent urachus. **B,** Urachal cyst. **C,** Vesicourachal diverticulum. (From Osborne CA, Johnston GR, Kruger JM, et al: Etiopathogenesis and biological behavior of feline vesicourachal diverticula. Vet Clin North Am Small Anim Pract 17:697, 1987.)

malformation and the presence of other concurrent anomalies.

Colourocystic Fistula

Communication between the urinary bladder and colon is a rare congenital defect that has been observed in a 5-week-old male domestic short-haired cat (Lawler and Monti, 1984). Colourocystic fistulas potentially predispose animals to urinary tract infections and urinary incontinence. Surgery design to obliterate the fistula without compromising the urinary bladder and colonic function would be of potential benefit.

Ectopic Uterine Horns Entering the Urinary Bladder

A 9-month-old female domestic short-haired cat with both uterine horns terminating into the urinary bladder has been reported (Jones, 1983). Clinical signs relating to this anomaly included dysuria, hematuria, and urinary incontinence.

Primary Neoplasia

Neoplasms of the urinary bladder are uncommon in puppies and kittens (Caywood et al, 1980a). Botryoid rhabdomyosarcomas are, however, commonly seen in young large-breed dogs younger than 18 months of age (Kelly, 1973). Botryoid rhabdomyosarcomas are embryonic mesenchymal tumors believed to arise from pluripotent stem cells originating from primitive urogenital ridge remnants (Snyder et al, 1992). These neoplasms are infiltrating tumors that arise from the trigone and project into the bladder lumen as botryoid (resembling a cluster of grapes) masses. Primary clinical signs of botryoid rhabdomyosarcomas include hematuria, dysuria, and stranguria and may be accompanied by secondary signs associated with urethral obstruction and/or hypertrophic osteoarthropathy. In dogs, botryoid rhabdomyosarcomas are locally invasive; however, distant metastases appear to be uncommon. Surgical resection alone has been reported to result in only short-term remissions of 3 months or younger (Kelly, 1973; Stamps and Harris, 1968). We observed long-term (greater than 5-year) remission in an 8-month-old male golden retriever, however, after radical surgical excision and ureteral transplantation. A partial response to combination chemotherapy utilizing doxorubicin, cyclophosphamide, and vincristine sulfate was observed in a female Doberman with local recurrence and distant metastases after surgical excision (Van Vechten et al, 1990).

CONGENITAL AND HEREDITARY ANOMALIES OF THE URETHRA
Aplasia and Hypoplasia

Urethral aplasia is a rare congenital anomaly characterized by complete absence of a patent urethra. Urethral aplasia and urinary bladder aplasia have been reported in a 4-month-old female mixed-breed dog with a life-long history of urinary incontinence (Pearson and Gibbs, 1971). In this case, both ureters were ectopic and terminated on the floor of the vagina. Urethral hypoplasia resulting in urinary incontinence has been described in immature female domestic short-haired cats (Holt and Gibbs, 1992). Early in life, cats with urethral hypoplasia typically develop severe urinary incontinence, which is most pronounced when the animal is recumbent or sleeping. Diagnosis is based on clinical signs and retrograde contrast vaginourethrography. Radiographic features include marked urethral shortening and vaginal aplasia. Urethral hypoplasia may be accompanied by other urogenital anomalies and is frequently complicated by urinary tract infection. Urinary incontinence may be resolved by surgical reconstruction of the bladder neck.

Urethrorectal Fistula

Most urethrorectal fistulas in puppies and kittens appear to be congenital (Osborne, 1977; Van Den Broek et al, 1988). Male puppies appear to be affected more frequently than female puppies, and there is an apparent breed predilection for English bulldogs. Breed or sex predispositions have not been reported in kittens. Abnormal urination patterns, usually observed early in life, are characterized by simultaneous passage of urine from the anus and the penis (male) or vulva (female) during micturition. Diagnosis is based on clinical signs and identification of a urethrorectal fistula by antegrade or retrograde contrast urethrography or retrograde colonography. Clinical signs are usually controlled by fistulectomy and eradication of secondary urinary tract infections.

Urethrogenital Malformations

Urinary incontinence is a common clinical manifestation of urethrogenital malformations in puppies and kittens associated with diseases of intersexuality, especially pseudohermaphroditism (Bredal et al, 1997; Holt et al, 1983). Urinary incontinence most likely is due to retention of urine in anomalous communications between the urethra and the genital tract and subsequent passive leakage of urine to the exterior. Diagnosis is based on history, physical examination, and contrast radiography (retrograde contrast urethrography and excretory urography). Urinary incontinence and pseudohermaphroditism may be reversible after surgical correction of urethrovaginal malformations.

Hypospadias

Hypospadias is an uncommon anomaly affecting predominantly male puppies and is characterized by ventral malposition of the urethral meatus (Áder and Hobson, 1978; Hayes and Wilson, 1986). Etiologic factors in puppies with hypospadias are unknown; however, the high prevalence of hypospadias in Boston terriers may suggest a genetic basis in some cases. Affected dogs are of variable age and may be asymptomatic or develop clinical signs of urinary incontinence, periurethral dermatitis, or recurrent urinary tract infection. Diagnosis is based on physical examination. The presence of an os penis in male dogs precludes surgical reconstruction in most cases; however, scrotal or perineal urethrostomy, combined with castration and removal of vestigial preputial and penile tissues, may be of cosmetic value.

Duplication

Duplication of the urethra is an uncommon congenital anomaly that has been encountered in puppies, but not kittens (Johnston et al, 1989; Longhofer et al, 1991; Wolf and Radecky, 1973). Complete urethral duplication occurs in both males and females and may be associated with concurrent duplication of descending colon, rectum, urinary bladder, vagina, and vulva in females and penis in males and with other urogenital anomalies (unilateral renal hypoplasia, bilateral cryptorchidism). Diagnosis is based on physical examination, contrast radiography, and exploratory celiotomy. Anomalies of urethral duplication may, in some cases, be amenable to surgical excerptation of the duplicated structure. Surgical reconstruction has rarely, however, been attempted in cases involving extensive duplication.

Ectopia

Urethral ectopia is a rare congenital anomaly characterized by abnormal position of the external urethral orifice. Clinical signs depend on the site of termination of the abnormal urethra and other urogenital anomalies. Life-long urinary incontinence was the predominant clinical feature in a 21-month-old female English bulldog with an ectopic urethra terminating in the cranial vagina and concurrent unilateral ectopia (Osborne and Hanlon, 1967). In contrast, a 2-month-old female domestic short-haired cat with an ectopic urethra terminating in the ventral rectum did not have urinary incontinence but did void urine through the anus (Lulich et al, 1987).

Prolapse

Prolapse of the mucosal lining of the distal portion of the urethra through the external urethral orifice occurs primarily in young male dogs 4 months to 5 years of age (Osborne and Sanderson, 1995). There is an apparent predilection for brachycephalic breeds, especially English bulldogs and Boston terriers. Diagnosis of urethral prolapse is based on characteristic historical and physical examination findings. The condition is usually recognized because of bleeding from the prolapsed urethra independent of micturition and intermittent or persistent licking of the penis. Treatment of urethral prolapse has traditionally involved surgery (Sinibaldi and Green, 1973). Clinical observations, however, suggest that, in some cases, urethral prolapse may be associated with only minor clinical signs or may be asymptomatic.

ACQUIRED DISORDERS OF THE URINARY TRACT
Renal Dysfunction
OVERVIEW

In our experience, acquired disorders are the most common cause of renal dysfunction in puppies and kittens. Causes of acquired renal dysfunction in immature animals are similar to those encountered in adults and may include infectious, inflammatory, toxic, ischemic, or neoplastic disease processes.

GLOMERULOPATHIES

Like their familial and congenital counterparts, acquired glomerulopathies are characterized by morphologic and/or functional alteration of glomeruli that, if progressive, may induce subsequent changes in renal tubules, interstitium, and blood vessels resulting in chronic generalized renal dysfunction (Brown, 1995). Acquired glomerulopathies usually develop secondary to systemic disorders in which the underlying disease processes damage not only the glomeruli but other major organs as well. Acquired glomerulopathies are infrequently encountered in young dogs and cats (Table 17–8) (Lulich et al, 1987; MacDougall et al, 1986). Diagnosis is based on clinical and laboratory evaluations similar to those described for familial glomerulopathies. Unlike familial disease, however, glomerulopathies acquired secondary to systemic disorders are potentially reversible. Identification and elimination of the primary disease process may halt progression of glomerular injury and, in some cases, result in its remission.

ACUTE TUBULAR NECROSIS

Acute tubular necrosis (acute intrinsic renal failure, nephrosis, vasomotor nephropathy) is a syndrome characterized by abrupt and sustained reductions in GFR associated with acute tubular degeneration (Grauer and Lane, 1995; Maxie and Prescott, 1993). Acute tubular necrosis is believed to result from a combination of vascular and tubular effects induced by renal hypo-perfusion (ischemia) or nephrotoxins. Acute tubular necrosis is a common cause of acquired renal dysfunction in young dogs and cats (see Table 17–8) (Kruger et al, 1995). Any condition predisposing to persistent or severe hypotension, hypovolemia, circulatory collapse, or renal hypoperfusion may induce acute tubular necrosis and renal failure (Grauer and Lane, 1995). We observed ischemia-induced acute tubular necrosis in a 7-day-old beagle puppy associated with respiratory arrest after aspiration of food. More commonly, acute tubular necrosis is associated with exposure to nephrotoxins (i.e., ethylene glycol; antimicrobial agents; radiographic contrast agents; heavy metals such as arsenic, mercury, lead, and zinc; plants such as Easter lily; herbicides; and nonsteroidal antiinflammatory drugs such as ibuprofen, phenylbutazone, and acetaminophen) (Grauer and Lane, 1995). Analgesic-induced acute renal failure was observed in two kittens after administration of a single dose of 25 to 50 mg of ibuprofen. Both kittens recovered after symptomatic and supportive care.

Clinical signs associated with acute tubular necrosis are variable and depend on the degree of renal parenchymal damage and extent of multisystem involvement. Mild nephrotoxic or ischemic renal injury is often self-limiting, and animals may be asymptomatic. Transient proteinuria, hematuria, pyuria, and abnormal num-

Table 17–8. Acquired Renal Disorders Identified in 36 Puppies and 15 Kittens Evaluated at Michigan State University*		NO. PUPPIES (%)	NO. KITTENS (%)
LOCATION	**LESION OR CLINICAL SYNDROME**		
Glomerular	Proliferative glomerulopathy	0	1 (7)
	Mesangioproliferative glomerulopathy	2 (5.5)	0
Tubular	Acute tubular necrosis	8 (22)	2 (13)
	Acute papillary necrosis	0	2 (13)
Tubulointerstitial	Acute interstitial nephritis	0	1 (7)
	Acute suppurative interstitial nephritis	2 (5.5)†	2 (13)†
	Pyogranulomatous nephritis	0	2 (13)‡
	Necrogranulomatous nephritis	0	1 (7)
	Pyelonephritis	10 (28)†	0
	Hypercalcemic nephropathy	1 (3)	0
	Chronic tubulointerstitial nephropathy	8 (22)	0
Unknown	Acute renal failure	3 (8)	3 (20)§
	Chronic renal failure	1 (3)	1 (7)
	Renal hemorrhage (trauma)	1 (3)	0

*Cases evaluated at the Michigan State University Veterinary Clinical Center and Animal Health Diagnostic Laboratory (1987 to 1993).
†Bacteria identified as the etiopathogenic agent.
‡Feline infectious peritonitis virus identified as the etiopathogenic agent.
§History of ibuprofen exposure in two of three cases.

ber of casts may be observed in urine sediment. In moderate to severe acute tubular necrosis, clinical signs characteristic of acute oliguric or nonoliguric renal failure and uremia are usually present. A diagnosis of toxic or ischemic acute tubular necrosis is based on history, physical examination, and laboratory findings. Treatment of acute tubular necrosis should be designed to eliminate or correct the specific cause if it is known. In cases of moderate to severe injury associated with acute renal failure, symptomatic and supportive therapy designed to minimize abnormalities in fluid, electrolyte, acid-base, and nutritional balance may allow life to be sustained until the body can restore adequate renal structure and functions.

TUBULOINTERSTITIAL DISEASES

Renal tubulointerstitial diseases include disorders such as acute generalized nephritis, chronic tubulointerstitial nephropathy, pyelonephritis, and hypercalcemic nephropathy (Maxie and Prescott, 1991). In our experience, tubulointerstitial diseases are the most common type of renal disease observed in young dogs and cats (see Table 17–8) (Kruger et al, 1995). Acute generalized nephritis refers to acute inflammatory diseases of the kidney that are characterized by interstitial inflammatory cell infiltrates, edema, and focal tubular degeneration (Finco and Brown, 1995). Acute generalized nephritis may be caused by systemic bacterial infections (e.g., bacterial endocarditis, bacterial septicemia, leptospirosis), systemic viral infection (e.g., canine herpesvirus, feline infectious peritonitis virus), immunologic disorders (e.g., systemic lupus erythematosus), and drugs (e.g., methicillin) (Finco and Brown, 1995; Maxie and Prescott, 1991). Systemic bacterial infections and feline infectious peritonitis virus were the most common etiologic agents identified in our series of puppies and kittens with acute nephritis (see Table 17–8) (Kruger et al, 1995). Clinical and laboratory abnormalities are indicative of acute renal failure and are indistinguishable from those associated with nephrotoxic or ischemic acute tubular necrosis. Diagnostic and therapeutic efforts should be directed at identifying and eliminating the primary cause in addition to providing supportive therapy for renal failure.

Chronic tubulointerstitial nephropathy is characterized by abnormally small, misshapen, irregular kidneys and microscopic findings of interstitial fibrosis, tubular atrophy, and mononuclear cell infiltration of the renal parenchyma (Finco and Brown, 1995). Kidneys affected by more advanced forms of chronic tubulointerstitial nephropathy are often referred to as "end-stage kidneys." In many cases, the underlying cause cannot be identified or localized to any particular portion of the nephron. In our experience, chronic tubulointerstitial nephropathy appears to be more common in young dogs than in young cats (see Table 17–8) (Kruger et al, 1995). Clinical findings of chronic tubulointerstitial nephropathy depend on the degree of renal injury and the severity of renal dysfunction. Animals with advanced disease usually present with clinical and laboratory findings characteristic of chronic renal failure and uremia and are indistinguishable from those caused by many congenital nephropathies. Histologic evaluation of renal biopsy samples may help differentiate chronic tubulointerstitial nephropathy from congenital forms of renal disease. Treatment is limited to symptomatic and supportive care (Polzin and Osborne, 1995a).

PYELONEPHRITIS

Pyelonephritis is the consequence of ascending bacterial urinary tract infections (Crowell et al, 1995). Congenital or acquired abnormalities of the urinary tract that compromise host defenses may represent important predisposing factors in the pathogenesis of pyelonephritis (Table 17–9). Urinary stasis or obstruction, vesicoureteral reflux, and anatomic abnormalities of the ureter or vesicoureteral junction are potentially important predisposing factors in young animals (Crowell et al, 1995). Pyelonephritis is a major cause of renal disease in young animals, especially puppies. In our series, pyelonephritis was the most common cause of renal disease in dogs younger than 6 months (see Table 17–8) (Kruger et al, 1995). In contrast, pyelonephritis was not diagnosed in any kitten during the same period. These observations may reflect the relatively high incidence of vesicoureteral reflux in young dogs and/or less effective host urinary tract defenses in dogs compared with cats. Bacterial infections of the kidney may be acute or chronic and focal or disseminated (Maxie and Prescott, 1991). Animals with advanced chronic generalized pyelonephritis typically have small, scarred kidneys, similar in gross appearance to those of animals with advanced chronic tubulointerstitial nephropathy.

Clinical findings associated with pyelonephritis depend on the degree of renal involvement and the duration of infection (Crowell et al, 1995). Acute generalized pyelonephritis may be associated with varying degrees of pyrexia,

Table 17–9	Host Defense Abnormalities Predisposing Immature Dogs and Cats to Complicating Bacterial Urinary Tract Infections

Altered Anatomic Barriers
Congenital
    Ectopic ureters
    Ureteroceles
    Ureteral duplication
    Urachal anomalies
    Exstrophy
    Colocystic fistula
    Urethrovaginal malformations
    Ectopic urethra
    Urethral duplication
    Urethral hypoplasia
    Epispadias/hypospadias
Acquired
    Urethrostomy
    Urethral stricture

Urine Retention
Urethral obstruction (partial or complete)
    Uroliths
    Urethral matrix-crystalline plugs
    Urethral stricture
    Ureterocele
    Neoplasia
Urachal diverticula
Detrusor atony or hypotony
    Spinal trauma
    Spinal dysraphism
    Chronic overdistention
    Dysautonomia

Damage to Urothelium
Trauma
    Palpation
    Catheterization
    Lavage
    Urolithiasis
Inflammation
Neoplasia

Altered Urine Volume or Composition
Decreased urine osmolality
    Renal failure
    Nephrogenic diabetes insipitus
    Postobstructive diuresis
    Fluid therapy
    Diuretic administration
    Urinary bladder lavage
Decreased urine volume
    Negative water balance
        Decreased water consumption
        Dehydration
    Primary oliguric renal failure
Glucosuria

Impaired Immune Responsiveness
Immunosuppressive drug administration
Congenital immunodeficiency
Uremia

lethargy, anorexia, vomiting, renal pain, leukocytosis, bacteriuria, pyuria, and casts. Finding white blood cell casts with bacteriuria is strongly suggestive of bacterial pyelonephritis. Manifestations of chronic generalized pyelonephritis are often subtle but may include polyuria, polydipsia, isosthenuria, recurrent asymptomatic bacteriuria, or recurrent urethrocystitis. If generalized involvement of both kidneys occurs, clinical signs and laboratory findings associated with renal failure may be present. A diagnosis of pyelonephritis is based on history, physical examination, and results of laboratory evaluations (complete blood count, serum biochemistries, urinalysis, quantitative urine culture) and radiographic or ultrasonographic studies. Treatment of bacterial pyelonephritis consists of antimicrobial therapy and the elimination of predisposing factors. Because eradication of bacteria from the kidney may be difficult, antimicrobial therapy is usually continued for 4 to 6 weeks (Crowell et al, 1995). In uremic animals, supportive therapy for renal failure should be provided.

Infection

Urinary tract infection (UTI) encompasses a variety of clinical entities whose common denominator is microbial invasion of any or all of its components. Bacteria are the most common uropathogen encountered in puppies and kittens, but UTI may also result from colonization of the urinary tract by mycoplasmas, ureaplasmas, fungi, viruses, and algae (Table 17–10). An uncomplicated UTI is one in which no underlying structural, neurologic, or functional abnormality can be identified. Complicated UTI occurs as a result of microbial invasion of the urinary system secondary to identifiable abnormalities that interfere with normal host defense mechanisms (see Table 17–9). Review of hospital records at the Michigan State University Veterinary Teaching Hospital revealed that over a 5-year period, UTIs were identified in 15 dogs and 1 cat younger than 6 months.

Our observations suggest that bacterial UTI is a common cause of urinary tract disease in dogs of all ages. In contrast, primary bacterial

Table 17–10	Canine and Feline Uropathogens

Bacteria	Fungi
Rods and cocci	*Candida* spp
Escherichia coli	*Torulopsis**
Staphylococcus spp	*Histoplasma*
Streptococcus spp	*Blastomyces**
Proteus spp	*Cryptococcus*
Klebsiella spp	*Coccidioides**
Pseudomonas spp	*Aspergillus* spp
Enterobacter spp	*Trichosporon* spp†
Pasteurella spp	*Cephalosporium*†
Others	Viruses
Spirochetes	Canine adenovirus 1*
Leptospira interrogans	Canine herpesvirus*
Rickettsia	Canine distemper virus*
Ehrlichia canis*	Feline calicivirus†‡
Rickettsia rickettsii*	Feline syncytia-forming virus†‡
Mycoplasmas	Feline immunodeficiency virus†‡
Mycoplasma spp*	Bovine herpesvirus 4†‡
Ureaplasma spp*	Parasites
Algae	*Capillaria* spp
Prototheca spp*	*Dioctophyma renale*

*Not reported in cats.
†Not reported in dogs.
‡Pathogenic role in feline urinary tract disease is uncertain.

UTIs are uncommon causes of urinary tract disease in kittens or adult cats younger than 10 years of age (Kruger et al, 1991). Over a 5-year period, we did not observe primary bacterial UTI in a cat younger than 6 months. A staphylococcal UTI was, however, observed in a 5-month-old domestic short-haired male cat after urethral catheterization for relief of urethral obstruction due to a matrix-crystalline urethral plug. Clinical manifestations of UTI are similar regardless of causative agent and are often indistinguishable from noninfectious causes. Bacterial UTIs confined to the lower urinary tract (urinary bladder and urethra) are typically associated with clinical signs of dysuria and pollakiuria and with urinalysis findings of pyuria, hematuria, and proteinuria (Osborne and Lees, 1995). Signs characteristic of upper urinary tract involvement depend on the degree of renal parenchymal involvement and duration of the disease. Other potential sequelae of bacterial UTI include septicemia, discospondylitis, chronic renal failure, urinary incontinence, and urinary obstruction due to formation of uroliths or matrix-crystalline urethral plugs. Most struvite uroliths in dogs and up to 10% of struvite uroliths in cats develop as a consequence of bacterial UTI with urease-producing microorganisms (Osborne et al, 1995b).

Establishing a diagnosis of bacterial UTI depends on routine laboratory evaluation consisting of urinalysis and quantitative urine culture. Although urinalysis findings of hematuria, pyuria, proteinuria, and bacteriuria are consistent with bacterial infection, caution must be used in establishing a diagnosis of bacterial UTI on the basis of urinalysis alone. The constellation of hematuria, pyuria, and proteinuria are nonspecific findings indicative of urinary tract inflammation that may result from infectious or noninfectious causes of urinary tract disease. Observation of bacteria in urine sediment is suggestive, but not conclusive, evidence for establishing a diagnosis of bacterial UTI. Use of quantitative urine cultures have largely circumvented problems of interpreting urine sediment findings and provide the most definitive means of confirming and characterizing bacterial UTI (Table 17–11) (Osborne and Lees, 1995).

Because most puppies and kittens with significant bacteriuria have a secondary UTI, survey and contrast radiography, ultrasonography, exfoliative cytology of urine sediment, and biopsy of urinary tract tissues may be of value for identifying predisposing factors. Antimicrobial agents remain the cornerstone of therapy for a bacterial UTI. Because compromised host defense mechanisms are extremely important factors in the pathogenesis of UTIs in puppies, identification and correction of the abnormali-

Table 17–11	Interpretation of Quantitative Urine Cultures in Dogs and Cats*					
COLLECTION METHOD	SIGNIFICANT		SUSPICIOUS		CONTAMINANT	
	Dog	Cat	Dog	Cat	Dog	Cat
Cystocentesis	10^3†	10^3	10^2 to 10^3	10^2 to 10^3	10^2	10^2
Catheterization	10^4	10^3	10^3 to 10^4	10^2 to 10^3	10^3	10^2
Voluntary voiding	10^5‡	10^4‡	10^4 to 9×10^4	10^3 to 10^4	10^4	10^3
Manual compression	10^5‡	10^4‡	10^4 to 9×10^4	10^3 to 10^4	10^4	10^3

*The data represent generalities. On occasion, a bacterial urinary tract infection may be detected in dogs and cats with fewer numbers of organisms (i.e., false-negative results).

†Numbers represent numbers of bacteria per milliliter of urine.

‡Caution: Contamination of midstream samples may result in colony counts of 10^5/ml or greater in some dogs and counts of 10^4/ml or greater in some cats (i.e., false-positive results).

ties are necessary prerequisites of successful long-term treatment. Once the causative agent is identified, antimicrobial agents should be selected on the basis of bacterial culture and susceptibility tests, safety, and potential expense. We emphasize that drug absorption, metabolism, and excretion may be substantially different in puppies and kittens compared with adults (Table 17–12) (Boothe and Tannert, 1992). Antimicrobial agents and dosing schedules routinely used in the treatment of UTIs in adults may be associated with serious adverse reactions or apparent therapeutic failures when empirically used for puppies and kittens (Table 17–13). Because of their safety, wide therapeutic index, and ability to achieve high urine concentrations, β-lactam antibiotics (i.e., penicillin, ampicillin, amoxicillin-clavulanic acid, and cephalosporins)

| Table 17–12 | Factors Affecting Drug Disposition in Immature Dogs and Cats |

Absorption
  Decreased or irregular gastrointestinal motility
  Increased intestinal permeability (neonates)
  Increased gastric pH
  Decreased muscle mass and blood flow

Distribution
  Larger volume of distribution
    Increased percentage of total body water
    Increased percentage of extracellular water
  Decreased plasma protein concentrations
  Decreased body fat

Metabolism and Excretion
  Decreased hepatic metabolism
  Decreased renal function
    Lower glomerular filtration rate
    Reduced renal blood flow
    Decreased renal tubular function

are recommended. Urine should be recultured 3 to 5 days after initiation of therapy to confirm sterilization of urine. Antimicrobial therapy should be continued until there is clinical and laboratory evidence of response as determined by clinical signs, urinalysis, and bacterial culture.

Mycoplasma and *Ureaplasma* organisms have been associated with naturally occurring or experimentally induced urinary tract disease in humans, dogs, sheep, and rats (Kruger and Osborne, 1993). In our experience, *Mycoplasma* UTIs in dogs younger than 6 months have been opportunistic infections that have invariably occurred as a sequela to preexisting lower urinary tract disease. The UTI is often preceded by indwelling urinary catheterization and administration of β-lactam antimicrobial agents. In two cases, *Mycoplasma* UTIs were associated with clinical signs of lower urinary tract disease (dysuria, urinary incontinence, and pyuria), which resolved after appropriate antimicrobial therapy. Although *Mycoplasma* and *Ureaplasma* organisms have been isolated from the genitourinary tract of cats, their role as causative agents in feline urinary tract disease is uncertain. Diagnosis of *Ureaplasma* or *Mycoplasma* UTIs requires isolation of the organisms from suitable urine or tissue samples. *Mycoplasma* and *Ureaplasma* organisms are fragile and fastidious with exacting growth requirements, which may vary considerably among *Mycoplasma* species. Successful recovery and identification of these organisms requires careful collection and transport of specimens and use of appropriate growth media and specific cultivation methods. Because many laboratories are not prepared to culture *Mycoplasma* and *Ureaplasma*, it is advisable to consult with laboratory staff for specific recommendations before collection and submission of samples.

Table 17–13 Antimicrobial Agents Available for Therapy of Urinary Tract Infection in Immature Dogs and Cats

ANTIMICROBIAL	METABOLISM/ ROUTE OF ELIMINATION	TOXICITY AND ADVERSE REACTIONS	THERAPEUTIC RECOMMENDATIONS
Penicillin G	Renal	Low toxicity	Parenteral routes preferred for neonates*; consider higher dose and longer intervals for patients <3 mo
Ampicillin/ amoxicillin	Renal	Low toxicity; may alter GI flora	Parenteral routes preferred for neonates*; consider higher dose and longer intervals for patients <3 mo
Amoxicillin- clavulanic acid	Renal	Low toxicity; may alter GI flora	Consider higher dose and longer intervals for patient <3 mo
Cephalosporins Cefadroxil (1st gen) Cefoxitin (2nd gen)† Ceftiofur (3rd gen)† Others†	Renal	Low toxicity; interaction with aminoglycosides?	Parenteral routes preferred for neonates*; consider higher dose and longer intervals for patients <3 mo
Fluoroquinolones Enrofloxacin Ciprofloxacin†	Renal; hepatic	Erosion of articular cartilage in dogs and cats <8 mo	Avoid prolonged high-dose therapy; consider lower dose and longer intervals for patients <5 mo
Trimethoprim- sulfadiazine	Renal; hepatic	KCS; hepatitis; anemia; leukopenia; pyrexia, polyarthritis	Consider lower dose and longer intervals for patients <5 mo
Aminoglycosides Gentamicin Amikacin†	Renal	Nephrotoxic; ototoxic; toxicity potentiated by pyrexia, dehydration, sepsis, furosemide, potassium depletion, and possibly by cephalosporins and NSAIDs	Avoid if possible; consider higher dose and longer interval; therapeutic drug monitoring recommended
Tetracyclines Tetracycline Oxytetracycline Doxycycline†	Renal; hepatic	Anabolic; chelate calcium; inhibit bone and enamel formation; discoloration of teeth; may alter GI flora	Avoid for patients <5 mo
Chloramphenicol	Hepatic	Dose-dependent bone marrow suppression	Avoid for patients <5 mo

GI = gastrointestinal; gen = generation; KCS = keratoconjunctivitis sicca; NSAIDs = nonsteroidal antiinflammatory drugs.
*Avoid intramuscular route because of small muscle mass and reduced blood flow in puppies and kittens.
†Not approved for use in dogs or cats in United States.

Urolithiasis

Urolithiasis may result from multiple congenital and/or acquired physiologic and pathologic processes (Osborne et al, 1995b). Thus, urolithiasis should not be conceived of as a single disease but rather as a sequela of one or more underlying abnormalities. Although urolithiasis tends to be a disease of middle to older aged animals, 1.6% of canine and 1.3% of feline uroliths analyzed at the Minnesota Urolith Center were obtained from animals 11 months of age or younger. Most urolith mineral types observed in adults have been encountered in puppies and kittens (Tables 17–14 and 17–15). Struvite, however, was the most common urolith mineral type identified, comprising approximately 65% of total uroliths analyzed. In our experience, most struvite uroliths encountered in immature animals have been induced by bacterial UTI with urease-producing microorganisms (Lulich et al, 1989).

Table
17–14

Table 17–14 Age Distribution of 391 Immature Dogs with Uroliths*

AGE (MONTHS)	Struvite	Calcium Oxalate	Calcium Apatite	Calcium Carb-Apat	Tricalcium Phosphate	Brushite	Uric Acid	Ammonium Urate	Sodium Urate	Xanthine	Cystine	Silica	Mixed‡	Compounds§	Other	TOTAL
≤1	15		1	2		1	1	1					1	1	1	24
1 < age ≤2	76	4	2	2			3	4					7	6		105
2 < age ≤3	40		1		1			4					1	4		50
3 < age ≤4	20		2					3					2	1		28
4 < age ≤5	10							6					1	2		19
5 < age ≤6	20							8	1		2			2		33
6 < age ≤7	12							3						1		18
7 < age ≤8	18	1	1					9			1		2			33
8 < age ≤9	11							10			1		3			22
9 < age ≤10	20	2						10					2	2		36
10 < age ≤11	13							9			1					23
Total	255	7	7	4	1	1	4	67	1	0	5	0	19	19	1	391

Carb-Apat = carbonate-apatite.

*Data from the University of Minnesota Urolith Center. Analyses performed by optical crystallography and x-ray diffraction.

†Urolith composed of 70% to 99% of mineral type listed.

‡Urolith contained less than 70% of predominant mineral; no nucleus or shell was detected.

§Urolith contained an identifiable nucleus and one or more surrounding layers of a different mineral.

Table 17–15 Age Distribution of 64 Immature Cats with Uroliths*

AGE (MONTHS)	MINERAL TYPE†															
	Struvite	Calcium Oxalate	Calcium Apatite	Calcium Carb-Apat	Tricalcium Phosphate	Brushite	Uric Acid	Ammonium Urate	Sodium Urate	Xanthine	Cystine	Silica	Mixed‡	Compounds§	Other	TOTAL
≤1	1															1
1 < age ≤2	4															4
2 < age ≤3	8	1											1			10
3 < age ≤4	7															7
4 < age ≤5	4	1		1				2			1					9
5 < age ≤6	4							1								5
6 < age ≤7	6		1					1								8
7 < age ≤8	3		1											1	2	7
8 < age ≤9	3							4		1						8
9 < age ≤10								1							1	2
10 < age ≤11	2														1	3
TOTAL	42	2	2	1	0	0	0	9	0	1	1	0	1	1	4	64

Carb-Apat = carbonate-apatite.
*Data from the University of Minnesota Urolith Center. Analyses performed by optical crystallography and x-ray diffraction.
†Urolith composed of 70% to 99% of mineral type listed.
‡Urolith contained less than 70% of predominant mineral; no nucleus or shell was detected.
§Urolith contained an identifiable nucleus and one or more surrounding layers of a different mineral.

Infection-induced struvite (magnesium ammonium phosphate) uroliths develop as a consequence of bacterial UTI with urease-producing microorganisms (especially staphylococci) (Osborne et al, 1995b). Clinical manifestations of urolithiasis vary and depend on (1) urolith number, location, size, shape, and surface characteristics; (2) local and systemic effects of underlying disease processes; and (3) presence of sequelae (UTI and urinary obstruction) (Osborne et al, 1995b). Most struvite uroliths are located in the urinary bladder and/or urethra and are typically associated with lower urinary tract signs. Uroliths located in the bladder neck or urethra may cause partial or complete urine outflow obstruction and signs of obstructive uropathy. Uroliths are usually suspected on the basis of characteristic findings obtained by history and physical examination. We emphasize, however, that most uroliths are not reliably detected by abdominal palpation. Urinalysis, urine culture, and radiography may be required to differentiate uroliths from other causes of congenital or acquired lower urinary tract disease (Table 17–16). Once urolithiasis has been confirmed, follow-up evaluation is essential to characterize the extent of disease and to identify predisposing abnormalities. Because quantitative stone analysis provides the most definitive diagnostic, prognostic, and therapeutic information, any uroliths removed or recovered from the urinary tract should be quantitatively analyzed to determine their mineral composition (Osborne et al, 1995b).

Objectives of management of infection-induced struvite urolithiasis include (1) relief of obstruction to urine outflow when necessary, (2) elimination of existing uroliths, (3) eradication or control of UTI, and (4) prevention of recurrence of uroliths (Osborne et al, 1995b). Surgery has been the traditional approach for management of all types of uroliths, especially in young dogs and cats. The combined use of short-term calculolytic diets (Prescription Diet Canine s/d, Hill's Pet Products) and antimicrobial agents has, however, successfully induced dissolution of urocystoliths presumed to be infection-induced struvite in immature dogs (Lulich et al, 1989). Despite the feasibility of medical dissolution of struvite uroliths in immature dogs and cats, consumption of calculolytic diets is associated with potential hazards. If initiated, calculolytic diets should not be given for more than approximately 4 weeks, and animals should be monitored carefully for evidence of nutritional deficiencies (especially protein malnutrition). Although a calculolytic diet designed to

Table 17–16	Problem-Specific Database for Urolithiasis in Immature Dogs and Cats

I. Medical history
   A. Note age, sex, and breed
   B. Note diet and use of supplements or drugs
   C. Note changes in micturition and/or character of urine
   D. Note if uroliths have been voided
II. Physical examination
   A. Palpate kidneys for number, size, shape, position, consistency, and pain
   B. Palpate urinary bladder for size, shape, consistency, position, and grating or nongrating masses
   C. Palpate urethra per rectum for size, shape, and urethral or periurethral masses
III. Complete urinalysis
IV. Quantitative urine culture
V. Complete blood count
VI. Serum biochemistries
   A. Urea nitrogen and creatinine concentrations
   B. Total protein and albumin concentrations
   C. Hepatic enzyme activities
VII. Survey abdominal radiographs
VIII. Characterize urinary tract abnormalities
   A. Urinary tract ultrasonography
   B. Consider excretory urography
   C. Consider contrast cystography
IX. Bladder or kidney biopsy during cystotomy or nephrotomy
X. Postsurgical survey abdominal radiographs
XI. Quantitative stone analysis

dissolve feline struvite uroliths (Prescription Diet Feline s/d, Hill's Pet Products) is not protein restricted, its use by immature cats may be associated with development of metabolic acidosis, anorexia, and dehydration (Osborne et al, 1995b). Eradication and/or control of UTI caused by urease-producing bacteria is the single most important factor in preventing recurrence of most infection-induced struvite uroliths. Because most bacterial UTIs in immature animals are associated with abnormal host defenses, identification and elimination of predisposing factors are essential for long-term prevention.

References and Supplemental Reading

Ader PL, Hobson HP: Hypospadias: A review of the veterinary literature and a report of three cases in the dog. J Am Anim Hosp Assoc 14:721, 1978.

Arant BS, Edelmann CM, Nash MA: The renal reabsorption of glucose in the development of canine kidney: A study of glomerulotubular balance. Pediatr Res 8:638, 1974.

Bauer SB, Perlmutter AD, Retik AB: Anomalies of the upper urinary tract. *In* Walsh PC, Retik AB, Stamey TA, et al (eds): Campbell's Urology, 6th ed. Philadelphia, WB Saunders, 1992, p 1357.

Bloedow AG: Familal renal disease in Samoyed dog. Vet Rec 108:167, 1981.

Boothe DM, Tannert K: Special considerations for drug and fluid therapy in the pediatric patient. Compend Contin Educ Pract Vet 14:313, 1992.

Bovée KC: Genetic and metabolic diseases of the kidney. *In* Bovée KC (ed): Canine Nephrology. Philadelphia, Harwal Publishing, 1984, p 339.

Bovée KC, Jezyk PF, Segal SC: Postnatal development of renal tubular amino acid reabsorption in canine pups. Am J Vet Res 45:830, 1984.

Bovée KC, Joyce T, Blazer-Yost B, et al: Characterization of renal defects in dogs with a syndrome similar to the Fanconi syndrome in man. J Am Vet Med Assoc 174:1094, 1979.

Bowles MH, Mosier DA: Renal amyloidosis in a family of beagles. J Am Vet Med Assoc 201:569, 1992.

Bredal WP, Thoresen SI, Kvellestad A, et al: Male pseudohermaphroditism in a cat. J Small Anim Pract 38:21, 1997.

Breitschwerdt EB, Verlander JW, Hribernik TN: Nephrogenic diabetes insipidus in three dogs. J Am Vet Med Assoc 179:235, 1981.

Brown CA, Crowell WA, Brown SA, et al: Suspected familial renal disease in chow chows. J Am Vet Med Assoc 196:1279, 1990.

Brown SA: Fanconi's syndrome: inherited and acquired. *In* Kirk RW (ed): Current Veterinary Therapy X. Philadelphia: WB Saunders, 1989, p 1163.

Brown SA: Primary diseases of glomeruli. *In* Osborne CA, Finco DR (eds): Canine and Feline Nephrology and Urology. Baltimore, Williams & Wilkins, 1995, p 368.

Brown SA, Rakich PM, Barsanti JA, et al: Fanconi syndrome and acute renal failure associated with gentamicin therapy in a dog. J Am Anim Hosp Assoc 22:635, 1986.

Brownie CF, Tess MW, Prasad RD: Bilateral renal agenesis in two litters of Shetland sheepdogs. Vet Hum Toxicol 30:483, 1988.

Burrows AK, Malik R, Hunt GB, et al: Familial polycystic kidney disease in bull terriers. J Small Anim Pract 35:364, 1994.

Casal ML, Giger U, Bovee KC, et al: Inheritance of cystinuria and renal defect in Newfoundlands. J Am Vet Med Assoc 207:1585, 1995.

Case LC, Ling GV, Franti CE, et al: Cystine-containing urinary calculi in dogs: 102 cases (1981–1989). J Am Vet Med Assoc 201:127, 1992.

Caywood DD, Osborne CA, Johnston GR: Neoplasia of the canine and feline urinary tracts. *In* Kirk RW (ed): Current Veterinary Therapy VII. Philadelphia, WB Saunders, 1980a, p 1203.

Caywood DD, Osborne CA, Stevens JB, et al: Hy-

pertrophic osteoarthropathy associated with an atypical nephroblastoma in a dog. J Am Anim Hosp Assoc 16:855, 1980b.

Chew DJ, DiBartola SP, Boyce JT, et al: Juvenile renal disease in Doberman pinscher dogs. J Am Vet Med Assoc 182:481, 1982a.

Chew DJ, DiBartola SP, Boyce JT, et al: Renal amyloidosis in related Abyssinian cats. J Am Vet Med Assoc 181:139, 1982b.

Christie BA: Vesicoureteral reflux in dogs. J Am Vet Med Assoc 162:772, 1973.

Cook SM, Dean DF, Golden DL, et al: Renal failure attributable to atrophic glomerulopathy in four related Rottweilers. J Am Vet Med Assoc 202:107, 1993.

Cort JH, McLance RA: The renal response of puppies to an acidosis. J Physiol 124:358, 1954.

Crawford MA: The urinary system: *In* Hoskins JD (ed): Veterinary Pediatrics. Philadelphia, WB Saunders, 1990, p 271.

Crowell WA, Hubbell JJ, Riley JC: Polycystic renal disease in related cats. J Am Vet Med Assoc 175:286, 1979.

Crowell WA, Neuwirth L, Mahaffey MB: Pyelonephritis. In Osborne CA, Finco DR (eds): Canine and Feline Nephrology and Urology. Baltimore, Williams & Wilkins, 1995, p 484.

DiBartola SP, Chew DJ, Boyce JT: Juvenile renal disease in related standard poodles. J Am Vet Med Assoc 183:693, 1983.

DiBartola SP, Chew DJ, Horton ML: Cystinuria in a cat. J Am Vet Med Assoc 198:102, 1991.

DiBartola SP, Chew DJ, Jacobs G: Quantitative urinalysis including 24-hour protein excretion in the dog. J Am Anim Hosp Assoc 16:537, 1980.

DiBartola SP, Tarr MJ, Webb DM, et al: Familial renal amyloidosis in Chinese shar pei dogs. J Am Vet Med Assoc 197:483, 1990.

Easley JR, Breitschwerdt EB: Glucosuria associated with renal tubular dysfunction in three basenji dogs. J Am Vet Med Assoc 168:938, 1976.

Eaton KA, Biller DS, DiBartola SP, et al: Autosomal dominant polycystic kidney disease in Persian and Persian-cross cats. Vet Pathol 34:117, 1997.

Eriksen K, Grondalen J: Familial renal disease of soft-coated wheaten terriers. J Small Anim Pract 25:489, 1984.

Fettman MJ, Allen TA: Developmental aspects of fluid and electrolyte metabolism and renal function in neonates. Compend Contin Educ Pract Vet 13:392, 1991.

Finco DR: Familial renal disease in Norwegian elkhound dogs: Physiologic and biochemical examinations. Am J Vet Res 37:87, 1976.

Finco DR, Brown CA: Primary tubulo-interstitial diseases of the kidney. *In* Osborne CA, Finco DR (eds): Canine and Feline Nephrology and Urology. Baltimore, Williams & Wilkins, 1995, p 386.

Finco DR, Duncan JR, Crowell WA, et al: Familial renal disease in Norwegian elkhound dogs: Morphologic examination. Am J Vet Res 38:941, 1977.

Fox MW: Inherited polycystic mononephrosis in the dog. J Hered 55:29, 1964.

Giesecke D, Tiemeyer W: Defect of uric acid uptake in Dalmatian dog liver. Experientia 40:1415, 1416, 1984.

Grauer GF, Lane IF: Acute renal failure: Ischemic and chemical nephrosis. In Osborne CA, Finco DR (eds): Canine and Feline Nephrology and Urology. Baltimore, Williams & Wilkins, 1995, p 441.

Guiguard JP: Renal function in the newborn infant. Pediatr Clin North Am 29:777, 1982.

Hanson JS: Patent urachus in a cat. Vet Med Small Anim Clin 67:379, 1972.

Hardy RM, Osborne CA: Water deprivation test in the dog: Maximal normal values. J Am Vet Med Assoc 174:479, 1979.

Hayes HM: Breed associations of canine ectopic ureter: A study of 217 female cases. J Small Anim Pract 25:501, 1984.

Hayes HM, Wilson GP: Hospital incidence of hypospadias in dogs in North America. Vet Rec 118:605, 1986.

Heller J, Capek K: Changes in body water compartments and inulin and PAH clearance in the dog during postnatal development. Physiol Bohemoslov 14:433, 1965.

Hobson HP, Ader PL: Exstrophy of the bladder in a dog. J Am Anim Hosp Assoc 15:103, 1979.

Holt PE, Gibbs C: Congenital urinary incontinence in cats: A review of 19 cases. Vet Rec 130:437, 1992.

Holt PE, Long SE, Gibbs C: Disorders of urination associated with canine intersexuality. J Small Anim Pract 24:475, 1983.

Holt PE, Moore AH: Canine ureteral ectopia: An analysis of 175 cases and comparison of surgical treatments. Vet Rec 136:345, 1995.

Hood JC, Robinson WF, Huxtable CR, et al: Hereditary nephritis in the bull terrier: Evidence for inheritance by an autosomal dominant gene. Vet Rec 126:456, 1990.

Hoppe A, Swenson L, Jönsson L, et al: Progressive nephropathy due to renal dysplasia in Shih Tzu dogs in Sweden: A clinical pathological and genetic study. J Small Anim Pract 31:83, 1990.

Horster M, Valtin H: Postnatal development of renal function: Micropuncture and clearance studies in the dog. J Clin Invest 50:779, 1971.

Hoskins JD, Abdelbaki YZ, Rost CR: Urinary bladder duplication in a dog. J Am Vet Med Assoc 181:603, 1982.

Hoskins JD, Turnwald GH, Kearney MT, et al: Quantitative urinalysis in kittens from four to thirty weeks after birth. Am J Vet Res 52:1295, 1991.

Jansen JH, Arnesen K: Oxalate nephropathy in a Tibetan spaniel litter. A probable case of primary hyperoxaluria. J Comp Pathol 103:79, 1990.

Jansen B, Thorner PS, Singh A, et al: Animal model of human disease: Hereditary nephritis in Samoyed dogs. Am J Pathol 116:175, 1984.

Jansen B, Tryphonas L, Wong J, et al: Mode of inheritance of Samoyed hereditary glomerulopathy: An animal model for hereditary nephritis in humans. J Lab Clin Med 107:551, 555, 1986.

Johnston SD, Bailie NC, Hayden DW, et al: Diphallia in a mixed-breed dog with multiple anomalies. Theriogenology 31:1253, 1989.

Jones AK: Unusual case of feline incontinence. Vet Rec 112:555, 1983.

Kaufmann ML, Osborne CA, Johnston GR, et al: Renal ectopia in a dog and cat. J Am Vet Med Assoc 190:73, 1987.

Keeler CE: The inheritance of predisposition of renal calculi in the Dalmatian. J Am Vet Med Assoc 96:507, 1940.

Kelly DF: Rhabdomyosarcoma of the urinary bladder in dogs. Vet Pathol 10:375, 1973.

Kilham L, Margolis G, Colby ED: Congenital infections of cats and ferrets by feline panleukopenia virus manifested by cerebellar hypoplasia. Clin Invest 17:465, 1967.

Klausner JS, Feeney DA: Vesicoureteral reflux. In Kirk RW (ed): Current Veterinary Therapy VIII. Philadelphia, WB Saunders, 1983, p 1041.

Kleinman LI: Renal sodium reabsorption during saline loading and distal blockade in newborn dogs. Am J Physiol 228:1403, 1975.

Kleinman LI, Lubbe RJ: Factors affecting the maturation of glomerular filtration rate and renal plasma flow in the newborn dog. J Physiol 223:395, 1972.

Klopfer U, Neumann F, Trainin R: Renal cortical hypoplasia in a keeshond litter. Vet Med Small Anim Clin 70:1081, 1975.

Krook L. The pathology of renal cortical hypoplasia in the dog. Nord Vet Med 9:161, 1957.

Kruger JM, Osborne CA: The role of uropathogens in feline lower urinary tract disease: Clinical implications. Vet Clin North Am Small Anim Pract 23:101, 1993.

Kruger JM, Osborne CA, Goyal SM, et al: Clinical evaluation of cats with lower urinary tract disease. J Am Vet Med Assoc 199:211, 1991.

Kruger JM, Osborne CA, Lulich JP, et al: The urinary system. In Hoskins JD (ed): Veterinary Pediatrics: Dogs and Cats from Birth to Six Months, 2nd ed. Philadelphia, WB Saunders, 1995, p 399.

Kucera J, Bulková T, Rychlá R, et al: Bilateral xanthine nephrolithiasis in a dog. J Small Anim Pract 38:302, 1997.

Lage AL: Nephrogenic diabetes insipidus in a dog. J Am Vet Med Assoc 163:251, 1973.

Lawler DV, Monti KL: Morbidity and mortality in neonatal kittens. Am J Vet Res 45:1455, 1984.

Lees GE, Wilson PD, Helman RG, et al: Glomerular ultrastructural findings similar to hereditary nephritis in 4 English cocker spaniels. J Vet Intern Med 11:80, 1997.

Longhofer SL, Jackson RK, Cooley AJ: Hindgut and bladder duplications in a dog. J Am Anim Hosp Assoc 27:97, 1991.

Lulich JP, Osborne CA, Lawler DF, et al: Urologic disorders of immature cats. Vet Clin North Am Small Anim Pract 17:663, 1987.

Lulich JP, Osborne CA, Johnson GR: Non-surgical correction of infection-induced struvite uroliths and a vesicourachal diverticulum in an immature dog. J Small Anim Pract 30:613, 1989.

MacDougall DF, Cook T, Steward AP, et al: Canine chronic renal disease: Prevalence and types of glomerulonephritis in the dog. Kidney Int 29:1144, 1986.

Maizels M: Normal development of the urinary tract. In Walsh PC, Retik AB, Stamey TA, et al (eds): Campbell's Urology, 6th ed. Philadelphia: WB Saunders, 1992, p 1301.

Marretta SM, Pask AJ, Green RW, et al: Urinary calculi associated with portosystemic shunts in six dogs. J Am Vet Med Assoc 178:133, 1981.

Maxie MG, Prescott JF: The urinary system. In Jubb KVF, Kennedy PC, Palmer N (eds): Pathology of Domestic Animals, vol 2, 4th ed. New York, Academic Press, 1991, p 447.

McAloose D, Casal M, Patterson DV, et al: Polycystic kidney and liver disease in two related West Highland white terrier litters. Vet Pathol 35:77, 1998.

McKenna SC, Carpenter JL: Polycystic disease of the kidney and liver in the Cairn terrier. Vet Pathol 17:436, 1980.

McKerrell RE, Blakemore WF, Heath MF, et al: Primary hyperoxaluria (L-glyceric aciduria) in the cat: A newly recognized inherited disease. Vet Rec 125:31, 1989.

McLoughlin MA, Hauptman JG, Spaulding K: Canine ureteroceles: A case report and literature review. J Am Anim Hosp Assoc 25:699, 1989.

Morton LD, Sanecki RK, Gordon DE, et al: Juvenile renal disease in miniature schnauzer dogs. Vet Pathol 27:455, 1990.

Murti GS: Agenesis and dysgenesis of the canine kidneys. J Am Vet Med Assoc 146:1120, 1965.

Noden DM, deLahunta A: The Embryology of Domestic Animals. Baltimore, Williams & Wilkins, 1985, p 47.

O'Brien TD, Osborne CA, Yano BL, et al: Clinicopathologic manifestations of progressive renal disease in Lhasa apso, Shih Tzu dogs. J Am Vet Med Assoc 180:658, 1982.

Odendaal JSJ: Diagnosis of a third kidney in a dog. Canine Pract 17:17, 1992.

O'Handley P, Carrig CB, Walshaw R: Renal and ureteral duplications in a dog. J Am Vet Med Assoc 174:484, 1979.

Osborne CA: Urethrorectal fistulas. In Kirk RW (ed): Current Veterinary Therapy VI. Philadelphia, WB Saunders, 1977, p 985.

Osborne CA, Hanlon GF: Canine congenital ureteral ectopia: Case report and review of literature. Anim Hosp 3:111, 1967.

Osborne CA, Johnston GR, Kruger JM, et al: Etiopathogenesis and biological behavior of feline vesicourachal diverticula. Vet Clin North Am Small Anim Pract 17:697, 1987.

Osborne CA, Johnston GR, Kruger JM: Ectopic ureters and ureteroceles. In Osborne CA, Finco DR (eds): Canine and Feline Nephrology and Urology. Baltimore, Williams & Wilkins, 1995a, p 608.

Osborne CA, Kroll RA, Lulich JP, et al: Medical management of vesicourachal diverticula in 15 cats with lower urinary tract disease. J Small Anim Pract 30:608, 1989.

Osborne CA, Lees GE: Bacterial infection of the canine and feline urinary tract. In Osborne CA, Finco DR (eds): Canine and Feline Nephrology and Urology. Baltimore, Williams & Wilkins, 1995, p 759.

Osborne CA, Lulich JP, Thumchai R, et al: Feline urolithiasis: Etiology and pathophysiology. Vet Clin North Am Small Anim Pract 26:217, 1996.

Osborne CA, Lulich JP, Bartges JW, et al: Canine and feline urolithiasis: Relationship of etiopathogenesis to treatment and prevention. In Osborne CA, Finco DR (eds): Canine and Feline Nephrology and Urology. Baltimore, Williams & Wilkins, 1995b, p 798.

Osborne CA, Sanderson SL: Medical management of urethral prolapse in male dogs. In Bonagura JD, Kirk RW (eds): Current Veterinary Therapy XII. Philadelphia, WB Saunders, 1995, p 1027.

Pearson H, Gibbs C: Urinary tract abnormalities in the dog. J Small Anim Pract 12:67, 1971.

Pearson H, Gibbs C, Hillson JM: Some abnormalities of the canine urinary tract. Vet Rec 77:775, 1965.

Percy DH, Carmichael LE, Albert DM, et al: Lesions in puppies surviving infections with canine herpesvirus. Vet Pathol 8:37, 1967.

Picut CA, Lewis RM: Comparative pathology of canine hereditary nephropathies: An interpretive review. Vet Res Commun 11:561, 1987a.

Picut CA, Lewis RM: Juvenile renal disease in Doberman pinschers; ultrastructural changes of the glomerular basement membrane. J Comp Pathol 97:587, 1987b.

Picut CA, Lewis RM: Microscopic features of canine renal dysplasia. Vet Pathol 24:156, 1987c.

Pollock S, Schoen SS: Urinary incontinence associated with congenital ureteral valves in a bitch. J Am Vet Med Assoc 159:332, 1971.

Polzin DJ, Osborne CA: Conservative medical management of chronic renal failure. In Osborne CA, Finco DR (eds): Canine and Feline Nephrology and Urology. Baltimore, Williams & Wilkins, 1995a, p 508.

Polzin DJ, Osborne CA: Pathophysiology of renal failure and uremia. In Osborne CA, Finco DR (eds): Canine and Feline Nephrology and Urology. Baltimore, Williams & Wilkins, 1995b, p 335.

Reusch C, Hoerauf A, Lechner J, et al: A new familial glomerulonephropathy in Bernese mountain dogs. Vet Rec 134:411, 1994.

Robinson JR: Ammonia formation by surviving kidney slices without specific substrates. J Physiol 124:1, 1954.

Robinson WF, Huxtable CR, Gooding JP: Familial nephropathy in cocker spaniels. Aust Vet J 62:109, 1985.

Robinson WF, Shaw SE, Stanley B, et al: Chronic renal disease in bull terriers. Aust Vet J 66:193, 1989.

Sinibaldi KR, Green RW: Surgical corrections of prolapse of the male urethra in three English Bulldogs. J Am Anim Hosp Assoc 9:450, 1973.

Snyder HM, D'Angio GJ, Evans AE, et al: Pediatric Oncology. *In* Walsh PC, Retik AB, Stamey TA, et al (eds): Campbell's Urology, 6th ed. Philadelphia: WB Saunders, 1992, p 1967.

Stamps P, Harris DL: Botryoid rhabdomyosarcoma of the urinary bladder of a dog. J Am Vet Med Assoc 153:1064, 1968.

Steward AP, MacDougall DF: Familial nephropathy in the cocker spaniel. J Small Anim Pract 25:15, 1984.

Tsan MF, Jones TC, Thornton GW, et al: Canine cystinuria: Its urinary amino acid pattern and genetic analysis. Am J Vet Res 33:2455, 1972.

Valli VEO, Baumal R, Thorner P, et al: Dietary modification reduces splitting of glomerular basement membrane and delays death due to renal failure in canine X-linked hereditary nephritis. Lab Invest 65:67, 1991.

Van Den Broek AHM, Else RW, Hunter MS: Atresia ani and urethrorectal fistula in a kitten. J Small Anita Pract 29:91, 1988.

Van Vechten M, Goldschmidt MH, Wortman JA: Embryonal rhabdomyosarcoma of the urinary bladder in dogs. Compend Contin Educ Pract Vet 12:783, 1990.

Vymetal F. Renal aplasia in beagles. Vet Rec 77:1344, 1965.

Welling LW, Grantham JJ: Cystic and developmental diseases of the kidney. *In* Brenner BM, Rector FC (eds): The Kidney, 4th ed. Philadelphia: WB Saunders, 1991, p 1657.

White RN, Tick NT, White HL: Naturally occurring xanthine urolithiasis in a domestic shorthair cat. J Small Anim Pract 38:299, 1997.

Wilcock BP, Patterson JM: Familial glomerulonephritis in Doberman pinscher dogs. Can Vet J 20:244, 1979.

Wolf A, Radecky M: Anomaly in a poodle puppy. Vet Med Small Anim Clin 68:732, 1973.

Zuber RM: Systemic amyloidosis in Oriental and Siamese cats. Aust Vet Pract 23:66, 1993.

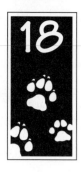

The Skeletal System

Peter K. Shires and Kurt S. Schulz

Several factors influence the incidences of the orthopedic conditions that occur in young dogs and cats exclusively. Until the physeal lines close, they represent the weakest and most active area in the bone-ligament-tendon-muscle unit. Metabolic or traumatic disturbances will be magnified by the intense activity present. Young animals tend to be less coordinated and more trusting than their elders, leading to their increased incidence of traumatic injuries. Because many orthopedic conditions become evident as a result of accelerated degenerative changes, frequently a recognized condition that exists at an early age does not become a clinical problem until later in life. As with any animal, these conditions can be subdivided according to origin as inheritable, developmental, infectious, neoplastic, nutritional, and traumatic. For the purposes of this discussion, a clinical subdivision is also used according to which part(s) of the animal's body are clinically affected.

OSTEOCHONDRITIS DISSECANS

Osteochondritis dissecans (OCD) may be involved in several developmental bone problems, including cervical vertebral instability, hip dysplasia, nonunited anconeal process, and fragmented coronoid process. Only the OCD manifestation of osteochondrosis is described here. Osteochondritis is the result of a delay of the ossification process of the normal developing cartilage. As this occurs, it causes a relative thickening of the cartilage layer in the affected area, with a concurrent defect in the underlying subchondral bone. This thickened cartilage represents a biomechanically deficient area on the

joint surface. Poor oxygenation and nutrition result in cell death of the deep layers. Normal or greater than normal stresses applied to the affected joint cause separation of layers of this cartilage from underlying layers. This separation frequently connects to the synovial space, allowing synovia to penetrate and dissect free the cartilaginous segment. The term *osteochondritis dissecans* refers to this stage of the process.

The free flap that is created may remain partially attached and in place in the defect, or it may float completely free in the synovial space. A free-floating cartilage flap undergoes dissolution and degradation unless it becomes attached to the joint capsule and revascularizes. In this situation, a portion of the cartilage may become calcified. If the flap remains attached within the defect, it prevents any filling of the defect by fibrocartilage. If the flap is detached, the defect may fill with minimal surface irregularities.

Signs of OCD are precipitated by the continued synovial irritation induced by the degrading cartilage flap and the defect. Articular surface incongruity adds to the problem through abnormal wear patterns and instability. Underlying and predisposing causes for OCD may include rapid growth and inherited and hormonal factors. Males are more commonly affected than females, and commonly affected dog breeds include Labrador retrievers, golden retrievers, Rottweilers, and German shepherds.

Treatment usually involves removal of cartilage flap and creation of vascular access to the area through holes drilled through the subchondral plate (forage) to help the defect heal. A good prognosis for normal joint function may be offered if degenerative joint disease is not advanced before surgery, whereas failure to treat OCD may result in moderate to severe degenerative joint disease later in life. Successful surgical treatment will not eliminate degenerative joint disease but in most cases will limit the incidence of crippling joint deterioration. Postoperative dietary adjustments to decrease protein and caloric intake have been recommended, although the efficacy of the dietary changes at this later stage of the disease is questionable. It may be more appropriate to recommend moderate caloric and protein intake at an early age in rapidly growing, large-breed puppies. Several syndromes are recognized according to the joint affected.

The Shoulder Joint

Signs of OCD in the shoulder joint are generally seen initially at about 6 months of age and are characterized by a partially weight-bearing lameness that worsens with exercise. A sudden onset of forelimb lameness may be induced by a period of intense activity. Orthopedic examination of the shoulder elicits a pain response, especially on full flexion or full extension. Joint effusion may be palpable and can be confirmed by a joint tap. Arthrocentesis commonly reveals low-grade nonsuppurative reaction with evidence of sepsis, although the volume of fluid may be increased. Radiographs show a flattening of the caudal medial aspect of the humeral head (Fig. 18–1). A free-floating joint

mouse may be visible in the caudal pouch of the joint capsule or within the bicipital bursa. The lesion can usually be seen in both shoulders, although dogs are frequently only symptomatic in one. A vaccum phenomenon has been associated with radiographs of shoulders with clinical OCD. This refers to a gaseous line within the joint space caused by negative pressure within the joint. Surgical removal of the flap and curettage or forage of the defect is recommended in cases with signs of lameness and pain (Berzon, 1979). Lesions seen radiographically, in the absence of lameness, indicate limited exercise as the only management unless lameness develops (Olsson, 1976).

The Stifle Joint

Osteochondritis dissecans occurs less commonly in the stifle joint than in the shoulder joint. A rear limb lameness can be localized to the stifle by palpation of joint effusion and pain on manipulation. Arthrocentesis confirms the presence of traumatic synovitis. Radiographs show a subchondral defect in the weight-bearing surface of the medial or lateral femoral condyle. The lateral condyle is more commonly affected (Figs. 18–2 and 18–3). Periarticular osteophytes can be seen in more chronic cases. Surgical removal of the cartilage flap and forage of the defect are recommended (Alexander et al, 1981). Postoperative rest is essential to allow healing before activity can be resumed. The prognosis is good for full return of function if degenerative changes are not too far advanced.

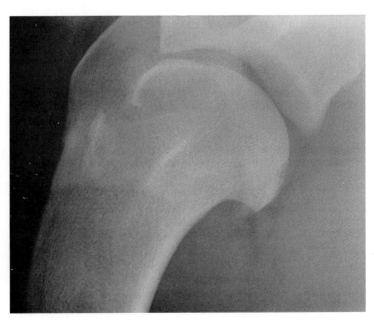

Figure 18–1. Lateral radiographic view of the humeral head showing a lucency in the subchondral bone characteristic of osteochondritis dissecans when associated with the clinical signs.

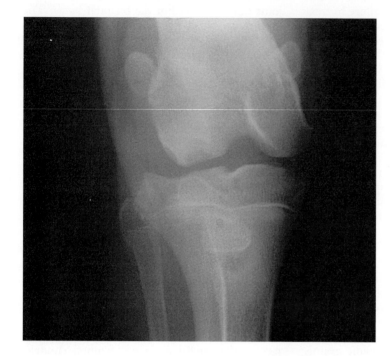

Figure 18–2. Posterior anterior radiographic view of the stifle showing a subchondral defect in the lateral femoral condyle, typical of osteochondrosis of the distal region of the femur.

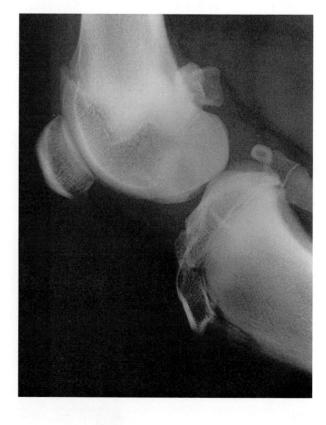

Figure 18–3. Lateral radiographic view of the stifle showing a lateral condylar subchondral defect, seen in cases of osteochondrosis.

The Hock Joint

Increasing numbers of OCD cases of the hock are being seen. Large breeds are affected; Labrador retrievers and Rottweilers are overrepresented (Olson, 1980). The diagnosis is frequently associated with an upright stance in the tarsus. An insidious onset of rear limb lameness is frequently reported. On physical examination, the dog is generally weight bearing but protects the limb. Palpation of the hock may induce a pain reaction. A joint tap confirms the presence of traumatic synovitis. Radiographs show a subchondral defect in the lateral aspect of the medial trochlear ridge. Osteochondritis dissecans of the lateral ridge has also been reported. The recommended treatment is removal of the cartilage flap and subchondral curettage or forage, although some authors have reported no difference in outcome whether or not surgery is performed. Non–weight-bearing exercise improves the cartilage rehabilitation postoperatively.

The Elbow Joint

Osteochondritis dissecans in the elbow joint is an uncommon diagnosis frequently confused with and diagnosed during exploration for a fragmented coronoid process. The lesion causes a low-grade elbow lameness with joint effusion and pain on manipulation of the affected elbow. Radiographically, a subchondral defect can occasionally be seen under the articular surface of the medial humeral condyle. The cartilage flap should be removed surgically and the defect curetted. Progressive arthritis can be slowed if the postoperative healing process of cartilage is allowed to proceed without excessive weight bearing.

CONGENITAL SHOULDER LUXATION

Small-breed and toy dog breeds have a tendency toward shoulder joint instability subsequent to a shallow glenoid cavity and flattened humeral head. In severely affected animals, this may lead to medial shoulder luxation at an early age associated with minor trauma. Miniature poodles and Pomeranians are commonly affected (Hohn et al, 1983). The forelimb is carried in flexion with the foot rotated outward. The shoulder can usually be luxated easily and is easily reduced. Radiographs confirm the luxation if a flexed and rotated view is taken of the shoulder. Conservative management with a flexion sling is rarely successful. Surgical repair is slightly more effi-cient in maintaining joint stability. The most commonly used technique requires the translocation of the biceps brachii tendon caudally under an osseous hinged flap of the lesser tubercle. The medial joint capsule is imbricated, and the surrounding musculature is tightened. The leg is protected in a sling at least 2 weeks postoperatively. The prognosis is guarded when joint laxity is a congenital problem (Vaughan and Jones, 1969). Reluxation is common and difficult to stabilize. Shoulder arthrodesis may be considered as a salvage procedure. Because this disorder has an inherited aspect, breeding is not recommended for affected dogs.

FRAGMENTED CORONOID PROCESS

The development of the coronoid process is infrequently disturbed during the growing stages in several giant and large dogs, particularly the Rottweiler, Labrador retriever, and German shepherd. Male dogs are more frequently affected than female dogs. It is presumed that the coronoid process is traumatized or overstressed before ossification has occurred, with the resultant fragmentation or fracture occurring (Berzon and Quick, 1980). The instability of the elbow joint that results is compounded by the presence of bone fragments within the joint, and the combination causes a progressive arthritis to be initiated (Lewis et al, 1989). This arthritis eventually causes pain and degenerative joint disease.

Puppies are usually presented with a fragmented coronoid process before they are 1 year of age. Puppies may show early unilateral or bilateral lameness associated with overexertion. Joint instability leads to palpable joint effusion that, if sampled, shows a traumatic synovitis reaction. Palpation of the medial aspect of the elbow joint may reveal soft tissue thickening and pain. Radiographs taken at this stage may show only the effusion and early periarticular degenerative lesions, most prominent at the proximal anconeal process and proximal cranial surface of the radius (Figs. 18–4 and 18–5). A lateral radiograph may also show sclerosis of the ulna at the radioulnar articulation. Similar radiographic findings may be seen in clinically unaffected elbows. Visualizing the coronoid process requires careful radiographic technique and positioning (Henry, 1984). Isolated fragments of bone can occasionally be seen at the site of the normal coronoid process. Suspicion of the disease is based on clinical signs and

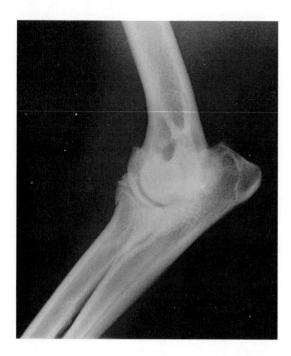

Figure 18–4. Lateral radiographic view of the elbow showing the periarticular osteophyte formation frequently associated with cases of fragmented medial coronoid process in dogs.

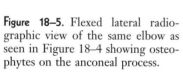

Figure 18–5. Flexed lateral radiographic view of the same elbow as seen in Figure 18–4 showing osteophytes on the anconeal process.

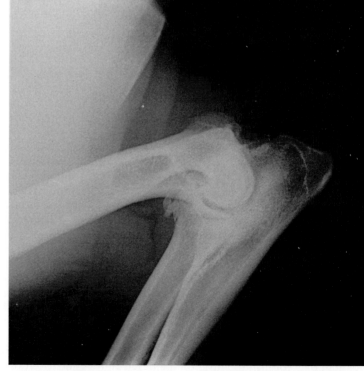

radiographic changes, whereas definitive diagnosis is based on surgical findings.

Recommended treatment includes removal of the bone fragments through a medial approach to the elbow joint. Surgical therapy may not decrease the incidence of postoperative lameness but has been shown to decrease the severity and duration of clinical signs. Continual progression of the arthritis can be expected postoperatively, although at a diminished rate. Conservative management of the elbow joint instability is advised, requiring body weight management, restricted exercise, and passive range of motion exercises. Eventual management of the arthritis is likely to be necessary, including analgesic medication and rest. Surgical fusion of the elbow joint is rarely necessary.

UNUNITED ANCONEAL PROCESS

An ununited anconeal process (UAP) occurs in the dog when the fourth ossification center of the ulna fails to unite with the ulnar diaphysis. This disease is seen most commonly in German shepherd and other large-breed dogs. The pathogenesis remains unknown; however, theories include osteochondrosis, trauma to immature cartilage, and congenital elbow incongruity. The anconeus should unite with the ulnar diaphysis by 4.5 months of age; therefore, a diagnosis of UAP should not be made before 5 months of age. Failure of the anconeal growth plate to close leads to elbow joint laxity and synovitis that produces arthritic changes. This condition is frequently inapparent until the secondary arthritis occurs. Affected dogs show a vague forelimb lameness that can be precipitated by exercise or manipulation of the joint. The elbow joint is usually swollen and painful at the extremes of the normal range of motion. A joint tap confirms the presence of traumatic arthritis. Radiographs of the elbow show an open growth plate in the anconeus after the normal age for closure has passed (Goring and Bloomberg, 1983). This is best demonstrated by a flexed lateral view (Fig. 18–6). The anconeal process may be smaller than expected, and occasionally it may be displaced or angulated. In older dogs, the clinical presentation is determined by the degree of arthritis, and the radiographic findings vary according to the level of arthritis present.

Treatment of the young dog is aimed at removing the anconeal process to reduce the irritation it precipitates within the elbow joint. The joint instability remains after surgical removal, and the development of arthritis progresses despite surgery. To slow this process, a management program is recommended that prevents the animal from becoming overweight, limits weight-bearing exercise, and promotes passive or non–weight-bearing joint movement (e.g., swimming). Analgesics are used in later stages of joint degeneration. As a salvage procedure, joint fusion can be considered in end-stage arthritis situations. The prognosis for limited use of the forelimb is good. Degeneration of the affected joint is inevitable, and the owners

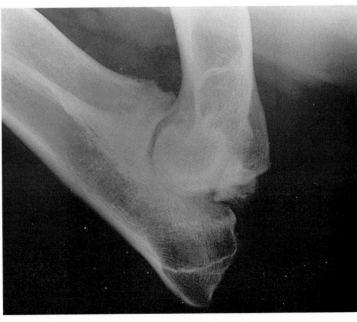

Figure 18–6. Flexed lateral radiographic view of a dog's elbow showing a chronic nonunited anconeal process.

should be counseled about the ramifications of this problem as it relates to normal function over a long period of time.

CONGENITAL ELBOW LUXATION (ELBOW DYSPLASIA)

An abnormal developmental pattern of the bones that constitute the elbow joint leads to a lateral displacement of the radius and ulna in relation to the humerus. The initiating factor is unknown, but several breeds of dogs are more commonly affected. Toy breeds like the Pomeranian and Yorkshire terrier are most commonly reported to have this condition, but larger dog breeds like the Airedale terrier have also been diagnosed with the problem. The problem is frequently bilateral, and numerous members of a litter may be affected. The early closure or complete absence of epiphyseal growth centers and failure of normal development of the articular ligaments result in an instability that translates into luxation as growth occurs. Conformational and degenerative abnormalities are present at an early age and become worse with growth and weight gains (Milton et al, 1979). The severity of the condition depends on the degree of laxity and joint malformation. Radiographs illustrate the type and extent of the malformation (Figs. 18–7 and 18–8).

Puppies and kittens generally show conformational abnormalities at an early age, around 4 to 6 weeks of age. The limited exercise and minimal body weight allow them to function adequately despite their abnormal appearance. With advancing age, the problem becomes more obvious. Gait abnormalities vary according to the severity of the condition but usually are weight bearing at first. The forelimbs are generally rotated inward with the elbows wide, the carpi close together, and the metacarpals angled laterally. Palpable elbow joint laxity can usually be demonstrated, especially under sedation or anesthesia. Radiographs of the elbows confirm the lack of normal joint anatomy and the luxation present. Treatment is usually surgical and varies according to the deficiency involved. Replacement of the elbow luxation and maintenance of joint congruity are the objectives of surgery. To accomplish these objectives, closed or open reduction is combined with extension splinting, transarticular pinning, collateral ligament reconstruction, joint capsule imbrication, and, occasionally, corrective osteotomies or orthopedic banding. The final result is generally a functional limb, but it

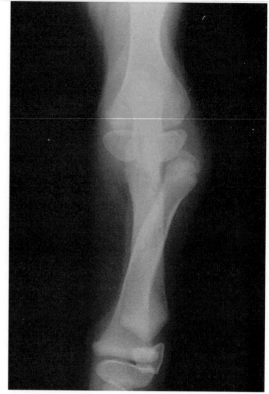

Figure 18–7. Anterior posterior radiographic view of the forearm of a puppy with congenital elbow dysplasia. Note the proximal radial luxation laterally.

is not cosmetic. The prognosis is guarded even in the best of cases because of the degenerative changes that usually develop. Smaller animals are less prone to degenerative arthritis and therefore do better than larger breeds. Because an inherited trait is likely to be involved, breeding these animals should be discouraged.

OTHER ELBOW ABNORMALITIES

Other diseases of the puppy elbow include patella cubiti and dystrophic calcification of the origin of the flexor tendons. Patella cubiti is a proximal displacement of the olecranon growth center. Affected puppies walk with a stilted, partially flexed gait, and radiographs reveal a proximally displaced olecranon. An ununited medial epicondyle of the humerus has been described in the German shepherd (Fox et al, 1983). This disease may actually be a traumatic or developmental calcification of the antebrachial flexor tendons at their origin on the medial epicondyle (Zontine et al, 1989) (Fig. 18–9).

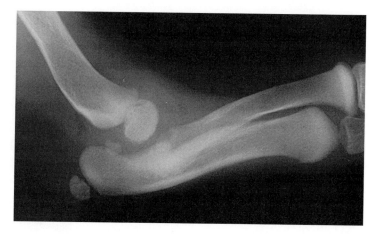

Figure 18–8. Lateral radiographic view of the forearm of a puppy with congenital elbow dysplasia. Note the malformation of the proximal region of the radius.

HYPERTROPHIC OSTEODYSTROPHY

Hypertrophic osteodystrophy (HOD) is a problem of rapidly growing large-breed puppies between 3 and 7 months of age. It is a metabolic bone disorder characterized by increased activity in the metaphyseal areas of the long bones. A history of lameness, lethargy, and anorexia is

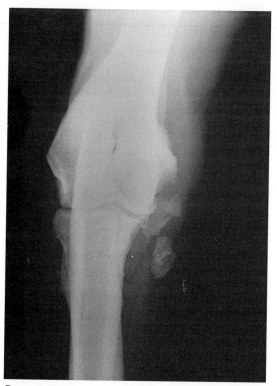

Figure 18–9. Anterior posterior radiographic view of the elbow of a dog with calcification of the antebrachial flexor tendons on the medial epicondyle of the humerus.

commonly reported. Other clinical findings may include fever and pain and swelling of the metaphyseal regions of the radius, ulna, and tibia (Alexander, 1978; Grondalen, 1976). Suggested causes of HOD include vitamin C deficiency, overnutrition, primary metabolic disease, and bacterial and viral (canine distemper) infection; however, the definitive cause remains unknown. The metaphyses enlarge due to increased bone formation at the growth plate and perichondrial ring. The rapid bone growth leaves a weakened metaphysis that is prone to microfractures during normal activity. The microfractures precipitate lysis and sclerosis during the healing process, which adds to the bulk and density of the bone in the metaphyses. Pain associated with palpation of the metaphyses of long bones is the most important finding associated with HOD. The diagnosis can be confirmed with radiographs of the metaphyses. An increased density of the metaphyseal bone is usually bordered by a lytic line parallel to and near the physeal line. This "double physeal line" is characteristic and diagnostic when accompanied by widening and periosteal bone proliferation at the metaphyses (Figs. 18–10 and 18–11).

A complete blood count may be normal or may demonstrate a high leukocyte count. Serum biochemistry results may reveal elevated calcium and phosphorus concentrations and generalized metabolic disturbances in electrolytes, glucose, and acid-base balance. Blood cultures have revealed secondary septicemia in severely affected cases (Schulz et al, 1991). Therapy varies with the severity of the disease. Mildly affected animals may recover spontaneously with rest and analgesics. More severely diseased animals may exhibit life-threatening secondary metabolic derangement and infection. In these cases, intensive care including fluid therapy and systemic antimicrobial agents is indicated. The prognosis is guarded because severe secondary metabolic derangements may be fatal, and, uncommonly, the disease may recur. Permanent osseous deformity can occur in those dogs that survive. Entire litters of puppies can be affected, and certain families appear to be more prone than others. Although no genetic trait is suspected, the bone metabolic character may be heritable, and affected animals are less desirable for breeding.

FORELIMB ANGULAR DEFORMITIES

The two-bone system of the forelimb precipitates asynchronous growth problems if the radius and ulna grow at different rates. The normal limb length is provided by growth from the proximal and distal physes of both bones. The proximal ulnar physis contributes 15% to longitudinal ulnar growth and the distal ulnar physis,

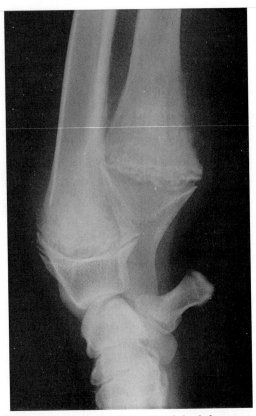

Figure 18–11. Lateral radiograph of the left carpus of a dog with hypertrophic osteodystrophy.

85%. The proximal radial physis contributes 40% and the distal physis 60% to radial length. Cessation of growth in either bone, except the proximal ulna, markedly affects the length and curvature of the antebrachium. As the physes are prone to injury in the young animal, these growth deformities are not uncommon.

Premature Closure of the Distal Ulnar Physis

The conical shape of the distal ulnar physis and its 85% contribution to ulnar length make injury common and the results of closure severe. In the young animal any significant trauma to the forelimb can precipitate early closure of the distal ulna. Owners should be cautioned of this possibility whenever a puppy or kitten experiences forelimb trauma. If the distal ulnar physis closes, then the most ulnar lengthening stops while the radius continues to grow. The result is a progressive bowing and twisting of the radius as the ulna acts as a bowstring, preventing normal antebrachial lengthening. Because the distal portion of the ulna is situated laterally, a

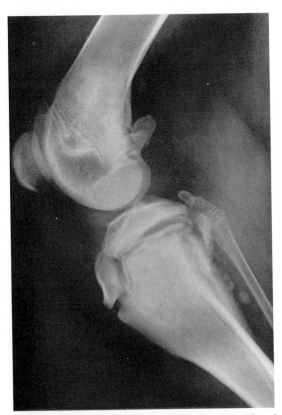

Figure 18–10. Lateral radiograph of the right stifle of a dog with hypertrophic osteodystrophy. Note the widened proximal tibial physis, periosteal proliferation, and transverse radiolucent band and sclerosis in the distal femoral metaphysis.

valgus deviation of the distal region of the limb develops from the carpus (Fig. 18–12). The radius is bowed cranially (Fig. 18–13), and the paw becomes supinated. The radiocarpal joint becomes subluxated caudolaterally, and the radial head may displace the humeral condyles from the semilunar notch. The severity of these changes depends on the age of the animal at the time of injury and or the potential size of the animal involved. Because the problem is progressive up to the time of skeletal maturity, various levels of deformation are recognized. The later stages of malarticulation precipitate severe osteoarthritic degeneration given time. The impression of bowing and curvature is easily confirmed with full-length radiographs of the radius and ulna that are compared with those of the opposite leg.

There are several methods of treating the early deformity cases in immature animals (other methods apply to older animals) (Fox, 1984a). The simplest is to perform an ulnar ostectomy, removing 2 cm of the ulna from the medial to distal third of the ulna. This permits

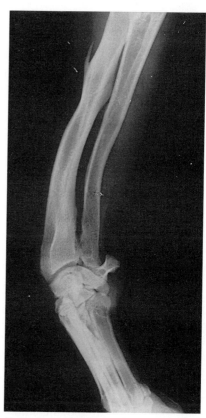

Figure 18–13. Lateral radiographic view of the foreleg of a dog showing remodeling of an old midshaft radius and ulnar fracture with bowing of the radius distally secondary to distal ulnar physeal closure.

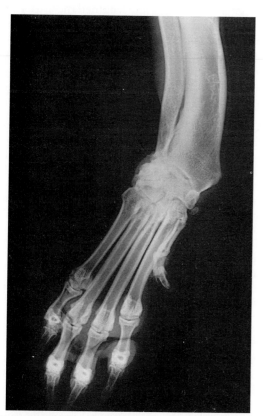

Figure 18–12. Anterior posterior radiographic view of the forelimb of a dog showing closure of the distal ulnar physis and lateral curvature of the distal region of the radius.

elongation of the radius as long as the ostectomy remains unbridged by fibrous callus or bone. Some recommend filling the defect with a free fat graft to slow healing between the cut ends of the ulna (Craig, 1981). Excision or oversewing of the periosteum may delay subsequent closure of the ostectomy site. A more definitive method uses distraction of the separated ulnar segments to actively obtain normal length and angulation of the radius and ulna. An external skeletal fixation device is attached to both fragments of the ulna, which is then osteotomized. Over a period of a few weeks, the fragments are progressively distracted to an anatomic position while the radius adjusts to the release in tension that the ulnar ostectomy has provided (DeCamp et al, 1986). This technique may be used in either the growing or skeletally mature dog. Mature dogs may also be treated by corrective wedge osteotomy. In this procedure the ulna is transected and a wedge of bone is removed from the radius so that either reversed replacement of this wedge or complete removal of this wedge allows for stabilization of the radius with more anatomic alignment of the antebrachium and carpus. All techniques can result in a functionally normal forelimb if successful. A less favorable prognosis is likely if the deformity persists due to elbow and radiocarpal malarticulation.

Premature Closure of the Distal Radial Physis

Less commonly, the distal radius may be injured and close prematurely. The closure is usually asymmetric, with one side of the radius continuing to grow when the other side closes. The resultant deformity is an angulation of the carpus and metacarpal bones toward the closed side. Infrequently, the entire distal radius closes, and the result is a straight but shortened radius with caudal bowing of the ulna and a lax elbow joint because of a lack of contact between the proximal radius and the humerus (Vandewater and Olmstead, 1983). Comparative radiographs delineate the problem, and early treatment in young immature animals allows correction before permanent damage results. Resection of the damaged portion of the physis and replacement with a free fat graft allows continued radial growth and self-correction of the angulation problem. The success rate of the procedure is limited by the inability of surgeons to readily recognize the closed portion of the physis. Recently a simple ostectomy procedure has been described that allows dynamic realignment of the elbow joint after surgery. A section of the proximal ulna is removed, and alignment is maintained with an intramedullary pin. The joint incongruity diminishes within a few days, and the ulna heals in the new position. Excellent function returns to the limb very rapidly. This simple procedure has had good results to date in several cases. Corrective osteotomies are frequently necessary to realign the mature antebrachium. Complete distal radial closure is treated in a fashion similar to the ulnar closures. An osteotomy of the radius and progressive distraction of the segments with an external fixator allows lengthening and re-establishment of joint congruity. The prognosis again depends on the degree of injury and the age and potential growth of the animal.

Proximal Radial Physeal Closure

Closure of the proximal radial physis results in a progressive separation of the radial head from the distal humerus. This laxity eventually causes a malarticulation and degenerative joint disease. A limb shortening is also evident in some cases. Radiographs confirm the radial closure and the deformity. Treatment by osteotomy and progressive distraction of the radial segments can be quite successful, or the ulnar ostectomy technique can be used for similar results. The prognosis for treated cases is good provided that the joint incongruity has not started a degenerative process in the elbow joint.

Synostosis of the Radius and Ulna

The asynchronous growth that results after fusion of the radius and ulna in growing animals reflects the different proportions of leg lengthening that are due to the distal and proximal ulna. The primary result of synostosis is the lack of lengthening of the proximal ulna (Carrig and Wortman, 1981). As the radius continues to grow, the radial head displaces the humerus out of the ulnar notch because the ulna does not keep up a similar growth rate, causing malarticulation and joint disease. The diagnosis can be confirmed with radiographs. Treatment is designed to progressively lengthen the ulna with an external fixator after an osteotomy has been performed. The prognosis is fair for normal function if the joint has not suffered severe arthritic changes.

RADIAL AGENESIS

A complete lack of development of the radius has been reported primarily in kittens, but also in puppies. The lack of medial support for the carpus results in a medial deviation of the paw that is recognizable early in life. The condition may be unilateral or bilateral. Signs depend on the degree of conformational deformity present. Diagnosis is easily confirmed with radiographs. Treatment is restricted to amputation for unilateral cases. The prognosis for ambulation in bilateral cases is poor. Because heritability has a role in the occurrence of this condition, these animals should not be bred.

CARPAL HYPEREXTENSION

Puppies that are raised in a confined situation may develop a period of carpal hyperextension. The condition probably reflects poor muscle tone or weakness (Alexander and Earley, 1984; Shires et al, 1985). The signs are generally confined to abnormalities in the carpal joint. The puppies walk on the plantar surface of the carpus in severe cases or with varying degrees of

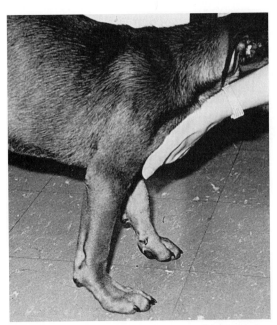

Figure 18–14. A 3-month-old Staffordshire terrier-cross puppy with hyperextension of the right carpus and mild bowing of the left carpus. Both conditions resolved with managed exercise.

overextension of the carpus in less severe cases (Fig. 18–14). The normal standing position should be close to a straight line between the elbows and the toes. No pathologic features have been associated with the condition, which appears to be self-limiting as the puppies mature (Shires et al, 1985). Treatment is confined to physical therapy, including exercise on a surface providing good traction. The exercise should be increased over a 1- to 3-week period. The prognosis is very good for immature puppies with carpal hyperextension.

HIP DYSPLASIA

Hip dysplasia is a common musculoskeletal complaint in large-breed dogs. Hip dysplasia does develop in small dogs also, but these cases are generally asymptomatic. A significant heritability factor has been found, but environmental influences determine the expression of the problem as a symptomatic disease. High activity levels, rapid body weight gains, poor muscle mass development, and adolescent incoordination all contribute to the hip laxity that develops in a growing puppy. The combination of congenital and environmental factors leads to coxofemoral subluxation and subsequent abnormal development of the acetabulum. Pain occurs due to joint capsule tearing and subchondral microfractures, causing the lameness seen in young puppies. If subluxation and dysplasia persist, affected dogs develop secondary osteoarthritis due to malarticulation.

Two clinical situations are generally seen. Dogs younger than 6 months of age usually present with a sudden onset of hindlimb lameness, frequently associated with some incident during play or exercise. Because awareness of hip dysplasia has become widespread, owners may present their animals for a complaint of an abnormal hindlimb gait or pain or difficulty standing. The hip joint is painful when manipulated, and arthrocentesis may confirm the presence of traumatic arthritis in the hip joint. Coxofemoral laxity is demonstrated by lateral force on the proximal portion of the femur (Barden sign) or by the Ortalani maneuver, which involves dorsolateral subluxation of the joint and subsequent relocation on abduction of the femur. Radiographs show varying degrees of hip dysplasia and subluxation of one or both hip joints. Specific radiographic changes on a dorsoventral view may include an increased space between the femoral head and acetabulum, divergence of the medial acetabular rim from the femoral head (Fig. 18–15), sclerosis at the sites of joint capsule insertion, and early degenerative joint disease. Osteoarthritic changes are not usually a feature at the early stages of hip dysplasia. Some animals may go through a subclinically quiescent period after the joint capsule scars and microfractures heal and before degenerative joint disease causes noticeable pain. Puppies may exhibit the juvenile signs of hip dysplasia without clinical signs later in life.

Numerous modes of therapy are recommended, but the appropriate treatment chosen is according to the individual case. Conservative therapy includes confinement of the dog to a cage or crate and the administration of analgesic drugs (aspirin at a dosage of 25 mg/kg bid for 2 to 3 days). This approach allows the periarticular structures to heal temporarily and the pain to subside. Joint laxity and dysplasia persist, and recurrence of the pain and lameness are likely when the animal becomes active again. Three methods are recommended to improve the femoral head/acetabulum coverage and thereby decrease the stress and laxity of the dysplastic hip. The subtrochanteric osteotomy is used to change the angle of the femoral neck, which is then held in its new position by a plate and screw fixation to the femur. Alternatively, the pelvic osteotomy allows the acetabulum to be rotated over the femoral head, and it, too, is

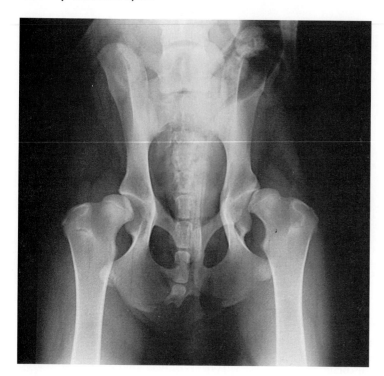

Figure 18–15. A ventrodorsal radiographic view of a dog's pelvis showing severe bilateral hip laxity and subluxation as a result of hip dysplasia.

secured in this position with a plate and bone screws (Slocum and Devine, 1986). Femoral neck lengthening uses wedge segments in the proximal femur to increase the medially directed forces on the femoral head into the acetabulum. Proponents of these surgical techniques advocate their use interchangeably, but the pelvic osteotomy has become more popular in veterinary surgery. The prognosis for pain-free limb function and a decreased or halted rate of joint degeneration is reported to be excellent. Candidates for this surgery should be without radiographic evidence of secondary degenerative joint disease and as young as possible, preferably before maturity. These surgical techniques provide the only corrective procedures that allow developmental changes to improve hip conformation with age. Bilateral surgeries may, however, be necessary.

Skeletally mature dogs generally have an osteoarthritis that precludes the use of any of the above surgical techniques with any real hope of success. In these cases, a total hip replacement (Olmstead, 1987) or a femoral head ostectomy offers the best chance of functional pain-free ambulation. Total hip replacement should, preferably, be restricted to dogs that have reached skeletal maturity. Because hip dysplasia is so common in large-breed and giant-breed dogs, the veterinarian should be aware of the potential for preventative measures applicable during the early growth stages. Owners of these puppies should be encouraged to limit activity to leash exercise of a moderate nature (Barr et al, 1987). Dietary control and avoidance of oversupplementation does not prevent the animal from reaching its full potential growth but does delay the growth spurt until the hip joints have matured sufficiently to withstand the stress of the weight gains. The natural tendency to think that bigger is better, especially in young growing dogs, should be avoided and counseled against. The heritable factor is recognized, and controlled breeding has been shown to reduce the incidence of hip dysplasia (Hutt, 1967; Lust et al, 1978). Breeding stock should be selected after radiographs taken at 2 years of age or older prove the absence of shallow hip joints.

LEGG-PERTHES (LEGG-CALVÉ-PERTHES) DISEASE

The condition known as Legg-Perthes disease is seen in toy-breed dogs, particularly the Yorkshire terrier. Aseptic necrosis of the femoral head starts developing at the time of physeal closure, which may be as early as 3 to 4 months of age in toy breeds. The cause of the condition is unknown. The aseptic necrosis is followed by collapse of the bone and eventual remodeling of the femoral head and neck. The end result is a grossly deformed femoral head, which leads to osteoarthritis in the hip joint (Ljunggren, 1967). Signs are not usually recognized until the arthritis develops, which can be as early as 6 months of age. Males are more commonly affected than females. A non–weight-bearing lameness develops, and manipulation of the hip joint causes a severe pain. Radiographs of the pelvis confirm the unilateral bony deformity of the femoral head (Fig. 18–16). Because these are toy-breed dogs, treatment by femoral head ostectomy is very rewarding. The dogs return to pain-free ambulation within a few weeks of surgery. Because a familial tendency is described, it would be wise to discourage breeding.

PATELLAR LUXATION

Congenital patellar luxation is most commonly seen as a medial displacement of the patella in toy-breed dogs. A medial or lateral luxation may occasionally occur in large-breed dogs. In medial displacement, the initiating factor probably is a lateral displacement of the femur by a congenital coxa vara of the femoral neck. This results in a medial displacement of the quadriceps muscle mechanism and the patella, which pulls the patella into a position medial to the trochlear groove and a medial patella luxation. The luxation results in abnormal stresses on the distal femur and proximal tibia during growth,

resulting in chronic conformational changes in the femur and tibia. A shallow trochlear groove, hypoplastic medial femoral condyle, hyperplastic lateral femoral condyle, and tibial and femoral rotation and bowing can all occur progressively. For grade 1 luxation, the patella is displaced out of the trochlea only when manually luxated. This results in no overt changes in the femur or tibia and is regarded as the mildest form of patellar luxation. In grade 4 luxation, the patella is permanently located out of the trochlear groove and cannot be replaced manually, resulting in severe changes in the distal femur and proximal tibia. All intervening stages depend on the chronicity of the congenital patellar luxation and severity of the underlying deformity (Table 18–1). Young cats have also been diagnosed with medial patellar luxation, but this is relatively rare.

The signs of medial patellar luxation are usually seen as short episodes of intermittent lameness. These episodes are related to the luxation that occurs in grade 2 cases, and the normal periods reflect a repositioning of the patella in the trochlear groove. The luxation is sometimes accompanied by pain, and the limb is carried until the patella relocates into the trochlea. In advanced cases, the dogs will be partially weight bearing, with the stifle rotated laterally and the hock pointed medially. The diagnosis can be confirmed by manual palpation of the patellar

Figure 18–16. A ventrodorsal radiographic view of a dog's pelvis showing severe unilateral remodeling changes in the femoral head and neck. A diagnosis of Legg-Perthes disease was made, and a femoral head and neck ostectomy was performed.

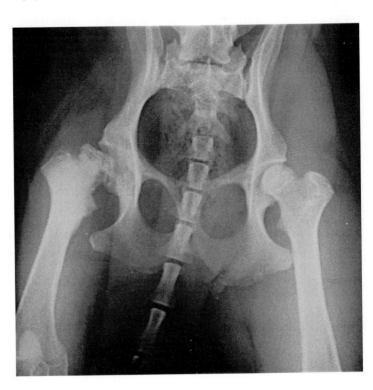

Table 18–1	Classification of Congenital Patellar Luxation	
GRADE OF LUXATION	**PRESENTING SIGN**	**CLINICAL FINDINGS ON PALPATION**
0	None	Patella cannot be luxated
1	Occasional yelp, usually none	Patella can be luxated manually but returns to the trochlear groove immediately
2	Short episodes of non–weight-bearing lameness and pain	When luxated, the patella will return to the trochlear groove only with the stifle in extension or on external rotation of the tibia
3	Frequent partial weight-bearing lameness	Patella will return to trochlear groove only if manually forced; reluxation is immediate
4	Constant weight-bearing lameness and bowed limbs	Patella cannot be replaced in trochlear groove

instability. Palpation techniques include inward rotation of the tibia and medial pressure on the patella. Once the patella is luxated, the depth of the trochlear groove may be assessed by palpation of the cranial distal femur. This procedure may need to be attempted with the dog standing and in lateral recumbency. Radiographs also confirm the luxation if the patella is displaced at the time of examination (Figs. 18–17 and 18–18). Secondary degenerative joint disease is rarely apparent in young dogs and only develops to a mild or moderate extent in chronic cases with the exception of grade 4 luxations.

As the condition worsens, it is preferable to correct the malalignment as soon as possible. Grade 1 luxations are not generally treated until they become grade 2 or worse. Corrective sur-

gery is recommended for grade 2 or worse luxations. A series of procedures is recommended according to the animal's needs. A medial capsulotomy is always used to release the medial fascial tension. A tibial crest transposition is used to correct the malalignment of the quadriceps/patella/tibial crest unit. The tibial crest is moved laterally and secured with two K-wires. The trochlea is examined and, if considered too shallow, it is deepened with a trochlearplasty, chondroplasty, or trochlear wedge recession. Where angular deformities exist in the distal femur and proximal tibia, wedge osteotomies can be used to straighten the bones appropriately. During closure, a lateral capsular imbrication helps to stabilize the patella and prevent medial luxation. Sutures between the fibula and

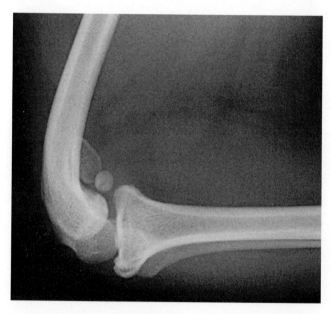

Figure 18–17. A lateral radiographic view of the hind leg of a dog with medial patellar luxation.

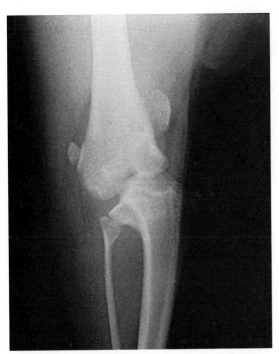

Figure 18–18. An anterior posterior radiographic view of the same leg seen in Figure 18–17 showing medial displacement of the patella, hypoplasia of the medial femoral condyle, curvature of the proximal tibia, and rotation of the tibia medially.

patella tendon can be used for this purpose as well. Descriptive details of these surgical procedures are provided elsewhere (Hulse and Shires, 1985). Although surgical correction does not halt the progression of degenerative joint disease, secondary osteoarthritis rarely leads to clinical lameness in dogs with mild to moderate patellar luxations. Because this condition is probably a heritable trait, breeding should be discouraged in affected animals.

Lateral patella luxation in large-breed dogs is treated in a similar manner to the medial patellar luxation but in an opposite fashion. The prognosis is similar for medial or lateral luxations with the same grade of patellar luxation.

ATLANTOAXIAL INSTABILITY

Several small breeds of dogs (Pomeranian, miniature poodle, Chihuahua) have shown a tendency to develop atlantoaxial instability in puppies without excessive trauma as the inciting cause (Shires, 1983). The anatomic abnormality is usually a congenital absence of the dens, unattached dens, angulated dens, or lack of ligamentous support between the atlas and axis. Head flexion during normal activity results in subluxa-

tion of the axis on the atlas and leads to variable degrees of spinal cord compression. If the dens is present or angled upward, the signs are proportionately more severe than would be seen when the dens is absent altogether. Affected puppies are usually presented with signs typical of a high cervical upper motor neuron disease. Ataxia in all four limbs may progress to quadriparesis or paralysis. Pain is usually seen with head movement. Radiographs confirm the diagnosis but flexed views should be avoided as this may further damage the spinal cord if a dens is present (Shires, 1983). Radiographs should be taken with the animal anesthetized; the neck must be protected during anesthesia (Fig. 18–19). The problem can be managed with a neck brace or by surgery.

Conservative management is generally a temporary measure to protect the neck until surgery is possible. Some dogs with mild cases have been braced for 3 to 4 weeks with no further breakdown of the atlantoaxial joint but many relapses at a later stage. Surgical treatment is to reattach the axis to the atlas. This can be accomplished by a dorsal approach and suture or wire fixation between the dorsal arch of C1 and the dorsal spine of C2. Dorsal stabilization using the nuchal ligament has also been described (LeCouteur et al, 1980). An alternative method is by a ventral approach using pins alone or in combination with methacrylate fixation of the bodies of the first and second cervical vertebrae. Ventral lag screw fixation of the first and second cervical vertebrae is also described. The prognosis is guarded and primarily depends on the neurologic status of the animal on admission. Animals with ataxia or paresis that are adequately stabilized can be expected to recovery fully. Breeding of these animals is not recommended.

CRANIOMANDIBULAR OSTEOPATHY

A genetic basis is suspected as the cause of craniomandibular osteopathy, which is a proliferative bone condition. The bones of the mandible, bullae, and occiput are most commonly affected (Alexander, 1985). Exuberant bony growth occurs on these bones that can lead to a functional impairment of mastication. In severe cases, fusion occurs between the vertical rami of the mandibles and the cranium. Puppies between 3 and 6 months of age are affected. The West Highland white and Scottish terrier breeds appear to be most commonly affected. In early cases, the signs are limited to pain

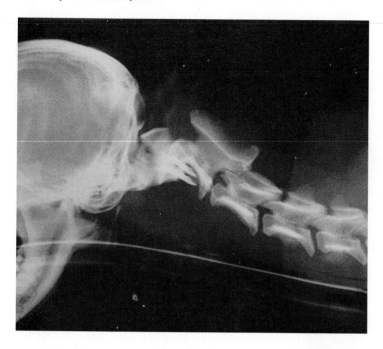

Figure 18–19. A lateral radiographic view of the upper cervical region of a dog with aplasia of the dens and atlantoaxial subluxation. Note the angulation of the canal at C1–C2 and the widened space between the dorsal arch of C1 and the spine of C2.

associated with opening the mouth. Intermittent fever, mandibular swelling, and salivation may also be seen. As the proliferation advances, mouth opening becomes restricted and eventually impossible. The diagnosis can be confirmed by radiographs of the skull that show proliferative sclerotic bone formation on the affected bones (Fig. 18–20).

Attempted medial therapy has included administration of corticosteroids and antimicrobial agents. Treatment is generally unrewarding, although the condition may be self-limiting. Unfortunately, in many cases, management of the puppy that is unable to open its mouth becomes impossible, and euthanasia is indicated. Surgical resection of segments of the mandible has been unrewarding because the proliferative process continued after surgery. The prognosis depends on the extent of the proliferation and rapidity of its development. Because a genetic basis for the condition is likely, affected animals are not considered breeding stock.

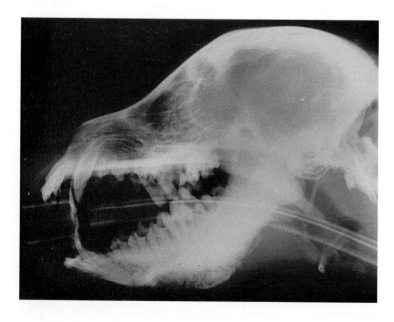

Figure 18–20. A lateral radiograph of the skull of a West Highland white terrier with proliferative bone on the mandible as a result of early craniomandibular osteoarthropathy.

PANOSTEITIS

Panosteitis is an inflammatory condition of the medullary canal that occurs in young, rapidly growing dogs (Barrett et al, 1986). The cause of the condition is unknown. More than one bone is usually affected, and the clinical sign is a shifting leg lameness. Puppies are usually presented at 6 to 8 months of age with a vague history of partial weight-bearing lameness (Burt and Wilson, 1972). Affected puppies are usually unwilling to play and are depressed. Appetite may be reduced. A diagnostic aid is the demonstration of pain associated with digital pressure applied directly on the long bones. Confirmation of the diagnosis is by observation of radiographic changes in the density of the bone in the medullary canal (Fig. 18–21). The canal often acquires a mottled appearance of varying densities. Treatment of panosteitis includes restriction of activity and administration of analgesic drugs. Typically, periods of increased and decreased lameness are observed. The condition usually resolves within 4 to 6 weeks.

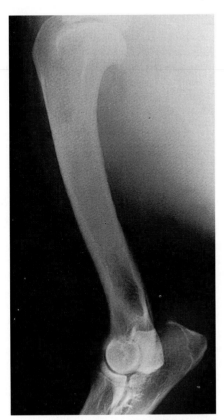

Figure 18–21. A lateral radiographic view of the humerus of a dog showing uneven increases in the density of the marrow cavity. When associated with pain on direct palpation of the bone, a diagnosis of panosteitis can be made.

BONE CYSTS

Bone cysts are fluid-filled defects occurring primarily in the distal extent of the long bones in dogs from 4 months to 4 years of age. The cysts are lined by fibrous connective tissue and rarely cause clinical signs until they become large or after a pathologic fracture through the lesion (Bierg et al, 1976). The cysts may be solitary or multiple, and affected breeds include German shepherd, Weimaraner, Irish wolfhound, and other large and giant breeds. Polyostotic bone cysts have been reported more often than monostotic cysts and may be associated with fibrous dysplasia. Polyostotic cysts also appear to cause clinical signs more frequently than monostotic cysts. The cause of bone cysts remains unknown but may be related to previous hemorrhage within the medullary canal with subsequent encapsulation and fluid transudation. Mature cysts have clearly defined radiographic features (Fig. 18–22). Pathologic fractures associated with bone cysts require rigid fixation and autogenous cancellous grafting. Therapy for nonfractured but clinical bone cysts may include drainage and autogenous grafting.

SWIMMER PUPPIES AND KITTENS

The condition of newborn puppies and kittens called swimmer puppy or kitten syndrome is similar to the myofibrillar hypoplasia syndrome seen in piglets. Although the cause is unknown, it has been suggested that viral or fungal infection in utero causes a muscular dystrophy in the developing fetus. Affected puppies and kittens are unable to stand at the expected developmental stage, usually after 10 days of age. The limbs, primarily the hindlimbs, project out sideways from the body, and forward movement is accomplished by lateral pedaling motions—hence "swimmer puppies and kittens."

Affected animals are frequently larger than littermates, and hyperlaxity of the affected joints is present. Their neurologic status is usually normal. Large puppies become dorsoventrally flattened, which is a permanent disfigurement. No other signs are associated with this disease, and affected animals usually begin to get up and walk over a 2- to 4-week period. The condition is self-correcting as the muscles develop and strengthen. Some veterinarians have suggested "hobbling" the hindlimbs together to prevent the splay-legged stance. Hobbling reduces the

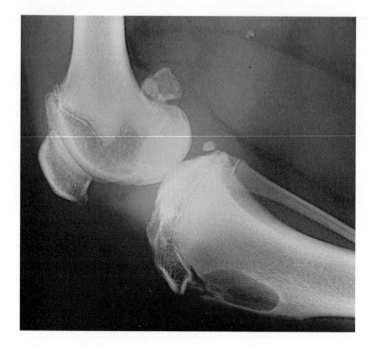

Figure 18–22. A lateral radiographic view of the stifle of a puppy showing a large bone cyst in the proximal region of the tibia.

permanent dorsoventral flattening but has no effect on the speed of functional improvement of the limbs.

MULTIPLE CARTILAGINOUS EXOSTOSES

A cartilaginous exostosis is a fragment of the growth plate that becomes detached from its normal location and remains on the surface of the newly formed bone. The chondrocytes continue to produce cartilage and bone until maturity is reached. Signs arise when the bony projections compromise adjacent normal structures. Affected puppies may have exostoses at multiple sites, which can be confirmed by radiography. Lesions appear as smooth or multilobular bony masses arising from normal cortical bone. If the bony outgrowths are causing a problem, they can be surgically removed. The prognosis for return of function is good if no permanent changes have occurred in the contiguous structures. Some authors have suggested a familial tendency and a possible association with osteosarcoma and chondrosarcoma.

OSTEOPETROSIS

Osteopetrosis is a rare inherited disease of dogs that results in a failure to resorb calcified cartilage. As a result, the bones are heavily mineralized. Australian shepherds and dachshunds are affected, and anemia secondary to obliteration of the medullary canal may occur (O'Brien et al, 1987). Osteopetrosis in a cat has also been reported. In 1- to 5-week-old puppies, the condition appears to resemble swimmer puppy. The limbs spread laterally, and the puppies usually rest on their sternebrae. Treatment is only supportive, and the condition carries a poor prognosis for recovery.

OSTEOMYELITIS, EPIPHYSITIS, AND SEPTIC ARTHRITIS

Septic arthritis is occasionally seen as a joint swelling in 1- to 6-week-old animals. The infection is usually recognized as an arthritis ("joint ill"), but this represents the end stage of a bacteremia originating from an infected umbilicus and localizing first near the end-arterial loops in the metaphysis of long bones. From there, infection spreads into the joint, and a symptomatic septic arthritis develops (Shires, 1990). Swollen, painful joints can be palpated in the affected young animal. The puppy or kitten is usually presented because it will not walk, cries when forced to walk, and has a depressed appetite and fever. A joint tap helps confirm the diagnosis when greater than 30,000 neutrophils/μl are seen in the synovial fluid (Harari, 1984). Aggressive antimicrobial therapy and joint lavage should be initiated early if the joints are to be salvaged. Systemic antimicrobial agents effective against gram-negative bacteria are appropriate until bacterial culture and sensitivity

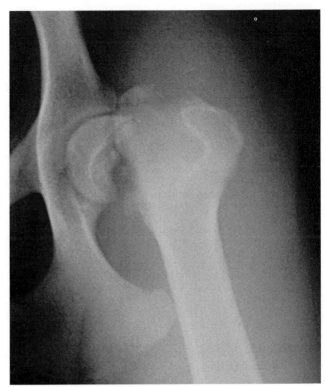

Figure 18–23. A ventrodorsal radiographic view of the hemipelvis and proximal portion of the femur of a 4-month-old puppy with a capital physeal fracture (Salter-Harris type II).

test results are available. Joint lavage with large volumes of sterile saline solution through an ingress-egress catheter system helps save some of the surviving cartilage. Non–weight-bearing exercise or passive physical therapy assists in cartilage rejuvenation and nutrition. Weight-bearing exercise must be severely curtailed for several weeks after the last signs of joint swelling have disappeared.

PHYSEAL FRACTURES

The weakest link in the bone-tendon-muscle unit is the growth plate. In the normal course of events, a severe traumatic injury to the young dog results in a physeal fracture (Fig. 18–23). The fracture line generally includes part of the weakest zone in the growth plate, which is the zone of hypertrophying cartilage. The consequences of a physeal fracture usually include complete or partial premature closure or partial closure of that growth plate (Shires, 1980). Premature closure has a pronounced impact in the radius and ulna (Fox, 1984a). Premature closure of the adjacent physis should be expected with any fracture in an immature animal; therefore, the owners should be advised of the potential problems associated with the eventual bone deformity.

Most expected problems are a direct result of reduced length of the affected bone. The magnitude of the discrepancy is dictated by the age of the animal at the time of trauma. Up to 20% of affected animals have a gait abnormality that usually leads to degenerative changes in the joints of the affected limb due to abnormal wear patterns. Some compensatory growth of the other long bones in the same extremity helps to offset the effects of the shortened bone. Prevention of physeal closure is not possible after the injury has occurred. Anatomic reconstruction and the use of implants that do not restrict bone lengthening minimize the effects of premature closure (Fox, 1984b). Some degree of additional length will be added to a bone after a fracture, even if the physis is bridged. The zone of hypertrophying cartilage continues to enlarge and mature despite the lack of new cartilage cells from the deeper layers. Bridging plates or sharply angled cross pins prevent this potential growth from occurring and worsen the effects of premature closure.

References and Supplemental Reading

Alexander JW: Hypertrophic osteodystrophy. Canine Pract 5:48, 1978.
Alexander JW: Craniomandibular osteopathy. *In* Slat-

ter DH (ed): Textbook of Small Animal Surgery, vol 2. Philadelphia, WB Saunders, 1985, p 2312.

Alexander JA, Earley TD: A carpal laxity syndrome in young dogs. J Vet Ortho 3:22, 1984.

Alexander JW, Richardson DC, Selcer BA: Osteochondritis diseases of the elbow, stifle and hock—A review. J Am Anim Hosp Assoc 17:51, 1981.

Barr ARS, Denny HR, Gibbs C: Clinical hip dysplasia in growing dogs: The long-term results of conservative management. J Small Anim Pract 28:243, 1987.

Barrett RB, Schall WB, Lewis RE: Clinical and radiographic features of canine eosinophilic panosteitis. J Am Anim Hosp Assoc 4:94, 1968.

Berzon JL: Osteochondritis diseases in the dog: Diagnosis and therapy. J Am Vet Med Assoc 175:796, 1979.

Berzon JL, Quick CB: Fragmented coronoid process: Anatomical, clinical and radiographic considerations with case analyses. J Am Anim Hosp Assoc 16:241, 1980.

Bierg DN, Goldschmidt M, Riser WH, et al: Bone cysts in dogs. J Am Vet Radiol Soc 17:202, 1976.

Breur GJ, Zerbe CA, Slocombe RF, et al: Clinical, radiologic, pathologic, and general features of osteochondrodysplasia in Scottish deerhounds. J Am Vet Med Assoc 195:606, 1989.

Burt JK, Wilson GP: A study of eosinophilic panosteitis (enostosis) in German shepherd dogs. Acta Radiol (Suppl 319):7, 1972.

Carrig CB, Wortman JA: Acquired dysplasias of the canine radius and ulna. Compend Contin Educ Pract Vet 3:557, 1981.

Craig E: Autogenous fat grafts to prevent recurrence following surgical correction of growth deformities of the radius and ulna in the dog. Vet Surg 10:69, 1981.

DeCamp CE, Haptman J, Knowlen G, et al: Periosteum and the healing of partial ulnar ostectomy in radius curvus of dogs. Vet Surg 15:185, 1986.

Fox SM: Premature closure of distal radial and ulnar physes in the dog. Part I. Pathogenesis and diagnosis. Compend Contin Educ Pract Vet 6:128, 1984a.

Fox SM: Premature closure of distal radial and ulnar physes in the dog. Part II. Treatment. Compend Contin Educ Pract Vet 6:212, 1984b.

Fox SM, Bloomberg MS, Bright RM: Developmental anomalies of the canine elbow. J Am Anim Hosp Assoc 19:605, 1983.

Goring RL, Bloomberg MS: Selected developmental abnormalities of the canine elbow: Radiographic evaluation and surgical management. Compend Contin Educ Pract Vet 5:178, 1983.

Grondalen J: Metaphyseal osteopathy in growing dogs. A clinical study. J Small Anim Pract 17:721, 1976.

Harari J: Osteomyelitis. J Am Vet Med Assoc 184:101, 1984.

Henry WB Jr: Radiographic diagnosis and surgical management of fragmented radial coronoid process in dogs. J Am Vet Med Assoc 184:799, 1984.

Hohn RB, Craig E, Anderson WD: Luxations of the shoulder joint. In Bojrab MJ (ed): Current Techniques in Small Animal Surgery, 2nd ed. Philadelphia, Lea & Febiger, 1983, p 726.

Hulse DA, Shires PK: The stifle joint. In Slatter DH (ed): Textbook of Small Animal Surgery, vol 2. Philadelphia, WB Saunders, 1985, p 2220.

Hutt FB: Genetic selection to reduce the incidence of hip dysplasia in dogs. J Am Vet Med Assoc 151:1041, 1967.

Kramers P, Fluckiger MA, Rahn BA, et al: Osteopetrosis in cats. J Small Anim Pract 29:153, 1988.

LeCouteur RA, McKeown D, Johnson J, et al: Stabilization of atlantoaxial subluxation in the dog using the nuchal ligament. J Am Vet Med Assoc 177:1011, 1980.

Lewis, DD, Parker RB, Hager DA: Fragmented medial coronoid process of the canine elbow. Compend Contin Educ Pract Vet 11:703, 1989.

Ljunggren G: Legg-Perthes disease in the dog. ACTA Orthop Scand Suppl 95:9, 1967.

Lust G, Farrell PW, Sheffy BE, et al: An improved procedure for genetic selection against hip dysplasia in dogs. Cornell Vet 68:41, 1978.

Manley PA, Romich JA: Miscellaneous orthopedic diseases. In Slatter DH (ed): Textbook of Small Animal Surgery, 2nd ed. Philadelphia, WB Saunders, 1993, p 1993.

Milton JL, Horne RD, Bartels JE, et al: Congenital elbow luxation in the dog. J Am Vet Med Assoc 175:542, 1979.

Montgomery M, Tomlinson J: Two cases of ectrodactyly and congenital elbow luxation in the dog. J Am Anim Hosp Assoc 21:781, 1985.

O'Brien SE, Riedesel EA, Miller LD: Osteopetrosis in an adult dog. J Am Anim Hosp Assoc 23:213, 1987.

Olmstead ML: Total hip replacement. Vet Clin North Am 17:943, 1987.

Olson NC, Mostosky UV, Flo GL, et al: Osteochondritis dissecans of the tarsocrural joint in three canine siblings. J Am Vet Med Assoc 176:635, 1980.

Olsson SE: Osteochondrosis—A growing problem to dog breeders. Gaines Prog 1:1, 1976.

Read RA, Armstrong SJ, O'Keefe JD, et al: Fragmentation of the medial coronoid process of the ulna in dogs: A study of 109 cases. J Small Anim Pract 31:330, 1990.

Roy RG, Wallace LJ, Johnston GR, et al: A retrospective evaluation of stifle osteoarthritis in dogs with bilateral medial patellar luxation and unilateral surgical repair. Vet Surg 21:475, 1992.

Schulz KS, Payne JT, Aronson E: Escherichia coli bacteremia associated with hypertrophic osteodystrophy in a dog. J Am Vet Med Assoc 199:1170, 1991.

Shires PK: Internal fixation of physeal fractures using the distal femur as an example. Compend Contin Educ Pract Vet 11:854, 1980.

Shires PK: Atlantoaxial instability. In Bojrab MJ (ed):

Current Techniques in Small Animal Surgery, 2nd ed. Philadelphia, Lea & Febiger, 1983, p 549.

Shires PK: Osteomyelitis. *In* Bojrab MJ (ed): Current Techniques in Small Animal Surgery, 3rd ed. Philadelphia, Lea & Febiger, 1990, p 909.

Shires PK, Hulse DA, Kearney JT: Carpal hyperextension in 2 month old pups. J Am Vet Med Assoc 186:49, 1985.

Slocum B, Devine T: Pelvic osteotomy technique for axial rotation of the acetabular segment in dogs. J Am Anim Hosp Assoc 22:331, 1986.

Van Bree H: Vacuum phenomenon associated with osteochondrosis of the scapulohumeral joint in dogs: 100 cases. J Am Vet Med Assoc 201:1916, 1992.

Vandewater A, Olmstead ML: Premature closure of the distal radial physis in the dog. Vet Surg 12:7, 1983.

Vaughan LC, Jones DGC: Congenital dislocation of the shoulder joint in the dog. J Small Anim Pract 10:1, 1969.

Wind AP, Packard ME: Elbow incongruity and developmental elbow diseases in the dog. J Am Anim Hosp Assoc 22:725, 1986.

Zontine WJ, Weitkamp RA, Lippincott CL: Redefined type of elbow dysplasia involving calcified flexor tendon attached to the medial humeral epicondyle in three dogs. J Am Vet Med Assoc 194:1082, 1989.

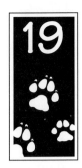

The Nervous and Neuromuscular Systems

Johnny D. Hoskins and G. Diane Shelton

The Nervous System

Johnny D. Hoskins

Numerous diseases affect the peripheral and central nervous systems of young dogs and cats. Most of these diseases are either inherited or caused by infectious agents. The veterinarian should appreciate special features of nervous system maturation as it relates to the young dog or cat. The peripheral and central nervous systems are not fully developed at birth, so their maturation presumably occurs as a function of several factors. There is continued differentiation of neuroblasts during at least the immediate postnatal period, with further arborization of cell processes. Myelination also continues until 6 weeks of age in puppies (Fox, 1967), and axon growth in peripheral nerves increases for at least the first 6 weeks of life (Braund et al, 1982). These processes appear to proceed at a somewhat variable rate among different dog and cat breeds.

PUPPY MATURATION

Puppies spend most of their time either sleeping or nursing during the first 2 weeks of life. Their sealed eyes and closed ear canals are two outward signs that actually reflect incompletely developed peripheral and central nervous systems. The gain or loss of certain responses is useful in the temporal monitoring of the maturation of the nervous system. Puppies can raise their heads at birth but not posture until 2 to 3 weeks of age. The rooting reflex, which begins disappearing at 4 days, causes the puppy to orient itself toward and push into any warm object near its head, and this warm object is most likely to be the mother or littermates. A puppy will also move toward the source of licking directed at its head and dorsum, using this as orientation toward its mother (Fox, 1965).

Immediately after birth, the puppy has little spontaneous movement and must receive stimulation from its mother's licking to begin breathing activities. Thereafter, activated sleep is prominent for the first week or longer. Activated sleep is characterized by jerking, tremor, crawling, scratching, and occasional vocalization. Quiet sleep does not appear until 1 to 2 weeks of age. Because of the inability to maintain its body heat, the puppy will huddle closely with its mother and littermates. During the first days of life, muscle tone is poorly developed, and there is an imbalance between the vertebral extensors and flexors. If the puppy is suspended by a hold at the base of the head, the puppy will respond during the first 4 to 5 days of life with the flexor dominance reflex by flexing the spine, tail, and limbs. From days 5 to 18, the extensor dominance reflex takes over so that the puppy extends the vertebral column and limbs, as if starting a backbend (Fox, 1965).

At the same time, maturation of the neuromuscular activities can be determined by other observatory factors. When moving, puppies rest on their abdomens and make stroking movements with their limbs on each side. Between 6 and 10 days of age, the forelimbs can support the weight of the puppy. Hindlimb support is expected between 11 and 15 days in normal, not overly fat puppies. Within a few days of being able to support its weight, the puppy is walking unsteadily around its environment. Another 4 weeks is needed before the puppy can quickly right itself.

In puppies younger than 18 days, the crossed extensor reflex is a normal reflex. The Magnus reflex, present from birth to 21 days of age, is normally seen only in puppies and not in adults (Fox, 1965). To test for the Magnus reflex, the body of the puppy is held and the nose is rotated to one side. The limbs on the side of the body opposite the side toward which the head was turned will be extended. The limbs on the other side will flex.

Reflex urination and defecation, in effect from birth through 21 days of age, requires that the mother be present to remove excreta from the puppy and to keep the sleeping area free of predator-attracting odors. The squatting urination posture for both male and female puppies is usually present by 28 days.

Visual and auditory responses continue to develop after birth. Initially the eyelids are sealed, and the auricular folds fill the auditory canal. With time, the eyelids separate and external ear canals open, usually between 5 and 14 days. Visual perception will still develop over time and is probably not complete until several months of age. Protective reflexes such as the light blink and corneal and palpebral reflexes are usually present before the eyelids actually separate. Startle reflex in response to sound is present at about 18 to 20 days of age (Scott and Fuller, 1965). With further maturation of the nervous system, a positive orientation to visual and auditory stimuli first occurs by 25 days of age, and specific recognition of familiar stimuli follows shortly (Fox, 1965).

KITTEN MATURATION

Although the processes of maturation of the kitten's and puppy's nervous systems and neuromuscular reflexes are often said to be similar, they are actually quite different (Beaver, 1992). In kittens, the sucking reflex begins about day 50 of gestation and ends by day 23 after birth. The crossed extensor reflex also begins by day 50 of gestation and continues up to 7 days after birth. The rooting reflex, present at birth, ends by day 16 (Beaver, 1992). Flexor dominance of the vertebral musculature in a suspended kitten is usually present from birth into adolescence and is commonly seen when a mother carries the kitten. Extensor dominance is much more variable in kittens than in puppies. Commonly, during the first 28 days, the kitten has an extended neck and flexed lower vertebral column.

The Landau reflex is first noted at birth and disappears by 19 days. To elicit this reflex, the kitten is suspended by the ventral midline in a normal dorsoventral relationship. The forelimbs and hindlimbs extend. The development of limb support is progressive in kittens, as it is in puppies. Forelimb support appears between 1 and 10 days of age, and the hindlimb support comes 4 days later (Beaver, 1980a).

Because the eyelids separate between 5 and 14 days after birth, the reflexes necessary to protect the eyes are in place earlier in kittens. The light blink reflex can develop as early as day 50 of gestation or as late as day 13 after birth (Beaver, 1992). It disappears in about 3 weeks. The pupillary response is present within 24 hours after the eyelids separate. Although slow at first, it will be adult-like within a few days. The palpebral reflex begins within the first few days after birth as a slow blink response and progresses to a more typical response by day 9. Depth perception is well developed by 4 weeks of age. Startle reflex in response to sudden noise can be present as early as day 3; however, it usually does not develop until shortly after the ear canals open. That occurs abruptly between days 6 and 17 (Beaver, 1980b).

Reflex urination and defecation disappear by 39 days of age, although kittens can voluntarily eliminate at 3 weeks. Another reflex, the air-righting reflex, develops as the kitten ages. This ability, which enables the cat to land on its feet, appears between 21 and 30 days of age, and it is perfected between 33 and 48 days (Carmichael, 1934; Warkentin and Carmichael, 1939).

NEUROLOGIC DISEASES

Numerous neurologic diseases have been recognized in puppies and kittens (Table 19–1). As in adults, neurologic lesions consistently cause characteristic neurologic deficits, thus allowing the veterinarian to predict the type of involvement—signs related to forebrain, cerebellar, vestibular, and spinal cord.

Forebrain Diseases: Change in Attitude, Seizures, Circling, Blindness, Compulsive Walking

Young dogs and cats with forebrain disease have expected neurologic deficits. Affected animals

Table 19–1 Neurologic and Muscular Diseases of Breeds of Young Dogs and Cats*

BREED	DISORDER	AGE AT ONSET	CLINICAL SIGNS
Afghan hound	Hereditary myelopathy	3–8 mo	Paraparesis progressing to tetraparesis
Airedale terrier	Cerebellar hypoplasia	<6 mo	Ataxia, hypermetria, intention tremor
Basset hoound	Cervical spondylopathy	<6 mo	Posterior ataxia progressing to tetraparesis
Beagle	Meningitis/vasculitis	<1 y	Hyperesthesia, stilted gait, ataxia
	Cerebellar degeneration	<4 wk	Cerebellar ataxia
Bernese mountain dog	Hypomyelination	<3 wk	Tremor
	Meningitis/vasculitis	<1 y	Cervical hyperesthesia, stilted gait, pyrexia
Birman cat	Distal axonopathy	8–10 wk	Posterior ataxia
Bluetick hound	Globoid cell leukodystrophy	3–6 mo	Paraparesis progressing to tetraparesis, tremor
Boston terrier	Hemivertebrae	Variable	Often subclinical; may cause hyperesthesia, ataxia, paresis
	Hydrocephalus	<6 mo	Depression, blindness, circling, ventrolateral strabismus, enlarged calvaria
Bouvier des Flandres	Laryngeal hemiplegia	4–6 mo	Exercise intolerance, stridor, dyspnea
Boxer	Progressive axonopathy	3–6 mo	Paraparesis progressing to tetraparesis, hyporeflexia
Brittany spaniel	Hereditary canine spinal muscular atrophy	4–6 mo	Crouching ataxic gait, proximal limb muscle atrophy, hyporeflexia
Bull mastiff	Cerebellar degeneration	6–9 wk	Ataxia, hypermetria, intention tremor
	Cervical spondylopathy	3–4 mo	Posterior ataxia, cervical hyperesthesia
Cairn terrier	Globoid cell leukodystrophy	3–6 mo	Paraparesis progressing to tetraparesis, blindness, tremor
	Chromatolytic neuronal degeneration	4–7 mo	Paraparesis progressing to tetraparesis, hyporeflexia, head tremor; cataplexy
Chihuahua	Hydrocephalus	<6 mo	Depression, blindness, circling, ventrolateral strabismus, enlarged calvaria
	Neuronal ceroid lipofuscinosis	12–15 mo	Dementia, ataxia, seizures
	Neuroaxonal dystrophy	7 wk	Tremor, ataxia, hypermetria
Chow chow	Dysmyelination	Birth to 4 wk	Ataxia, tremor
	Cerebellar hypoplasia	Birth to 4 wk	Ataxia, dysmetria, tremor
	Myotonia	2–4 wk	Muscle stiffness, myotonic dimple
Cocker spaniel	Multisystem neuronal degeneration	6–10 mo	Seizures, tremor, ataxia, aggression
	Congenital vestibular disease	Birth	Ataxia, rolling, head tilt

Table continued on following page

Table 19–1

Neurologic and Muscular Diseases of Breeds of Young Dogs and Cats* *Continued*

BREED	DISORDER	AGE AT ONSET	CLINICAL SIGNS
Collie	Dermatomyositis	<6 mo	Facial dermatitis, masticatory muscle atrophy
	Cerebellar degeneration	4–8 wk	Posterior/truncal ataxia, hypermetria, intention tremor
	Neuroaxonal dystrophy	2–4 mo	Truncal ataxia, hypermetria, intention tremor
Dachshund	Sensory neuropathy	Birth to 4 wk	Ataxia, decreased pain sensation, self-mutilation
	Narcolepsy-cataplexy	<6 mo	Excess sleep, postural collapse (cataplexy)
Dalmatian	Congenital deafness	Birth	Deafness
	Reflex myoclonus	2–6 wk	Muscular hypertonicity exacerbated by exercise
	Cavitating leukodystrophy	3–6 mo	Paraparesis progressing to tetraparesis; behavioral abnormalities; visual loss
Doberman pinscher	Narcolepsy-cataplexy	<6 mo	Excess sleep, postural collapse (cataplexy)
	Congenital vestibular disease	3–12 wk	Head tilt, ataxia, circling, nystagmus
English bulldog	Hydrocephalus	6 mo	Depression, blindness, circling, ventrolateral strabismus, enlarged calvaria
	Sacrocaudal malformation	Birth	Paraparesis, urinary-fecal incontinence
	Hemivertebrae	Variable	Often subclinical; may cause hyperesthesia, ataxia, paresis
English pointer	Sensory neuropathy	<6 mo	Distal limb anesthesia and self-mutilation
English setter	Congenital deafness	Birth	Deafness
	Neuronal ceroid lipofuscinosis	12–15 mo	Dementia, ataxia, seizures
German shepherd	Congenital vestibular disease	3–4 wk	Head tilt, ataxis
	Giant axonal neuropathy	15 mo	Paraparesis, areflexia, decreased pelvic limb pain sensation
	Spinal muscular atrophy	<4 wk	Valgus deformity of thoracic limb(s) due to flexor contracture; tetraparesis
German short-haired pointer	GM_1 gangliosidosis	6–12 mo	Dementia, blindness, seizures
Golden retriever	X-linked muscular dystrophy	8–10 wk	Stilted gait, muscle atrophy/hypertrophy, dysphagia
	Hypomyelinating polyneutropathy	<7 wk	Pelvic limb ataxia and weakness, hyporeflexia
Gordon setter	Hereditary cortical cerebellar abiotrophy	6–24 mo	Ataxia, dysmetria
Great Dane	Cervical spondylopathy	6 mo to 2 y	Posterior ataxia progressing to tetraparesis
Irish setter	Hereditary quadriplegia and amblyopia	Birth to 5 wk	Tetraplegia, tremor, nystagmus, seizures

| Table 19–1 | Neurologic and Muscular Diseases of Breeds of Young Dogs and Cats* *Continued* |

BREED	DISORDER	AGE AT ONSET	CLINICAL SIGNS
Irish terrier	X-linked muscular dystrophy	8–10 wk	Stilted gait, dysphagia
Jack Russell terrier	Myasthenia gravis	6 wk	Episodic weakness
	Hereditary ataxia	2–6 mo	Paraparesis progressing to tetraparesis, ataxia, dysmetria
Kerry blue terrier	Hereditary cerebellar cortical and extrapyramidal nuclear abiotrophy	9–16 wk	Ataxia, hypermetria, tremor, hypertonia
Korat cat	GM$_1$ gangliosidosis	4–8 wk	Tremor, ataxia, blindness, seizures
Labrador retriever	Myopathy	3–4 mo	Stiff gait, cervical ventroflexion, patellar hyporeflexia
	Reflex myoclonus	2–4 wk	Muscular hypertonicity, extensor rigidity, opisthotonos—exacerbated by exercise
	Spongiform encephalopathy	4–6 mo	Dysmetria, tremor, extensor rigidity
	Narcolepsy-cataplexy	<6 mo	Excess sleep, postural collapse (cataplexy)
	Cavitating leukodystrophy	4 mo to adult	Ataxia, blindness, depression
Lhasa apso	Lissencephaly	<18 mo	Depression, poor housetraining, seizures
Maltese	Idiopathic tremor	6 mo to 5 y	Generalized tremor
	Hydrocephalus	<1 y	Seizures, depression, poor housetraining
Manx cat	Sacrocaudal malformation	Birth	Paraparesis, urinary-fecal incontinence
Old English sheepdog	Congenital deafness	Birth	Deafness
	Metabolic myopathy	<1 y	Episodic weakness, stiff pelvic limb gait
Poodle	Atlantoaxial subluxation	6–18 mo	Hyperesthesia, ataxia, tetraparesis
	Sphingomyelinosis	4–6 mo	Ataxia, tremor, hypermetria
	Narcolepsy-cataplexy	<6 mo	Excess sleep, postural collapse (cataplexy)
Portuguese water dog	GM$_1$ gangliosidosis	<5 mo	Tremor, ataxia, dysmetria, nystagmus
Pug	Meningitis	<3 y	Seizures, depression, circling, head pressing, blindness, cervical hyperesthesia
Rottweiler	Neuroaxonal dystrophy	1–2 y	Ataxia, hypermetria, head tremor
	Spinal muscular atrophy	<4 wk	Paraparesis progressing to tetraparesis, hyporeflexia, head tremor

Table continued on following page

Table 19–1

Neurologic and Muscular Diseases of Breeds of Young Dogs and Cats* *Continued*

BREED	DISORDER	AGE AT ONSET	CLINICAL SIGNS
Samoyed	Hypomyelination	<3 wk	Tremor, inability to stand
	X-linked muscular dystrophy	8–10 wk	Stilted gait, muscle atrophy/ hypertrophy, dysphagia
Scottish terrier	Scottie cramp	2–18 mo	Muscle stiffness following exercise
Siamese cat	GM$_1$, GM$_2$ gangliosidosis	3–6 mo	Ataxia, tremor, tetraparesis
	Mucopolysaccharidosis	6–8 wk	Stunted growth, broad face, corneal clouding; para- paresis may develop later
	Sphingomyelinosis	4–6 mo	Ataxia, tremor, hypermetria
	Congenital strabismus and nystagmus	Birth	Strabismus, nystagmus
Siberian husky	Laryngeal paralysis	<1 y	Exercise intolerance, dyspnea, stridor
Silky terrier	Glucocerebrosidosis	6–8 mo	Ataxia, tremor
Smooth-haired fox terrier	Masthenia gravis	4–8 wk	Episodic weakness
	Hereditary ataxia	2–6 mo	Posterior ataxia, thoracic limb hypermetria
Springer spaniel	Hypomyelination	Birth to 4 wk	Ataxia, tremor
	Fucosidosis	6–18 mo	Behavioral changes, ataxia
	Myasthenia gravis	6 wk	Episodic weakness
Swedish Lapland	Hereditary neuronal abiotrophy	5–7 wk	Ataxia progressing to tetraplegia, atrophy of distal limb muscles, hyporeflexia
Tibetan mastiff	Hypertrophic neuropathy	2–3 mo	Paraparesis progressing to tetraparesis, hyporeflexia
Weimaraner	Spinal dysraphism	Birth to 4 wk	Simultaneous advancement of pelvic limbs
	Hypomyelination	Birth to 4 wk	Ataxia, tremor
West Highland white terrier	Globoid cell leukodystrophy	3–6 mo	Paraparesis progressing to tetraparesis, blindness, tremor
Yorkshire terrier	Atlantoaxial subluxation	<1 y	Tetraparesis, cervical hyperesthesia
	Hepatic encephalopathy	<1 y	Ataxia, seizures, head pressing, circling, blindness

Modified from Kornegay JN (ed): Neurologic Disorders, vol 5, Contemporary Issues in Small Animal Practice. New York, Churchill Livingstone, 1986, p 1.

*This table does not include most individual case reports or diseases that have been discussed only briefly in chapters and/or proceedings.

tend to be depressed or have atypical behavior, walk compulsively or circle to the side of the lesion, have contralateral postural reaction and visual field deficits, and may have seizures.

HYDROCEPHALUS

Excessive accumulation of cerebrospinal fluid (CSF) within or outside the ventricular system of the brain is characterized as *internal hydrocephalus* or *external hydrocephalus*, respectively. Most cases of congenital hydrocephalus in young dogs and cats are of the internal type. Congenital and acquired hydrocephalus is more common in young dogs than in young cats. Congenital hydrocephalus usually results from structural defects that either obstruct CSF outflow or impede absorption. Maltese, Yorkshire terrier, English bulldog, Chihuahua, Manchester terrier, Lhasa apso, Pomeranian, toy poodle, Cairn terrier, Boston terrier, pug, and Pekingese have a higher risk of congenital hydrocephalus than other dog breeds (Selby et al, 1979). Many cases of congenital hydrocephalus appear to progress after birth. For example, continued enlargement of the lateral ventricles is evident on sequential computed tomographic studies during the first 2 years of life in hydrocephalic

Maltese dogs (Simpson, 1989). A definite hereditary basis for congenital hydrocephalus has not been proved for any toy or brachycephalic dog breed. One report suggested that Siamese cats might inherit hydrocephalus as a recessive trait (Silson and Robinson, 1969).

Acquired hydrocephalus rarely occurs in young animals, except possibly in young cats. Acquired hydrocephalus has been recognized in young cats with encephalitis due to the feline infectious peritonitis virus (Krum et al, 1975; Tamke et al, 1998). This might occur because of impaired outflow of CSF due to ventriculitis and arachnoiditis.

Young dogs and cats with congenital or acquired hydrocephalus have variable clinical signs, with some having minimal signs and others having marked neurologic dysfunction referable to forebrain disease. Clinical findings typically include a dome-shaped calvarium (Fig. 19–1), open fontanelle, compulsive walking, head pressing, attitudinal changes, blindness, and seizures. In less affected animals, behavioral changes and difficulty in house training may occur. Some affected animals may have ventrolateral strabismus and be rather small for their age. The progression of neurologic dysfunction is also variable. The presence of an open fonta-

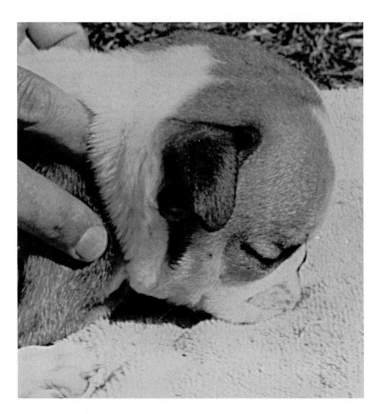

Figure 19–1. Bulldog puppy with a dome-shaped calvarium.

nelle should not be considered as diagnostic of congenital hydrocephalus because it may occur as a normal variant in otherwise healthy dogs.

A diagnosis of congenital hydrocephalus is suggested by the clinical findings. Ultrasonography is useful in demonstrating ventricular enlargement in dogs with persistent fontanelles (Rivers and Walter, 1992; Spaulding and Sharp, 1990). Dilation of the ventricular system may be confirmed by computed tomography. Nuclear scintigraphy may be used to evaluate the patency of the ventricular system and CSF shunt procedures used in long-term treatment (Kay et al, 1986). Cerebrospinal fluid should be evaluated in suspected dogs with congenital and acquired hydrocephalus to determine if encephalitis is present.

Dogs with minimal or no neurologic dysfunction may not require treatment. Many young dogs with congenital hydrocephalus remain relatively free of clinical signs with prolonged alternate-day glucocorticoids (dexamethasone, 0.1 mg/kg orally) (Averill, 1978; Sato et al, 1973). Unfortunately, puppies younger than 2 to 4 months may not respond to glucocorticoids as well as those that are older (Fukata and Arakawa, 1955; Hoerlein and Gage, 1978). Diuretics like furosemide generally offer limited improvement in puppies with any clinical signs. Surgical CSF drainage requires permanent placement of a ventriculovenous or ventriculoperitoneal shunt. Potential complications of such CSF shunt procedures include infection and occlusion or change in position of the catheter (Few, 1966; Gage and Hoerlein, 1968; Kay

et al, 1986). Young dogs with progressive underlying encephalitis are unlikely to benefit long term from CSF shunt procedures.

LISSENCEPHALY

Lissencephaly is characterized by marked reduction in the number of or absence of cerebral gyri (Fig. 19–2) (Frauchiger and Fankhauser, 1957; Greene et al, 1976; Zaki, 1976). A hereditary basis is suspected for wire-haired fox terriers, Irish setters, and Lhasa apsos. Lissencephaly may also occur concomitantly with cerebellar hypoplasia in wire-haired fox terriers and Irish setters (de Lahunta, 1983). Most affected animals are symptomatic at birth or shortly after. Signs in Lhasa apsos include alternating depression and excitability, aggression toward the owners, postural reaction and visual deficits, difficulty in housetraining, and seizures (Greene et al, 1976; Zaki, 1976). Computed tomography or magnetic resonance imaging may be useful in delineating the absence of gyri. There is no effective therapy.

CRANIAL DYSRAPHISM

Cranial dysraphism includes conditions such as anencephaly, exencephaly, cranium bifida, encephalocele, meningocele, and cyclopia. Anencephaly is a condition in which the brain is absent at birth, or, more commonly, only the basal nuclei and cerebellum are developed (Field and Wanner, 1975; Frauchiger and Fankhauser, 1957; Sekeles, 1981). In exencephaly,

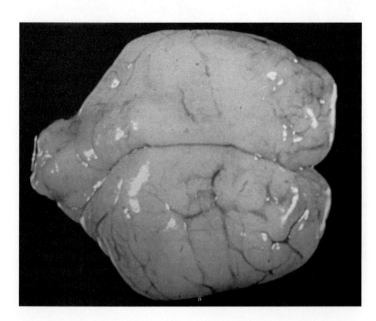

Figure 19–2. Cerebrum from a 3-day-old female mixed-breed puppy with depression and spina bifida noted soon after birth. The lack of cerebral sulci is consistent with lissencephaly. (Courtesy of Drs. John Santilli and Scott Plummer.)

the brain is exposed due to a congenital cleft in the skull (cranium bifida). In the case of encephalocele and meningocele, the brain or meninges actually protrude through the congenital cleft in the skull (Field and Wanner, 1975; Griffiths, 1971; Khera, 1973, 1979; Scott et al, 1974; Sekeles, 1981; Zook et al, 1983). Encephalocele and other craniofacial anomalies may be inherited in Burmese cats through a simple autosomal recessive mode (Zook et al, 1983). Cyclopia is a developmental anomaly characterized by a single orbital fossa, with either complete or partial agenesis of the eye. Affected puppies and kittens often are born dead or die soon after birth. Those anomalies involving the skull and brain generally are obvious. The animals that survive the immediate postnatal period generally have neurologic deficits related to forebrain disease. Euthanasia is generally appropriate because of secondary complications that arise. Simple cranial meningocele may be amenable to surgery.

NARCOLEPSY-CATAPLEXY

Narcolepsy is a condition associated with excessive daytime sleep, whereas cataplexy refers to periods of acute muscular hypotonia often seen in association with narcolepsy (Aldrich, 1992; Motoyama et al, 1989). Affected dogs often have abnormal sleep patterns. Rapid eye movement (REM) sleep rather than the expected initial period of nonrapid eye movement activity marks the onset of sleep in affected dogs. Excessive movement has also been associated with REM sleep in both dogs and cats (Hendricks et al, 1989). An apparent simple autosomal recessive mode of inheritance has been suggested in Doberman pinschers and Labrador retrievers with narcolepsy-cataplexy. Multiple cases have also been recognized in miniature poodle, dachshund, beagle, Saint Bernard, Airedale terrier, Afghan hound, Irish setter, Welsh corgi, Alaskan malamute, Rottweiler, English springer spaniel, and giant schnauzer dogs. Narcolepsy-cataplexy may also occur in the cat (Knecht et al, 1973). Dogs with narcolepsy-cataplexy may have abnormal sleep patterns as early as a few weeks of age (Baker et al, 1983). Doberman pinschers and Labrador retrievers usually have abnormal sleep patterns initially by 4 months of age. Although the abnormal sleep patterns may be severe early in life, they tend to ameliorate in adulthood. In those breeds without an established pattern of inheritance, initial abnormal sleep patterns have been noted between 10 weeks and 7 years of age.

Cataplexy is generally the most pronounced sign in affected dogs, perhaps in part because most owners (Shores and Redding, 1987) may not notice excessive sleepiness. Cataplectic attacks are characterized by periods of acute flaccid paralysis lasting from a few seconds to 20 minutes (Baker et al, 1983). Cataplectic attacks can involve all skeletal muscles or only those of the forelimbs or hindlimbs. Such attacks may number only a few episodes or hundreds per day. A typical attack is accompanied by components of REM sleep, such as rapid eye movements, twitches of distal muscles, weak vocalizations, and facial grimaces. Affected dogs remain conscious and still visually track objects during the attack. In most cases, feeding, playing, or attempts at sexual intercourse induce cataplexy in dogs. Petting the affected dog or making loud noises appears to speed resolution of the attack (Foutz et al, 1980).

Signs of narcolepsy-cataplexy are relatively specific but may be confused with other causes of transient weakness or loss of consciousness, such as myasthenia gravis and syncope. Intravenous physostigmine (0.025 to 0.1 mg/kg) may increase the frequency and severity of cataplectic attacks for up to 45 minutes, so it may be useful in identifying mildly affected dogs (Guilleminault and Baker, 1986). The food-elicited cataplexy test can be used to assess the severity of cataplectic attacks. Suspected dogs are encouraged to eat 10 pieces of food placed in a row. The time required to eat all of the pieces and the number of attacks noted during this period are recorded. Whereas unaffected dogs will eat all 10 pieces of food within 45 seconds without evidence of cataplexy, cataplectic dogs may require 2.5 to 30 minutes and may have from 2 to 20 complete or partial cataplectic attacks (Guilleminault and Baker, 1986).

Treatment of affected dogs generally is directed toward the cataplectic attacks. The tricyclic antidepressants (imipramine, 0.5 to 1.0 mg/kg orally three times a day) usually reduce the severity of cataplexy because of their anticholinergic effects (Hendricks and Hughes, 1989). Arousal-promoting agents can be used to relieve the excessive sleepiness if necessary. Any monoamine oxidase inhibitors should be avoided, as cardiovascular side effects may be pronounced. Owners should be told that complete elimination of cataplectic attacks might not be possible. Affected dogs should not be used for breeding.

METABOLIC DISORDERS

Hepatic encephalopathy and renal encephalopathy may cause deficits indicative of multifocal central nervous system involvement that is referable principally to forebrain disease. The most common neurologic signs include blindness, ataxia with associated head pressing, hysteria, seizures, ptyalism, and behavioral changes. Puppies with glycogen storage diseases, idiopathic hepatic lipidosis, or idiopathic hypoglycemia usually have clinical involvement by 1 to 3 months of age. The primary manifestations are signs related to the hypoglycemia. Signs of hypoglycemia generally occur only when the blood glucose concentration falls below 40 mg/dl. Signs may include tachycardia, tremor, nervousness, vocalization, irritability, and intense hunger. These signs may be absent if the fall in glucose concentration has occurred gradually, in which case neuroglucopenic signs (e.g., visual disturbances, mental dullness, depression or stupor, and seizures) will predominate.

Cerebellar Diseases: Ataxia, Dysmetria, Intention Tremor

CEREBELLAR ABIOTROPHIES

Cerebellar abiotrophies are a group of generally inherited, slowly progressive diseases of the cerebellum reported in many dog breeds—Kerry blue terrier, Gordon setter, rough-coated collie, Australian kelpie, Airedale terrier, Bernese running dog, Bernese mountain dog, Finnish harrier, Brittany spaniel, bull mastiff, border collie, Irish setter, beagle, Samoyed, wire-haired terrier, Labrador retriever, golden retriever, Great Dane, chow chow, Rhodesian ridgeback—and in cats. A simple autosomal recessive mode of inheritance has been suggested for most of the cerebellar abiotrophies. Neurologic deficits from cerebellar abiotrophies generally are not present immediately after birth but are noticed after 6 to 8 weeks of age and may not even be noticed until 2 years of age. A diagnosis of cerebellar abiotrophy is suggested by the presence of unexplained progressive neurologic dysfunction referable to the cerebellum. A diagnosis may be established by cerebellar biopsy in some dogs. Molecular genetic markers may eventually allow identification of affected dogs or carriers. There is no treatment for dogs with cerebellar abiotrophies, but some affected animals may be acceptable pets for several months, if not longer.

CANINE CEREBELLAR HYPOPLASIA

Numerous breed-related reports of cerebellar hypoplasia have been described in dogs. The cerebellum may appear to be malformed at birth or may contain uniform types of cerebellar hypoplasia in which clinical signs of cerebellar dysfunction are present soon after birth (de Lahunta, 1983; Knecht et al, 1979). Truncal ataxia, hypermetria, and intention tremor are most commonly first seen around 2 weeks of age when affected puppies begin to walk. The presence of nonprogressive signs of cerebellar dysfunction in a young dog is always suggestive of cerebellar hypoplasia. Computed tomography and cisternography (optic thecography) may be used to demonstrate lesions (Schmid et al, 1992). There is no treatment for affected dogs, but some may be acceptable pets.

FELINE CEREBELLAR HYPOPLASIA

Cerebellar hypoplasia in kittens is associated most commonly with in utero infection of pregnant cats with the panleukopenia virus (Johnson et al, 1967; Kilham and Margolis, 1966; Kilham et al, 1967). The panleukopenia virus induces cerebellar hypoplasia because of its cytopathic effect on rapidly dividing cells of the cerebellum. As a results, the cerebella of affected kittens generally are grossly small, and cerebellar folds are narrow. Multiple breeds of cats have been affected with cerebellar hypoplasia due to in utero panleukopenia virus infection. All kittens of some litters are affected, whereas only one kitten or a portion of the litter is affected in others. Affected kittens have signs of cerebellar involvement that are first noted when the animal begins to walk or eat solid food around 2 to 4 weeks of age. Apparent clinical improvement may be noted in some kittens. Establishing a definitive diagnosis may be difficult. Serologic assay for antibodies to the panleukopenia virus is not helpful. Magnetic resonance imaging studies can be helpful in identifying cerebellar hypoplasia and associated anomalies in affected kittens. Although there is no treatment for cerebellar hypoplasia, affected kittens are usually acceptable pets.

HYPOMYELINOGENESIS-DYSMYELINOGENESIS

Reduced (hypomyelinogenesis) and abnormal (dysmyelinogenesis) myelinogenesis of the central nervous system have been reported in several dog breeds—chow chow, Welsh springer spaniel, Samoyed, weimaraner, lurcher, golden retriever, Dalmatian, Australian silky terrier, schnauzer, and Bernese mountain dog (Cummings et al, 1986; Duncan et al, 1983; Griffiths et al, 1981a,b; Kornegay et al, 1987; Palmer et al, 1987; Vandevelde et al., 1978, 1981). The altered myelinogenesis in springer spaniels is inherited through an X-linked mode. Most affected dogs have generalized tremor by 2 to 3 weeks of age. In each case, only myelinogenesis of the central nervous system is affected. The generalized tremor tends to lessen at rest or during sleep and becomes more pronounced during excitement and movement. Generalized tremor often resolves in affected chow chow and Weimaraner dogs by 8 to 12 months of age, whereas in springer spaniel and Samoyed dogs there is a tendency to be more severely affected and not show significant improvement. Biopsy of the brain allows for a definitive diagnosis, if desired. Magnetic resonance imaging may be used to demonstrate the myelin paucity. There is no treatment, but spontaneous improvement may be anticipated in chow chows and Weimaraners. Affected springer spaniels may be unable to eat and thus require special attention.

Congenital Peripheral Vestibular Disease: Ataxia, Head Tilt, Nystagmus

Congenital peripheral vestibular dysfunction has been described in Siamese and Burmese cats (de Lahunta, 1983) and in a number of dog breeds, including German shepherd (Stirling and Clark, 1981), English cocker spaniel (Bedford, 1979), Doberman pinscher (Fig. 19–3) (Chrisman, 1982; Forbes and Cook, 1991), beagle (de Lahunta, 1983), and Shetland sheepdog (Simpson, 1983). The absence of signs of central vestibular disease in affected animals suggests that a neurologic problem resides within the peripheral labyrinth. Affected animals usually have signs such as head tilt, circling, and rolling at birth or within a few weeks. There is spontaneous improvement, if not resolution, of these signs in some animals by the time they are 6 months to 1 year of age. No specific treatment is indicated. Some affected dogs may also have deafness.

Spinal Cord Diseases: Paraparesis, Tetraparesis

ATLANTOAXIAL SUBLUXATION

Agenesis or hypoplasia of the dens, nonunion of the dens with the axis, absence of the transverse ligament of the atlas, and dorsal angulation of the odontoid process with compression of the spinal cord have been associated with atlantoaxial subluxation in young dogs and cats. Congen-

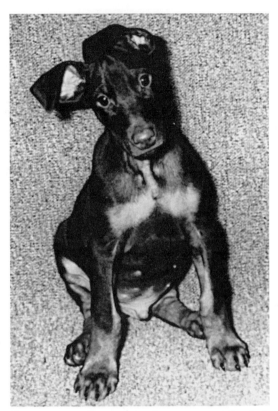

Figure 19–3. Doberman pinscher puppy with head tilt of suspected congenital origin.

ital lesions are seen most commonly in young toy or miniature breeds of dogs. Traumatic atlantoaxial subluxation may occur in any breed of dog or cat. Although signs may be noted within the first few months of life, affected dogs often are clinically normal until they are at least 1 year of age. Clinical signs vary from mild cervical pain to tetraparesis or tetraplegia. Deficits may occur with sudden onset or progress insidiously.

Survey radiographs should be obtained with the animal awake to lessen the likelihood of further movement of the axis. Dorsal displacement of the axis relative to the atlas can usually be demonstrated on a lateral cervical radiograph. This displacement results in loss of the normal parallel relationship of the dorsal laminae of the atlas and axis. A ventrodorsal view allows study of the cranial aspect of the axis in cases of abnormalities of the dens (Fig. 19–4). Conservative therapy, including external splinting or casting, generally is ineffective on a long-term basis. Various surgical techniques have been described, utilizing either a dorsal or a ventral approach (Schulz, 1997; Thomas, 1991; Thomson and Read, 1996).

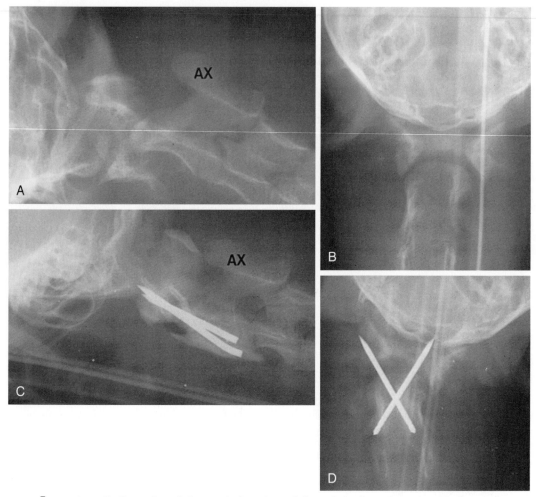

Figure 19–4. Radiographs of the cervical region of the spine of a miniature pinscher with cervical hyperesthesia and atlantoaxial subluxation taken before (**A** and **B**) and after (**C** and **D**) stabilization with pins placed across the joint ventrally. Note the marked dorsal luxation of the axis (AX) relative to the atlas preoperatively, with subsequent reduction. The odontoid process is absent. (Courtesy of Dr. Steve Lane.)

SPINAL DYSRAPHISM

Spinal dysraphism refers to congenital abnormalities involving the spinal, cord, vertebral column, and skin subsequent to faulty closure of the neural tube. Most lesions occur in the caudal lumbar, sacral, or caudal portions of the spine (Lemire, 1969). Defective fusion of the vertebral arch (spina bifida) is the most common vertebral lesion (Kitchen et al, 1972; Wilson et al, 1979). Meninges (meningocele) or roots (myelocele) or both (meningomyelocele) may protrude through this vertebral defect (Clark and Carlisle, 1975; Parker et al, 1973). The tethering effect of lesions such as meningocele on nerve roots contributes to clinical signs seen in affected animals (Plummer et al, 1993). Sa-

crocaudal vertebral dysgenesis is often observed in affected animals, particularly in Manx cats (James et al, 1969). Sacrocaudal vertebral dysgenesis is inherited as an autosomal dominant trait and may be lethal in some homozygote Manx cats (Leipold et al, 1974).

Several congenital spinal cord lesions are associated with spinal dysraphism. Spinal clefts (myeloschisis) may communicate with a dilated central canal (hydromyelia) or cystic spaces within the spinal parenchyma (syringomyelia) (James et al, 1969; Wilson et al, 1979). These spinal cord lesions may occur in the absence of vertebral and meningeal lesions (Child et al, 1986; Johnson et al, 1992). Intraarachnoid cysts also may occur because of spinal dysraphism (Bentley et al, 1991).The spinal cord may terminate further caudally in the vertebral canal or be divided in half by a bony spicule or fibrous band (diastematomyelia) (James et al, 1969). Other vertebral changes such as hemivertebra and vertebral stenosis also may occur concomitant with spinal dysraphism (Shell et al, 1988). The spinal dysraphism observed in Weimaraner dogs is transmitted by a codominant gene with reduced penetrance and variable expressivity (Engel and Draper, 1982a,b; McGrath, 1965).

Spinal dysraphism is most common in Manx cats (James et al, 1969; Leipold et al, 1974) and brachycephalic breeds of dogs, such as the bulldog (Parker et al, 1973; Wilson et al, 1979). Neurologic dysfunction generally is present from birth and has a nonprogressive course (James et al, 1969). Because the caudal lumbar, sacral, and caudal spinal cord segments are affected most commonly, lower motor neuron dysfunction in the distribution of the sciatic, pudendal, and caudal nerves predominates. There often is mild paraparesis, with loss of the flexion and perineal reflexes, and urinary-fecal incontinence. The tail may be absent or extremely short. Meningoceles may be palpated or exposed in cases where there are dermal clefts (rachischisis) (Frye and McFarland, 1965). Hair overlying dysraphic lesions is sometimes whorled. Cervicothoracic lesions may cause torticollis, scoliosis, or both (Child et al, 1986; Johnson et al, 1992).

Most vertebral anomalies can be identified on survey radiographs (Parker et al, 1973; Wilson et al, 1979). The dorsal spine and vertebral arch are absent in spina bifida. Meningoceles may be found with myelography. Simple meningoceles can be excised surgically. Most anomalous spinal cord lesions cannot be surgically corrected. Hindlimb paralysis and urinary-fecal incontinence persist.

OSTEOCHONDROMATOSIS

Osteochondromatosis, also referred to as multiple cartilaginous exostoses, hereditary multiple exostoses, and hereditary deforming osteochondromatosis, is characterized by benign proliferations of cartilage and bone that typically arise from long bones, ribs, or vertebrae in young dogs (Bichsel et al, 1985; Chester, 1971; Gambardella et al, 1975; Prata et al, 1975). Those arising from vertebrae may compress the spinal cord, resulting in spinal pain or paresis caudal to the spinal cord lesion. The thoracic and lumbar vertebrae are affected most commonly in dogs within the first 6 months of life (Bichsel et al, 1985). There is no definite gender

or breed predilection, although a familial relationship is probable (Chester, 1971; Gee and Doige, 1970). Surgical excision may be curative (Prata et al, 1975).

CERVICAL VERTEBRAL INSTABILITY

Cervical vertebral instability, also known as wobbler syndrome, cervical spondylomyelopathy, caudal cervical vertebral malformation-malarticulation, or caudal cervical spondylomyelopathy, occurs most commonly in Doberman pinschers and Great Danes (Olsson et al, 1982; Read et al, 1983; VanGundy, 1988). Other breeds of dogs that may be affected include the Saint Bernard, Weimaraner, Labrador retriever, German shepherd, basset hound, boxer, Rhodesian ridgeback, Dalmatian, Samoyed, Old English sheepdog, bull mastiff, Irish setter, and borzoi. Males appear to be affected more frequently than females. Combined osseous and soft tissue lesions at C6–C7 and, less commonly, C5–C6, C4–C5, and C3–C4 often lead to chronic spinal cord compression. The incidence of this disease in certain breeds suggests a heritable basis, a simple recessive mode in Great Danes (Selcer and Oliver, 1975) and Doberman pinschers (Mason, 1979). An autosomal recessive mode of inheritance has also been suggested in borzois.

Great Danes with cervical vertebral instability generally are younger than 2 years, whereas Doberman pinschers often are middle aged. Either breed may be 6 months old or younger at the time signs are first noted. Both basset hounds and bull mastiffs are generally younger than 1 year, whereas borzois are generally older female adults. Signs in affected dogs range from simple neck pain to tetraplegia. Gait deficits in the hindlimbs usually are noticed first and remain more severe. Vertebral changes that may be observed on survey radiographs include dorsal displacement of the caudal vertebra of the involved interspace, stenosis of the vertebral canal at the cranial vertebral orifice, and enlargement of the articular facets (Denny et al, 1977; Mason, 1977; Olsson et al, 1982). Survey radiographic changes do not necessarily predict the actual site of spinal cord compression. This should be demonstrated by myelography. Ventrodorsal views are required to demonstrate lateral spinal cord compression due to articular facet enlargement. Advanced imaging techniques such as computed tomography may be helpful in defining the degree and location of spinal cord compression, especially when combined with myelography, and in differentiating cervical vertebral instability from other causes of caudal cervical spinal cord compression.

Confinement for several days and use of anti-inflammatory medications usually result in improvement in mildly affected dogs; however, if long-term improvement is to be gained, surgical management is required. Any of several surgical procedures directed at decompression, stabilization, or both may be attempted to correct the underlying spinal cord compression. Neurologic deterioration may occur subsequent to any of the surgical procedures. Some dogs that initially improve may eventually deteriorate months or even years later owing to involvement of an adjacent disc space. Recovered animals of the high-risk breeds should not be used for breeding.

CONGENITAL VERTEBRAL ANOMALIES

Any congenital vertebral anomaly can result in abnormal curvature of the spine. Lateral deviation is referred to *scoliosis*, whereas dorsal or ventral curvature is termed *kyphosis* (Fig. 19–5) or lordosis. Spinal curvature also may be acquired in association with congenital spinal cord lesions. *Hemivertebrae* are shortened or misshapen vertebrae that result when the right and left halves of the vertebral body develop asymmetrically or fail to fuse (Bailey, 1975; Walker, 1979). Hemivertebrae occur most commonly in the thoracic spine of screw-tailed brachycephalic breeds (e.g., English and French bulldogs, Chinese pugs, and Boston terriers). Thoracic hemivertebrae are inherited through an autosomal recessive mode in German short-haired pointers (Kramer et al, 1982). Although most thoracic spine lesions are subclinical, spinal pain or paresis may occur. Myelography

should be used to confirm chronic spinal cord compression. Decompressive surgery should be combined with some form of stabilization in affected animals.

Block vertebrae result when there is incomplete segmentation of two or more adjacent vertebrae because of ossification of the portion of the sclerotome intended to become the intervertebral disc (Bailey, 1975; Walker, 1979). These vertebrae usually are stable, and the vertebral canal is not narrow. *Butterfly vertebrae* result because of persistence or sagittal cleavage of the notochord (Bailey, 1975). The latter leads to a sagittal cleft dorsoventrally through the vertebral body. On a dorsoventral radiographic view, such a vertebra resembles a butterfly with wings spread. Brachycephalic dog breeds are affected most commonly. Although most of these vertebral anomaly lesions are subclinical, spinal pain or paresis may occur. Myelography should be used to determine whether chronic spinal cord compression is present. Decompressive surgery may be combined with some form of stabilization in affected animals.

DEGENERATIVE SPINAL CORD DISEASES

Hereditary Ataxia. An inherited, progressive, generalized ataxia has been described to occur in young smooth-haired fox terriers (Bjorck et al, 1962) and Jack Russell terriers (Hartley and Palmer, 1973). Hereditary ataxia is inherited as an autosomal recessive trait in smooth-haired fox terriers. The inheritance pattern in Jack Russell terriers is unknown. There is demyelination in certain spinal cord tracts in both breeds. Hindlimb ataxia and dysmetria are noted between 2 and 6 months of age. The forelimbs are affected to a lesser degree. Some

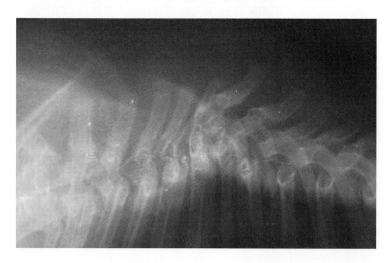

Figure 19–5. Lateral radiograph of the cranial thoracic spinal region of a 5-week-old female basenji with paraplegia. There is marked kyphosis at the level of T5 and T6, presumably due to hemivertebrae at these sites.

dogs have been maintained for as long as 25 months before euthanasia.

Degenerative Myelopathies. Degenerative myelopathies have been described in several breeds of dogs other than smooth-haired fox terriers and Jack Russell terriers, including English foxhounds, Finnish harriers, beagles, boxers, German shepherds, poodles, Afghan hounds, Dutch Kooiker dogs, and Australian cattle dogs. The degenerative myelopathy of Afghan hounds is presumed to have a simple autosomal recessive inheritance pattern (Averill and Bronson, 1977; Cockrell et al, 1973; Cummings and de Lahunta, 1978). The inheritance pattern in the other breeds is unknown. The myelopathic lesion in the Afghan hound is most pronounced in the dorsal funiculi of the caudal cervical spinal cord, all funiculi in the thoracic segments, and the ventral funiculi of the lumbar area. Paraparesis is noted between 3 and 13 months of age and progresses to paraplegia within 3 to 7 days. The forelimbs become involved 1 to 2 weeks after hindlimb involvement; however, some motor function is retained, and pain sensation is depressed caudal to the cranial thoracic area. Attitude, cranial nerve function, and spinal reflexes remain normal.

Demyelination in Miniature Poodles. Several miniature poodles with progressive demyelination involving principally the spinal cord have been reported (Douglas and Palmer, 1961; McGrath, 1960). The condition is presumed to be inherited, but no inheritance pattern has been established. Paraparesis is noted between 2 and 4 months of age; tetraplegia develops within several weeks.

Axonopathy of Birman Cats. Posterior ataxia was noted in three female Birman cats at 8 to 10 weeks of age (Moreau et al, 1991). The tarsi were plantigrade and adducted. Mild hypermetria was noted in all limbs. The kittens were euthanized shortly after the original clinical examination. Degeneration of axons and myelin was noted in both the central and peripheral nervous systems. A distal axonopathy with a heritable basis was suspected.

Multifocal Neurologic Diseases: Multiple Signs

Young animals relatively often have neurologic deficits that cannot be localized to a single neurologic site. In these cases, multiple lesions are generally present, and the animals are said to have multifocal neurologic disease. These diseases include inflammation, metabolic dysfunction, certain toxicities, and inherited diseases. Several viruses may cause meningoencephalitis in young dogs. These include canine distemper virus, canine herpesvirus, canine parvovirus type 2, adenovirus type 1, and parainfluenza. Of these viruses, canine distemper virus and canine herpesvirus are the most common. Feline infectious peritonitis is the most common viral cause of encephalitis in young cats.

CANINE DISTEMPER

Neurologic signs of classic canine distemper often follow polysystemic disease within 1 to 3 weeks, but some puppies have no initial systemic involvement. Young dogs with canine distemper–induced encephalitis often have progressive, worsening seizures and changes in attitude. Those with cerebellopontine lesions often have signs suggestive of cerebellar or vestibular dysfunction. Others may have signs isolated to spinal cord involvement. Signs of acute visual disturbance may predominate in some dogs because of optic neuritis or lesions affecting the central visual pathways. As with any disease causing meningitis, there may be marked hyperesthesia. All of these signs may occur alone or concomitantly. Signs usually progress over a period of days to weeks and may persist in some dogs for months. Although many dogs die, others improve significantly so that they are functional animals, if not fully recovered. Recovered animals may develop myoclonus, a rhythmic contraction of a single, or multiple, muscles.

Canine distemper and congenital portosystemic shunts should be considered in any young dog with unexplained neurologic dysfunction, even if there is no concomitant systemic disease. Although vaccination generally affords protection, some dogs with excellent vaccination histories still develop canine distemper, presumably because of a lack of immunocompetence (Thomas et al, 1993). Serum antibody titers can be positive in many dogs, but it is difficult to be sure whether this has resulted from recent or past exposure or because of vaccination. There may be lymphocytic pleocytosis and increased protein levels on CSF evaluation, but many dogs have no changes. Increases in IgG and IgM in CSF generally are indicative of active infection, except in cases where globulins have originated hematogenously and reached the CSF nonspecifically through a damaged blood-brain barrier. In the latter case, CSF titers to other viruses to which the dog has been vaccinated also should be positive. Inclusion bodies may infrequently be identified in mononuclear cells in CSF (Alleman et al, 1992). Because of a lack of immunocompetence, some dogs with the neurologic form of canine distemper do not develop positive CSF titers. A definitive diagnosis may not ultimately be made until necropsy, when demyelination or neuronal necrosis and intranuclear inclusions are seen microscopically.

There are no antiviral drugs for the treatment of canine distemper. Broad-spectrum antimicrobial agents are used to control secondary bacterial infections, and fluids, electrolytes, and nutritional supplements are indicated for supportive therapy. Chronic anticonvulsant therapy may be indicated for dogs with seizures. The prognosis is guarded for most cases of acute canine distemper, especially if neurologic signs are present and progressing, but control of secondary infections and supportive therapy improve the chances for recovery and having a better quality of life in the future.

CANINE HERPESVIRUS INFECTION

Canine herpesvirus causes severe illness and death in puppies younger than 3 weeks of age. Older puppies show respiratory signs and seizures with subsequent recovery. Puppies that recover usually have latent canine herpesvirus infections, and some may develop neurologic signs such as ataxia, blindness, and seizures. Treatment of affected puppies is usually supportive.

FELINE INFECTIOUS PERITONITIS

A pyogranulomatous inflammatory cell infiltrate may occur in the meninges, choroid plexus, and superficial neuropil of the CNS in cats with feline infectious peritonitis. Feline infectious peritonitis virus–induced vasculitis may lead to brain edema, hemorrhage, and thrombosis in some affected cats. Some affected cats develop acquired hydrocephalus, hydromyelia, or both (Tamke et al, 1988). Signs of neurologic dysfunction are usually seen in cats younger than 2 years (Barlough and Summers, 1984). Signs of neurologic dysfunction include paraparesis, nystagmus, and seizures. These signs are invariably progressive, eventually causing death or necessitating euthanasia. On CSF evaluation, there usually are high levels of protein and a moderate to marked pleocytosis (either lymphocytes or neutrophils may predominate). Treatment of cats with the neurologic form of feline infectious peritonitis usually incorporates long-term antiinflammatory use of corticosteroids.

BREED-ASSOCIATED MENINGITIS

Several syndromes of meningitis, with or without significant encephalitis and vasculitis, have been described in specific breeds of young dogs. A condition termed *pug encephalitis* has been recognized in young Chinese pug dogs (de Lahunta, 1983). Affected dogs have primary signs of forebrain disease, including seizures, attitude change, and circling. There is a marked, predominantly mononuclear pleocytosis on CSF evaluation. Some dogs improve transiently with the administration of glucocorticoids, but most dogs continue to deteriorate and are euthanized. The cause of this condition is unknown.

Meningitis-vasculitis syndrome, primarily affecting the spinal cord, has been described in beagles (Scott-Moncrieff et al, 1992) and Bernese mountain dogs (Meric et al, 1986). The meningitis-vasculitis syndrome is also referred to as juvenile polyarteritis syndrome. Cervical hyperesthesia is the most prominent neurologic sign in these dogs. Fever, ataxia, and paresis also may occur. Affected beagles may have nonregenerative anemia and neutrophilic leukocytosis. Suppurative pleocytosis and increased protein levels are noted on CSF evaluation. Signs may lessen or resolve with the administration of glucocorticoids (1.1 mg/kg orally twice daily initially followed by 0.25 to 0.5 mg/kg every other day) but typically recur when administration is discontinued. A similar form of *nonseptic, suppurative meningitis* has been described in young, large-breed dogs (Meric et al, 1985).

INFECTIOUS MENINGOENCEPHALITIS

Signs of bacterial, protothecal, rickettsial, or fungal meningoencephalitis are indistinguishable from those of other causes of meningoencephalitis in young dogs and cats. Other causes include granulomatous meningoencephalitis, steroid-responsive meningitis and necrotizing vasculitis of the meningeal arteries, canine distemper virus infection in young dogs, and neosporosis, and central nervous system toxoplasmosis and feline infectious peritonitis meningoencephalitis in cats. The diagnosis of meningitis also includes consideration of traumatic-induced intervertebral disc protrusion, spinal fracture, diskospondylitis, polymyositis, and polyarthritis.

LYSOSOMAL STORAGE DISEASES

Several lysosomal storage diseases in which there is an inherited deficiency of enzymes necessary for hydrolysis of proteins, polysaccharides, and complex lipids occur in young dogs and cats. Clinical effects of the lysosomal storage diseases are due to the deleterious effects on cell function that result from intracellular accumulation of substrate. Most of the lysosomal storage diseases are inherited as autosomal recessive traits. The more important lysosomal storage diseases, the defective enzyme, and breeds that are affected are listed in Table 19–2.

The lysosomal storage diseases cause signs of multifocal neurologic involvement, although some affected animals may at least initially have deficits suggesting focal lesions. Common signs include change in attitude, seizures, tetraparesis, intention tremor, and blindness. Signs generally are noted within the first several months of life and are progressive over the first year. Lysosomal storage diseases should be considered in young dogs and cats with signs of multifocal neurologic involvement. A definitive diagnosis is made through quantitation of the deficient enzyme in tissue or by cell culture system. Sup-plementation of the defective enzyme may be accomplished through bone marrow transplantation (Taylor et al, 1986).

NEUROAXONAL DYSTROPHY

Neuroaxonal dystrophy has been infrequently found in collie sheepdogs, Rottweilers, Chihuahuas, and a family of domestic cats. Signs of cerebellar involvement, including hypermetria, ataxia, and intention tremor, were noted in collie sheepdogs between 2 and 4 months of age. An autosomal recessive mode of inheritance was suggested. Ataxia, dysmetria, head tremor, menace deficits, nystagmus, and exaggerated spinal reflexes were noted in all limbs of Rottweilers between 1 and 2 years of age and slowly progressed. Chihuahua littermates were 7 weeks old when tremor and hypermetria were noted. Ataxia, dysmetria, and head tremor were noted in affected domestic kittens by 5 weeks of age and gradually progressed. These kittens also had a lighter haircoat than that of normal littermates.

SPONGIFORM ENCEPHALOPATHIES

Several spongiform encephalopathies in which there were signs of multifocal neurologic dys-

Table 19–2	Lysosomal Storage Diseases of Young Dogs and Cats	
DISEASE	**BREEDS AFFECTED**	**DEFICIENT ENZYME**
Ceroid lipofuscinosis	Siamese cat Dogs: English setter, cocker spaniel, Chihuahua, dachshund, Saluki, border collie	Unknown, perhaps p-phenylenediamine
Fucosidosis	English springer spaniel	α-L-Fucosidase
GM$_1$ gangliosidosis	Cats: domestic short-haired, Siamese, Korat Dogs: beagle, English springer spaniel, Portuguese water dog	β-Galactosidase
GM$_2$ gangliosidosis	Cats: domestic short-haired, Korat Dogs: German short-haired pointer, Japanese spaniel	β-Hexosaminidase
Globoid cell leukodystrophy	Domestic short-haired cat Dogs: Cairn and West Highland white terriers, poodle, bluetick hound, beagle, basset hound, Pomeranian	β-Galactocerebrosidase
Glucocerebrosidosis	Dalmatian	β-Glucosidase
Glycogenosis	Cats: domestic short-haired, Norwegian Forest Silky terrier dog	α-Glucosidase
Mannosidosis	Cats: domestic short-haired, Persian	α-Mannosidase
Metachromatic leukodystrophy	Domestic short-haired cat	Arylsulfatase (?)
Mucopolysaccharidosis I	Domestic short-haired, Siamese, Korat cats	α-L-Iduronidase
Mucopolysaccharidosis VI	Siamese cat	Arylsulfatase B
Sphingomyelinosis	Cats: domestic short-haired, Siamese, Balinese Dogs: German shepherd, poodle	Sphingomyelinase

function and marked vacuolation of central nervous system white matter have been described in young dogs and cats. Two Egyptian Mau kittens had developed paraparesis and hypermetria at 7 weeks of age (Kelly and Gaskell, 1976). These signs progressed, and one of the kittens also had seizures. A syndrome characterized by signs of cerebellar dysfunction and episodes of extensor rigidity has been described in two Labrador retriever littermates (Zachary and O'Brien, 1985; O'Brien and Zachary, 1985). Signs were observed initially at 4 months of age and progressed. Analogous syndromes have been described in a litter of Samoyeds (Mason et al, 1979) and a silky terrier puppy (Richards and Kakulas, 1978). The primary sign in the Samoyeds was tremor. Myoclonus predominated in the silky terrier. A syndrome of progressive paraparesis and loss of visual acuity has been characterized in multiple related Dalmatians (Bjerkas, 1977). These neurologic signs were noted between 3 and 6 months of age. The forelimbs eventually became paretic. A similar syndrome has been noted in two related Labrador retriever dogs with cortical blindness, dullness, and loss of learned habits.

NEURONAL DEGENERATION

Neuronal degeneration that causes pronounced multifocal neuronal loss has been described in young cocker spaniels (Jaggy and Vandevelde, 1988). Four dogs from separate litters exhibited ataxia and tremor by several months of age. Signs of mental dullness (apathy and loss of house training) or aggression were noted. All dogs were traced to a common ancestor, but a mode of inheritance was not defined. Neuronal degeneration affecting the cerebrum and cerebellum was described in two miniature poodle littermates (Cummings and de Lahunta, 1988). At 7 weeks of age, the puppies were unable to right themselves, rolled, were opisthotonic, made dysmetric movements with their limbs, and had vertical nystagmus and head tremor. Paraparesis progressing to tetraparesis, ataxia, head tremor, and inconsistent loss of spinal reflexes has been noted in multiple Cairn terriers (Cummings et al, 1988c, 1991; Palmer and Blakemore, 1989). Signs typically are noted initially at about 5 months of age and progress.

Seizures

Seizures may be characterized as being generalized or focal in origin. Generalized seizures originate from the forebrain and are associated with symmetric clinical dysfunction. Focal seizures are relatively specific for a certain area of the brain. Focal motor seizures are exhibited by tonic movements on the side of the body contralateral to the seizure focus. Focal motor seizures ultimately may become generalized. Temporolimbic seizures are exhibited by behavioral changes, including aggression, biting at imaginary objects (fly biting), and tail chasing. Seizures may also be characterized as to whether the cause is an intracranial or extracranial disease. Intracranial diseases of young dogs and cats include mostly inflammatory and anomalous conditions that affect the forebrain as well as idiopathic epilepsy. Extracranial causes that have a predilection for young animals are metabolic disorders such as hypoglycemia and hepatic encephalopathy due to congenital portosystemic shunts.

Idiopathic epilepsy occurs in several breeds of dogs, including the beagle, Belgian Tervuren shepherd, German shepherd, and keeshond. In these breeds, the idiopathic epilepsy originates at a young age and appears to have a heritable basis (Cunningham and Farnbach, 1988). A genetic predisposition to seizures is suspected in several other dog breeds (Oliver, 1980). A heritable basis has not been reported in any breed of cats. Dogs and cats with idiopathic epilepsy are clinically normal between periods of seizure activity. The age at onset of idiopathic epilepsy varies widely; a range of 4 months to 5 years has been recognized.

The diagnostic evaluation of young dogs and cats with seizure activity varies with the suspected underlying cause. Extracranial causes of seizure activity should be ruled out first before intracranial causes are pursued, just as the veterinarian is always encouraged to do with the older dog or cat. Specific treatments for particular diseases that can cause seizures were discussed earlier. There is no set frequency of seizures that necessitates anticonvulsant therapy; as a general rule, dogs and cats younger than 6 months will continue to have increasing seizure activity, so anticonvulsant medication is given much earlier to these animals than to the older animals.

The preferred anticonvulsant for long-term management of seizures in dogs is either oral phenobarbital or potassium bromide. The dosages may vary with age and concurrent diseases. The author's therapeutic approach for the initial administration of phenobarbital to young dogs is 0.5 mg/kg once daily for animals younger than 3 months, 1 mg/kg twice daily for animals between 3 and 6 months of age, and 2 mg/kg twice daily for animals older than 6 months. Serum levels should be measured 2 weeks after therapy is initiated. The therapeutic range is 15 to 40 μg/ml; a value between 30 and 40 μg/ml is preferred. Serum levels in excess of the therapeutic range may, however, be required for some dogs.

Oral potassium bromide may be given to puppies at 12 weeks of age or older, possibly even as young as 8 weeks. Because potassium bromide does not undergo hepatic metabolism, there should be limited problems in giving potassium bromide to puppies at such a young age. Monotherapy with oral potassium bromide is recommended at 40 to 80 mg/kg per day as a starting dose but may need to be increased to 120 mg/kg per day for some dogs. This agent is usually given once a day, but the total dosage can also be divided and administered twice a day if the puppy is experiencing gastrointestinal upsets. Serum bromide levels should be monitored at 4 and 8 weeks after initiation of the potassium bromide therapy and then every 2 months. Therapeutic serum bromide levels should range between 1.5 and 3.5 mg/ml.

Either phenobarbital (in a similar regimen to that for young dogs) or diazepam (0.5 to 1.0 mg/kg orally daily, divided into two or three doses) may be used for chronic seizure control in young cats. When phenobarbital or diazepam is not effective, several other anticonvulsants may be used alone or in combination. These include primidone, sodium valproate, and clonazepam. The author routinely suggests that anticonvulsant medication be slowly withdrawn after 5 to 6 months if the puppy or kitten has remained seizure free.

The Neuromuscular System[*]

G. Diane Shelton

Neuromuscular diseases are disorders of the motor unit and include neuropathies (disorders of the neuron including the cell body, axon, Schwann cell, and myelin), junctionopathies (disorders of neuromuscular transmission), myopathies (disorders of the muscle fiber), and neuromyopathies (disorders of both neurons and muscle fibers). Diseases associated with each of these components have been described in dogs and cats younger than 6 months. The primary clinical sign in all of these disorders is generalized or localized muscle weakness. Weakness may be manifested by functional abnormalities including paresis or paralysis, gait abnormalities, exercise-related weakness, dysphagia, dysphonia, dyspnea, or regurgitation. Muscle atrophy, hypotrophy, and hypertrophy and skeletal deformities may be present. The diagnosis of neuromuscular disease depends on the physical and neurologic examination, electrophysiologic testing, and examination of muscle and nerve biopsy specimens. With the exception of disorders having an infectious or immune-mediated cause, neuromuscular disorders of early onset are predominantly familial and carry a poor prognosis for recovery.

NEUROPATHIES
Neuronal Cell Body Lesions

Hereditary Motor Neuron Diseases. Inherited motor neuron diseases in animals are characterized by progressive degeneration of ventral horn cells of the spinal cord and brainstem. This has been extensively studied in Brittany spaniels (Lorenz et al, 1979; Cork et al, 1979) and described as a dominantly inherited lower motor neuron disease recognized in three forms: accelerated (weakness noted by 1 month of age with tetraparesis by 3 to 4 months of age), intermediate (weakness noted at 4 to 6 months of age with tetraparesis at 2 to 3 years of age), and chronic (slowly progressive). With the exception of the chronic form, with which dogs may survive well into adult life, the prognosis is poor, and tetraparesis and tetraplegia develop within 1 to 6 months of age. Other affected breeds include English pointers (Inada et al, 1978), Swedish Lapland dogs (Sandefelt et al, 1973), and Rottweilers (Shell et al, 1987a,b). In Rottweilers, clinical signs have been described at 4 weeks of age with mildly progressive tetraplegia, tremors, megaesopha-

*Portions of this work appear in Shelton GD: Neuromuscular disorders affecting young dogs and cats. Vet Neurol Neurosurg 199: http://neurovet.org, 2000.

gus, generalized muscle atrophy, and pelvic limb extensor rigidity (Fig. 19–6). One affected kitten has been described with weakness present at 4 weeks of age (Vandevelde et al, 1976). Inherited motor neuron diseases are untreatable.

Sensory Neuronopathy. Several breeds of dogs have been affected with loss of neuronal cell bodies and sensory nerve fibers, including long-haired dachshunds and English pointers (Duncan and Cuddon, 1989). Inheritance has been described as autosomal recessive in both breeds. In the English pointers, a deficiency in growth or differentiation of primary sensory neurons may be involved. Loss of primary sensory neurons is associated with a notable reduction in staining of substance P, an excitatory agent that mediates nociception. This loss is most apparent in the superficial laminae of the spinal dorsal horns. Clinical signs of sensory dysfunction predominate, including pelvic limb ataxia, loss of conscious proprioception, depressed pain sensation, patellar hyporeflexia, and self-mutilation. Self-mutilation may be the predominant clinical sign beginning before 6 months of age.

Neuronopathies

Progressive Axonopathy in Boxers. An autosomal recessive neuropathy with clinical signs of progressive ataxia, diminished or absent reflexes, proprioceptive loss, decreased muscle tone, and weakness beginning in the pelvic limbs and progressing to the thoracic limbs has been described in boxers beginning at 1 to 2 months of age (Griffiths et al, 1980). Axons in both the peripheral and central nervous systems are enlarged. Pelvic limb ataxia may be present as early as 2 months of age. Hyporeflexia is

present with retention of flexion. A central axonopathy has also been described in young Labrador retrievers (de Lahunta et al, 1994).

Laryngeal Paralysis–Polyneuropathy Complex. Generalized polyneuropathy associated with laryngeal paralysis and megaesophagus has been described in several young Dalmatian dogs (Braund et al, 1994). Although the mode of inheritance was not determined, an autosomal recessive pattern was suspected. Onset of clinical signs was at 4 to 6 months of age, with respiratory distress and loss of endurance, progressive laryngeal stridor, voice changes, dyspnea, cyanosis during episodes of severe dyspnea, and collapse. The prognosis is guarded to poor. No specific treatments are available, and controlled breeding is suggested. A laryngeal paralysis–polyneuropathy complex has also recently been described in young Rottweiler dogs with inspiratory stridor beginning at 11 to 13 weeks of age (Mahony et al, 1998). Other breeds described with hereditary forms of laryngeal paralysis include the Bouvier des Flandres (Venker-van Haagen et al, 1981) and possibly young Siberian huskies and young husky crossbreeds.

Schwann Cell Defects

Inherited Hypertrophic Neuropathy. Hypertrophic neuropathy has been described as an autosomal recessive motor neuropathy in Tibetan mastiffs (Cooper et al, 1984). Pathologic findings include a reduced density of myelinated fibers, widespread demyelination, and primitive onion-bulb formation with relatively little axonal degeneration in peripheral nerves and roots. Actin-like filaments accumulate in the Schwann cell cytoplasm. Results of initial studies indicate

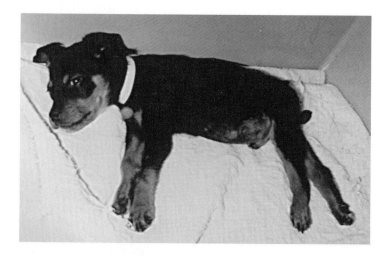

Figure 19–6. A 6-week-old Rottweiler puppy with hereditary motor neuron disease. There was rapidly progressive recumbency and tetraplegia with pelvic limb extensor rigidity. (Courtesy of Dr. Elizabeth Shull.)

a Schwann cell defect. Clinical signs appear in animals from 7 to 10 weeks of age and include rapidly progressive generalized weakness, hyporeflexia, hypotonia, and dysphonia. Electrodiagnostic studies reveal moderate to severe reduction in nerve conduction velocities. The prognosis is guarded, and there is no treatment available.

Hypomyelinating Polyneuropathy in Golden Retrievers. Hypomyelination of the peripheral nervous system has been described in Golden Retriever littermates (Braund et al, 1989). Clinical signs of pelvic limb ataxia were present between 5 to 7 weeks of age with abduction of pelvic limbs and increased flexion of the hocks, resulting in a crouched appearance. Mild pelvic limb muscle atrophy and weakness were described in the dogs with a "bunny hopping" gait when they ran. Motor nerve conduction velocities were markedly reduced. Histopathologic and morphometric analyses documented hypomyelination. No treatment is available. In animals studied for 1 year, no progression or improvement of clinical signs was described.

Neuropathies Associated with Inborn Errors of Metabolism

Niemann-Pick Disease. A primary polyneuropathy may be associated with Niemann-Pick disease, an autosomal recessive lysosomal storage disease characterized by a deficiency of sphingomyelinase. Three Siamese cats between 2 and 5 months of age with this disease have been described (Cuddon et al, 1989). Neurologic signs include progressive tetraparesis and ataxia, a palmigrade/plantigrade stance, fine generalized tremors, and diminished or absent reflexes. Moderate hepatosplenomegaly has also been described. There is widespread infiltration of virtually every body system with distended granular macrophages. The disease is progressive and fatal, with no treatment available.

Primary Hyperoxaluria. Profound weakness (Fig. 19–7) and renal failure have been described in related cats from Britain associated with primary hyperoxaluria (L-glyceric aciduria), analogous to primary hyperoxaluria type II in humans (McKerrel et al, 1989) Clinical signs became apparent at 5 months of age. An autosomal recessive mode of inheritance has been suggested. All reported cats died before 1 year of age despite symptomatic therapy for acute renal failure.

Glycogen Storage Disease Type IV. A deficiency of the glycogen-branching enzyme has been reported in three young related Norwegian Forest cats (Fyfe et al, 1992). Clinical signs, including generalized muscle tremors and weakness progressing to tetraplegia, became apparent at about 5 months of age. Severe generalized muscle atrophy and contractures were present at the time of euthanasia. Accumulations of abnormal glycogen and severe degeneration were noted in the central nervous system, peripheral nervous system, skeletal muscle, and heart.

DISORDERS OF NEUROMUSCULAR TRANSMISSION

Myasthenia Gravis

Myasthenia gravis (MG) is a disorder of neuromuscular transmission resulting from either a deficiency of acetylcholine receptors (congenital MG) or an autoimmune response against the receptor (acquired MG). Both forms of MG can occur in dogs up to 6 months of age. Congenital MG has been described in the Jack Russell terrier (Wallace and Palmer, 1984), springer spaniel (Johnson et al, 1975), and smooth-coated fox terrier (Miller et al, 1983). Onset of clinical weakness is at 6 to 9 weeks of age. Regurgitation from megaesophagus is a variable finding. Acquired MG with similar clinical signs may occur

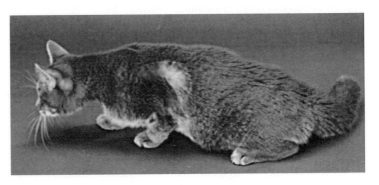

Figure 19–7. A 1-year-old female domestic short-haired cat with primary hyperoxaluria and markedly elevated urinary excretion of L-glyceric acid. Clinical signs of renal failure occurred at 5 months of age with onset of profound weakness at 11 months of age. Weakness may precede the renal failure in some cases. (Courtesy of Dr. Danielle Gunn-Moore.)

in puppies at 3 to 4 months of age (G. D. Shelton, unpublished data, 1999). In acquired MG, dogs are normal before onset of clinical signs.

Diagnosis of congenital MG is made by improvement in muscle strength on intravenous administration of the short-acting anticholinesterase drug edrophonium chloride (Tensilon, 0.1 mg/kg IV). Demonstration of a decrement in the muscle action potential after repetitive nerve stimulation that reverses with anticholinesterase drugs also supports the diagnosis. Confirmation of the diagnosis is made by biochemical quantification of the acetylcholine receptor content within fresh frozen intercostal muscle tissue. The diagnosis of acquired MG is made by demonstration of the presence of serum acetylcholine receptor antibodies by immunoprecipitation radioimmunoassay (Shelton et al, 1997).

The mainstay of treatment for congenital MG has been anticholinesterase drugs. Pyridostigmine bromide (Mestinon, 0.5 to 3 mg/kg orally two to three times daily) may be effective in controlling clinical signs, although drug resistance with chronic treatment may occur. Treatment for acquired MG is similar, with some dogs requiring the addition of corticosteroids (0.5 mg/kg orally once daily). Prognosis is guarded to poor in congenital MG and good to guarded in acquired MG, depending on severity of the disease and concurrent aspiration pneumonia.

Other Disorders of Neuromuscular Transmission

Although uncommon in dogs, ingestion of the preformed exotoxin of *Clostridium botulinum* may result in mild weakness to severe flaccid tetraplegia with absent spinal reflexes and weakness of the facial muscles, pharynx, esophagus, and jaw. Diagnosis is suggested by historical, clinical, and electrodiagnostic evaluation and confirmed by identification of the toxin in the material ingested or in the serum, feces, or vomitus of affected animals. Treatment is primarily supportive and the prognosis usually favorable in dogs.

Tick paralysis, caused by a neurotoxin generated by some species of ticks, results in a flaccid, afebrile ascending motor paralysis in dogs with recumbency in 24 to 72 hours. Reflexes are lost, with preservation of pain sensation. With tick removal and supportive care, there is usually recovery within 1 to 3 days.

Chronic organophosphate (OP) toxicity may result in persistent ventroflexion of the neck in cats and generalized weakness in dogs and cats, without the classic autonomic signs of vomiting, diarrhea, salivation, and miosis. Diagnosis is based on a history of recent use of OP, low plasma acetylcholinesterase levels, and a decremental response to repetitive nerve stimulation. Treatment consists of bathing to remove any residual OP and oral diphenhydramine (4 mg/kg every 8 hours). Recovery usually takes 3 to 6 weeks.

MYOPATHIES
Muscular Dystrophies

Muscular dystrophy (MD) is a general term that refers to a large group of inherited and progressively debilitating muscle disorders characterized by degeneration of skeletal muscle. In humans, more than 20 diseases have been characterized based on genetic as well as clinical features (Ozawa et al, 1998). Both X-linked and autosomal recessive inheritance patterns have been described in humans. In dogs and cats, X-linked forms have been well documented.

Canine X-linked Muscular Dystrophy. X-linked muscular dystrophy has been described in several breeds, including the golden retriever (Kornegay et al, 1988), Irish terrier (Wentink et al, 1972), Samoyed (Presthus and Nordstoga, 1989), miniature schnauzer (Paola et al, 1993), Belgian Groenendaeler shepherd (van Ham et al, 1993), Rottweiler (Winand et al, 1994), German short-haired pointer (Schatzberg et al, 1998), and Pembroke corgi (Woods et al, 1998). Clinical signs first appear at 6 to 9 weeks of age and include progressive weakness, stiff gait, muscle atrophy, and contractures. Serum creatine kinase levels are markedly elevated, and these elevations may be detected as early as 1 to 2 days of age. Characteristic morphologic lesions present in muscle biopsy specimens include muscle necrosis, phagocytosis, regeneration, hypertrophy, endomysial fibrosis, and myofiber mineralization. Clinically, the diagnosis of X-linked muscular dystrophy is made by demonstration of the absence of the protein dystrophin by immunocytochemical or molecular methods. The prognosis is poor because no specific treatment is available. Cardiomyopathy has consistently been present in X-linked muscular dystrophy, and older dystrophic dogs may die of heart failure (Valentine et al, 1989).

Feline X-linked Muscular Dystrophy. A hypertrophic form of X-linked muscular dystrophy has been described in young domestic short-hair cats (Carpenter et al, 1989; Gashen

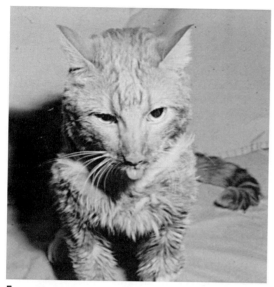

Figure 19–8. A 1-year-old male domestic short-haired cat with hypertrophic feline muscular dystrophy. Clinical signs of muscle hypertrophy and weakness were present since approximately 3 months of age. Glossal hypertrophy was present with inability to close the mouth and groom efficiently. (Courtesy of Dr. Stephen Atwater.)

et al, 1992). In contrast to the atrophy present in dogs, the disease in cats is characterized by marked generalized muscular hypertrophy with potentially lethal complications (Gashen et al, 1994). Clinical signs are present at approximately 3 months of age and include muscular hypertrophy, stiffness, and decreased agility. Glossal hypertrophy may be present with inability to close the mouth and groom (Fig. 19–8).

Regurgitation may be present due to severe hypertrophy of the diaphragm. The serum creatine kinase level is markedly elevated. Characteristic morphologic lesions are present in muscle biopsy specimens. Dystrophin is markedly decreased although not totally absent in immunocytochemical assays. The prognosis is poor, and no treatment is available.

Distal Myopathy in Rottweiler Dogs. Although not studied as completely as X-linked dystrophic disorders, a familial distal myopathy has recently been described in young Rottweiler dogs (Hanson et al, 1998). Although an exact inheritance pattern has not been determined, multiple dogs may be affected in a litter. All dogs confirmed to date to be affected were bred in southern California. Clinical signs are present at 6 to 8 weeks of age and include distal appendicular weakness evidenced by postural abnormalities ranging from splayed digits (Fig. 19–9) and hyperflexion of the hocks to a plantigrade and palmigrade stance (Fig. 19–10). Diagnosis is confirmed by electrophysiologic testing and histologic evaluation of distal muscles, including the gastrocnemius. No specific treatment is available.

Metabolic Myopathies

Mitochondrial Myopathy. A myopathy characterized by poor exercise tolerance and development of severe metabolic acidosis and lactic and pyruvic acidemia after exercise has been described in Clumber (Herrtage and Houlton, 1979) and Sussex (Houlton and Herrtage, 1980) spaniels. Biochemical analysis in the

Figure 19–9. Forelimbs of a 4-month-old male Rottweiler puppy with distal myopathy. There was progressive weakness and gait abnormality present since initial ambulation. Note the splaying of the forepaw digits.

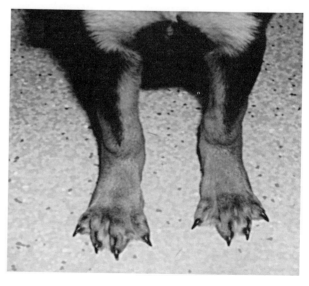

Sussex spaniel demonstrated a defect in pyruvate oxidation due to a deficiency of pyruvate dehydrogenase. A mitochondrial myopathy with altered cytochrome c oxidase activities and reduced mitochondrial mRNA has also been described in Old English sheepdog littermates with exercise intolerance (Breitschwerdt et al, 1992; Vijayasarathy et al, 1994). Evaluation of mitochondrial disorders requires demonstration of elevated resting or postexercise plasma lactate and pyruvate concentrations and light and electron microscopic study of muscle biopsy sections. Precise characterization depends on specialized biochemical assays and molecular studies.

Defects of Glycogen Metabolism. Glycogen metabolism disorders, uncommon in young dogs and cats, result from inborn errors of glycogen metabolism and accumulation of glycogen-like material within muscle and other tissues. A defect of the debranching enzyme amylo-1,6-glucosidase (glycogenosis type III) has been reported in German shepherds and Akitas, with muscular weakness evident at 2 months of age (Rafiquzzaman et al, 1976; Ceh et al, 1976). Abdominal distention may also be present owing to hepatomegaly resulting from deposition of glycogen-like material. An autosomal recessively inherited form of phosphofructokinase deficiency (type VII glycogen storage disease) has been described in young English springer spaniels (Giger et al, 1986) at approximately 8 months of age. Clinical signs were composed predominantly of compensated hemolytic anemia and intravascular hemolysis with hemoglobinuria without overt muscle weakness.

Although the serum creatine kinase concentration may be mildly elevated, the lack of prominent muscle weakness is probably related to the high oxidative potential of canine muscle. A similar condition occurs in American cocker spaniels. Molecular testing is available for detection of affected dogs and clinically normal carriers.

Myotonic Myopathies

A state in which active muscle contraction persists after voluntary effort or stimulation has stopped is referred to as myotonia. Congenital forms of myotonia with onset of clinical signs at about 2 months of age have been described in the chow chow (Farrow and Malik, 1981), Staffordshire terrier (Shires et al, 1983), and Great Dane (Honhold and Smith, 1986) and more recently at 5 months of age in two domestic short-haired cats (Toll et al, 1998). Stiffness is usually present after rest and characteristically disappears after exercise (the "warming-out" phenomenon). Hypertrophy of the proximal limb muscles, tongue, and neck may be present. Dimples result after percussion of muscles. The diagnosis is usually confirmed by the presence of characteristic trains of repetitive discharges that wax and wane in frequency to produce a "dive-bomber" sound. Muscle biopsy specimens are usually normal or show only mild myopathic changes.

Recently, a myotonic disorder with dimpling and characteristic electrophysiologic abnormalities (myotonic discharges) has been observed in miniature schnauzers at approximately 6 weeks

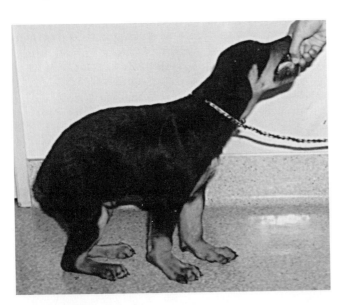

Figure 19–10. A 4-month-old male Rottweiler puppy with distal myopathy. A palmigrade and plantigrade stance was present from the time of initial ambulation. The abnormal stance and gait did not improve with maturation. Ulcerations may develop on the palmar and plantar surfaces as affected dogs grow and increase in weight.

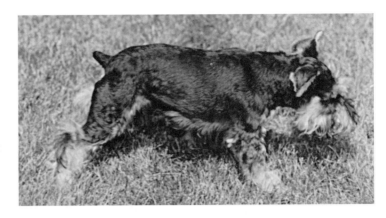

Figure 19–11. A 4-month-old miniature schnauzer puppy with congenital myotonia. Stiffness and muscle hypertrophy were evident at 6 weeks of age. Stiffness increased after activity. Myotonic dimpling was present and typical myotonic discharges were present on electromyographic evaluation. (Courtesy of Dr. Michael Podell.)

of age (Fig. 19–11). Marked hypertrophy of proximal limb muscles is present, and the tongue muscle stiffens and protrudes from the mouth (Fig. 19–12). Dysphagia and excessive salivation are common. Facial dysmorphism, described as a beak shape to the jaw, has been present in some affected dogs. An unusual finding is the presence of stiffness after exercise instead of improvement with exercise. Muscle morphology has been unremarkable. No treatment is currently available.

Other Hereditary Myopathies

Hereditary Myopathy of Labrador Retrievers. Hereditary myopathy in Labrador retrievers is characterized clinically by weakness, a marked deficiency in skeletal muscle mass, abnormal posture and gait, and exercise intolerance (Kramer et al, 1976). Tendon reflexes are generally reduced or absent with normal proprioception. Both males and females are affected, and animals with black and yellow coat colors have been affected as well. Clinical signs, aggravated by cold, excitement, and exercise, are evident by 3 months of age and usually stabilize between 6 months and 1 year of age. Inheritance was shown to be by a simple autosomal recessive mode (Kramer et al, 1981).

The serum creatine kinase level may be within normal limits or mildly elevated. Electromyographic evaluation may show spontaneous activity, including fibrillation potentials, positive sharp waves, and bizarre high-frequency discharges. The nerve conduction velocity is normal, and there is no decremental response to repetitive nerve stimulation. The diagnosis of this myopathy is confirmed by eval-

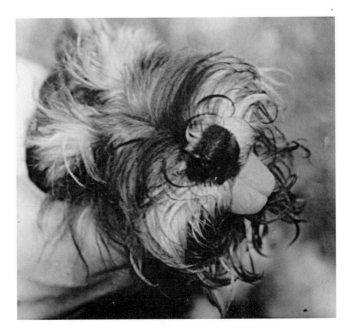

Figure 19–12. A 4-month-old miniature schnauzer puppy with congenital myotonia. Spontaneous contractions of the tongue muscle resulted in the tongue's protruding from the dog's mouth and in some cases curling up.

uation of fresh frozen muscle biopsy sections, including fiber typing. Although the original report of this myopathy described a type II muscle fiber deficiency (Kramer et al, 1976), a wide range of morphologic features may be observed in muscle biopsy material from affected dogs. Typical neuropathic features have been present in some cases, and in others myopathic features predominate. The underlying cause of this disorder, whether myopathic or neuropathic in origin, has not yet been determined. No treatment is currently available. Although affected dogs are not suitable for work, they may be acceptable house pets because clinical signs stabilize at 6 months to 1 year of age. Because the molecular defect in this disorder has not yet been identified and a test is not available for identification of heterozygous carriers, breeders should eliminate parents or siblings of affected puppies from their breeding program.

Nemaline Rod Myopathy. Nemaline rods have been described in association with a congenital myopathy in a family of cats (Cooper et al, 1986) and in a blue merle border collie (Delauche et al, 1998). The onset of clinical signs in the reported cats began at about 6 months of age and consisted of mild weakness and reluctance to be handled, progressing to tremor and muscle atrophy. Clinical signs in the border collie, evident at 14 weeks of age, consisted of tremors, exercise intolerance, stiff and stilted gait, and muscle atrophy (Fig. 19–13). Histochemical evaluation of fresh frozen muscle biopsy sections is required for diagnosis because rods are not visible by routine paraffin

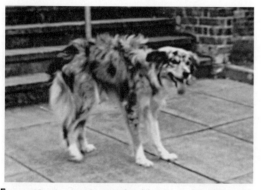

Figure 19–13. A 10-month-old intact female border collie dog with congenital nemaline rod myopathy. Exercise intolerance and stiff, stilted gait began at 3 months of age and progressed to severe tetraparesis and muscle atrophy. (Courtesy of Dr. Agnes Delauche.)

sections stained with hematoxylin and eosin (Fig. 19–14). Weakness is progressive, and no treatment is currently available. Nemaline rods were also described in association with a severe progressive myopathy in a young silky terrier with clinical signs evident at 12 weeks of age, including dysphagia, choking, stiff hindlimb gait, and hunched stance (Huxtable et al, 1994).

Central Core Myopathy. An inherited myopathy, beginning at about 6 months of age, has been described in Great Danes in the United Kingdom (Fig. 19–15). Clinical signs begin at about 6 months of age, with progressive muscle wasting and exercise intolerance that is exacerbated by excitement to include generalized body tremors and collapse (Targett et al, 1994). The diagnosis of central core myopathy depends on evaluation of muscle biopsy sections that show well-defined dark-staining central areas within many myofibers consistent with central cores. No specific treatment is currently available.

Hypertonic Myopathies. An electrically silent hypertonic myopathy beginning at about 3 months of age has been described in Cavalier King Charles spaniels in the United Kingdom (Herrtage and Palmer, 1983; Wright et al, 1987), and muscle biopsy specimens were evaluated from two affected littermates from Australia (G. D. Shelton, unpublished data, 1999). All described dogs had a history of exercise-induced and excitement-induced "collapse" that was preceded by "deer-stalking" movements. An increase in extensor tone of muscles of all four limbs was evident during the time of collapse, with recovery occurring in about 10 minutes. Treatment with diazepam did not result in improvement. Progression of the disorder has not been reported; in fact, stabilization or some improvement may occur. Although mitochondrial and membranous abnormalities have been found morphologically within muscle biopsy specimens, the pathogenesis of this condition remains obscure.

A hypertonic disorder characterized by myoclonus and extensor rigidity has been described in Labrador retrievers (Fox et al, 1984). Clinical signs, occurring at 6 weeks of age, included intermittent stimulus-sensitive contractions of the appendicular and axial muscles and generalized contractions initiated by voluntary movements. Therapeutic trials with diazepam and clonazepam were not effective (Fox et al, 1984).

Muscular hypertonicity (Scotty cramp) associated with postural and locomotive difficulties and characterized by paroxysms of muscular hypertonicity has been described in Scottish terri-

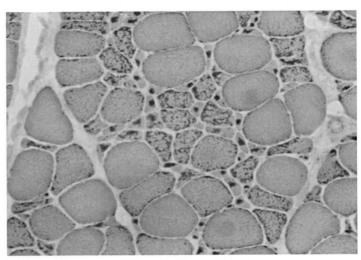

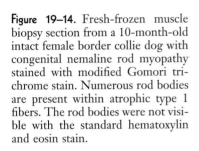

Figure 19–14. Fresh-frozen muscle biopsy section from a 10-month-old intact female border collie dog with congenital nemaline rod myopathy stained with modified Gomori trichrome stain. Numerous rod bodies are present within atrophic type 1 fibers. The rod bodies were not visible with the standard hematoxylin and eosin stain.

ers (Myers et al, 1969; Clemmons et al, 1980). Clinical signs may be observed in puppies at 6 to 8 weeks of age. Marked pelvic limb extensor rigidity may cause the dog to fall when running, and severity may be such that ambulation is impossible. An autosomal recessive mode of inheritance is suggested. Administration of methylsergide (0.1 to 0.6 mg/kg orally) is effective in identifying mildly affected dogs, with cramping evident within 2 hours, and its effect lasts for 8 hours. Diazepam (0.5 to 1.5 mg/kg orally three times daily) may be used to treat affected dogs.

Miscellaneous Noninflammatory Myopathies. There are scattered reports of other inherited myopathies in the literature. An autosomal recessive myopathy has been described in Devon Rex cats (Robinson, 1992; Malik et al, 1993). Clinical signs are observed between 1 and 6 months of age and include generalized appendicular weakness, ventroflexion of the neck, megaesophagus, and dorsal protrusion of the scapulae with normal reflexes and normal creatine kinase values. Dystrophic changes have been described in muscle biopsy sections. To date, the pathogenetic mechanisms responsible for Devon Rex myopathy remain unknown. A familial polysystemic disorder involving dyserythropoiesis, polymyopathy, and cardiac abnormalities has also been described in three related springer spaniel dogs (Holland et al, 1991). The list will continue to grow as newly recognized breed-specific myopathies are described.

Inflammatory Myopathies

Masticatory Muscle Myositis. Masticatory muscle myositis is an immune-mediated, focal inflammatory myopathy that selectively affects the muscles of mastication and can occur in

Figure 19–15. A 10-month-old intact female Great Dane with central core myopathy. Weakness and muscle atrophy were present since 5 months of age. Diagnosis was made by demonstration of typical central cores within myofibers. (Courtesy of Dr. Clare Rusbridge.)

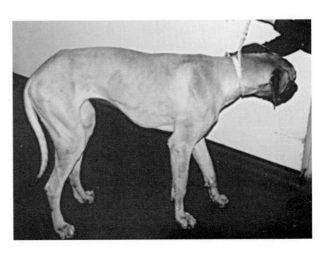

dogs younger than 6 months. Clinical signs include some combination of masticatory muscle atrophy or swelling and abnormal jaw function, manifested generally by restricted jaw mobility. The serum creatine kinase concentration may be normal or mildly elevated. Laboratory diagnosis is made by detection of circulating antibodies against type 2M fibers, a unique fiber type present only in the muscles of mastication (Shelton and Cardinet, 1989). Evaluation of a muscle biopsy specimen is necessary for confirmation of the diagnosis and also for prognosis as determined by the amount of myofiber destruction and fibrosis present. Immunosuppressive doses of corticosteroids should be administered until jaw function returns to normal and serum creatine kinase level is within the reference range. The dosage should then be decreased until the lowest alternate-day dosage is reached that keeps the animal free of clinical signs. This dosage should be continued for an additional 4 to 6 months because clinical signs will recur if treatment is stopped too soon or if an inadequate dosage was initially used.

Dermatomyositis in Collie Dogs and Shetland Sheepdogs.

Familial canine dermatomyositis has been report in the collie dog (Kunkle et al, 1985) and in Shetland sheepdogs (Hargis et al, 1985). Clinical signs of dermatitis predominate, beginning at approximately 8 to 10 weeks of age. Clinical signs of muscle disease, including generalized muscle atrophy, stiff gait, dysphagia, and megaesophagus, may occur in severely affected dogs, and mildly affected dogs may be asymptomatic. Dermatomyositis has been shown to have an autosomal dominant inheritance pattern in the collie dog.

Infectious Polymyositis.

Inflammatory myopathy, polyneuropathy, and multifocal neurologic disease may be found in young puppies infected with *Toxoplasma gondii* and *Neospora caninum* (Dubey, 1985; Hay et al, 1990). Clinical signs may be present as early as 4 weeks of age and include progressive paraparesis and "bunny hopping" gait with progression to pelvic limb hyperextension (Fig. 19–16) and muscle atrophy. Progression to pelvic limb hyperextension is more likely when infection develops before 4 months of age (Hass et al, 1989). Serum creatine kinase concentration is usually elevated. Evaluation of serum and CSF for both *N. caninum* and *T. gondii* antibodies should confirm an infection. Muscle and peripheral nerve biopsy specimens should confirm the presence of polymyositis and peripheral neuropathy. Occasionally, organisms are found within muscle biopsy

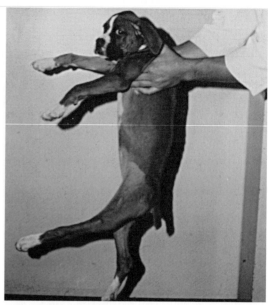

Figure 19–16. Typical posture of a young puppy with pelvic limb hyperextension as a result of infection before 4 months of age with either *Toxoplasma gondii* or *Neospora caninum*. Prognosis for resolution of pelvic limb hyperextension after treatment is guarded. (Courtesy of Dr. Terrell Holliday.)

sections. Treatments have included clindamycin (Greene et al, 1985) and sulfadiazine and trimethoprim (Dubey and Yeary, 1977). Although improvement in neurologic function may be noted, resolution of pelvic limb hyperextension has not been reported.

References and Supplemental Reading

THE NERVOUS SYSTEM

Adams RD, Victor M: Principles of Neurology, 3rd ed. New York, McGraw-Hill Book Co, 1985, p 434.

Aldrich MS: Narcolepsy. Neurology 42(Suppl 6):34, 1992.

Alleman AR, Christopher MM, Steiner DA, et al: Identification of intracytoplasmic inclusion bodies in mononuclear cells from the cerebrospinal fluid of a dog with canine distemper. Vet Pathol 29:84, 1992.

Alroy J, Orgad U, Ucci AA, et al: Neurovisceral and skeletal GM₁ gangliosidosis in dogs with β-galactosidase deficiency. Science 229:470, 1985.

Amann JF, Tomlinson J, Hankison JK: Myotonia in a chow chow. J Am Vet Med Assoc 187:415, 1985.

Anvik JO, Lewis R: *Actinomyces* encephalitis associated with hydrocephalus in a dog. Can Vet J 17:42, 1976.

Appleby EC, Longstaffe JA: Ceroid lipofuscinosis in two Saluki dogs. J Comp Pathol 92:375, 1982.

Averill DR Jr: Diagnosis and treatment of hydrocephalus in the dog. Proc Kal Kan Symposium Treatment of Dog and Cat Diseases, Columbus, Ohio, 1978, p 28.

Averill DR Jr, Bronson RT: Inherited necrotizing myelopathy of Afghan hounds. J Neuropathol Exp Neurol 36:734, 1977.

Bailey CS: An embryological approach to the clinical significance of congenital vertebral and spinal cord abnormalities. J Am Anim Hosp Assoc 11:426, 1975.

Baker HJ: Inherited metabolic disorders of the nervous system in dogs and cats. In Kirk RW (ed): Current Veterinary Therapy V. Philadelphia, WB Saunders, 1974, p 700.

Baker HJ, Reynolds GD, Walkley SU, et al: The gangliosidoses: Comparative features and research applications. Vet Pathol 16:635, 1979.

Baker HJ, Wood PA, Wenger DA, et al: Sphingomyelin lipidosis in a cat. Vet Pathol 24:386, 1987.

Baker TL, Mitler MM, Foutz AS, et al: Diagnosis and treatment of narcolepsy in animals. In Kirk RW (ed): Current Veterinary Therapy VIII. Philadelphia, WB Saunders, 1983, p 755.

Barlough JE, Summers BA: Encephalitis due to feline infectious peritonitis virus in a twelve-week-old kitten. Feline Pract 14:43, 1984.

Baumgartner WK, Krakowka S, Koestner A, et al: Acute encephalitis and hydrocephalus in dogs caused by canine parainfluenza virus. Vet Pathol 19:79, 1982.

Beaver BV: Neuromuscular development of Felis catus. Lab Anim 14:197, 1980a.

Beaver BV: Sensory development of Felis catus. Lab Anim 14:199, 1980b.

Beaver BV: Somatosensory development in puppies. Vet Med Small Anim Clin 77:39, 1982.

Beaver BV: Feline Behavior: A Guide for Veterinarians. Philadelphia, WB Saunders, 1992, p 276.

Becker C-M: Disorders of the inhibitory glycine receptor: the spastic mouse. FASEB J 4:2767, 1990.

Bedford BGC: Congenital vestibular disease in the English cocker spaniel. Vet Rec 105:530, 1979.

Bentley JF, Simpson ST, Hathcock JT: Spinal arachnoid cyst in a dog. J Am Anim Hosp Assoc 27:549, 1991.

Bichsel P, Lang J, Vandevelde M, et al: Solitary cartilaginous exostoses associated with spinal cord compression in three large-breed dogs. J Am Anim Hosp Assoc 21:619, 1985.

Bjerkas I: Hereditary "cavitating" leukodystrophy in Dalmatian dogs. Acta Neuropathol (Berl) 40:163, 1977.

Bjorck G, Mair W, Olsson S-E, Sourander P: Hereditary ataxia in fox terriers. Acta Neuropathol (Berl) Suppl 1:45, 1962.

Black PML: Normal pressure hydrocephalus. Current understanding of diagnostic tests and shunting. Postgrad Med 71:57, 1982.

Blakemore WF: GM$_1$-gangliosidosis in a cat. J Comp Pathol 82:179, 1972.

Blakemore WF, Palmer AC: Nervous disease in the Chihuahua characterised by axonal swellings. Vet Rec 117:498, 1985.

Bland Van den Berg P, Baker MK, Lange AL: A suspected lysosomal storage disease in Abyssinian cats. Part 1: Genetic, clinical, and clinical pathological aspects. J S Afr Vet Assoc 48:195, 1977.

Blaxter AC, Lievesley P, Gruffydd-Jones T, et al: Periodic muscle weakness in Burmese kittens. Vet Rec 118:619, 1986.

Bollo E, Zurbriggen A, Vandevelde M, et al: Canine distemper virus clearance in chronic inflammatory demyelination. Acta Neuropathol (Berl) 72:69, 1986.

Botteron C, Zurbriggen A, Griot C, et al: Canine distemper virus-immune complexes induce bystander degeneration of oligodendrocytes. Acta Neuropathol (Berl) 83:402, 1992.

Boysen BG, Tryphonas L, Harries, NW: Globoid cell leukodystrophy in the blue tick hound dog. 1. Clinical manifestations. Can Vet J 15:303, 1974.

Braund KG, McGuire JA, Lincoln CE: Age-related changes in peripheral nerves of the dog. II. A morphologic and morphometric study of cross-sectional nerve. Vet Pathol 19:379, 1982.

Breazile JE: Neurologic and behavioral development in the puppy. Vet Clin North Am 8:31, 1978.

Breazile JE, Blaugh BS, Nail N: Experimental study of canine distemper myoclonus. Am J Vet Res 27:1375, 1966.

Brown JR: The Dandy-Walker syndrome. In Vinken PJ, Bruyn GW (eds): Handbook of Clinical Neurology. Amsterdam, North Holland Publishing 1977, p 623.

Brown RJ, Trevethan WP, Henry VL: Multiple osteosarcoma in a Siamese cat. J Am Vet Med Assoc 160:433, 1972.

Bundza A, Lowden JA, Charlton KM: Niemann-Pick disease in a poodle dog. Vet Pathol 16:530, 1979.

Carmichael L: The genetic development of the kitten's capacity to right itself in the air when falling. J Genet Psychol 44:453, 1934.

Carmichael S, Griffiths IR, Harvey MJA: Familial cerebellar ataxia with hydrocephalus in bull mastiffs. Vet Rec 112:354, 1983.

Carpenter MR, Harter DH: A study of congenital feline cerebellar malformations. An anatomic and physiologic evaluation of genetic defects. J Comp Neurol 105:51, 1956.

Center SA, Hornbuckle WE: Congenital portosystemic shunts in cats. In Kirk RW (ed): Current Veterinary Therapy IX. Philadelphia, WB Saunders, 1986, p 825.

Chester DK: Multiple cartilaginous exostoses in two generations of dogs. J Am Vet Med Assoc 159:895, 1971.

Child G, Higgins RJ, Cuddon PA: Acquired scoliosis associated with hydromyelia and syringomyelia in two dogs. J Am Vet Med Assoc 189:909, 1986.

Chrisman CL: Problems in Small Animal Neurology. Philadelphia, WB Saunders, 1982, p 263.

Chrisman CL, Cork LC, Gamble DA: Neuroaxonal dystrophy of Rottweiler dogs. J Am Vet Med Assoc 184:464, 1984.

Clark L, Carlisle CH: Spina bifida with syringomyelia and meningocoele in a short-tailed cat. Aust Vet J 51:392, 1975.

Clark RG, Hartley WJ, Burgess GS, et al: Suspected inherited cerebellar neuroaxonal dystrophy in collie sheep dogs. N Z Vet J 30:102, 1982.

Cockrell BY, Herigstad RR, Flo GL, et al: Myelomalacia in Afghan hounds. J Am Vet Med Assoc 162:362, 1973.

Cook JR, Oliver JE Jr: Atlantoaxial luxation in the dog. Compend Contin Educ Pract Vet 3:242, 1981.

Cordy DR, Snelbaker HA: Cerebellar hypoplasia and degeneration in a family of Airedale dogs. J Neuropathol Exp Neurol 11:324, 1952.

Core DM, Hoff EJ, Milton JL: Hindlimb hyperextension as a result of Toxoplasma gondii polyradiculitis. J Am Anim Hosp Assoc 19:713, 1983.

Cork LC, Munnell JF, Lorenz MD, et al: GM$_2$ ganglioside lysosomal storage disease in cats with β-hexosaminidase deficiency. Science 196:1014, 1977.

Cornwell HJC, Thompson H, McCandlish IAP, et al: Encephalitis in dogs associated with a batch of canine distemper (Rockborn) vaccine. Vet Rec 112:54, 1988.

Csiza CK, de Lahunta A, Scott FW, et al: Spontaneous feline ataxia. Cornell Vet 62:300, 1972.

Csiza CK, Scott FW, de Lahunta A, et al: Feline viruses. XIV. Transplacental infections in spontaneous panleukopenia of cats. Cornell Vet 61:423, 1971a.

Csiza CK, Scott FW, de Lahunta A, et al: Immune carrier state of feline panleukopenia virus-infected cats. Am J Vet Res 32:419, 1971b.

Cummings JF, Cooper BJ, de Lahunta A, et al: Canine inherited hypertrophic neuropathy. Acta Neuropathol (Berl): 53:137, 1981a.

Cummings JF, de Lahunta A: Hereditary myelopathy of Afghan hounds, a myelinolytic disease. Acta Neuropathol (Berl) 42:173, 1978.

Cummings JF, de Lahunta A: A study of cerebellar and cerebral cortical degeneration in miniature poodle pups with emphasis on the ultrastructure of Purkinje cell changes. Acta Neuropathol (Berl) 75:261, 1988.

Cummings JF, de Lahunta A, Gasteiger EL: Multisystemic chromatolytic neuronal degeneration in Cairn terriers. J Vet Intern Med 5:91, 1991.

Cummings JF, de Lahunta A, Mitchell WJ Jr: Ganglioneuritis in the dog: A clinical and light- and electron-microscopic study. Acta Neuropathol (Berl) 60:29, 1983.

Cummings JF, de Lahunta A, Moore JJ III: Multisystemic chromatolytic neuronal degeneration in a Cairn terrier pup. Cornell Vet 78:301, 1988a.

Cummings JF, de Lahunta A, Suter MM, et al: Canine protozoan polyradiculoneuritis. Acta Neuropathol (Berl) 76:46, 1988b.

Cummings JF, de Lahunta A, Winn SS: Acral mutilation and nociceptive loss in English pointer dogs. Acta Neuropathol (Berl) 53:119, 1981b.

Cummings JF, George C, de Lahunta A, et al: Focal spinal muscular atrophy in two German Shepherd pups. Acta Neuropathol 79:113, 1989.

Cummings JF, Summers BA, de Lahunta A, et al: Tremors in Samoyed pups with oligodendrocyte deficiencies and hypomyelination. Acta Neuropathol (Berl) 71:267, 1986.

Cummings JF, Wood PA, de Lahunta A, et al: The clinical and pathologic heterogeneity of feline alpha-mannosidosis. J Vet Intern Med 2:163, 1988c.

Cummings JF, Wood PA, Walkley SU, et al: GM$_2$ gangliosidosis in a Japanese spaniel. Acta Neuropathol (Berl) 67:247, 1985.

Cunningham JG: Canine seizure disorders. J Am Vet Med Assoc 158:589, 1971.

Cunningham JG, Farnbach GC: Inheritance and idiopathic canine epilepsy. J Am Anim Hosp Assoc 24:421, 1988.

de Lahunta A: Veterinary Neuroanatomy and Clinical Neurology, 2nd ed. Philadelphia, WB Saunders, 1983.

de Lahunta A, Fenner WR, Indrieri RJ, et al: Hereditary cerebellar cortical abiotrophy in the Gordon setter. J Am Vet Med Assoc 177:538, 1980.

Denny HR, Gibbs C, Gaskell CJ: Cervical spondylopathy in the dog—a review of thirty-five cases. J Small Anim Pract 18:117, 1977.

Denny HR, Gibbs C, Waterman A: Atlanto-axial subluxation in the dog: A review of thirty cases and an evaluation of treatment by lag screw fixation. J Small Anim Pract 29:37, 1988.

Douglas SW, Palmer AC: Idiopathic demyelination of brain-stem and cord in a miniature poodle puppy. J Pathol Bacteriol 82:67, 1961.

Drake JC, Hime JM: Two syndromes in young dogs caused by Toxoplasma gondii. J Small Anim Pract 8:621, 1967.

Dubey JP, Carpenter JL, Speer CA, et al: Newly recognized fatal protozoan disease of dogs. J Am Vet Med Assoc 192:1269, 1988.

Dubey JP, Lindsay DS: Transplacental Neospora caninum infection in cats. J Parasitol 75:765, 1989a.

Dubey JP, Lindsay DS: Transplacental Neospora caninum infection in dogs. Am J Vet Res 50:1578, 1989b.

Dubey JP, Lindsay DS, Lipscomb TP: Neosporosis in cats. Vet Pathol 27:335, 1990.

Duncan ID: Abnormalities of myelination of the central nervous system associated with congenital tremor. J Vet Intern Med 1:10, 1987.

Duncan ID, Griffiths IR: A sensory neuropathy affecting long haired Dachshund dogs. J Small Anim Pract 23:381, 1982.

Duncan ID, Griffiths IR, Munz M: The pathology of a sensory neuropathy affecting long haired Dachshund dogs. Acta Neuropathol (Berl) 58:141, 1982.

Duncan ID, Griffiths IR, Munz M: "Shaking pups": A disorder of central myelination in the spaniel dog. III. Quantitative aspects of glia and myelin in the spinal cord and optic nerve. Neuropathol Appl Neurobiol 9:355, 1983.

Eger CE, Robinson WF, Huxtable CRR: Primary

aldosteronism (Conn's syndrome) in a cat; a case report and review of comparative aspects. J Small Anim Pract 24:293, 1983.

Emerson R, D'Souza BJ, Vining EP, et al: Stopping medication in children with epilepsy. Predictors of outcome. N Engl J Med 304:1125, 1981.

Engel HN, Draper DD: Comparative prenatal development of the spinal cord in normal and dysraphic dogs: Embryonic stage. Am J Vet Res: 43:1729, 1982a.

Engel HN, Draper DD: Comparative prenatal development of the spinal cord in normal and dysraphic dogs: Fetal stage. Am J Vet Res: 43:1735, 1982b.

Ewing GO, Suter PF, Bailey CS: Hepatic insufficiency associated with congenital anomalies of the portal vein in dogs. J Am Anim Hosp Assoc 10:463, 1974.

Farnbach GC: Serum concentrations and efficacy of phenytoin, phenobarbital, and primidone in canine epilepsy. J Am Vet Med Assoc 184:1117, 1984.

Farrell DF, Baker HJ, Herndon RM, et al: Feline GM₁ gangliosidosis: Biochemical and ultrastructural comparisons with the disease in man. J Neuropathol Exp Neurol 32:1, 1973.

Fenner WR: Seizures. In Kornegay JN (ed): Neurologic Disorders, vol 5, Contemporary Issues in Small Animal Practice. New York, Churchill Livingstone, 1986, p 41.

Few AB: The diagnosis and surgical treatment of canine hydrocephalus. J Am Vet Med Assoc 149:286, 1966.

Field B, Wanner RA: Cerebral malformation in a Manx cat. Vet Rec 96:42, 1975.

Fletcher TF, Kurtz HJ, Low DG: Globoid cell leukodystrophy (Krabbe type) in the dog. J Am Vet Med Assoc 149:165, 1966.

Forbes S, Cook JR Jr: Congenital peripheral vestibular disease attributed to lymphocytic labyrinthitis in two related litters of Doberman pinscher pups. J Am Vet Med Assoc 198:447, 1991.

Foutz AS, Mitler MM, Dement WC: Narcolepsy. Vet Clin North Am Small Anim Pract 10:65, 1980.

Fox JG, Averill DR, Hallett M, et al: Familial reflex myoclonus in Labrador retrievers. Am J Vet Res 45:2367, 1984.

Fox MW: Conditioned reflexes and innate behaviour of the neonate dog. J Small Anim Pract 4:85, 1963.

Fox MW: Canine Behavior. Springfield, IL, Charles C Thomas, 1965, p 137.

Fox MW: Postnatal development of the EEG in the dog. I. Introduction and EEG techniques. J Small Anim Pract 8:71, 1967.

Fox MW, Inman OR, Himwich WA: The postnatal development of the spinal cord of the dog. J Comp Neurol 130:233, 1967.

Frauchiger E, Fankhauser R: Vergleichende Neuropathologie des Menschen und der Tiere. Berlin, Springer, 1957, p 33.

Frey H-H, Loscher W: Pharmacokinetics of antiepileptic drugs in the dog: A review. J Vet Pharmacol Ther 8:219, 1985.

Frye FL: Spina bifida occulta with sacro-coccygeal agenesis in a cat. Anim Hosp 3:238, 1967.

Frye FL, McFarland LZ: Spina bifida with rachischisis in a kitten. J Am Vet Med Assoc 146:481, 1965.

Fukata T, Arakawa A: Dexamethasone treatment of hydrocephalus in dogs. Mod Vet Pract 66:256, 1985.

Gage ED, Hoerlein BF: Surgical treatment of canine hydrocephalus by ventriculoatrial shunting. J Am Vet Med Assoc 153:1418, 1968.

Gambardella PC, Osborne CA, Stevens JB: Multiple cartilaginous exostoses in the dog. J Am Vet Med Assoc 166:761, 1975.

Gee BR, Doige CE: Multiple cartilaginous exostoses in a litter of dogs. J Am Vet Med Assoc 156:53, 1970.

Good R: Untersuchungen uber eine Kleinhirn-rindenatrophie beim Hund. Dissertation, University of Bern, 1962.

Green PD, Little RB: Neuronal ceroid-lipofuscin storage in Siamese cats. Can J Comp Med 38:207, 1974.

Greene CE, Cook JR, Mahaffey EA: Clindamycin for treatment of toxoplasma polymyositis in a dog. J Am Vet Med Assoc 187:631, 1985.

Greene CE, Gorgacz EJ, Martin CL: Hydranencephaly associated with feline panleukopenia. J Am Vet Med Assoc 767, 1982.

Greene CE, Vandevelde M, Braund K: Lissencephaly in two Lhasa apso dogs. J Am Vet Med Assoc 169:405, 1976.

Griffiths IR: Abnormalities in the central nervous system of a kitten. Vet Rec 89:123, 1971.

Griffiths IR: Progressive axonopathy of boxer dogs. In Kirk RW (ed): Current Veterinary Therapy X. Philadelphia, WB Saunders, 1989, p 828.

Griffiths IR, Duncan ID, McCulloch M: Shaking pups: A disorder of central myelination in the spaniel dog. II. Ultrastructural observations on the white matter of the cervical spinal cord. J Neurocytol 10:847, 1981a.

Griffiths IR, Duncan ID, McCullough M, et al: A disorder of central myelination in the spaniel dog. I. Clinical, genetic, and light microscopic observations. J Neurol Sci 50:423, 1981b.

Guilleminault C, Baker TL: Canine narcolepsy. An animal model of human narcolepsy cataplexy syndrome. In Asbury AK, McKhann GM, McDonald WI (eds): Diseases of the Nervous System. Clinical Neurobiology. London, William Heinemann Medical Books Ltd, 1986, p 873.

Harari J, Padgett GA, Grace J: Cerebellar agenesis in two canine littermates. J Am Vet Med Assoc 182:622, 1983.

Harcourt RA: Polyarteritis in a colony of beagles. Vet Rec 102:519, 1978.

Hartley WJ: Lower motor neuron disease in dogs. Acta Neuropathol (Berl) 2:334, 1963.

Hartley WJ: A post-vaccinal inclusion body encephalitis in dogs. Vet Pathol 11:301, 1974.

Hartley WJ, Barker JSF, Wanner RA, et al: Inherited

cerebellar degeneration in the rough coated collie. Aust Vet Pract 8:79, 1978.

Hartley WJ, Palmer AC: Ataxia in Jack Russell terriers. Acta Neuropathol (Berl) 26:71, 1973.

Harvey JW, Calderwood Mays MB, Gropp KE, et al: Polysaccharide storage myopathy in canine phosphofructokinase deficiency (type VII glycogen storage disease). Vet Pathol 27:1, 1990.

Haskins ME, Jezyk PF, Desnick, et al: Animal model of human disease. Mucopolysaccharidosis VI. Maroteaux-Lamy syndrome. Arylsulfatase B–deficient mucopolysaccharidosis in the Siamese cat. Am J Pathol 105:191, 1981.

Haskins ME, McGraft JT: Meningiomas in young cats with mucopolysaccharidosis. J Neuropathol Exp Neurol 42:664, 1983.

Haupt KH, Prieur DJ, Hargis AM, et al: Familial canine dermatomyositis: Clinicopathologic, immunologic, and serologic studies. Am J Vet Res 46:1870, 1985a.

Haupt KH, Prieur DJ, Moore MP, et al: Familial canine dermatomyositis: Clinical, electrodiagnostic and genetic studies. Am J Vet Res 46:1861, 1985b.

Hazewinkel HAW, Goedegebuure SA, Poulos PW, et al: Influences of chronic calcium excess on the skeletal development of growing Great Danes. J Am Anim Hosp Assoc 21:377, 1985.

Heavner JE: Congenital hydrocephalus secondary to in utero infection. Vet Med Small Anim Clin 73:157, 1978.

Hedhammar A, Wu FM, Krook L, et al: Overnutrition and skeletal disease. An experimental study in growing Great Dane dogs. Cornell Vet 64 (Suppl)5:1, 1974.

Hendricks JC, Hughes C: Treatment of cataplexy in a dog with narcolepsy. J Am Vet Med Assoc 194:791, 1989.

Hendricks JC, Lager A, O'Brien D, et al: Movement disorders during sleep in cats and dogs. J Am Vet Med Assoc 194:686, 1989.

Higgins RJ, Krakowka SG, Metzler AE, et al: Primary demyelination in experimental canine distemper virus–induced encephalomyelitis in gnotobiotic dogs. Sequential immunologic and morphologic findings. Acta Neuropathol (Berl) 58:1, 1982.

Higgins RJ, Vandevelde M, Braund KG: Internal hydrocephalus and associated periventricular encephalitis in young dogs. Vet Pathol 14:236, 1977.

Hoerlein BF, Gage ED: Hydrocephalus. In Hoerlein BF (ed): Canine Neurology. Diagnosis and Treatment, 3rd ed. Philadelphia, WB Saunders, 1978, p 747.

Hoover DM, Little PB, Cole WD: Neuronal ceroid-lipofuscinosis in a mature dog. Vet Pathol 21:359, 1984.

Hoshino K, Pompeiano O: Selective discharge of pontine neurons during the postural atonia produced by an anticholinesterase in the decerebrate cat. Arch Ital Biol 114:224, 1976.

Izumo S, Ikuta F, Igata A, et al: Morphological study on the hereditary neurogenic amyotrophic dogs: Accumulation of lipid compound-like structures in the lower motor neuron. Acta Neuropathol (Berl) 61:270, 1983.

Jaggy A, Gaillard C, Lang J, et al: Hereditary cervical spondylopathy (wobbler syndrome) in the Borzoi dog. J Am Anim Hosp Assoc 24:453, 1988.

Jaggy A, Vandevelde M: Multisystem neuronal degeneration in cocker spaniels. J Vet Intern Med 2:117, 1988.

James CC, Lassman LP, Tomlinson BE: Congenital anomalies of the lower spine and spinal cord in Manx cats. J Pathol 97:269, 1969.

Johnson BJ, Castro AE: Isolation of canine parvovirus from a dog brain with severe necrotizing vasculitis and encephalomalacia. J Am Vet Med Assoc 184:1398, 1984.

Johnson GC, Krakowka S, Axthelm MK: Prolonged viral antigen retention in the brain of a gnotobiotic dog experimentally infected with canine distemper virus. Vet Pathol 24:87, 1987.

Johnson GR, Oliver JE Jr, Selcer R: Globoid cell leukodystrophy in a beagle. J Am Vet Med Assoc 167:380, 1975.

Johnson KH: Globoid leukodystrophy in the cat. J Am Vet Med Assoc 157:2057, 1970.

Johnson L, Rolsma M, Parker A: Syringomyelia, hydromyelia and hydrocephalus in two dogs. Prog Vet Neurol 3:82, 1992.

Johnson RH, Margolis G, Kilham L: Identity of feline ataxia virus with feline panleukopenia virus. Nature 214:175, 1967.

Jones BR: Hereditary myotonia in the chow chow. Vet Ann 24:286, 1984.

Jones BR, Johnstone AC, Cahill JL, et al: Peripheral neuropathy in cats with inherited primary hyperchylomicronaemia. Vet Rec 119:268, 1986.

Joseph RJ, Carrillo JM, Lennon VA: Myasthenia gravis in the cat. J Vet Intern Med 2:75, 1988.

Juul-Jensen P: Frequency of recurrence after discontinuance of anticonvulsant therapy in patients with epileptic seizures. Epilepsia 5:352, 1964.

Karbe E: Animal model of human disease. GM_2 gangliosidosis (amaurotic idiocies) types I, II, and III. Am J Pathol 71:151, 1973.

Kay ND, Holliday TA, Hornof WJ, et al: Diagnosis and management of an atypical case of canine hydrocephalus using computed tomography, ventriculoperitoneal shunting, and nuclear scintigraphy. J Am Vet Med Assoc 188:423, 1986.

Kay WJ: Epilepsy in cats. J Am Anim Hosp Assoc 11:77, 1975.

Kay WJ, Aucoin DP: Seizure disorders. In Davis LE (ed): Handbook of Small Animal Therapeutics. New York, Churchill Livingstone, 1985, p 505.

Kelly DF, Gaskell CJ: Spongy degeneration of the central nervous system in kittens. Acta Neuropathol (Berl) 35:151, 1976.

Khera KS: Teratogenic effects of methylmercury in the cat: Note on the use of this species as a model for teratogenic studies. Teratology 8:293, 1973.

Khera KS: A teratogenicity study on hydroxyurea and diphenylhydantoin in cats. Teratology 20:447, 1979.

Kilham L, Margolis G: Viral etiology of spontaneous ataxia of cats. Am J Pathol 48:991, 1966.

Kilham L, Margolis G, Colby ED: Congenital infections of cats and ferrets by feline panleukopenia virus manifested by cerebellar hypoplasia. Lab Invest 17:465, 1967.

Kitchen H, Murray RE, Cockrell BY: Spina bifida, sacral dysgenesis, and myelocele. Animal model: Manx cats. Am J Pathol 68:203, 1972.

Knecht CD, Lamar CH, Schaible, et al: Cerebellar hypoplasia in chow chows. J Am Anim Hosp Assoc 15:51, 1979.

Knecht CD, Oliver JE, Redding R, et al: Narcolepsy in a dog and cat. J Am Vet Med Assoc 162:1052, 1973.

Koppang N: Neuronal ceroid-lipofuscinosis in English setters. J Small Anim Pract 10:639, 1970.

Kornegay JN: Cerebellar vermian hypoplasia in dogs. Vet Pathol 23:374, 1986.

Kornegay JN: The X-linked muscular dystrophies. In Kirk RW, Bonagura JD (eds): Current Veterinary Therapy XI. Philadelphia, WB Saunders, 1992, p 1042.

Kornegay JN, Goodwin MA, Spyridakis LK: Hypomyelination in Weimaraner dogs. Acta Neuropathol (Berl) 72:394, 1987.

Kramer JW, Schiffer SP, Sande RD, et al: Characterization of heritable thoracic hemivertebra of the German shorthaired pointer. J Am Vet Med Assoc 181:814, 1982.

Kraviec DR: Cataplexy in a dog. Compend Contin Educ Pract Vet 5:450, 1983.

Krum S, Johnson K, Wilson J: Hydrocephalus associated with the noneffusive form of feline infectious peritonitis. J Am Vet Med Assoc 167:746, 1975.

Lappin MR, Greene CE, Winston S, et al: Clinical feline toxoplasmosis. Serologic diagnosis and therapeutic management of 15 cases. J Vet Intern Med 3:139, 1989.

LeCouteur RA, McKeown D, Johnson J, et al: Stabilization of atlantoaxial subluxation in the dog, using the nuchal ligament. J Am Vet Med Assoc 177:1011, 1980.

Leifer CE, Peterson ME: Hypoglycemia. Vet Clin North Am Small Anim Pract 14:873, 1984.

Leipold HW, Huston K, Blauch B, et al: Congenital defects of the caudal vertebral column and spinal cord in Manx cats. J Am Vet Med Assoc 164:520, 1974.

Lemire RJ: Variations in development of the caudal neural tube in human embryos (Horizons XIV–XXI). Teratology 2:361, 1969.

Lincoln JD, Pettit GD: Evaluation of fenestration for treatment of degenerative disc disease in the caudal cervical region of large dogs. Vet Surg 14:240, 1985.

Lowenthal AC, Cummings JF, Wenger DA, et al: Feline sphingolipidosis resembling Niemann-Pick disease type C. Acta Neuropathol (Berl) 81:189, 1990.

Luttgen PJ, Braund KG, Storts RW: Globoid cell leukodystrophy in a basset hound. J Small Anim Pract 24:153, 1983.

Malik R, Mepstead K, Yang F, et al: Hereditary myopathy of Devon rex cats. J Small Anim Pract 34:539, 1993.

March PA, Knowles K, Thalhammer JG: Reflex myoclonus in two Labrador retriever littermates: A clinical, electrophysiological, and pathological study. Prog Vet Neurol 4:19, 1993.

Mason K: A hereditary disease in Burmese cats manifested as an episodic weakness with head nodding and neck ventroflexion. J Am Anim Hosp Assoc 24:147, 1988.

Mason RW, Hartley WJ, Randall M: Spongiform degeneration of the white matter in a Samoyed pup. Aust Vet Pract 9:11, 1979.

Mason TA: Cervical vertebral instability (wobbler syndrome) in the Doberman. Aust Vet J 53:440, 1977.

Mason TA: Cervical vertebral instability (wobbler syndrome) in the dog. Vet Rec 104:142, 1979.

Matz ME, Shell L, Braund K: Peripheral hypomyelinization in two golden retriever littermates. J Am Vet Med Assoc 197:228, 1990.

McGrath JT: Neurologic Examination of the Dog, 2nd ed. Philadelphia, Lea & Febiger, 1960, p 207.

McGrath JT: Spinal dysraphism in the dog. With comments on syringomyelia. Vet Pathol (Suppl) 2:1, 1965.

McKerrell RE, Braund KG: Hereditary myopathy in Labrador retrievers: Clinical variations. J Small Anim Pract 28:479, 1987.

McKerrell RE, Braund KG: Hereditary myopathy of Labrador retrievers. In Kirk RW (ed): Current Veterinary Therapy X. Philadelphia, WB Saunders, 1989, p 820.

Meric SM, Child G, Higgins RJ: Necrotizing vasculitis of the spinal pachyleptomeningeal arteries in three Bernese mountain dog littermates. J Am Anim Hosp Assoc 22:459, 1986.

Meric SM, Perman V, Hardy R: Corticosteroid responsive meningitis in ten dogs. J Am Anim Hosp Assoc 21:667, 1985.

Mitchell WJ, Summers BA, Appel MJG: Viral expression in experimental canine distemper demyelinating encephalitis. J Comp Pathol 104:77, 1991.

Montali RJ, Strandberg JD: Extraperitoneal lesions in feline infectious peritonitis. Vet Pathol 9:109, 1972.

Montgomery DL, Storts RW: Hereditary striatonigral and cerebello-olivary degeneration of the Kerry blue terrier. Vet Pathol 20:143, 1983.

Moreau PM, Vallat JM, Hugon J, et al: Peripheral and central distal axonopathy of suspected inherited origin in Birman cats. Acta Neuropathol (Berl) 82:143, 1991.

Morgan JP: Congenital anomalies of the vertebral column of the dog: A study of the incidence and significance based on a radiographic and morphologic study. J Am Vet Radiol Soc 9:21, 1968.

Motoyama M, Kilduff TS, Lee BSM, et al: Restriction fragment length polymorphism in canine narcolepsy. Immunogenetics 29:124, 1989.

Nesbit JW, Lourens DC, Williams MC: Spastic paresis in two littermate pups caused by *Toxoplasma gondii*. J S Afr Vet Assoc 52:243, 1981.

Neuwelt EA, Johnson WG, Blank NK, et al: Characterization of a new model of GM$_2$-gangliosidosis (Sandhoff's disease) in Korat cats. J Clin Invest 76:482, 1985.

Newsholme SJ, Gaskell CJ: Myopathy with core-like structures in a dog. J Comp Pathol 97:597, 1987.

Nimmo Wilkie JS, Hudson EB: Neuronal and generalized ceroid-lipofuscinosis in a cocker spaniel. Vet Pathol 19:623, 1982.

Njoku CO, Esievo KA, Bida SA, et al: Canine cyclopia. Vet Rec 102:60, 1978.

O'Brien DP, Zachary JF: Clinical features of spongy degeneration of the central nervous system in two Labrador retriever littermates. J Am Vet Med Assoc 186:1207, 1985.

Oliver JE Jr: Seizure disorders in companion animals. Compend Contin Educ Pract Vet 2:77, 1980.

Oliver JE Jr: Seizure disorders and narcolepsy. *In* Oliver JE Jr, Hoerlein BF, Mayhew IG (eds): Veterinary Neurology. Philadelphia, WB Saunders, 1987, p 285.

Oliver JE Jr, Lewis RE: Lesions of the atlas and axis in dogs. J Am Vet Med Assoc 9:304, 1973.

Olsson S-E, Stavenborn M, Hoppe F: Dynamic compression of the cervical spinal cord. A myelographic and pathologic investigation in Great Dane dogs. Acta Vet Scand 23:65, 1982.

Oppelt WW, Patlak CS, Rall DP: Effect of certain drugs on cerebrospinal fluid production in the dog. Am J Physiol 206:247, 1964.

Palmer AC: Myasthenia gravis. Vet Clin North Am Small Anim Pract 10:213, 1980.

Palmer AC, Blakemore WF: A progressive neuronopathy in the young Cairn terrier. J Small Anim Pract 30:101, 1989.

Palmer AC, Blakemore WF, Wallace ME, et al: Recognition of "trembler," a hypomyelinating condition in the Bernese mountain dog. Vet Rec 120:609, 1987.

Palmer AC, Payne JE, Wallace ME: Hereditary quadriplegia and amblyopia in the Irish setter. J Small Anim Pract 14:343, 1973.

Palmer AC, Wallace ME: Deformation of cervical vertebrae in basset hounds. Vet Rec 80:430, 1967.

Parker AJ, Park RD, Byerly CS, et al: Spina bifida with protrusion of spinal cord tissue in a dog. J Am Vet Med Assoc 163:158, 1973.

Percy DH, Carmichael LE, Albert DM, et al: Lesions in puppies surviving infection with canine herpesvirus. Vet Pathol 8:37, 1971.

Plummer SB, Bunch SE, Khoo LA, et al: Tethered spinal cord and intradural lipoma with a meningocele in a Manx-cross cat. J Am Vet Med Assoc 203:1159, 1993.

Prata RG, Stoll SG, Zaki FA: Spinal cord compression caused by osteocartilaginous exostoses of the spine in two dogs. Vet Med Assoc 166:371, 1975.

Presthus J, Lindboe CF: Polymyositis in two German wirehaired pointer littermates. J Small Anim Pract 29:239, 1988.

Presthus J, Nordstoga K: Congenital myopathy in a

litter of Samoyed dogs. Prog Vet Neurol 4:37, 1993.

Rac R, Giesecke PR: Lysosomal storage disease in Chihuahuas. Aust Vet J 51:403, 1975.

Raffe MR, Knecht CD: Cervical vertebral malformation in bull mastiffs. J Am Anim Hosp Assoc 14:593, 1978.

Raffe MR, Knecht CD: Cervical vertebral malformation—A review of 36 cases. J Am Anim Hosp Assoc 16:881, 1980.

Read DH, Harrington DD, Keenan TW, et al: Neuronal-visceral GM$_1$ gangliosidosis in a dog with β-galactosidase deficiency. Science 194:442, 1976.

Read RA, Robins GM, Carlisle CH: Caudal cervical spondylomyelopathy (wobbler syndrome) in the dog: A review of thirty cases. J Small Anim Pract 24:605, 1983.

Redding RW: Electrophysiologic diagnosis. Electroencephalography. *In* Oliver JE Jr, Hoerlein BF, Mayhew IG (eds): Veterinary Neurology. Philadelphia, WB Saunders, 1987, p 111.

Regnier AM, Ducos de Lahitte MJ, Delisle MB, et al: Dandy-Walker syndrome in a kitten. J Am Anim Hosp Assoc 29:514, 1993.

Reidarson TH, Metz AL, Hardy RM: Thoracic vertebral ostochondroma in a cat. J Am Vet Med Assoc 192:1102, 1988.

Rendano VT, Smith LL: Cervical vertebral malformation-malarticulation (wobbler syndrome)—The value of the ventrodorsal view in defining lateral spinal cord compression in the dog. J Am Anim Hosp Assoc 17:627, 1981.

Renegar WR, Stoll SG: The use of methylmethacrylate bone cement in the repair of atlantoaxial subluxation stabilization failures—Case report and discussion. J Am Anim Hosp Assoc 15:313, 1979.

Richards RB, Kakulas BA: Spongiform leucoencephalopathy associated with congenital myoclonia syndrome in the dog. J Comp Pathol 88:317, 1978.

Richter K, Lorenzana R, Ettinger SJ: Traumatic displacement of the dens in a cat: Case report. J Am Anim Hosp Assoc 19:751, 1983.

Rivers WJ, Walter PA: Hydrocephalus in the dog: Utility of ultrasonography as an alternate diagnostic imaging technique. J Am Anim Hosp Assoc 28:333, 1992.

Sahar A, Hochwald GM, Kay WJ, et al: Spontaneous canine hydrocephalus: Cerebrospinal fluid dynamics. J Neurol Neurosurg Psychol 34:308, 1971.

Sanders DB, Howard JF Jr: AAEE Minimonograph #25: Single-fiber electromyography in myasthenia gravis. Muscle Nerve 9:809, 1986.

Sandstrom B, Westman J, Ockerman PA: Glycogenosis of the central nervous system in the cat. Acta Neuropathol (Berl) 14:194, 1969.

Sato O, Hara M, Asai T, et al: The effect of dexamethasone on the production rate of cerebrospinal fluid in the spinal subarachnoid space of dogs. J Neurosurg 39:480, 1973.

Saunders GK, Wood PA, Myers RK, et al: GM$_1$ gangliosidosis in Portuguese water dogs: Pathologic and biochemical findings. Vet Pathol 25:265, 1988.

Savell CM: Cerebral ventricular tap: An aid to diagnosis and treatment of hydrocephalus. J Am Anim Hosp Assoc 10:500, 1974.

Schmid V, Lang J, Wolf M: Dandy-Walker-like syndrome in four dogs: Cisternography as a diagnostic aid. J Am Anim Hosp Assoc 28:355, 1992.

Schulz KS: Application of ventral pins and polymethylmethacrylate for the management of atlantoaxial instability: Results in nine dogs. Vet Surg 26:17, 1997.

Schwartz-Porsche D: Epidemiological, clinical, and pharmaceutical studies in spontaneously epileptic dogs and cats. Proc Am Coll Vet Intern Med, 1986, p 11.

Schwartz-Porsche D, Loscher W, Frey H-H: Therapeutic efficacy of phenobarbital and primidone in canine epilepsy: A comparison. J Vet Pharmacol Therap 8:113, 1985.

Scott FW, de Lahunta A, Schultz RD, et al: Teratogenesis in cats associated with griseofulvin therapy. Teratology 11:79, 1974.

Scott JP, Fuller JL: Dog Behavior: The Genetic Basis. Chicago, University of Chicago Press, 1965, p 468.

Scott-Moncrieff JCR, Snyder PW, Glickman LT, et al: Systemic necrotizing vasculitis in nine young beagles. J Am Vet Med Assoc 201:1553, 1992.

Seim HB: Wobbler syndrome in the Doberman pinscher. In Kirk RW (ed): Current Veterinary Therapy X. Philadelphia, WB Saunders, 1989, p 858.

Seim HB, Withrow SJ: Pathophysiology and diagnosis of caudal cervical spondylo-myelopathy with emphasis on the Doberman pinscher. J Am Anim Hosp Assoc 18:241, 1982.

Sekeles E: Craniofacial and skeletal malformations in a cat. Feline Pract 11:28, 1981.

Selby LA, Hayes HM, Becker SV: Epizootiologic features of canine hydrocephalus. Am J Vet Res 40:411, 1979.

Selcer EA, Selcer RR: Globoid cell leukodystrophy in two West Highland white terriers and one Pomeranian. Compend Contin Educ Pract Vet 6:621, 1984.

Selcer RR, Oliver JE Jr: Cervical spondylopathy—Wobbler syndrome in dogs. J Am Anim Hosp Assoc 11:175, 1975.

Sharp NJH, Kornegay JN, Van Camp SD, et al: An error in dystrophin mRNA processing in golden retriever muscular dystrophy, an animal homologue of Duchenne muscular dystrophy. Genomics 13:115, 1991.

Shell LG, Carrig CB, Sponenberg DP, et al: Spinal dysraphism, hemivertebra, and stenosis of the spinal canal in a Rottweiler puppy. J Am Anim Hosp Assoc 24:341, 1988.

Shelton SB, Bellah J, Chrisman C, et al: Hypoplasia of the odontoid process and secondary atlantoaxial luxation in a Siamese cat. Prog Vet Neurol 2:209, 1991.

Shores A: Neurologic examination of the canine neonate. Compend Contin Educ Pract Vet 5:1033, 1983.

Shores A, Redding RW: Narcoleptic hypersomnia syndrome responsive to protriptyline in a Labrador retriever. J Am Anim Hosp Assoc 23:455, 1987.

Shull RM, Munger RJ, Spellacy E, et al: Animal model of human disease. Canine α-L-iduronidase deficiency. Am J Pathol 109:244, 1982.

Silson M, Robinson R: Hereditary hydrocephalus in the cat. Vet Rec 84:477, 1969.

Simpson S: Diseases of the vestibular system. In Kirk RW (ed): Current Veterinary Therapy VIII. Philadelphia, WB Saunders, 1983, p 726.

Simpson ST: Hydrocephalus. In Kirk RW (ed): Current Veterinary Therapy X. Philadelphia, WB Saunders, 1989, p 842.

Simpson ST, Braund KG: Myotonic dystrophy-like disease in a dog. J Am Vet Med Assoc 186:495, 1985.

Sisk DB, Levesque DC, Wood PA, et al: Clinical and pathologic features of ceroid lipofuscinosis in two Australian cattle dogs. J Am Vet Med Assoc 197:361, 1990.

Sorjonen DC, Cox NR, Swango LJ: Electrophoretic determination of albumin and gamma globulin concentrations in cerebrospinal fluid of dogs with encephalomyelitis attributable to canine distemper virus infection: 13 cases (1980–1987). J Am Vet Med Assoc 195:977, 1989.

Sorjonen DC, Shires PK: Atlantoaxial instability: A ventral surgical technique for decompression, fixation, and fusion. Vet Surg 10:22, 1981.

Spaulding KA, Sharp NJH: Ultrasonographic imaging of the lateral cerebral ventricles in the dog. Vet Radiol 31:59, 1990.

Steiss JE, Pook HA, Clark EG, et al: Sensory neuronopathy in a dog. J Am Vet Med Assoc 190:205, 1987.

Stirling J, Clarke M: Congenital peripheral vestibular disorder in two German shepherd dogs. Aust Vet J 57:200, 1981.

Stockard CR: An hereditary lethal for localized motor and preganglionic neurons with a resulting paralysis in the dog. Am J Anat 59:1, 1936.

Summers BA, Greisen HA, Appel MJG: Canine distemper encephalomyelitis: Variation with virus strain. J Comp Pathol 94:65, 1984.

Tamke PG, Petersen MG, Dietze AE, et al: Acquired hydrocephalus and hydromyelia in a cat with feline infectious peritonitis: A case report and brief review. Can Vet J 29:997, 1988.

Taylor RM, Farrow BRW: Ceroid-lipofuscinosis in border collie dogs. Acta Neuropathol (Berl) 75:627, 1988.

Taylor RM, Farrow BRH, Healy PJ: Canine fucosidosis: Clinical findings. J Small Anim Pract 28:291, 1987.

Taylor RM, Farrow BRH, Stewart GJ: Correction of enzyme deficiency by allogenic bone marrow transplantation following total lymphoid irradiation in dogs with lysosomal storage disease (fucosidosis). Transplant Proc 18:326, 1986.

Thomas JB, Robertson D: Hereditary cerebellar abiotrophy in Australian Kelpie dogs. Aust Vet J 66:301, 1989.

Thomas WB: Surgical management of atlantoaxial subluxation in 23 dogs. Vet Surg 20:409, 1991.

Thomas WB, Sorjonen DC, Steiss JE: A retrospective evaluation of 38 cases of canine distemper encephalomyelitis. J Am Anim Hosp Assoc 29:129, 1993.

Thomson MJ, Read RA: Surgical stabilisation of the atlantoaxial joint in a cat. VCOT 9:36, 1996.

Tonttila P, Lindberg LA: Ett fall av cerebellar ataxia hos finsk stovare. Suomen Elainlaakarilehti 77:135, 1971.

Trotter EJ, de Lahunta A, Geary JC, et al: Caudal cervical vertebral malformation-malarticulation in Great Danes and Doberman pinschers. J Am Vet Med Assoc 168:917, 1976.

Valentine BA, Cooper BJ, de Lahunta A, et al: Canine X-linked muscular dystrophy. An animal model of Duchenne muscular dystrophy: Clinical studies. J Neurol Sci 88:69, 1988.

Vandevelde M, Braund KG, Walker TL, et al: Dysmyelination of the central nervous system in the chow-chow dog. Acta Neuropathol (Berl) 42:211, 1978.

Vandevelde M, Fankhauser R, Bischel P, et al: Hereditary neurovisceral mannosidosis associated family of Persian cats. Acta Neuropathol (Berl) 58:64, 1981.

Vandevelde M, Fatzert R: Neuronal ceroid-lipofuscinosis in older dachshunds. Vet Pathol 17:686, 1980.

Vandevelde M, Zurbriggen A, Steck A, et al: Studies on the intrathecal humoral immune response in canine distemper encephalitis. J Neuroimmunol 11:41, 1986.

Van De Water NS, Jolly RD, Farrow BRH: Canine Gaucher disease—The enzymatic defect. Aust J Exp Biol Med Sci 57:551, 1979.

VanGundy TE: Disc-associated wobbler syndrome in the Doberman pinscher. Vet Clin North Am Small Anim Pract 18:667, 1988.

Walker TL: Spinal curvature in the dog. Canine Pract 6:44, 1979.

Walkley SU, Baker HJ, Rattazzi MC, et al: Neuroaxonal dystrophy in neuronal storage disorders: Evidence for major GABAergic neuron involvement. J Neurol Sci 104:1, 1991.

Walvoort HC, van Nes JJ, Stokhof AA, et al: Canine glycogen storage disease type II: A clinical study of four affected Lapland dogs. J Am Anim Hosp Assoc 20:279, 1984.

Ware Wa, DiBartola SP, Couto CG: Atypical portosystemic shunt in a cat. J Am Vet Med Assoc 188:187, 1986.

Warkentin J, Carmichael L: A study of the development of the air righting reflex in cats and rabbits. J Genet Psychol 55:67, 1939.

Wheeler SJ: Sensory neuropathy in a border collie puppy. J Small Anim Pract 28:281, 1987.

Wilson JW, Kurtz HJ, Leipold HW, et al: Spina bifida in the dog. Vet Pathol 16:165, 1979.

Woodard JC, Collins GH, Hessler JR: Feline hereditary neuroaxonal dystrophy. Am J Pathol 74:551, 1974.

Woods CB: Hyperkinetic episodes in two Dalmatian dogs. J Am Anim Hosp Assoc 13:255, 1977.

Wouda W, Vandevelde M, Oettle P, et al: Sensory neuronopathy in dogs: A study of four cases. J Comp Pathol 93:437, 1983.

Wright JA, Smyth JBA, Brownlie SE, et al: A myopathy associated with muscle hypertonicity in the Cavalier King Charles spaniel. J Comp Pathol 97:559, 1987.

Wright NG: Recent advances in canine virus research. J Small Anim Pract 14:241, 1973.

Yamagami T, Umeda M, Kamiya S, et al: Neurovisceral sphingomyelinosis in a Siamese cat. Acta Neuropathol (Berl) 79:330, 1989.

Yasuba M, Okimoto K, Iida M, et al: Cerebellar cortical degeneration in beagle dogs. Vet Pathol 25:315, 1988.

Zachary JF, O'Brien DP: Spongy degeneration of the central nervous system in two canine littermates. Vet Pathol 22:561, 1985.

Zaki FA: Lissencephaly in Lhasa apso dogs. J Am Vet Med Assoc 169:1165, 1976.

Zaki FA, Kay WJ: Globoid cell leukodystrophy in a miniature poodle. J Am Vet Med Assoc 163:248, 1973.

Zook BC, Sostaric BR, Draper DJ, et al: Encephalocele and other congenital craniofacial anomalies in Burmese cats. Vet Med Small Anim Clin 78:695, 1983.

THE NEUROMUSCULAR SYSTEM

Braund KG, Mehta JR, Toivio-Kinnucan M, et al: Congenital hypomyelinating polyneuropathy in two golden retriever littermates. Vet Pathol 26:202, 1989.

Braund KG, Shores A, Cochrane S, et al: Laryngeal paralysis-polyneuropathy complex in young Dalmations. Am J Vet Res 55:534, 1994.

Breitschwerdt EB, Kornegay JN, Wheeler SJ, et al: Episodic weakness associated with exertional lactic acidosis and myopathy in Old English sheepdog littermates. J Am Vet Med Assoc 201:731, 1992.

Carpenter JL, Hoffman EP, Romanul FCA, et al: Feline muscular dystrophy with dystrophin deficiency. Am J Pathol 135:909, 1989.

Ceh L, Hauge JG, Svenkerud R, et al: Glycogenosis type III in the dog. Acta Vet Scand 7:210, 1976.

Clemmons RM, Peters RI, Meyers KM: Scotty cramp: A review of cause, characteristics, diagnosis, and treatment. Compend Contin Educ Pract Vet 2:385, 1980.

Cooper BJ, deLahunta A, Cummings JF, et al: Canine inherited hypertrophic neuropathy: Clinical and electrodiagnostic studies. Am J Vet Res 45:1172, 1984.

Cooper BJ, deLahunta A, Gallagher E, et al: Nemaline myopathy in cats. Muscle Nerve 9:618, 1986.

Cork LC, Gfiffin JW, Munnell JF, et al: Hereditary

canine spinal muscular atrophy. J Neuropathol Exp Neurol 38:209, 1979.

Cuddon PA, Higgins RJ, Duncan ID, et al: Polyneuropathy in feline Niemann-Pick disease. Brain 112:1429, 1989.

deLahunta A, Ingram JT, Cummings JF, et al: Labrador retriever central axonopathy. Prog Vet Neurol 5:117, 1994.

Delauche AJ, Cuddon PA, Podell M, et al: Nemaline rods in canine myopathies: 4 case reports and literature review. J Vet Intern Med 12:424, 1998.

Dubey JP: Toxoplasmosis in dogs. Canine Pract 12:7, 1985.

Dubey JP, Yeary RA: Anticoccidial activity of 2-sulfamoyl-4,4-diaminodiphenylsulfone, sulfadiazine, pyrimethamine and clindamycin in cats infected with *Toxoplasma gondii*. Can Vet J 18:51, 1977.

Duncan ID, Cuddon PA: Sensory neuropathy. *In* Kirk RW (ed): Current Veterinary Therapy X. Philadelphia, WB Saunders, 1989, p 822.

Farrow BRH, Malik R: Hereditary myotonia in the chow chow. J Small Anim Pract 22:451, 1981.

Fox JG, Averill DR, Hallett M, et al: Familial reflex myoclonus in Labrador retrievers. Am J Vet Res 45:2367, 1984.

Fyfe JC, et al: Glycogen storage disease type IV: Inherited deficiency of branching enzyme activity in cats. Pediatr Res 32:719, 1992.

Gashen FP, Haugh PG, Swendrowski MA: Hypertrophic feline muscular dystrophy—A unique clinical expression of dystrophin deficiency. Feline Pract 22:23, 1994.

Gashen FP, Hoffman EP, Gorospe JRM, et al: Dystrophin deficiency causes lethal muscle hypertrophy in cats. J Neurol Sci 110:149, 1992.

Giger U, Reilly MP, Asakura T, et al: Autosomal recessive inherited phosphofructokinase deficiency in English springer spaniel dogs. Anim Genet 17:12, 1986.

Greene CE, Cook JR, Mahaffey EA: Clindamycin for treatment of *Toxoplasma* polymyositis in a dog. J Am Vet Med Assoc 187:631, 1985.

Griffiths IR, Duncan ID, Barker J: A progressive axonopathy of boxer dogs affecting the central and peripheral nervous systems. J Small Anim Pract 21:29, 1980.

Hanson SM, Smith MO, Walker TL, et al: Juvenile-onset distal myopathy in Rottweiler dogs. J Vet Intern Med 12:103, 1998.

Hargis AM, Haupt KH, Prieur DJ, et al: A skin disorder in three Shetland sheepdogs: Comparison with familial canine dermatomyositis of collies. Compend Contin Educ Pract Vet 7:306, 1985.

Hass JA, Shell L, Saunders G: Neurological manifestations of toxoplasmosis: A literature review and case summary. J Am Anim Hosp Assoc 25:253, 1989.

Hay WH, Shell LG, Lindsay DS, et al: Diagnosis and treatment of *Neospora caninum* infection in a dog. J Am Vet Med Assoc 197:87, 1990.

Herrtage ME, Houlton JEF: Collapsing Clumber spaniels. Vet Rec 105:334, 1979.

Herrtage ME, Palmer AC: Episodic falling in the Cavalier King Charles spaniel. Vet Rec 112:458, 1983.

Holland CT, Canfield PJ, Watson ADJ, et al: Dyserythropoiesis, polymyopathy and cardiac disease in three related English springer spaniels. J Vet Intern Med 5:151, 1991.

Honhold N, Smith DA: Myotonia in the Great Dane. Vet Rec 119:162, 1986.

Houlton JEF, Herrtage ME: Mitochondrial myopathy in the Sussex spaniel. Vet Rec 106:206, 1980.

Huxtable CR, Chadwick B, Eger C, et al: Severe subacute progressive myopathy in a young silky terrier. Prog Vet Neurol 5:21, 1994.

Inada S, Sakamoto H, Haruta K, et al: A clinical study on hereditary progressive neurogenic muscular atrophy in pointer dogs. Jpn J Vet Sci 40:539, 1978.

Johnson RP, Watson DJ, Smith J, et al: Myasthenia in springer spaniel littermates. J Small Anim Pract 16:641, 1975.

Kornegay JN, Tuler SM, Miller DM, et al: Muscular dystrophy in a litter of golden retriever dogs. Muscle Nerve 11:1056, 1988.

Kramer JW, Hegreberg GA, Bryan GM, et al: A muscle disorder of Labrador retrievers characterized by deficiency of type II muscle fibers. J Am Vet Med Assoc 169:817, 1976.

Kramer JW, Hegreberg GA, Hamilton MJ: Inheritance of a neuromuscular disorder of Labrador retriever dogs. J Am Vet Med Assoc 179:380, 1981.

Kunkle GA, Chrisman CL, Gross TL, et al: Dermatomyositis in collie dogs. Compend Contin Educ Pract Vet 7:185, 1985.

Lorenz MD, Cork LC, Griffin JW, et al: Hereditary spinal muscular atrophy in Brittany spaniels: Clinical manifestations. J Am Vet Med Assoc 75:833, 1979.

Mahoney OM, Knowles KE, Braund KG, et al: Laryngeal paralysis-polyneuropathy complex in young Rottweilers. J Vet Intern Med 12:330, 1998.

Malik R, et al: Hereditary myopathy of Devon Rex cats. J Small Anim Pract 34:539, 1993.

McKerrell RE, Blakemore WF, Heath MF, et al: Primary hyperoxaluria (L-glyceric aciduria) in the cat: A newly recognized inherited disease. Vet Rec 125:31, 1989.

Miller LM, Lennon VA, Lambert EH, et al: Congenital myasthenia gravis in 13 smooth fox terriers. J Am Vet Med Assoc 182:694, 1983.

Myers KM, Lund JE, Padgett GA, et al: Hyperkinetic episodes in Scottish terrier dogs. J Am Vet Med Assoc 155:129, 1969.

Ozawa E, Noguchi S, Mizuno Y, et al: From dystrophinopathy to sarcoglycanopathy: Evolution of a concept of muscular dystrophy. Muscle Nerve 21:421, 1998.

Paola JP, Podell M, Shelton GD: Muscular dystrophy in a miniature schnauzer. Prog Vet Neurol 4:14, 1993.

Presthus J, Nordstoga K: Probable X-linked myopathy in a Samoyed litter. Ann Symp Eur Soc Vet Neurol 3:52, 1989.

Robinson R: "Spasticity" in the Devon Rex cat. Vet Rec 132:302, 1992.

Rafiquzzaman M, Svenkerud R, Strande A, et al: Glycogenosis in the dog. Acta Vet Scand 17:196, 1976.

Sandefeldt E, Cummings JF, de Lahunta A, et al: Hereditary neuronal abiotrophy in the Swedish Lapland dog. Cornell Vet 63(Suppl 3):1, 1973.

Schatzberg S, Olby N, Steingold S, et al: The molecular basis of German short-haired pointer muscular dystrophy. J Vet Intern Med 12:208a, 1998.

Shell LG, Jortner BS, Leib MS: Spinal muscular atrophy in two Rottweiler littermates. J Am Vet Med Assoc 190:878, 1987a.

Shell LG, Jortner BS, Leib MS: Familial motor neuron disease in Rottweiler dogs: Neuropathologic studies. Vet Pathol 24:135, 1987b.

Shelton GD, Cardinet GH III: Canine masticatory muscle disorders. In Kirk RW (ed): Current Veterinary Therapy X. Philadelphia, WB Saunders, 1989, p 816.

Shelton GD, Schule A, Kass PH: Risk factors for acquired myasthenia gravis in dogs: 1,154 cases (1991–1995). J Am Vet Med Assoc 211:1428, 1997.

Shires PK, Nafe LA, Hulse DA: Myotonia in a Staffordshire terrier. J Am Vet Med Assoc 183:229, 1983.

Targett MP, Franklin RJM, Olby NJ, et al: Central core myopathy in a Great Dane. J Small Anim Pract 35:100, 1994.

Toll J, Cooper B, Altschul M: Congenital myotonia in 2 domestic cats. J Vet Intern Med 12:116, 1998.

Valentine BA, Cummings JE, Cooper BJ: Development of Duchenne-type cardiomyopathy: Morphologic studies in a canine model. Am J Pathol 135:671, 1989.

Vandevalde M, Greene CE, Hoff EJ: Lower motor neuron disease with accumulation of neurofilaments in a cat. Vet Pathol 13:428, 1976.

van Ham LML, Desmidt M, Tshamala M, et al: Canine X-linked muscular dystrophy in Belgian Groenendaeler shepherds. J Am Anim Hosp Assoc 29:570, 1993.

Venker-van Haagen AJ, Hartmen W, Goedegebuure SA: Spontaneous laryngeal paralysis in young Bouviers. J Am Anim Hosp Assoc 17:75, 1981.

Vijayasarathy C, Giger U, Prociuk U, et al: Canine mitochondrial myopathy associated with reduced mitochondrial mRNA and altered cytochrome c oxidase activities in fibroblasts and skeletal muscle. Comp Biochem Physiol 109:887, 1994.

Wallace ME, Palmer AC: Recessive mode of inheritance in myasthenia gravis in the Jack Russell terrier. Vet Rec 114:350, 1984.

Wentink GH, van der Linde-Sipman JS, Meijer AEFH, et al: Myopathy with possible recessive X-linked inheritance in a litter of Irish terriers. Vet Pathol 9:328, 1972.

Winand N, Pradham D, Cooper B, et al: Molecular characterization of severe Duchenne-type muscular dystrophy in a family of Rottweiler dogs. In Proceedings of the Molecular Mechanisms of Neuromuscular Disease. Tuczon, AZ, Muscular Dystrophy Association, 1994.

Woods P, Sharp N, Schatzberg S: Muscular dystrophy in Pembroke corgis and other dogs. Proc Am Coll Vet Intern Med Forum 16:301, 1998.

Wright JA, Smyth JBA, Brownlie SE, et al: A myopathy associated with muscle hypertonicity in the Cavalier King Charles spaniel. J Comp Pathol 97:559, 1987.

The Reproductive System

Augustine T. Peter

Most puppies and kittens attain puberty between 8 and 19 months of age, with a range of 6 to 22 months. Although most puppies and kittens are not capable of reproducing at 6 months of age, it is relevant to discuss the prepuberal changes that occur in their organs of reproduction. The process of gonadal descent into the scrotum is unique to males. Veterinarians are asked to diagnose cases of ambiguous external genitalia. A discussion of the abnormalities of phenotypic sex is appropriate here. The major topics covered in this chapter are normal and abnormal processes of testicular descent, abnormalities of phenotypic sex, postnatal development of gonads, prepuberal gonadectomy, and puppy vaginitis.

TESTICULAR DESCENT

Process

The process of normal testicular descent is as follows. During fetal development, each testis, covered by the visceral peritoneum, moves to a position caudoventral to the inguinal canal from its original location (the caudal pole of the metanephric kidney). The gubernaculum (a mesenchymal structure composed of fibroblasts, fine collagen fibers, and a mucoid intercellular substance containing large amounts of mucopolysaccharides) extends from the caudal part of the testis into the inguinal canal. The peritoneum covers the abdominal part of the gubernaculum and invades the extraabdominal portion of the gubernaculum at the level of the future deep inguinal ring, forming an invagination into the genital swelling (Baumans et al, 1981; Wensing, 1975, 1980). As the testis

approaches the internal ring of the inguinal canal, the caudal part of the gubernaculum enlarges enormously ("welling reaction") (Wensing, 1968), dilating the inguinal canal and extending into the scrotum (Fig. 20–1).

The following theories have been proposed for the transinguinal migration of the testis in

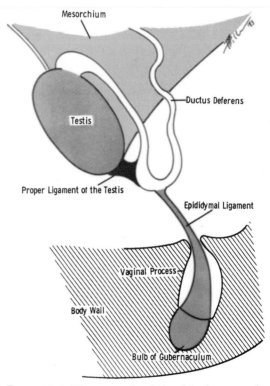

Figure 20–1. The normal relationship between the vaginal process, epididymal ligament, and gubernaculum. (Courtesy of S.B. Adams.)

463

domestic animals based on theories from human medicine (Sizonenko, 1988): the traction hypothesis, pulling of the testis by the epididymis, and the abdominal pressure theory. It is also believed that the changes in the length and thickness of the gubernaculum facilitate the passage of the testis through the inguinal canal and into the scrotum. The gubernaculum (before its regression) may even be mistaken for the descended testis. There are indications that testosterone plays a role in the initiation of gubernacular regression (Wensing, 1988). Eventually the gubernaculum differentiates, forming the proper ligament of the testis and the ligament of the tail of the epididymis. The enlargement of the gubernaculum is a major phenomenon antecedent to and persisting during the transabdominal movement (Hullinger and Wensing, 1985a). The factor or factors controlling this reaction, however, remain unknown (Hullinger and Wensing, 1985b).

Timing

In puppies, the process of testicular descent into the scrotum is completed after birth; however, the timing of the process is unclear (Ashdown, 1963). The first report on this subject described the testicular descent as occurring sometime in the neonatal period, but usually a few weeks after birth (Skoda, 1913). A subsequent report suggested that the scrotum is not yet formed at birth and that the testes lie in the inguinal position (Kunzel, 1954). Another report indicated that the vaginal process reaches the scrotum at birth and that the testes are still in the abdomen (Zietzschmann and Krolling, 1955). Based on his work with 12 puppies (from birth to 30 days of age), Arthur (1956) confirmed that in most puppies the testes remain in the abdomen at birth. He suggested that testicular descent is normally completed within 7 to 10 days after birth.

Michel (1968) stated, rather unspecifically, that passage of the testis through the inguinal canal takes place long after birth. According to Wensing (1968), the testis passes through the inguinal canal 3 to 4 days after birth. In the views of Meyer (1977) and Arbeiter (1975), testicular descent occurs at 30 to 33 days after birth, whereas Schorner (1975) dates it at the time of birth. Others have also been of the opinion that puppies are born with undescended testicles (Burke, 1979; Donovan, 1963). It is widely believed that the process of testicular descent is completed a week after birth and that the testes are palpable in the scrotum around 5

to 7 weeks of age (Burke, 1979). In a detailed study of 87 puppies from four breeds of dogs, Baumans and others (1981) concluded that the testis passes through the inguinal canal on the third or fourth day after birth and reaches its final scrotal location on the thirty-fifth day after birth. Based on these reports, it can be concluded that the testicular descent is completed within 7 weeks after birth.

It is generally accepted that in puppies the testes may be retracted easily by the action of the external cremaster muscle. If the testes of a puppy can be retracted beyond the possibility of palpation, a single examination may be insufficient to establish a firm diagnosis of failure of testicular descent. After its descent into the vaginal process, the testis can also be drawn through the external ring and remain in that location permanently (Whitney, 1961).

In kittens, the testes are fully descended into the scrotum at birth (Scott and Scott, 1957). Despite their normal descent into the scrotum, they may move up and down in the inguinal canal, and they do not remain permanently in the scrotum until 10 to 14 weeks of age (Christiansen, 1984).

Failure

Failure of the testis to descend into the scrotum is a developmental defect, and either one or both testes may fail to descend to their normal position in the scrotum, creating a condition known as *cryptorchidism* (Osterhoff, 1977). After partial descent, the testis can remain in the abdominal region or inguinal canal or can reach an ectopic subcutaneous location. In certain cases, the testis (including the epididymis) may be in the abdomen, or the testis may be in the abdomen with a portion of the epididymis in the inguinal canal. In instances of ectopic subcutaneous testis, the incompletely descended testes have passed from the abdominal cavity through the inguinal canal but have not reached the scrotum and lie under the skin between scrotum and the inguinal canal.

In colts with undescended testes, the anatomic location of the vaginal process may be variable (Stickle and Fessler, 1978). In puppies, it may also be possible for the vaginal process to be everted into the inguinal canal (Fig. 20–2) or inverted into the abdomen (Fig. 20–3), as has been suggested for colts. In addition to a portion of the gubernaculum testis, an everted vaginal process may contain the tail of the epididymis or a loop of ductus deferens (Fig. 20–4). In puppies with undescended testes, the right testis

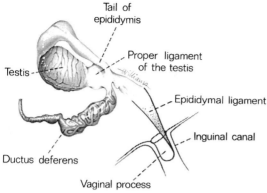

Figure 20–2. Everted vaginal process containing a portion of the gubernaculum. (From Stickle RL, Fessler JF: Retrospective study of 350 cases of equine cryptorchidism. J Am Vet Med Assoc 172:343, 1978. Reprinted with permission.)

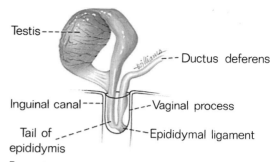

Figure 20–4. Everted vaginal process containing the tail of epididymis and proximal ductus deferens. (From Stickle RL, Fessler JF: Retrospective study of 350 cases of equine cryptorchidism. J Am Vet Med Assoc 172:343, 1978. Reprinted with permission.)

is usually retained in the inguinal region (Bloom, 1954; Brodey and Martin, 1958; Cox et al, 1978). In kittens, on the other hand, abdominal retention of the testis is more common than inguinal retention.

Incidence

The incidence of permanent testicular retention in dogs is estimated for the general population to be less than 0.1% (Rhoades and Foley, 1977). In a survey taken from a small animal practice (Dunn et al, 1968), 194 of 1494 male dogs examined failed to have both testes in the scrotum, yielding an incidence of 13.0%. In 30 of these cases, however, the animals were younger than 6 months at the initial examination, and the testes subsequently descended. An addi-

tional 27 dogs with undescended testes were never reevaluated. Removal of these 57 dogs from the calculations leaves an incidence of 9.5% for testicular retention in a small animal practice, which is comparable with the estimate from a subsequent study (Reif and Brodey, 1969).

Cause

Failure of testicular descent is considered by many authors to be hereditary, but its mode of inheritance remains to be firmly established. Most authors now consider the condition to be a simple recessive trait, although some believe that there is a possibility of multiple gene effect (Rehfeld, 1971; Rhoades and Foley, 1977).

It is generally agreed that the failure of testicular descent is due to a hereditary recessive trait. The condition is common in dwarf and brachycephalic dog breeds, and in these breeds it is believed to be inherited as a sex-limited recessive trait. Breeding trials in boxers and cocker spaniels also confirmed the sex-limited inheritance. The type of inheritance may not be similar for different grades of testicular retention. For example, the unilateral testicular retention in an inbred family of Saint Bernards was considered to be the result of a simple recessive trait. Although the type of inheritance for the condition has not been fully documented, it is thought to be genetically related (Leipold, 1978).

Although it is difficult to eliminate this condition by using only intact dogs (dogs with both testicles descended) as stud animals, this method will help to reduce the number of carriers. To reduce the incidence of the condition, a report developed by the British Veterinary Medical Association (1955) recommended *not* using the fol-

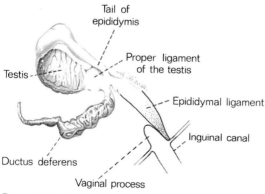

Figure 20–3. Inverted vaginal process. (From Stickle RL, Fessler JF: Retrospective study of 350 cases of equine cryptorchidism. J Am Vet Med Assoc 172:343, 1978. Reprinted with permission.)

lowing animals for breeding: (1) those with testicular retention, (2) their littermates, and (3) their parents. Even this degree of stringency may not completely eliminate the defect because carriers for this trait can be produced after several generations. The condition would appear should two carriers then be mated. Nevertheless, abstention from breeding known carriers should reduce the incidence.

Absence of Testis

One or both of the testes may be congenitally absent in a puppy (Bloom, 1954). These conditions are referred to as monorchidism or anorchidism, respectively. The term *monorchidism* is used colloquially to denote the presence of only one testis in the scrotum, but strictly speaking it should be used to indicate the condition in which only one testis is present in the animal. Estimation of peripheral testosterone concentrations before and after human chorionic gonadotrophin treatment may help in the diagnosis. Surgical exploration may not provide useful information because the possible positions of the retained testis within the abdomen may vary widely.

Complications

When both testes are retained, the animal is sterile. Spermatogenesis does not occur due to the high temperature of the undescended testis. In unilateral testicular retention, the testis inside the scrotum will have normal spermatogenesis. Surgical transfer of the descended testis experimentally into the inguinal canal or the abdominal cavity results in degeneration of the germinal epithelium with the formation of polynuclear giant cells. Regeneration occurs when the testis is replaced in the scrotum (Schlotthauer and Bollman, 1942). Grossly, before puberty an undescended testicle is similar in size and appearance to a normal testis. Microscopically, before puberty the retained testis is similar to the testis present in its normal position in the scrotum. After puberty and with increasing age, the retained testis becomes smaller and flabby, and the tunica albuginea is often thickened and wrinkled. The blood vessels and nerves are normal, but the vas deferens may be tortuous. In the adult animal the most conspicuous microscopic difference is the absence of spermatogenesis and a single layer of sustentacular cells (Sertoli's cells) lining the seminiferous tubules. The production of the male hormone testosterone by the interstitial cells (Leydig's cells) continues in the undescended testicle. There are reports of the condition affecting the general health or disposition of the animal, with common symptoms being unreliable character, nervousness, and increased fat deposition (Moss, 1962; Wolff, 1981).

One notable feature is the tendency of some ectopic testes to become the site of neoplasm formation. A 5:1 incidence of Sertoli's cell tumor and a 3:1 incidence of seminoma have been reported in the retained testis versus scrotal testis (Reif and Brodey, 1969). It has also been suggested that hip dysplasia, patellar dislocation, defects of the penis and prepuce, and umbilical hernia are associated with testicular retention (Pendergrass and Hayes, 1975).

Diagnosis

When a prepuberal dog is presented with one or both testicles not lying in the scrotum, it is difficult to determine if it is a case of delayed testicular descent or retained testis. Obviously, the smaller the puppy, the more difficult the palpation. While palpating small puppies, it is preferable to use the index and middle finger (one placed on each side of the penis), and the testes are located by gentle traction in a front-to-back direction (Burke, 1979). For sound diagnosis and prognosis, more information is needed about the period of life during which spontaneous testicular descent can occur and about the mobility of the testicles in young puppies. Most veterinarians believe that the testes are palpable within the scrotum by 6 to 8 weeks of age and that a definitive diagnosis should not be made until the dog is 6 months of age (Burke, 1979; Rhoades and Foley, 1977). The possibility of ectopic testis, anorchidism, or monorchidism must also be considered.

Prognosis

Any attempt to induce descent of the undescended testis by hormonal treatment is unethical. In this regard, injections of testosterone have been relatively ineffective. In a few cases, intramuscular administration of human chorionic gonadotrophin (1000 IU given intramuscularly to 20- to 30-pound puppies 4 to 6 months of age) has been helpful. Repeated administration of human chorionic gonadotrophin (1000 IU given weekly for 3 to 6 weeks for 7- to 8-week-old puppies) may be helpful in certain cases. Therapy, even if successful, does not correct the genetic flaw. Dogs with a retained testis should not be used for breeding because this perpetuates the genetic defect. The owner should be informed of the increased risk of testicular neoplasia, the secondary effects of feminization, possible skin changes, and possible changes in temperament. Prophylactic castration may be recommended because of the increased risk of testicular neoplasia as the animal grows older (Rhoades and Foley, 1977).

ABNORMALITIES OF PHENOTYPIC SEX

Disorders of sexual differentiation involving chromosomes, gonads, and phenotype can result in intersexuality. In abnormalities of phenotypic sex, the chromosomal and gonadal sex agree, but there is some ambiguity in the genitalia. Affected animals are either female or male pseudohermaphrodites. A pseudohermaphrodite has the gonads of one sex with the internal or external genitalia of the opposite sex and is defined as male or female according to the gonadal sex. That is, a female pseudohermaphrodite has ovaries; a male pseudohermaphrodite has testes.

Male Pseudohermaphroditism

Male pseudohermaphroditism occurs when genetic males differentiate partly or completely as phenotypic females. Puppies with unambiguous male external genitalia and varying degrees of malformation of the penis, prepuce, and scrotum, but with female internal genitalia, are included in the male pseudohermaphrodite group. Human and veterinary literature describes the following four conditions that fall in this category: various forms of hypospadias, persistent müllerian duct syndrome, 5α-reductase deficiency, and testicular feminization (George, 1992; Meyers-Wallen and Patterson, 1986).

Hypospadias

Hypospadias is an abnormality in the location of the urinary meatus, which is normally ventral and proximal to the normal site in the glans penis. Thus, the urinary orifice may be in the glans, the penile shaft, the prescrotal junction, or the perineum. The abnormality occurs as a result of incomplete closure of the urethral folds, which may be due to inadequate fetal testosterone or dihydrotestosterone production.

Persistent Müllerian Duct Syndrome

Dogs affected by persistent müllerian duct syndrome are usually bilaterally or unilaterally cryptorchid but otherwise appear to be normal males externally. Internally both testes are attached to the cranial ends of a bicornuate uterus. The testes may be in an ovarian position or within the inguinal ring or scrotum. If they are in a scrotal position, the cranial uterine horn may be palpable. The cranial portions of the vagina and prostate are often present (Brown et al, 1976).

Deficiency of 5α-Reductase

A deficiency of 5α-reductase, the enzyme that converts testosterone to dihydrotestosterone, results in the syndrome of pseudovaginal, perineoscrotal hypospadias (George, 1992). This condition has not been reported in the veterinary literature. It is believed that the condition is inherited as an autosomal recessive trait in humans. Individuals of this phenotype have wolffian duct structures (epididymis and vas deferens), and their urogenital sinus and external genitalia are of a female type. The labioscrotal folds (genital swellings) do not fuse, and the urogenital sinus does not close, resulting in perineoscrotal hypospadias and a blind pouch that resembles a vagina (George, 1992). In such humans, the peripheral levels of dihydrotestosterone are lower than in normal humans.

Testicular Feminization

Testicular feminization is divided into two categories: complete, believed to result from a defect in the androgen cytosol receptor (Kaufman et al, 1976), and incomplete, due to a deficiency of the binding protein for dihydrotestosterone (Griffin et al, 1976). The affected individuals are genetic males. It is believed that the condition is inherited as an X-linked recessive trait. Humans with testicular feminization syndrome have a normal male karyotype, bilateral testes, and female external genitalia. At puberty, these individuals become externally feminized as would be expected for normal females. The internal genital tract is absent except for gonads that have the histologic features of undescended testes (normal or increased Leydig's cells and seminiferous tubules without spermatogenesis). Occasionally, remnant structures of müllerian or wolffian origin can be identified in the paratesticular fascia or in fibrous bands extending from the testis. The testes may be located in the abdomen, along the course of the inguinal canal, or in the labia majora. Domestic species with complete testicular feminization are apparently normal females that fail to show behavioral or physical signs of estrus by the expected time of puberty (Meyers-Wallen et al, 1989).

In incomplete testicular feminization, subjects resemble individuals with the complete disorder but have some ambiguity of the external genitalia and experience some degree of virilization as well as feminization at puberty (Madden et al, 1975; Morris and Mahesh, 1963). The testes are in the abdomen or in the inguinal canal and are indistinguishable on histologic grounds from those seen in cases of complete testicular feminization. Partial fusion of the labioscrotal folds and a variable degree of clitoromegaly are distinctive features of the external genitalia. The vagina is short and ends blindly. Wolffian duct structures are present; this latter feature, together with the partial virilization of the external genitalia, separates the phenotype from that of complete testicular feminization (Peter et al, 1993).

POSTNATAL DEVELOPMENT OF GONADS

Testes

Kittens. The testes in kittens weigh approximately 20 mg each at birth (Fig. 20–5) and increase to 150 mg at 12 weeks of age and 500 mg at 20 weeks of age. During this period, the diameter of the seminiferous tubules also starts to increase. At birth the diameter of the seminiferous tubules is 60 to 90 μm, and it reaches 110 μm by 20 weeks of age. In the early stages of development, the intertubular tissue consists of vascular mesenchyme with abundant interstitial cells. Spermatogenesis is evident at 20 weeks of age, and at 30 weeks of age the spermatids appear in the testis (Scott and Scott, 1957).

Near the time of birth, a surge of fetal testosterone organizes and masculinizes the higher center(s) that will later direct male feline sexual behavior; however, the Leydig cells remain inactive after this surge until the kitten is about 3 months of age. By 3.5 months of age there is sufficient testosterone to initiate the growth of penile spines, which reach full size between 6 and 7 months of age (Beaver, 1992). Growth or regression of the spines has been positively correlated with androgen-dependent mating activity (Aronson and Cooper, 1967). By 5 months the kitten's spermatogenetic cells are mature enough for early spermatogenesis, but usually another 1 or 2 months must pass before spermatozoa can be found in the seminiferous tubules.

Puppies. Development of the testis, epididymis, and prostate gland in 53 male beagles was

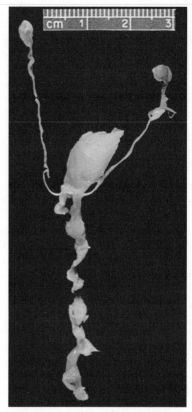

Figure 20–5. Reproductive structures of a 1-day-old male kitten.

examined histologically with periodic acid–Schiff (PAS) hematoxylin stain from birth to sexual maturity (Kawakami et al, 1991). The diameter of the testes was less than 100 μm until 20 weeks of age and then increased markedly between 22 and 28 weeks of age. Only Sertoli's cells and gonocytes (or spermatogonia) were detected in the seminiferous tubules before 16 weeks of age. Spermatocytes and spermatids appeared in the tubules at 20 and 22 weeks of age, respectively. Shed spermatocytes and round spermatids were seen in the lumen of the ductus epididymis, and a PAS-positive secretion was especially present in the ducts of the cauda epididymis at 24 weeks of age (Fig. 20–6).

Ovaries

Kittens. The developing prenatal or early neonatal kitten that is not exposed to testosterone develops a female nervous system and, at puberty, displays female behavioral characteristics. The onset of puberty in the cat varies considerably, depending on several factors. For

CAPUT   CORPUS   CAUDA

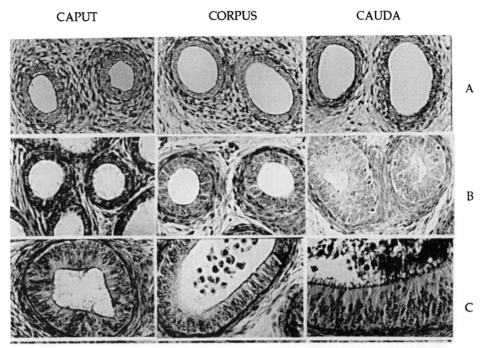

A

B

C

Figure 20–6. Histologic changes of caput (left), corpus (middle), and cauda (right) of epididymis of puppies. (PAS hematoxylin stain; original magnification × 100.) **A**, At birth. **B**, At 16 weeks of age. **C**, At 24 weeks of age. Note the germ cells in the lumen of corpus and cauda epididymis and PAS-positive secretion in the lumen of cauda. (From Kawakami E, Tsutsui T, Ogasa A: Histological observations of the reproductive organs of the male dog from birth to sexual maturity. J Vet Med Sci 53:241, 1991. Reprinted with permission.)

a domestic cat, the first signs of estrus appear between 3.5 and 12 months of age, usually between 5 and 9 months. Environmental factors can affect the onset of puberty. Most female cats born early in the season or exposed when young either to tomcats or cycling females or to increasing amounts of light show the first signs of estrus before similar individuals born later or not exposed to these factors (Beaver, 1992).

Puppies. In puppies, primordial oocytes surrounded by epithelial cells of the follicle are seen at 4 days of age (Raps, 1948). The primary follicle with a layer of granulosa cells appears around 15 days of age (Gilbert and Bosu, 1987). At 2 months, the ovary measures 5 mm in diameter (Fig. 20–7). At 6 months (around the time of puberty), an antrum has formed in many follicles. The germinal epithelium is present at 2 days after birth, and it appears that the cuboidal cells that are part of the germinal epithelium disappear during the first few weeks and start to reappear around 11 weeks of age. Around 17 days after birth, the tunica albuginea develops as a layer of thick collagenous connective tissue below the germinal epithelium. Cortical growth

reaches its maximum during this time. The only recognizable change in the tubular genitalia observed during the first 6 months of life is an increase in size (Pineda et al, 1973).

PREPUBERAL GONADECTOMY

Prepuberal gonadectomy involves the surgical removal of the gonads in sexually immature animals. In the United States, surgical removal of the ovaries and/or uterus or of the testicles of dogs and cats has long been a basis of population control and a part of many routine veterinary health maintenance programs for animals not intended for breeding purposes (Johnston, 1991). Terms used to describe such surgery in females include *oophorectomy* and *ovariectomy* (removal of one or both ovaries) and *ovariohysterectomy, oophorohysterectomy,* and *spaying* (removal of the ovaries and uterus). Terms used to describe such surgery in males include *orchidectomy* and *orchiectomy* (removal of one or both testicles). *Castration* (removal of the gonads) and *gonadectomy* (removal of one or both ovaries or testicles) describe the surgical removal of the gonads of either sex. *Sterilization* refers to procedures

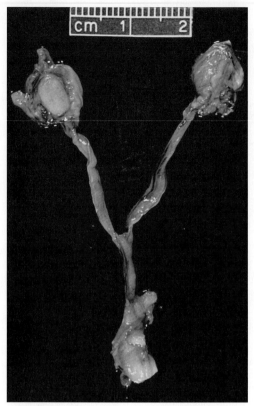

Figure 20–7. Reproductive structures of a 2-month-old female puppy.

by which an animal is made incapable of reproduction, including gonadectomy, vasectomy, and salpingectomy, and it does not necessarily imply complete removal of gonadal tissue. Neutering implies removing or inactivating the gonads of either sex. The term *neuter* also refers to an animal that may have been of either sex before bilateral gonadectomy (Johnston, 1991). The terms *spay* and *neuter* have been widely used (perhaps incorrectly) in describing the ovariohysterectomy procedure in the female (spaying) and the orchidectomy procedure in the male (neutering) (Olson et al, 1991). This discussion uses the terms *neutering* and *castration* to refer to the procedure of removing the gonads of either sex.

Overpopulation of unwanted dogs and cats is a major concern (American Veterinary Medical Association Animal Welfare Forum, 1993). Neutering is still the mainstay weapon in the war against a burgeoning pet population. Neutering of cats and dogs as young as 2 months is now being studied as an alternative to allowing sexually intact animals to leave an animal shelter (Carter, 1990). Although prepuberal neutering

was recommended in the early 1900s (Smithcors, 1957), at the present time most dogs and cats are neutered when they are 5 to 8 months of age (Guard, 1953; Henderson and Dilon, 1985; Knecht and Archibald, 1984; Olson et al, 1986; Stone, 1985). This wait allows the animals to have one estrous cycle. In some instances, females are neutered after they have had a litter. The reason for the selection of this age is not known. The nonavailability in the past of safe anesthetic agents has been suggested as the primary factor for delaying the procedure until around 6 months of age (Lieberman, 1982). Current anesthetic techniques and surgical equipment, however, allow dogs and cats to be neutered as early as 8 to 10 weeks of age with a wide margin of safety. Anesthesia of pediatric patients (Faggella and Aronsohn, 1993; Grandy and Dunlop, 1991; Robinson, 1983) and surgical techniques for neutering 6- to 14-week-old kittens (Aronsohn and Faggella, 1993) have been described. These studies have indicated that the anesthetic and surgical risk in neutering pediatric kittens is minimal, provided that proper precautions and techniques are used. The surgical and anesthetic management of puppies and kittens has been described (Hosgood, 1992).

Possible Disadvantages

Possible disadvantages of neutering include urinary incontinence in females (Joshua, 1965), stunted growth, obesity (Chalifoux et al, 1981; Jagoe and Serpell, 1988), perivulvar dermatitis (Jagoe and Serpell, 1988; Joshua, 1965; Knecht and Archibald, 1984), vaginitis (Knecht and Archibald, 1984; Olson et al, 1986), and behavioral changes (Chalifoux et al, 1981; Stone, 1985). An association between early spaying and urinary incontinence is still questionable. Thrusfield (1985) has suggested that there is a positive association between urinary incontinence and spaying in bitches (34 of 791 spayed and 7 of 2427 entire had urinary incontinence) 6 months of age and older. Complete penile extrusion was not possible at 22 months of age when castration was performed in kittens at 7 weeks of age (Root et al, 1996a). The proximal radial physeal closure was significantly delayed in prepuberally gonadectomized female kittens (Root et al, 1997). One of the most common complaints by owners is that of obesity in neutered bitches. Findings of one survey (Edney and Smith, 1986) suggest that neutered bitches were about twice as likely to be obese as intact females. Further research is needed in this area. It is believed that perivulvar dermatitis may be a direct consequence of retarded development of the external genitalia, which can also be related to obesity; both problems may be associated with early neutering.

Possible Advantages

Many possible advantages of early neutering have been suggested. For example, it has been suggested that the surgical process of early neutering is less stressful for the patient and is followed by quick recovery (Lieberman, 1987). The time required for the surgery is also shorter. Animals that undergo early neutering are believed to be more people-oriented pets; to be calmer, gentler, and less likely to wander; and to retain persistent juvenile behavior (which is seemingly desirable). Health advantages have also been cited. For instance, early neutering reduces the risk of mammary tumors in dogs (Schneider et al, 1969). In one study, more than 100 puppies and kittens were neutered between 8 and 10 weeks of age with no undesirable effects reported in the following 2 years (Lieberman, 1982). Recent work has dispelled an earlier perception that prepuberal gonadectomy results in unfavorable traits in male and female puppies (Salmeri and Bloomberg, 1989). Observation of puppies up to 15 months of age indicated that immaturity of the external genital organs at the time of surgery was not associated with any clinical problems.

Owners of cats neutered at 6 to 12 weeks of age were pleased with their cat's behavior at 4, 10, and 14 years after surgery. Only 3% of the cats were reported to spray urine intermittently (Kellington and Hannawalt, 1985). Prepuberal neutering has resulted in a reduced incidence of mammary neoplasia in dogs (Taylor et al, 1976). Bitches neutered before their first estrous cycle, after one estrous cycle, and after two or more estrous cycles had a mammary cancer risk of 0.5, 0.8%, and 26%, respectively.

Work by Herron (1971) suggested that the preputial separation from the penis is a prerequisite for castration because 4 of 10 cats castrated at 5 months of age had adhesions of the prepuce to the penis. It is believed that testosterone is essential for keratinizing the epithelium, allowing the normal separation of the glans penis from the layer of cells lining the prepuce to form the balanopreputial fold. Early castration of the cat has been shown to cause arrest of the normal development of the balanopreputial fold (Retter and Lellevre, 1913). The association of early castration and preputial adhesions of the penis needs to be evaluated further in cats and dogs.

Additional Comments

Early neutering appears to be a feasible means of reducing unwanted pregnancies; however, further long-term studies in dogs and cats are needed. Although there is no evidence to suggest that the outcome of neutering done at 7 weeks is different from that of neutering done at 7 months of age (Herron, 1972; Reed, 1993; Salmeri et al, 1991a), long-term studies are called for. More important, the effects of early neutering on bone strength, urethral development and function, and immunocompetence require further investigation (Cardwell, 1993; Salmeri et al, 1991b). The pros and cons of early surgical neutering are stirring up heated debates and spurring some studies into the purported side effects (Carter, 1990). It is probably too early to reach a valid conclusion about the merits of early surgical neutering (Jagoe and Serpell, 1988; Lieberman, 1987); however, the concept of early neutering should command concerted attention (Lieberman, 1982) because 10% to 25% of the offspring of U.S. dogs and cats are destroyed annually because they lack owners (Olson et al, 1991). Results of many recent studies seem to support prepuberal gonadectomy. It did not influence mortality or morbidity (Howe, 1997), heat production (Root, et al, 1996b), or physical and behavioral development (Stubb et al, 1996). Inclusion of a prepuberal gonadectomy program in the veterinary curriculum will allow students to understand the pet overpopulation problem and the unique role of the veterinarian in combating this problem (Howe and Slater, 1997).

PUPPY VAGINITIS

Puppies often develop vaginitis before their first estrus. Although juvenile vaginitis is not normal, it usually subsides after the first estrus and may not require treatment. Cases of several weeks' duration, however, may require treatment (Olson, 1980).

Diagnosis

Vaginal culture specimens should be taken from any animal suspected of having vaginitis. This can be done using a sterile culturette or a sterilized cotton-tipped applicator, which is passed through an otoscope cone (Fig. 20–8) or vaginal speculum. A guarded culture system can also be

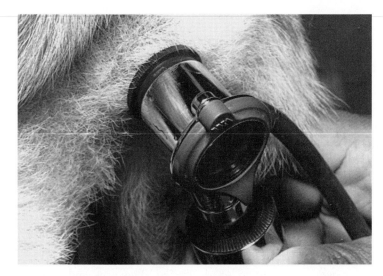

Figure 20–8. Examination of the vagina using an otoscope cone.

used to obtain anterior vaginal culture specimens. Puppies younger than 6 months harbor significantly more coagulase-positive staphylococci than do older animals (Olson, 1976). The types of bacteria found in the prepuberal posterior vaginal swabs are listed in Tables 20–1 and 20–2. Once a potential pathogen is isolated, antimicrobial sensitivity testing should be performed to formulate proper antimicrobial therapy.

Treatment

Conservative medical therapy usually allows vaginal inflammation and discharge to resolve spontaneously at puberty. Conservative therapy includes cleaning the perivulvar area to prevent moist dermatitis. In some cases, a urinary antiseptic such as methenamine mandelate reduces clinical signs (Brown, 1992). Antimicrobial

treatment is based on the sensitivity results obtained by vaginal culture. For puppies with primary bacterial infections, antimicrobial agents may be infused directly into the vagina. Intravaginal infusions of antimicrobial agents may be administered daily in conjunction with systemic antimicrobial therapy.

Prevention

Although the means for dissemination of vaginal bacteria is unknown, animals grouped together seem to harbor similar vaginal bacteria (Olson, 1976). The perineal area of puppies should be kept clean. This is all the more important for puppies with excess hair in the area around the external genitalia and for puppies with poor external genital conformation ("tucked-in vulva"). In the latter condition, there is a good chance for mucus to collect in

Table 20–1	Classification of Vaginal Isolates from 20 Puppies, 1 to 11 Weeks Old		
TYPE OF ISOLATE	NO. OF ISOLATES	PERCENTAGE OF TOTAL ISOLATES	PUPPIES WITH ISOLATE (%)
Escherichia coli	9	18.0	45.0
Coagulase-positive staphylococci	13	26.0	65.0
Coagulase-negative staphylococci	6	12.0	30.0
α-Hemolytic staphylococci	3	6.0	15.0
β-Hemolytic staphylococci	6	12.0	30.0
Nonhemolytic staphylococci	4	8.0	20.0
Proteus	3	6.0	15.0
Bacillus	3	6.0	15.0
Corynebacterium	2	4.0	10.0
Pseudomonas	1	2.0	5.0

From Olson PNS, Mather EC: Canine vaginal and uterine bacterial flora. J Am Vet Med Assoc 172:709, 1978. Used with permission.

Table 20-2	Classification of Vaginal Isolates from 21 Puppies, 12 Weeks to 6 Months Old		
TYPE OF ISOLATE	NO. OF ISOLATES	PERCENTAGE OF TOTAL ISOLATES	PUPPIES WITH ISOLATE (%)
Escherichia coli	8	17.0	38.1
Coagulase-positive staphylococci	14	29.8	66.7
Coagulase-negative staphylococci	5	10.6	23.8
α-Hemolytic staphylococci	4	8.5	19.0
β-Hemolytic staphylococci	3	6.4	14.3
Nonhemolytic staphylococci	2	4.3	9.5
Proteus	1	2.1	4.8
Bacillus	3	6.4	14.3
Corynebacterium	2	4.3	9.5
Micrococcus	3	6.4	14.3
Neisseria	1	2.1	4.8
Klebsiella	1	2.1	4.8

From Olson PNS, Mather EC: Canine vaginal and uterine bacterial flora. J Am Vet Med Assoc 172:709, 1978. Used with permission.

the vagina, which leads to vaginitis. Surgical correction is possible for the poor vulvar conformation. In general, clipping the hair in the perivulvar area and keeping the puppies in clean surroundings will reduce the incidence of puppy vaginitis.

References and Supplemental Reading

NORMAL AND ABNORMAL TESTICULAR DESCENT

Arbeiter K: Zum Maldescensus Testis beim Hund. Tierarztl, Praxis 3:129, 1975.

Arthur GH: A study of some aspects of descent of the testicles and cryptorchidism in domesticated animals. Fellowship thesis. London, Royal College of Veterinary Surgeons, 1956.

Ashdown RR: The diagnosis of cryptorchidism in young dogs: A review of the problem. J Small Anim Pract 4:261, 1963.

Baumans V, Dijkstra G, Wensing CJG: Testicular descent in the dog. Zentralbl Veterinarmed 10:97, 1981.

Bloom F: Testis and epididymis. In Bloom F: Pathology of the Dog and Cat. Evanston, IL, American Veterinary Publications, 1954, p 215.

British Veterinary Medical Association: Cryptorchidism in the dog. Vet Rec 67:472, 1955.

Brodey RS, Martin JE: Sertoli cell neoplasms in the dog: The clinicopathological and endocrinological findings in thirty-seven dogs. J Am Vet Med Assoc 133:49, 1958.

Burke TJ: Descent of testes. Canine Pract 6:16, 1979.

Christiansen J: Parturition and newborn kittens. In Christiansen J: Reproduction in the Dog and Cat. Philadelphia, Bailliere Tindall, 1984, p 287.

Cox VS, Wallace LJ, Jessen CR: An anatomic and genetic study of canine cryptorchidism. Teratology 18:233, 1978.

Donovan EF: Castration of cryptorchid dogs. Mod Vet Pract 44:84, 1963.

Donovan EF: Inheritances of monorchidism. Mod Vet Pract 46:32, 1965.

Dunn ML, Foster WJ, Goddard KM: Cryptorchidism in dogs: A clinical survey. J Am Anim Hosp Assoc 4:180, 1968.

Hullinger RL, Wensing CJG: Descent of the testis in the fetal calf. Acta Anat 121:63, 1985a.

Hullinger RL, Wensing CJG: Testicular organogenesis in the fetal calf: Interstitial endocrine (Leydig) cell development. Acta Anat 121:99, 1985b.

Kunzel E: Zum Kryptorchidismus des Hundes. Zentralbl Veterinarmed 1:782, 1954.

Leipold HW: Nature and causes of congenital defects of dogs. Vet Clin North Am 8:47, 1978.

Meyer P: Palpatorische Befunde zum Descensus: Testis beim Deutsche Kunhaar. Dtsch Tierarztl Wochenschr 79:590, 1977.

Michel G: Embryologie: Kompendium der vet. In Schwarzl E (ed): Kompendium der Veterinaranatomie. Jena, Gustav Fischer, 1968.

Moss LC: Monorchidism in the dog. Mod Vet Pract 43:56, 1962.

Osterhoff DR: Canine cryptorchidism. J S Afr Vet Med Assoc 48:145, 1977.

Pendergrass TW, Hayes HM Jr: Cryptorchism and related defects in dogs: Epidemiologic comparisons with man. Teratology 12:51, 1975.

Rehfeld CE: Cryptorchidism in a large beagle colony. J Am Vet Med Assoc 158:1864, 1971 (abstract).

Reif JS, Brodey RS: The relationship between cryptorchidism and canine testicular neoplasia. J Am Vet Med Assoc 155:2005, 1969.

Rhoades JD, Foley CW: Cryptorchidism and intersexuality. Vet Clin North Am 7:789, 1977.

Schlotthauer CF, Bollman JL: The effect of artificial cryptorchidism on the prostate gland of dogs. Am J Vet Res 3:202, 1942.

Schorner G: Gestorter Descensus Testis beim Ruden und therapeutische. Wien Tierarzt Mon Schr 62:11, 1975.

Scott MG, Scott PP: Post-natal development of the

testicle and epididymis in the cat. Proc Physiol Soc 7:40, 1957.

Sizonenko PC: Cryptorchidism: Introductory remarks. Horm Res 30:137, 1988.

Skoda K: Arch Wiss Prakt Tierheilk 39:328, 1913.

Stickle RL, Fessler JF: Retrospective study of 350 cases of equine cryptorchidism. J Am Vet Med Assoc 172:343, 1978.

Wensing CJG: Testicular descent in some domestic mammals. I. Anatomical aspects of testicular descent. Proc K Ned Akad Wet Ser C Biol Med Sci 71:423, 1968.

Wensing CJG: Descent of the testis. *In* Getty R (ed): Sisson and Grossman's The Anatomy of the Domestic Animals. Philadelphia, WB Saunders, 1975, p 147.

Wensing CJG: The developmental anomalies, including cryptorchidism. *In* Morrow DA (ed): Current Therapy in Theriogenology. Philadelphia, WB Saunders, 1980, p 585.

Wensing CJG: The embryology of testicular descent. Horm Res 30:144, 1988.

Whitney LF: Non-inherited monorchidism in dogs. Vet Med 56:204, 1961.

Wolff A: Castration, cryptorchidism, and cryptorchidectomy in dogs and cats. Vet Med Small Anim Clin 76:1739, 1981.

Zietzschmann O, Krolling O: Lehrbuch der Entwick-lungsgeschichte der Haustiere, 2nd ed. Berlin, P Parey, 1955, p 400.

Abnormalities of Phenotypic Sex

Brown TT, Burek JD, McEntee K: Male pseudohermaphroditism, cryptorchism and Sertoli cell neoplasia in three miniature schnauzers. J Am Vet Med Assoc 169:821, 1976.

George FW: Sexual differentiation. *In* Griffin JE, Ojeda SR (eds): Textbook of Endocrine Physiology. New York, Oxford University Press, 1992, p 118.

Griffin JE, Punyashthiti K, Wilson JD: Dihydrotestosterone binding by cultured human fibroblasts: Comparison of cells from control subjects and from patients with hereditary male pseudohermaphroditism due to androgen resistance. J Clin Invest 57:1342, 1976.

Kaufman M, Straisfeld C, Pinsky L: Male pseudohermaphroditism presumably due to target organ unresponsiveness to androgens: Deficient 5 alpha-dihydrotestosterone binding in cultured skin fibroblasts. J Clin Invest 58:345, 1976.

Madden JD, Walsh PC, MacDonald PC, et al: Clinical and endocrinological characterization of a patient with the syndrome of incomplete testicular feminization. J Clin Endocrinol Metab 41:751, 1975.

Meyers-Wallen VN, Patterson DF: Disorders of sexual development in the dog. *In* Morrow DA (ed): Current Therapy in Theriogenology, 2nd ed. Philadelphia, WB Saunders, 1986, p 567.

Meyers-Wallen VN, Wilson JD, Griffin TE, et al: Testicular feminization in a cat. J Am Vet Med Assoc 195:631, 1989.

Morris JM, Mahesh VB: Further observations on the syndrome "testicular feminization." Am J Obstet Gynecol 87:731, 1963.

Peter AT, Markwelder D, Asem EK: Phenotypic feminization in a genetic male dog caused by nonfunctional androgen receptors. Theriogenology 40:1093, 1993.

Postnatal Development of Gonads

Aronson LR, Cooper ML: Penile spines of the domestic cat: Their endocrine behavior relations. Anat Rec 157:71, 1967.

Beaver BV: Feline Behavior: A Guide for Veterinarians. Philadelphia, WB Saunders, 1992, p 121.

Gilbert RO, Bosu WTK: Clinical reproductive endocrinology of the dog and cat. *In* Drazner FH (ed): Small Animal Endocrinology. New York, Churchill Livingstone, 1987, p 341.

Kawakami E, Tsutsui T, Ogasa A: Histological observations of the reproductive organs of the male dog from birth to sexual maturity. J Vet Med Sci 53:241, 1991.

Pineda MH, Kainer RA, Fulkner LC: Dorsal median post-cervical fold in the canine vagina. Am J Vet Res 34:1487, 1973.

Raps G: The developmental of the dog ovary, from birth to 6 months of age. Am J Vet Res 9:61, 1948.

Scott MG, Scott PP: Post-natal development of the testicle and epididymis in the cat. J Physiol 136:40, 1957.

Prepuberal Gonadectomy

Aronsohn MG, Faggella AM: Surgical techniques for neutering 6- to 14-week-old kittens. J Am Vet Med Assoc 202:53, 1993.

American Veterinary Medical Association Animal Welfare Forum: Overpopulation of unwanted dogs and cats. J Am Vet Med Assoc 202:903, 1993.

Cardwell DL: Pros and cons associated with early-age neutering. J Am Vet Med Assoc 202:1789, 1993 (letter).

Carter CN: Pet population control: Another decade without solutions? J Am Vet Med Assoc 197:192, 1990.

Chalifoux A, Fanjoy P, Niemi G, et al: Early spay-neutering of dogs and cats. Can Vet J 22:381, 1981 (letter).

Edney ATB, Smith PM: Study of obesity in dogs visiting veterinary practices in the United Kingdom. Vet Rec 118:391, 1986.

Faggella AM, Aronsohn MG: Anesthetic techniques for neutering 6- to 14-week-old kittens. J Am Vet Med Assoc 202:56, 1993.

Grandy JL, Dunlop CI: Anesthesia of pups and kittens. J Am Vet Med Assoc 198:1244, 1991.

Guard WF: Surgical Principles and Techniques. Columbus, OH, WF Guard, 1953, p 175.

Henderson RA, Dilon AR: The male genital system. *In* Gouley IM, Vasseur PB (eds): General Small Animal Surgery. Philadelphia, JB Lippincott, 1985, p 673.

Herron MA: A potential consequence of prepuberal feline castration. Feline Pract 1:17, 1971.

Herron MA: The effect of prepuberal castration on the penile urethra of the cat. J Am Vet Med Assoc 160:208, 1972.

Hosgood G: Surgical and anesthetic management of puppies and kittens. Compend Contin Educ Pract Vet 14:345, 1992.

Howe LM: Short-term results and complications of prepuberal gonadectomy in cats and dogs. J Am Vet Med Assoc 211:57, 1997.

Howe LM, Slater MR: Student assessment of the educational benefits of a prepuberal gonadectomy program (preliminary findings). J Vet Med Educ 24:12, 1997.

Jackson EKM: Contraception in the dog and cat. Br Vet 1140:132, 1984.

Jagoe JA, Serpell JA: Optimum time for neutering. Vet Rec 122:447, 1988 (letter).

Johnston SD: Questions and answers on the effects of surgically neutering dogs and cats. J Am Vet Med Assoc 198:1206, 1991.

Joshua JO: The spaying of bitches. Vet Rec 77:642, 1965.

Kellington E, Hannawalt EH: Study of the Effects of Early Spaying and Neutering. Medford, OR, SPCA Report, May 1985.

Knecht C, Archibald J: Female genital system. In Archibald J, Catcott EJ (eds): Canine and Feline Surgery. Santa Barbara, CA, American Veterinary Publications, 1984, p 249.

Lieberman LL: Advantages of early spaying and neutering. J Am Vet Med Assoc 181:42, 1982.

Lieberman LL: A case for neutering pups and kittens at two months of age. J Am Vet Med Assoc 191:518, 1987.

Lieberman LL: The optimum time for neutering surgery of dogs and cats. Vet Rec 122:369, 1988 (letter).

Madewell BR, Theilen GH: Tumors of the mammary gland. In Theilen GH, Madewell BR (eds): Veterinary Cancer Medicine. Philadelphia, Lea & Febiger, 1987, p 328.

Olson PN, Moulton C, Nett TM, et al: Pet overpopulation: A challenge for companion animal veterinarians in the 1990s. J Am Vet Med Assoc 198:1151, 1991.

Olson PN, Nett TM, Bowen RA, et al: A need for sterilization, contraceptives, and abortifacients: Abandoned and unwanted pets. I. Current methods of sterilizing pets. Compend Contin Educ Pract Vet 8:87, 1986.

Reed L: Pros and cons associated with early neutering. J Am Vet Med Assoc 202:1789, 1993 (letter).

Retter E, Lellevre A: Influence de la castration sur l'evolution et les transformations cellulaires. Cpt Rd Seances Soc Biol 74:1403, 1913.

Robinson EP: Anesthesia of pediatric patients. Compend Contin Educ Pract Vet 5:1004, 1983.

Root MV, Johnston SD, Johnston GR, et al: The effect of prepuberal and postpuberal gonadectomy on penile extrusion and urethral diameter in the domestic cats. Vet Radiol Ultrasound 140:279, 1996a.

Root MV, Johnston SD, Olson PN: Effect of prepuberal and postpuberal gonadectomy on heat production measured by indirect calorimetry in male and female domestic cats. Am J Vet Res 27:37, 1996b.

Root MV, Johnston SD, Olson PN: The effect of prepuberal and postpuberal gonadectomy on radial physeal closure in male and female domestic cats. Vet Radiol Ultrasound 38:42, 1997.

Salmeri KR, Olson PN, Bloomberg MS: Elective gonadectomy in dogs: A review. J Am Vet Med Assoc 198:1183, 1991a.

Salmeri KR, Bloomberg MS: Prepubertal gonadectomy in the dog: Effects on skeletal growth and physical development. Vet Surg 18:61, 1989 (abstract).

Salmeri KR, Bloomberg MS, Scruggs SL, et al: Gonadectomy in immature dogs: Effects on skeletal, physical, and behavioral development. J Am Vet Med Assoc 198:1193, 1991b.

Schneider R, Dorn CR, Taylor D: Factors influencing canine mammary cancer development and postsurgical survival. J Natl Cancer Inst 43:1249, 1969.

Smithcors JF: Evolution of the Veterinary Art. Kansas City, MO, Veterinary Medicine Publishing, 1957, p 54.

Stone EA: The uterus. In Slatter DH (ed): Small Animal Surgery. Philadelphia, WB Saunders, 1985, p 1661.

Stubb WP, Bloomberg MS, Scruggs et al: Effects of prepuberal gonadectomy on physical and behavioral development in cats. J Am Vet Med Assoc 209:1864, 1996.

Taylor GN, Shabestari L, Williams J, et al: Mammary neoplasia in a closed beagle colony. Cancer Res 36:2740, 1976.

Theran P: Early-age neutering of dogs and cats. J Am Vet Med Assoc 202:914, 1993.

Thrusfield MV: Association between urinary incontinence and spaying in bitches. Vet Rec 116:695, 1985.

Puppy Vaginitis

Brown SA: Urogenital disorders. In Lorenz SID, Cornelius LM, Ferguson DC (eds): Small Animal Medicine Therapeutics. Philadelphia, JB Lippincott, 1992, p 313.

Olson PNS: Canine Vaginal Flora. Master's thesis. University of Minnesota, St. Paul, 1976.

Olson PNS: Canine vaginitis. In Kirk RW (ed): Current Veterinary Therapy VII. Philadelphia, WB Saunders, 1980, p 1219.

Olson PNS, Mather EC: Canine vaginal and uterine bacterial flora. J Am Vet Med Assoc 172:708, 1978.

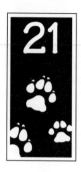

21

Nutrition and Nutritional Problems

Johnny D. Hoskins

THE GROWING PUPPY AND KITTEN

Nutritional requirements, feeding, and health care of puppies and kittens from birth to 6 months of age are substantially different during their growth stages. Growth is a demanding time in a puppy's or kitten's life, involving heredity, hormonal regulation, health concerns, and solid nutrition. Puppies and kittens will fail to grow to the size determined by their hereditary factors unless they consume sufficient food of adequate quality. If poor-quality, unbalanced, commercially prepared diets or homemade diets of single food items or indiscriminate mixtures of single food items are fed to the animals during their growth periods, nutrition-related disorders often occur. Additionally, supplementation of poor or questionable diets with specific nutrients such as cysteine, fatty acids, calcium, phosphorus, vitamin A, vitamin D, or organ tissues may create dietary imbalances that could lead to a number of nutritional disorders, especially during the demanding period of growth. Proper nutrition, therefore, equals good health and performance of puppies and kittens from birth to 6 months of age.

FEEDING THE PUPPY

During the first 2 to 3 weeks of their lives, healthy puppies should only eat and sleep. Nursing should be vigorous and active, with each puppy receiving sufficient milk from its mother. If the mother is healthy and well nourished, the puppy's nutritional needs for its first 3 to 4 weeks of life should be provided completely by her. Signs that the puppy is not receiving sufficient milk are the puppy's constant crying, extreme inactivity, and failure to gain sufficient weight. A puppy should demonstrate at least a 10% weight gain per day.

The transition from mother's milk to a growth diet should be a gradual process, beginning at about 3 weeks of age (4 weeks of age for toy and miniature breeds); however, if necessary, supplemental feeding may be started as soon as the puppy fails to show sufficient weight gain (Sheffy, 1978). During the transition to the growth diet, the puppy can be offered a mixture of a good-quality puppy food designed for growth and water as a thick gruel (a mixture of one part dry food blended with three parts water or two parts canned food blended with one part water). To get the puppy eating, the gruel is placed in a shallow food dish or force-fed with a commercial dosing syringe. The puppy is encouraged to lap the gruel by touching its lips to the food, or the feeder can put a finger into the gruel and then into the puppy's mouth. Once the puppy is eating the gruel well, the amount of water in the gruel should be gradually reduced until the water is omitted.

By 6 weeks of age, the puppy should be getting at least 25% of its requirements from the weaning diet. The puppy may be permanently separated from its mother as soon as it learns to eat readily and drink satisfactorily. Most puppies are completely weaned at 7 to 8 weeks of age, depending somewhat on the dog's size and breed. Early weaning and separation from littermates before 6 weeks of age can, however, cause malnutrition or numerous behavioral problems later in life. Because of this, complete weaning should not be attempted until puppies are at least 6 weeks old and close human contact has been established.

The primary challenges of feeding growing puppies are providing adequate energy and essential nutrients and avoiding a too rapid growth rate. An appropriate growth food provides adequate nutrients and energy in a volume that can be easily consumed by the puppy. Supplementation with meat, table scraps, or other items is not recommended, because it is likely to create a finicky eater, nutritional deficiencies or excesses, or both. Because the puppy's eating habits are still in the developmental stage, it is important that a good-quality growth-formulated puppy food be fed daily at regular intervals and that fresh water in a clean bowl be available at all times.

Feeding the weaned puppy should always be directed to attaining the moderate growth rate for the breed (Hedhammar, 1980; Lewis et al, 1987). The feeding chart in Table 21–1 is a convenient guide for determining the amount of food to feed daily to puppies for average growth rate, according to size and age (Lewis et al, 1987; Sheffy, 1978). Instead of making food available to the puppy at all times (free-choice feeding), time-limited meal feeding is recommended. At each feeding, the puppy should be given 15 to 20 minutes to eat all that it wants, and the remaining food should then be removed. From the time of weaning to 4 to 6 months of age (9 months for giant breeds), puppies are best fed at least three times a day at regular intervals. Thereafter, puppies should be fed twice a day on a regular schedule.

FEEDING THE LARGE AND GIANT BREED PUPPY

Some large and giant breeds of dogs (those weighing over 30 kg at maturity) have the genetic capacity to grow rapidly and will do so if provided with a food that meets or exceeds their nutrient and energy needs. A too rapid growth rate is not compatible with normal skeletal

Table 21–1	Recommended Daily Caloric Requirements for Maintenance of Average Growing Puppies of Different Body Weights and Ages		
BODY WEIGHT		**DAILY KILOCALORIE REQUIREMENTS***	
Kilograms	Pounds	Weaning to 3 Mo†	3–6 Mo‡
1	2.2	268	214
2	4.4	464	373
3	6.6	649	520
4	8.8	808	646
5	11.0	915	732
7	15.4	1167	934
9	19.8	1394	1115
11	24.3	1670	1336
13	28.7	1929	1543
15	33.1	2179	1743
17	37.5	2415	1932
19	41.9	2640	2112
21	46.3	2856	2285
23	50.7	3062	2450
25	55.1		2618
27	59.5		2785
29	63.9		2945
31	68.3		3104
33	72.8		3250
35	77.2		3422
37	81.6		3551

*These values only approximate the daily energy needs. The reduction in kilocalories required per unit of body weight occurs gradually as the puppy approaches maturity. Requirements vary with environmental conditions, activity, and temperament. The amount fed should be adjusted to maintain optimal body weight and condition. This may require substantially more or less food than the amount indicated.

†Values represent two times the maintenance energy requirement of the adult per unit of body weight.

‡Values represent 1.6 times the maintenance energy requirement of the adult per unit of body weight.

growth, however, and may result in certain types of developmental bone diseases.

Several studies have shown that diet and feeding management have an important influence on the development of osteochondrosis and hypertrophic osteodystrophy in large and giant breeds of dogs (Brawner et al, 1996; Goodman et al, 1997). Puppies fed a diet with a reduced-fat content for lower caloric intake and medium levels of calcium and phosphorus (0.8% and 0.67% as fed, respectively) grew at a satisfactory rate. After 4 months of age, these puppies were larger and had appropriate skeletal development.

Beginning at weaning and continuing until they reach maturity, large and giant breeds of dogs should be fed for a moderate growth rate. This can be accomplished by limiting food intake or by feeding a growth-formulated puppy food for large and giant breeds. If osteochondrosis or hypertrophic osteodystrophy occurs, nutritional management should be to reduce caloric intake by reducing the amount of food that is fed or feeding a growth-formulated puppy food for large and giant breeds.

FEEDING THE KITTEN

Love, care, and attention are important factors in raising well-adjusted kittens, but a quality diet is the most essential factor in the kitten's physical development. During their first 4 weeks of life, healthy kittens should nurse vigorously and actively. If the mother is healthy and well nourished, the nutritional needs of the kittens for the first 4 weeks of life should be filled completely by her. Each kitten should receive sufficient milk from its mother. Kittens not receiving sufficient milk cry constantly, are restless or extremely inactive, and fail to achieve the expected weight gain of 10 to 15 g/d.

Kittens should be encouraged to begin eating solid food at 4 weeks of age. At this time, the kitten can be offered a mixture of a good-quality kitten food designed for growth and milk or water as a thick gruel (a mixture of one part dry food blended with three parts milk or two parts canned food blended with one part milk). The gruel is fed to kittens from a shallow bowl or force-fed with a commercial dosing syringe. The feeder can encourage the kitten to eat the gruel by smearing some of the gruel on the kitten's lips, being careful not to get any in the nose, or can place a finger in the gruel and then into the kitten's mouth. This usually encourages the kitten to eat and leads to eating the solid food from a bowl at an early age. Once the kitten is eating the gruel well, the amount of milk or water in the gruel should be gradually reduced until the kitten is consuming only solid food. The kitten may be permanently separated from the mother as soon as it learns to eat readily and drink satisfactorily. Most kittens are completely weaned at 6 to 8 weeks of age. Early weaning and separation from littermates before 6 weeks of age can result in behavioral problems such as slowness to learn and more suspicious, cautious, and aggressive actions (Hart, 1972).

The food that is given the weaned kitten should be one specifically formulated for growth. Feeding between 3 to 3.5 oz of dry food per day or 8 to 10 oz of canned food per day usually meets the growth requirements of most kittens. Any supplementation with meat, table scraps, or other items is not recommended, because it will create dietary imbalances, finicky eaters, or nutritional deficiencies or excesses. Because the kitten's eating habits are still in the formative stage after weaning, it remains important that easily digested, high-quality, caloric-dense food be provided daily and that fresh water in a clean bowl be available at all times. Cow's or goat's milk is often fed to kittens after weaning and is a good food provided that it does not cause diarrhea. Milk should never be given in place of fresh water.

Kittens should be fed all the food that they are willing to consume. The average amount of food needed during growth is presented in Table 21–2 (Lewis et al, 1987). Excessive caloric intake and an excessively rapid growth rate are seldom problems of growing kittens. Most kittens are nonvoracious noninhibited eaters that nibble at food frequently when it is always available. Kittens fed unlimited amounts of food (free-choice feeding), regardless of its form (dry or canned), eat every few hours. Free-choice feeding or at least three times per day is preferred during a kitten's growth period.

At 12 weeks of age, the kitten's energy needs are three times greater than those of an adult cat, or more than 840 kJ/kg of body weight. As kittens mature past 6 months of age, their growth rate slows and their food needs decrease. Their energy needs are still greater than those of adult cats, or approximately 378 kJ/kg of body weight.

Male kittens tend to grow more rapidly and for a longer time than female kittens. A female kitten's growth rate slows down at 7 months, but she continues to grow through her ninth month. A male kitten's growth slows down at 9 months, but he continues to grow through his twelfth month.

| Table 21–2 | Recommended Daily Caloric Requirements for Maintenance of Average Growing Kittens of Different Body Weights and Ages | | | |

| BODY WEIGHT | | DAILY KILOCALORIE REQUIREMENTS* | |
Kilograms	Pounds	Weaning to 3 Mo†	3–6 Mo‡
0.5	1.1	125	65
0.75	1.6	188	98
1.0	2.2	250	130
1.5	3.3	375	195
2.0	4.4	500	260
3.0	6.6		390
4.0	8.8		520
5.0	11.0		650

*These values only approximate the daily energy needs. Requirements vary with environmental conditions, activity, and temperament. The amount fed should be adjusted to maintain optimal body weight and condition. This may require substantially more or less food than the amount indicated.

†Values represent 250 kilocalories per kg of body weight per day for kittens from weaning to 3 months of age.

‡Values represent 130 kilocalories per kg of body weight per day for kittens from 3 to 6 months of age.

RAISING PUPPIES AND KITTENS

Successful raising of puppies and kittens requires providing them with a suitable environment; the correct quantity and quality of nutrients for growth; a regular schedule of feeding, sleeping, grooming, and exercise; and the stimulus that provokes micturition and defecation (Sheffy, 1978).

Newborn puppies and kittens are unable to effectively control their body temperature (Bjorck, 1982). During their first 4 weeks of life, they gradually change from being largely poikilothermic to being homeothermic. For the first week of life, their body temperature is directly related to the environmental temperature, and a steady ambient temperature of 30° to 32° C (86° to 90° F) is needed. Over the next 3 weeks, the ambient temperature can be gradually lowered to 24° C (75° F). Humidity should be maintained at 55% to 60%. It is equally important that sudden changes in environmental conditions be avoided and that disturbances be minimized outside of socialization, exercise, and hygiene activities.

Feeding puppies and kittens that still require mother's milk can be rewarding. The most obvious alternative to a mother raising her own young is for another nursing mother to act as a foster mother. Although this is a more satisfactory arrangement than trying to raise orphaned puppies and kittens by hand, the chances of having access to a foster mother at the right stage of lactation and with sufficient resources to raise a litter are poor.

If a foster mother is not available, it is necessary to feed the puppies or kittens a replacement food that is a prototype of a nutritive substance formulated to meet the optimum requirements of the puppy or kitten. Mother's milk is the preferred food. Several homemade or commercially prepared milk replacers for raising puppies and kittens are listed in Table 21–3. Commercially prepared milk replacers are best because they more closely compare with mother's milk (Baines, 1981; Bjorck, 1982; Remillard et al, 1993). These milk replacers generally provide 4.2 to 5.2 kJ of metabolizable energy per milliliter of milk replacer. The caloric need for most puppies and kittens of nursing age is 92.4 to 109.2 kJ per 100 g of body weight. These amounts of milk replacer should be given in equal portions three or four times daily. For the pies and kittens are listed in Table 21–3. Comwarmed before each feeding to about 37.8° C (100° F) or to a temperature near the animal's body temperature.

After each feeding, the abdomen should be enlarged but not overdistended. When a milk replacer is used, less than the prescribed amount should be given per feeding for the first feedings. The amount is then gradually increased to the recommended feeding level by the second or third day. The amount of milk replacer is increased accordingly as the puppy or kitten gains weight and a favorable response to feeding occurs. Puppies should gain 2 to 4 g/kg per day (1 to 2 g/lb per day) of their anticipated adult weight for the first 5 months of their lives (Lewis et al, 1987). Kittens should weigh at birth 80 to 140 g (most weighing around 100

Table 21-3 Milk Replacers for Nursing Puppies and Kittens

Commercial prepared formula for puppies or kittens
  Begin Milk Replacer for Puppies (Performer
    Brand, St. Joseph, MO)
  Begin Milk Replacer for Kittens (Performer
    Brand)
  Esbilac Powder for Puppies (Pet-Ag Inc, Elgin,
    IL)
  Esbilac Liquid for Puppies (Pet-Ag Inc)
  GME Powder for Puppies (a goat's milk formula;
    Pet-Ag Inc)
  Kitten Milk Replacer Formula (Eukanuba, The
    Iams Co., Dayton, OH)
  Kittylac Powder for Kittens (Landco Corp, Post
    Falls, ID)
  KMR Liquid for Kittens (Pet-Ag Inc)
  KMR Powder for Kittens (Pet-Ag Inc)
  Multi-Milk for Multi-Animals (milk replacer for
    animals with lactose intolerance; Pet-Ag Inc)
  Nurturall Liquid for Puppies (Veterinary
    Products Laboratories, Phoenix, AZ)
  Nurturall Powder for Puppies (Veterinary
    Products Laboratories)
  Nurturall Liquid for Kittens (Veterinary Products
    Laboratories)
  Nurturall Powder for Kittens (Veterinary
    Products Laboratories)
  Puppylac Powder for Kittens (Landco Corp)
  Puppy Milk Replacer Formula (Eukanuba, The
    Iams Co.)
  Veta-Lac Powder for Puppies (Vet-A-Mix,
    Shenandoah, IA)
  Veta-Lac Powder for Kittens (Vet-A-Mix)

Homemade prepared formula for puppies
  120 ml of cow's or goat's milk
  120 ml of water
  2–4 egg yolks
  1–2 tsp vegetable oil
  1000 mg calcium carbonate

Homemade prepared formula for kittens
  90 ml of condensed milk
  90 ml of water
  120 ml of plain yogurt (not low fat)
  3 large or 4 small egg yolks

to 120 g) and gain 50 to 100 g weekly (Lewis et al, 1987).

The milk replacer should always be prepared according to the manufacturer's directions, and all feeding equipment should be kept scrupulously clean. A good way of handling prepared milk replacer is to prepare only a 48-hour supply at a time and divide this into the portions required for each feeding. Once milk replacer is prepared, it is best stored in the refrigerator at 4° C.

The easiest and safest way of feeding prepared milk replacer to puppies and kittens of nursing age is by nipple bottle, dosing syringe, or tube (Lewis et al, 1987; Sheffy, 1978). Nipple bottles made especially for feeding orphaned puppies or kittens or bottles equipped with premature infant nipples are preferred. When a nipple bottle is used, the bottle should be held so that the puppy or kitten does not ingest air. The hole in the nipple should be such that when the bottle is inverted, milk slowly oozes from the nipple. It may be necessary to enlarge the nipple hole with a hot needle to get milk to ooze from the inverted bottle. A drop of milk should be squeezed onto the tip of the nipple, and the nipple should then be inserted into the puppy's or kitten's mouth. The milk should never be squeezed out of the bottle while the nipple is in the animal's mouth; doing so may result in laryngotracheal aspiration of the milk into the lungs. In addition, prepared milk replacer should never be fed to a puppy or kitten that is chilled or that does not have a strong sucking reflex. Only when the sucking reflex is present should nipple bottle feeding be attempted.

Tube feeding is the fastest way to feed orphaned puppies or kittens. Most owners can do it easily with a little training. A number 5 French infant feeding tube may be used for puppies or kittens weighing less than 300 g, and a number 8 to 10 French infant feeding tube may be used for puppies or kittens weighing over 300 g. Once weekly, the feeding tube should be marked clearly to indicate the depth of insertion to ensure gastric delivery. The distance from the last rib to the tip of the nose can be measured and marked off on the feeding tube as a guide. The tube should be placed into the stomach and not the distal esophagus for feeding. When feeding, a syringe should be filled with warm prepared milk replacer and fitted to the feeding tube, and any air in the tube or syringe expelled. The animal's mouth should be opened slightly; with the animal's head held in the normal nursing position, the feeding tube should be gently passed to the marked area. If an obstruction is felt or coughing occurs before the mark is reached, the tube is in the trachea. If this does not happen, the prepared milk replacer should be slowly administered over a 2-minute period to allow sufficient time for slow filling of the stomach. Regurgitation of milk replacer rarely occurs; if it does, the feeding tube should be withdrawn and feeding should be interrupted until the next scheduled meal.

During the first 3 weeks of life, a vital aspect of caring for puppies and kittens of nursing age is to simulate, after feeding, the mother's tongue action on the anogenital area, which provokes reflex micturition and defecation. Application of this stimulus has to be taken over by the person tending the puppies or kittens. The necessary result can be achieved by swabbing the anogenital area with dry or moistened cotton or with soft tissue paper to manually stimulate the elimination reflex. It is sometimes possible to effect the same response simply by running a forefinger along the abdominal wall. This stimulation should be regularly provided after each feeding. After they reach about 3 weeks of age, puppies and kittens are usually able to relieve themselves without simulated stimulation.

Most puppies and kittens benefit from gentle handling before feeding to allow for some exercise and to promote muscular and circulatory development. In addition, at least once a week, the person tending the nursing puppy or kitten should wash the animal gently with a soft moistened cloth for general cleansing of the skin, simulating the cleansing licks of the mother's tongue.

As mentioned before, the puppy or kitten should be encouraged to begin eating solid food at 3 to 4 weeks of age. Once the puppy or kitten is eating satisfactorily from a bowl, the amount of prepared milk replacer being given should be gradually reduced until only the puppy or kitten food designed for growth is being fed at least three times a day.

NUTRITIONAL PROBLEMS OF THE GROWING PUPPY AND KITTEN

Malnutrition

Malnutrition is especially common during the time when puppies and kittens depend entirely on the mother for their nutritional needs. The nursing puppy and kitten have similar nutritional requirements, and their survival depends on their mother's ability to care for them; their ability to digest, absorb, and utilize nutrients; and the gradually increasing plane of nutrition provided.

Several factors can contribute to malnutrition in the nursing puppy or kitten (Baines, 1981; Bjorck, 1982). The puppy or kitten may ingest insufficient milk because the mother dies or disowns her young, because the mother cannot adequately care for a large litter, or because of partial or complete lactation failure by the mother due to illness, mastitis, metritis, or underdeveloped mammae. In addition, the puppy or kitten may be born prematurely or underdeveloped; it may be so weak and sick that it cannot suckle normally, or it may have congenital defects that preclude sufficient milk intake. Failure to provide an appropriate growth-formulated diet at 3 to 4 weeks of age and older can result in nutrient intake inadequate to meet the needs of growth.

Immediate recognition of a malnourished puppy or kitten is usually based on its smaller and lighter appearance, its feeble attempts to feed, or its inability to attain adequate weight gain for its age. High-pitched constant crying or inactivity accompanied by a weak sucking reflex is an advanced indication that the nursing puppy or kitten is receiving insufficient milk. Reduced body tone and muscle strength may be evident on handling. Coexisting congenital defects that are not immediately life threatening may be detected on physical examination also.

The treatment of malnutrition in the nursing puppy and kitten generally requires that proper nourishment be provided (Baines, 1981). Complications that are frequently encountered during the management of malnutrition are diarrhea, dehydration, hypoglycemia, and hypothermia (Mosier, 1977). If diarrhea occurs during feeding of adequate amounts of properly prepared commercial milk replacer, the amount of solid intake should be reduced immediately by half. This can be done by diluting the milk replacer to a 4:1 ratio with water or preferably with a mixture of equal parts of multiple electrolyte solution and 5% dextrose in water solution. As the condition of feces improves, the amount of solids should be gradually increased to the recommended level.

Hypoglycemia and dehydration occur quickly when a malnourished puppy or kitten is not fed adequately. To help alleviate dehydration and mild hypoglycemia, an equal mixture of warm multiple electrolyte solution and 5% dextrose in water solution should be administered parenterally until the puppy or kitten responds. No type of milk replacer should be given to a weak and severely chilled puppy or kitten that displays a diminished sucking reflex or a rectal temperature below 35° C (95° F).

It is important to maintain the rectal body temperature above 35° C (95° F). Warming of the puppy or kitten should be done slowly over a period of 1 to 3 hours, depending on the degree of chilling. Until the rectal temperature is about 100° F, only warmed fluid solutions should be given. Once the rectal temperature is about 100° F, warmed milk replacer may be substituted for the mixed fluid solution.

Nutritional Secondary Hyperparathyroidism

Nutritional secondary hyperparathyroidism is a common skeletal disorder that occurs as a result of the disturbance in mineral homeostasis induced by nutritional imbalances. The disorder occurs most frequently in the puppy or kitten during growth and is caused primarily by diets composed exclusively of meat or organ tissues, which are inherently deficient in calcium and/or contain a much greater amount of phosphorus than calcium (Bray, 1984; Capen and Martin, 1983). As a result, a transient decrease in serum calcium concentration occurs.

In response to the dietary calcium deficiency, the parathyroid glands enlarge and release increased amounts of parathormone (Crager and Nachreiner, 1993). The elevated levels of parathormone promote the acceleration of osteoclastic resorption of bone with release of calcium that increases the blood calcium levels to the low normal range. In addition, parathormone prevents the mineralization of osteoid formed by the osteoblasts, diminishes renal tubular resorption of phosphate, and increases tubular resorption of calcium. Continued ingestion of a calcium-deficient diet sustains the state of compensatory hyperparathyroidism, leading to progressive development of the bone disorder.

Puppies and kittens younger than 6 months of age are more susceptible to nutritional secondary hyperparathyroidism and develop severe skeletal lesions (Capen and Martin, 1983). Kittens fed exclusively a meat or organ tissue diet, such as beef heart or liver, develop abnormal locomotion within 4 weeks (Fig. 21–1). Signs include inability or reluctance to stand and walk, localized lameness, and uncoordinated gait due to weak bones and laxity of ligaments. The skeletal problem becomes progressively more severe after 5 to 14 weeks. Kittens become quiet and reluctant to play. They assume a sitting position or are in sternal recumbency, with the hind legs abducted at the pelvis. Any activity may create a weight-bearing lameness as a result of incomplete or folding pathologic fractures of one or more bones. Collapsed vertebral fractures with compression of the spinal cord and paralysis are common in advanced cases. Constipation due to collapsed, narrow pelvis occurs.

Lameness is more likely the identifying problem in growing puppies and may vary from a slight weight-bearing limp to complete inability to walk. Affected puppies may have enlargement and thickening of the ends of long bones, particularly of the distal radius and ulna (Fig. 21–2). The bones are painful on palpation, and pathologic fractures of long bones and vertebrae frequently occur.

The radiographic signs of nutritional secondary hyperparathyroidism generally vary with the severity of the skeletal disorder (Capen and Martin, 1983). There is usually evidence of generalized skeletal demineralization as indicated by the extremely poor bone density, often with very little difference between skeletal and soft tissue. The cortex of long bones is greatly thinned, and the medullary cavity is widened. Epiphyses of the long bones may be wide and appear moth-eaten (Fig. 21–3). Multiple fractures that may take the form of compression, folding, or complete fractures are evident. Other radiographic signs include lamellation of the bony cortices, loss of lamina dura dentes of the alveolar sockets, and bowing deformities of the long bones.

The serum calcium and phosphorus concentrations of affected puppies or kittens are usually in the low normal range for their age, but the serum alkaline phosphatase activity is increased. Serum immunoreactive parathormone concentrations are increased, often to greater than 1000 μEq/ml, or 2000 ng/L (normal value is 43 to 213 μEq/ml, or less than 900 ng/L) (Feldman and Krutzik, 1981).

The primary treatment of nutritional secondary hyperparathyroidism is to feed exclusively a nutritionally balanced, commercially prepared growth diet. Calcium and vitamin D supplementation are to be avoided. Supportive nursing care is provided to prevent ensuing complications such as decubitus ulcers, constipation, and additional fractures. The affected puppy or kitten should be closely confined for 4 to 8 weeks or until the mineralization of the skeleton has improved. Fractures should be supported or repaired until calluses become radiodense and the general mineral density and cortical bone thickness approach the norm. When the appropriate growth diet is being provided, these improvements of the skeleton can be easily monitored with serial survey radiographs. The healed pelvic fractures may lead to subsequent health problems such as gait abnormality, dystocia, and obstipation. Neurologic damage from vertebral fractures may leave the puppy or kitten with permanent neurologic deficits. With adequate nutrition and time for bone repair, however, the affected puppy's or

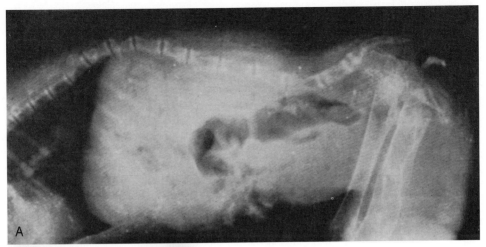

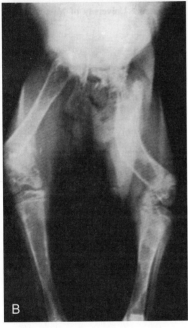

Figure 21–1. Nutritional secondary hyperparathyroidism. **A**, Extreme calcium depletion in a kitten manifested by radiolucent vertebrae, pelvis, and femurs. **B**, Note the thin cortices, decreased mineralization, and folding fractures of the femurs. (From O'Donnell JA, Hayes KC: Nutrition and nutritional disorders. *In* Holzworth J [ed]: Diseases of the Cat: Medicine and Surgery, vol 1. Philadelphia, WB Saunders, 1987, p 34.)

kitten's skeleton can, in most situations, recover to a nearly normal state (Krook et al, 1971).

Hypervitaminosis D

Vitamin D, or its most active metabolite 1,25-dihydroxyvitamin D_3, is one of several factors necessary for calcium homeostasis. Excessive long-term ingestion of vitamin D or any of its active metabolites can be fatal. In puppies and kittens, sources of excessive vitamin D are usually inappropriate dietary supplementation or the ingestion of day-blooming jessamine *(Cestrum diurnum)*, a house plant, or vitamin D–containing rodenticide.

Hypervitaminosis D produces hypercalcemia and hyperphosphatemia. Metastatic calcification of soft tissues occurs when the numerical product of the serum calcium and phosphorus levels exceeds 70. The signs in puppies and kittens are caused by hypercalcemia and, in advanced cases, the uremia caused by hypercalcemic nephropathy (Howerth, 1983; Spangler et al, 1979). Signs include vomiting, diarrhea, limb stiffness, failure to gain weight, rapid respiration, muscular weakness, anorexia, polyuria, and polydipsia. In addition to the hypercalcemia and hyperphosphatemia, low levels of serum alkaline phosphatase activity, isosthenuria, azotemia, and glucosuria are usually present.

The diagnosis of hypervitaminosis D is usually based on the dietary history of excessive

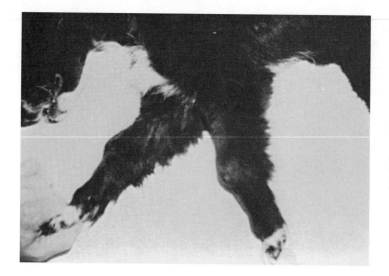

Figure 21–2. Nutritional secondary hyperparathyroidism. Note the enlargement and thickening of the distal radius and ulna in a growing puppy. (Courtesy of Dr. C. B. Chastain, University of Missouri, Columbia.)

ingestion of vitamin D or its various active forms, along with physical findings and hypercalcemia. Serum 25-hydroxyvitamin D_3 and 1,25-dihydroxyvitamin D_3 can also be assayed commercially. Treatment of hypervitaminosis D requires removal of the excess source of the vitamin. Because vitamin D is stored in the liver, complete removal of vitamin D from the diet may be required until the amount in the liver is reduced. Diuresis with sterile saline solution and furosemide aids in producing calciuria (Kruger et al, 1986). The prognosis is guarded, and the resolution of soft tissue calcification will be slow and probably incomplete.

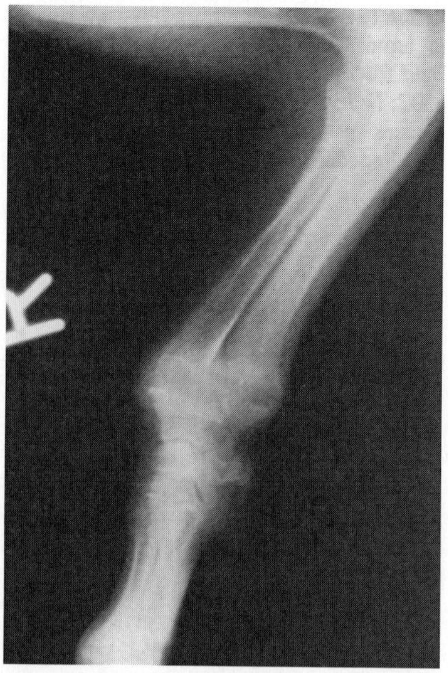

Secondary Hypercalcitoninism of Dietary Origin

Factors that promote increased serum calcium concentration indirectly stimulate calcitonin secretion. Calcitonin is a polypeptide hormone produced by the thyroid gland's parafollicular cells to decrease serum calcium and phosphorus levels. It also inhibits osteoclastic resorption of bone and decreases renal hydroxylation of vitamin D. Calcitonin inhibits renal resorption of calcium and phosphorus. Its physiologic role serves as a protective mechanism to prevent hypercalcemia after the excessive ingestion of calcium.

In puppies fed excessive dietary calcium, parafollicular cell hyperplasia occurs (Hedhammar et al, 1974). Although above-normal serum levels of calcitonin have not been unequivocally demonstrated, decreased numbers of osteoclasts and impaired remodeling of bones suggest hypercalcitoninism. Excessive dietary magnesium could cause similar effects.

Articular and physeal cartilaginous changes associated with secondary hypercalcitoninism include irregularities of retained cartilage cores with disturbances in endochondral ossification (Hedhammar et al, 1974). Induced osseous lesions result from retarded maturation and remodeling of trabecular and cortical bone. The effects of retarded bone remodeling caused by

Figure 21–3. Nutritional secondary hyperparathyroidism. Lateral radiograph of forelimb showing enlarged and widened epiphyses of the distal radius and ulna in the same puppy as in Figure 21–2. (Courtesy of Dr. C. B. Chastain, University of Missouri, Columbia.)

excessive dietary calcium are more obvious in some areas than others. Among the more obvious gross changes are abnormal alignment of the radius and ulna, posterior ataxia, stunted growth, stenosis of the spinal canal, osteochondrosis, and retained cartilage cores in the distal ulna.

When secondary hypercalcitoninism is caused by excessive dietary calcium, high normal or abnormally high serum calcium levels are present. Serum phosphorus levels are usually low. Serum alkaline phosphatase, blood urea nitrogen, and creatinine concentrations are often increased.

The diagnosis of secondary hypercalcitoninism of dietary origin may be readily apparent after correlation of a dietary history of calcium or magnesium supplementation with physical examination and radiographic findings. Bone biopsy material reveals a reduction in osteoclasts, and thyroid and parathyroid gland biopsy materials show hyperplasia of parafollicular cells and inactivity of chief cells, respectively. Older puppies are less severely affected. Biopsy specimens and serum chemistry profiles should be collected while possibly affected dogs are still consuming the suspected imbalanced diet. Improvement occurs rapidly when affected animals begin to consume a balanced diet without additional vitamin or mineral supplementation.

Rickets

Rickets is caused by a vitamin D deficiency in which the normal process of skeletal ossification is disturbed. Its occurrence in the growing puppy and kitten is no longer a common problem in most countries. The necessity of vitamin D and calcium in proper amounts and proportions in the diets of growing puppies is appreciated by breeders (Hedhammar, 1980), and thus rickets is uncommonly seen.

Dog breeders are still concerned about any signs related to rickets, especially broadening of metaphyseal regions of long bones and bulging costochondral junctions (Hedhammar, 1980). These changes are often referred to as rickets-like, because they resemble rickets in its skeletal appearance but do not represent defective ossification of developing cartilage and newly formed bones, as is made evident by radiographic and histologic findings.

Broadening of the metaphyseal regions of long bones is, to some extent, a normal physiologic event during skeletal development—necessary for adequate bone growth to occur. During periods of rapid growth, especially in giant breeds of dogs (those weighing more than 30 kg as adults), broadening of the metaphyseal regions is sometimes so pronounced that it is difficult to distinguish the physiologic changes of the metaphyses from pathologic processes, including rickets. Physiologic broadening of the metaphyses regresses when the puppy is mature, and there are, in most situations, no signs of impaired skeletal development.

Diagnosis of vitamin D deficiency requires a thorough dietary history in addition to observation of the skeletal abnormalities. Treatment consists of feeding a nutritionally balanced, commercially prepared growth diet without vitamin D supplementation or vitamin D supplementation at not more than 500 IU/kg of diet or 10 to 20 IU/kg of body weight daily. Additional amounts may result in vitamin D toxicity.

Thiamine Deficiency

Thiamine deficiency occurs most commonly in growing kittens fed either all-fish or commercially prepared diets (Loew et al, 1970; Smith and Proutt, 1944) and occasionally in dogs fed only cooked meat diets. In the metabolic energy pathways of mammals, thiamine in the form of thiamine pyrophosphate is a coenzyme involved in the oxidative decarboxylation of pyruvate and α-ketoglutarate and in the transketolation of glucose, processes concerned with the utilization of carbohydrates. The storage of thiamine in the body is limited. In thiamine deficiency, the transformation reaction of pyruvate to acetyl coenzyme A into the Krebs cycle is compromised, and plasma levels of pyruvate and lactate increase. Consequently, energy metabolism is compromised.

Thiamine deficiency as seen in the cat predominantly affects the nervous system, the alimentary tract, and the cardiovascular system. Initially the cat, although acting as if interested in food, does not eat (Everett, 1944). It may also salivate, lose weight, vomit, and show generalized progressive muscular weakness. After a few days, the cat suddenly experiences neurologic disturbances—impaired postural and vestibuloocular reflexes, spasticity, dilatation of the pupils with slow response to light, circling, dysmetria, and spinal hypersensitivity. At this point, when handled, the kitten often experiences a rapid succession of short clonic convulsions in which it is rigid and has ventriflexion of the head and neck (Fig. 21–4). Spasticity of the limbs and spinal hypersensitivity follow, so that the cat seems to walk on its toes. A tap on the dorsum may elicit a sudden extensor thrust. The

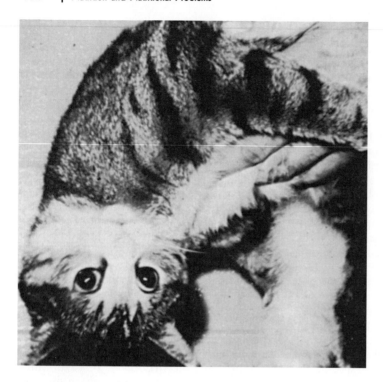

Figure 21–4. Ventriflexion of the head and neck and dilation of pupils in a cat afflicted with thiamine deficiency. Cats afflicted with potassium depletion show similar postural reactions on handling. (From Loew FM, Martin CL, Dunlop RH, et al: Naturally occurring and experimental thiamine deficiency in cats receiving commercial cat food. Can Vet J 11:109, 1970.)

retinal vessels are dilated, and sometimes there are retinal hemorrhages. The cardiac disturbances may include alternating slowing and acceleration of the heart rate, as well as sinus irregularity and ectopic rhythm (Toman et al, 1945). If not treated, the kitten that has reached the convulsive stage progresses into a semicomatose state of continual crying and opisthotonos. Extensor limb rigidity is maintained, and the kitten dies within 24 to 48 hours.

Diagnosis of thiamine deficiency is based on the dietary history and signs of the affected animal and its responsiveness to thiamine administration. Plasma pyruvate and lactate concentrations may be increased. Reduced activity of erythrocyte transketolase, a thiamine-requiring enzyme in the energy pathway, can also be used to confirm thiamine deficiency, but this assay is not readily available.

Specific treatment for thiamine deficiency is with thiamine, 25 to 50 mg per dose given by intramuscular or subcutaneous administration daily for 2 to 3 days. A marked improvement is generally seen in 2 or 3 days if therapy is initiated in the early phases of the deficiency, but residual ataxia may last for 2 or more weeks. Severe neurologic damage may occur with any delay in diagnosis and therapy; therefore, prompt action is desirable. If anorexia persists, enteral nutrition should be provided. Once the kitten is eating and improvement is noted in its

neurologic status, commercial vitamin preparation of multiple B complex may be continued until complete recovery occurs.

To prevent thiamine deficiency, owners should avoid feeding their kittens raw fish such as smelt, bullhead, herring, catfish, carp, and others that contain the active heat-labile enzyme thiaminase in their viscera (Jubb et al, 1956). In addition, kittens and puppies should not be fed improperly processed or stored commercially prepared diets (Baggs et al, 1978); owners should be encouraged to feed only nutritionally complete, commercially prepared diets. As a general rule, commercially prepared dry foods should be fed within 6 months of manufacture.

Potassium Depletion

Hypokalemia in kittens and puppies generally develops only when there is depletion of total body potassium stores, such as occurs from excessive gastrointestinal or renal losses of potassium or when extracellular potassium is redistributed into cells, as may occur in metabolic alkalosis or during insulin administration. Decreased dietary intake of potassium rarely causes hypokalemia directly but may contribute to an overall body potassium deficit (Dow et al, 1987a).

Kittens affected with persistent hypokalemia

are characterized by a sudden onset of generalized muscle weakness with persistent ventriflexion of the neck, a crouched posture, stilted gait, and apparent muscular pain (Dow et al, 1987b). Kittens with persistent hypokalemia generally have a serum potassium concentration of 3.1 mEq/L or less, an elevated serum creatine kinase activity (500 to 10,000 IU/L), and mild to moderate increases in serum creatinine and/or blood urea nitrogen concentrations (Dow et al, 1987b).

Most of the clinical effects of the persistent hypokalemia in affected cats resolve over several days after the daily addition of potassium to the diet and parenteral administration of potassium-supplemented multiple-electrolyte solution. Fluid administration is not recommended unless necessary because it may worsen the hypokalemia in some cats, leading to paralysis and death. In severely hypokalemic cats, short-term intravenous infusion of potassium-containing solutions, which deliver 0.5 to 1.0 mEq of potassium per kg per hour, is suggested if necessary. Serum potassium concentrations should be monitored closely when concentrated potassium solutions are administered to these kittens; the serum potassium concentrations have a tendency to rebound after 1 to 2 days of aggressive parenteral and oral administration of potassium (Dow et al, 1987b).

The ensuring of continued adequate dietary intake of potassium is essential in the long-term management of severely hypokalemic kittens, particularly because kittens not continually treated often develop recurrent hypokalemia. Periodic determinations of serum potassium concentration are recommended to monitor the adequacy of potassium supplementation and to avoid hyperkalemia or hypokalemia.

Taurine Deficiency

Taurine deficiency occurs most commonly in growing kittens that are receiving inadequate amounts of dietary taurine (Berson et al, 1976). Taurine is an essential amino acid for cats but not for dogs. It is normally present in bile as taurocholic acid and in high concentrations in the retina and olfactory bulb. In dogs, sufficient taurine synthesis occurs as a result of the actions of the sulfur-containing amino acids methionine and cysteine. Cats, however, unlike dogs, conjugate cholic acid exclusively with taurine and are unable to alternate between taurine and glycine conjugations in producing bile (Hayes and Sturman, 1982; Rabin et al, 1976). The kitten, therefore, has a continual dietary requirement

for taurine to replace fecal losses, which occur because of its incomplete recovery by the enterohepatic circulation.

Inadequate taurine intake by adult cats produces central retinal degeneration that can cause irreversible blindness (Hayes et al, 1975). Dietary taurine deficiency can also suppress reproductive performance in queens, causing fetal resorption or abortion, stillbirths, or the birth, at term, of underweight kittens with low survival rate (Sturman et al, 1985). Surviving kittens from taurine-deficient mothers may grow at a slower than normal rate and show a number of neurologic abnormalities, including paresis and a peculiar gait characterized by excessive abduction, abnormal hind limb development, and an apparent thoracic kyphosis (Sturman et al, 1986). In addition, milk from taurine-deficient mothers has only 10% of the taurine content of milk from mothers whose diets contain supplemental taurine.

Diagnosis of taurine deficiency in a growing kitten is based on the dietary history and clinical signs of the affected animal and on clinical responsiveness to taurine supplementation (da Costa and Hoskins, 1990). Plasma taurine concentration (normal being greater than 50 nM/ml) can be obtained from several commercial laboratories.

Treatment of kittens with clinical signs and low plasma taurine concentrations involves oral administration of purified taurine, 500 mg twice a day, or feeding a taurine-fortified diet (1000 to 1200 mg taurine per kg of dry diet or 2000 to 2500 mg taurine per kg of canned diet) to the lactating queen or growing kitten for 4 to 6 weeks.

Steatitis

Steatitis, also known as pansteatitis and "yellow fat disease," is an inflammatory disorder of the body fat. The disorder primarily affects growing cats of either sex. Most cats that develop steatitis are fed commercial or home-prepared diets that contain large amounts of fish-based ingredients—red tuna or other fish (Cordy and Stillinger, 1953; Gaskell et al, 1975). These diets may contribute to a vitamin E deficiency (Cordy, 1954).

Vitamin E, known chemically as α-tocopherol, is a biologically active antioxidant that is synthesized by plants and found in vegetable oils. Its presence in fish-based diets may be lowered or destroyed by oxidation of the contained unsaturated fats. The ingestion of large amounts of dietary unsaturated fats without sufficient antioxidants (vitamin E and/or other synthetic antioxidants) results in peroxidation of body fat with subsequent fat necrosis and steatitis. Most commercially prepared cat foods manufactured today are supplemented with vitamin E or other artificial antioxidants, and thus the incidence of steatitis has decreased. It still occurs occasionally, however, especially when home-prepared diets that contain a large amount of fish are fed (Gaskell et al, 1975).

Steatitis usually occurs after the cat has been receiving a fish-based diet for weeks or months. The owner usually first notices that the cat is eating poorly and is unwilling to move about and jump onto its favorite place or be handled. It is evident that the cat is sore and will not tolerate even the lightest stroking over its dorsum. Abdominal palpation may be so painful to the animal that the procedure cannot be performed. When steatitis is advanced, the subcutaneous fat feels firm and lumpy or granular, especially in the groin area. Frequently, the cat has a high fever that persists in spite of antimicrobial therapy.

If steatitis is not treated, the cat's leukocyte count tends to increase progressively and may reach 70,000 to 100,000 leukocytes/μl. The leukocytosis mostly involves the neutrophils, but the eosinophil count is sometimes increased. Radiographically, the subcutaneous fat of the abdomen and thorax may have a mottled appearance. Biopsy specimens should be taken from the area of greatest tenderness, usually the groin or back. In early stages of steatitis the fat, although lumpy or granular, is not discolored; later it becomes yellowish or grayish white, and ultimately it assumes an orange color and may contain small brownish nodules. The colorations are imparted by the collection of ceroid, the inert peroxidation product of the unsaturated fatty acids deposited in adipose tissue.

Histologically, fat necrosis with inflammatory infiltrate of large numbers of neutrophils and fewer mononuclear cells (lymphocytes, plasma cells, and macrophages) is evident (Fig. 21–5). The ceroid pigment may be found intracellularly (in macrophages, fat cells, and giant cells) and extracellularly. In addition, macrophages in liver, spleen, and lymph nodes may also contain the pigment (Cordy and Stillinger, 1953).

Treatment consists most importantly of a change in diet. Fish products should be removed from the diet and replaced by a nutritionally balanced, commercially prepared cat food. Initially, the cat may need to be coaxed to eat because the painful and inflamed subcutaneous tissues do not permit administration of flu-

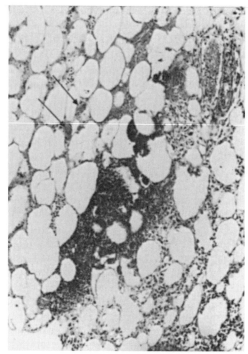

Figure 21–5. Photomicrograph showing steatitis due to vitamin E deficiency. Note that the adipose tissue demonstrates interstitial inflammatory cells, necrosis, and aggregates of peroxidized lipid-ceroid (arrows). (From O'Donnell JA, Hayes KC: Nutrition and nutritional disorders. *In* Holzworth J [ed]: Diseases of the Cat: Medicine and Surgery, vol 1. Philadelphia, WB Saunders, 1987, p 27.)

ids by the subcutaneous route or frequent handling. Daily oral doses of α-tocopherol acetate, 10 to 20 IU twice a day, are given until the signs of steatitis have subsided. Antiinflammatory doses of corticosteroids may be given to reduce the discomfort from the painful and inflamed fat. The response to treatment is gradual, recovery requiring weeks or even months, as a result of the difficulty in getting the cat to eat. If the cat does not eat, it will slowly deteriorate until it dies or is euthanized by the discouraged owner.

References and Supplemental Reading

Baggs RB, de Lahunta A, Averill DR: Thiamine deficiency encephalopathy in a specific-pathogen-free cat colony. Lab Anim Sci 28:323, 1978.

Baines FM: Milk substitutes and the hand rearing of orphan puppies and kittens. J Small Anim Pract 22:555, 1981.

Berson EL, Hayes KC, Rabin AR, et al: Retinal degeneration in cats fed casein. II. Supplementation with methionine, cysteine, or taurine. Invest Ophthalmol 15:52, 1976.

Bjorck G: Care and feeding of the puppy in the postnatal and weaning period. *In* Nutrition and Behavior in Dogs and Cats. New York, Pergamon Press, 1982, p 25.

Brawner WR, Hathcock JT, Goodman SA, et al: Body composition of growing Great Dane puppies fed diets varying in calcium and phosphorus concentration evaluated by dual energy x-ray absorptiometry. Am Coll Vet Radiol 12:1, 1996.

Bray NC: Nutritional secondary hyperparathyroidism in a kitten. Feline Pract 14:31, 1984.

Capen CC, Martin SL: Calcium-regulating hormones and diseases of parathyroid glands. *In* Ettinger SJ (ed): Textbook of Veterinary Internal Medicine, vol 2, 2nd ed. Philadelphia, WB Saunders, 1983, p 1550.

Cordy DR: Experimental production of steatitis (yellow fat disease) in kittens fed a commercial canned cat food and prevention of the condition by vitamin E. Cornell Vet 44:310, 1954.

Cordy DR, Stillinger CJ: Steatitis ("yellow fat disease") in kittens. North Am Vet 34:714, 1953.

Crager CS, Nachreiner RF: Increased parathyroid hormone concentration in a Siamese kitten with nutritional secondary hyperthyroidism. J Am Anim Hosp Assoc 29:331, 1993.

da Costa PD, Hoskins JD: The role of taurine in cats: Current concepts. Compend Contin Educ Pract Vet 12:1235, 1990.

Dow SW, Fettman MJ, LeCouteur RA, et al: Potassium depletion in cats: Renal and dietary influences. J Am Vet Med Assoc 191:1569, 1987a.

Dow SW, LeCouteur RA, Fettman MJ, et al: Potassium depletion in cats: Hypokalemic polymyopathy. J Am Vet Med Assoc 191:1563, 1987b.

Everett GM: Observations on the behavior and neurophysiology of acute thiamine deficient cats. Am J Physiol 141:439, 1944.

Feldman EC, Krutzik S: Case reports of parathyroid levels in spontaneous canine parathyroid disorders. J Am Anim Hosp Assoc 17:393, 1981.

Gaskell CJ, Leedale AH, Douglas SW: Pansteatitis in the cat: A report of four cases. J Small Anim Pract 16:117, 1975.

Goodman SA, Montgomery RD, Lauten SD, et al: Orthopedic observations in Great Dane puppies fed diets varying in calcium and phosphorus content: A preliminary report. Proceedings of the 24th Annual Veterinary Orthopedic Society, San Francisco, 1997, p 51.

Hart BL: Feline behavior. Feline Pract 2:6, 1972.

Hayes KC, Carey RE, Schmidt SY: Retinal degeneration associated with taurine deficiency in the cat. Science 188:949, 1975.

Hayes KC, Sturman JA: Taurine deficiency: A rationale for taurine depletion. *In* Huxtable RJ, Pa-

santes-Morales H (eds): Taurine in Nutrition and Neurology. New York, Plenum Publishing, 1982, p 79.

Hedhammar A: Nutrition as it relates to skeletal disease. Proceedings of the 4th Kal Kan Symposium, 1980, p 41.

Hedhammar A, Wu F, Krook L, et al: Overnutrition and skeletal disease. An experimental study in growing Great Dane dogs. Cornell Vet 64(suppl 5):1, 1974.

Howerth EW: Fatal soft tissue calcification in suckling puppies. J S Afr Assoc 54:21, 1983.

Jubb KV, Saunders LZ, Coates HV: Thiamine deficiency encephalopathy in cats. J Comp Pathol 66:217, 1956.

Krook L, Lutwak L, Henrikson P, et al: Reversibility of nutritional osteoporosis: Physicochemical data on bones from an experimental study in dogs. J Nutr 101:233, 1971.

Kruger JM, Osborne CA, Polzin DJ: Treatment of hypercalcemia. *In* Kirk RW (ed): Current Veterinary Therapy IX. Philadelphia, WB Saunders, 1986, p 75.

Lewis LD, Morris ML Jr, Hand MS: Small Animal Clinical Nutrition III. Topeka, KS, Mark Morris Associates, 1987.

Loew FM, Martin CL, Dunlop RH, et al: Naturally-occurring and experimental thiamine deficiency in cats receiving commercial cat food. Can Vet J 11:109, 1970.

Mosier JE: Causes and treatment of neonatal deaths. *In* Kirk RW (ed): Current Veterinary Therapy VI. Philadelphia, WB Saunders, 1977, p 44.

Rabin B, Nicolosi RJ, Hayes KC: Dietary influence on bile acid conjugation in the cat. J Nutr 106:1241, 1976.

Remillard RL, Pickett JP, Thatcher CD, et al: Comparison of kittens fed queen's milk with those fed milk replacers. Am J Vet Res 54:901, 1993.

Sheffy BE: Nutrition and nutritional disorders. Vet Clin North Am 8:7, 1978.

Smith DC, Proutt LM: Development of thiamine deficiency in the cat on a diet of raw fish. Proc Soc Exp Biol Med 56:1, 1944.

Spangler WL, Gribble DH, Lee TC: Vitamin D intoxication and the pathogenesis of vitamin D nephropathy in the dog. Am J Vet Res 40:73, 1979.

Sturman JA, Gargano AD, Messing JM, et al: Feline maternal taurine deficiency: Effect on mother and offspring. J Nutr 116:655, 1986.

Sturman JA, Moretz RM, French JH, et al: Taurine deficiency in developing cat: Persistence of the cerebellar external granule cell layer. J Neurosci Res 13:405, 1985.

Toman JEP, Everett GM, Oster RH, et al: Origin of cardiac disorders in thiamine-deficient cats. Proc Soc Exp Biol Med 58:65, 1945.

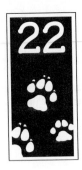

Toxicology

Johnny D. Hoskins and Steven S. Nicholson

Poisoning or suspected poisoning of the young dog and cat is a clinical entity that frequently confronts the owner and the veterinarian. The common occurrence of poisoning is probably a function of the animal's restriction to a confined environment, sensitivity to toxicants, access to toxicants, and developmental behavior—chewing habits and curious natures. Plants, insects, compounds, or formulations that are widely available and that have the potential to cause toxic effects are more likely to be involved in poisonings.

COMMON TOXICANTS INVOLVED IN POISONING

Immediate recognition and treatment of poisonings or suspected poisonings can often save the life of the young dog or cat. Recognition or suspicion of poisoning is usually based on the owner's seeing the animal ingest the toxicant or spill the toxicant on itself, or on the owner's giving or applying the toxicant to the animal or observing the evidence that the animal came in contact with the toxicant by ingestion or dermal application. There is often, however, no clear evidence of exposure to a toxicant. Therefore, the veterinarian needs to act on the suspected poisoning based on clinical suspicion that a toxicant is involved.

Many of the toxicants or suspected toxicants that are involved in poisonings of young dogs and cats are listed in Tables 22–1, 22–2, and 22–3. By no means are all possible toxicants included in these tables, but only those that are suspected most frequently.

Available to the veterinarian for additional information concerning various toxicants and their dangerous effects is the ASPCA National Animal Poison Control Center (allied agency of the University of Illinois College of Veterinary Medicine). The Poison Control Center provides a telephone service to answer questions about known or suspected cases of animal poisoning or chemical contamination on a 24-hour-a-day, 365-day-a-year basis. The current poison hotline service for veterinarians and animal owners can be reached via telephone at 888–426–4435 (fee of $45 per case; credit cards only, no extra charge for follow-up calls) or 900–680–0000. There is no charge when the call involves a product covered by the Animal Product Safety Service. Also useful to the veterinarian and animal owner is the National Pesticide Telecommunications Network (can be reached via telephone at 800–858–7877). The U.S. Environmental Protection Agency and Oregon State University sponsor this service, and it provides information about pesticide products and poisonings, toxicology, environmental chemistry, and other pesticide-related issues.

TREATMENT OF POISONINGS

General Treatment Procedures. The primary goal of therapy for a poisoning is to provide immediate treatment to the affected animal(s). The procedures used, in a general way, are presented in Table 22–4. The most important aspect of the immediate treatment of poisoning is to ensure adequate physiologic function. All the antidotal procedures available to the veterinarian are of no avail if the animal has lost one or all of its vital physiologic

Text continued on page 507

Table 22-1 Major Toxic Components, Synonyms or Trade Names, Clinical Effects, and Therapy for Common Toxic Agents

AGENTS	MAJOR TOXIC COMPONENTS	SYNONYMS OR TRADE NAMES	CLINICAL EFFECTS	THERAPY
Avicides (bird-killing agents)	4-Aminopyridine	Avitrol	Hyperexcitability, salivation, tremors, muscle incoordination, seizures, cardiac and/or respiratory failure	Emesis or gastric lavage. Activated charcoal. Control the seizures. Cardiopulmonary support as needed
	3-Chloro-*p*-toluidine	Starlicide	CNS depression, muscular weakness, cyanosis, mild methemoglobinemia, Heinz bodies	Emesis or gastric lavage. Activated charcoal. No specific antidote
Insecticides	Organophosphates	Vapona (dichlorvos), Dipterex or Neguvon (trichlorofon), Cygon (dimethoate), Ruelene (crufomate), Cythion (malathion), Bladan (parathion), Korlan (ronnel), Spectracide (diazinon), Dursban (chlorpyrifos), Dyfonate (fonofos), Imidan (phosmet), D-Syston (disulfoton), Co-Ral (coumaphos), Warbex (famphur), Thimet (phorate), Spotton (fenthion)	Acetylcholinesterase inhibition: vomiting, diarrhea, dyspnea, cyanosis, miosis, hypermotility, abdominal cramping (in extreme cases, tetany followed by weakness and paralysis), seizures	Atropine sulfate. Diphenhydramine. Organophosphates—2-PAM. Wash skin with soap and water. Activated charcoal. Control the seizures. Supportive treatment otherwise
	Carbamates	Sevin (carbaryl), Lannate (methomyl), Baygon (propoxur), Ficam (bendiocarb), Temik (aldicarb), Furadan (carbofuran)	Acetylcholinesterase inhibition: vomiting, diarrhea, dyspnea, cyanosis, miosis, hypermotility, abdominal cramping (in extreme cases, tetany followed by weakness and paralysis), seizures	Atropine sulfate. Diphenhydramine. Carbamates—2-PAM (pralidoxime contraindicated). Wash skin with soap and water. Activated charcoal. Control the seizures. Supportive treatment otherwise
	Methoprene	Several products	No toxic effects yet described	Gastric lavage if ingested. Activated charcoal. Symptomatic treatment otherwise
	Fenoxycarb	Several products	No toxic effects yet described	Wash thoroughly with direct stream of water for 15 min if in eyes. Gastric lavage if ingested. Activated charcoal
	Pyrethrins, synthetic pyrethroids, and piperonyl butoxide	Several products	Nausea, vomiting, diarrhea, stupor, salivation, pallor, tremors, convulsions, and respiratory arrest with heavy doses	Gastric lavage or emesis. Activated charcoal. Oxygen, sedatives as needed. IV fluids and electrolytes. Bathe with detergent and flush eyes with water. Control the seizures

Table continued on following page

Table 22-1

Major Toxic Components, Synonyms or Trade Names, Clinical Effects, and Therapy for Common Toxic Agents *Continued*

AGENTS	MAJOR TOXIC COMPONENTS	SYNONYMS OR TRADE NAMES	CLINICAL EFFECTS	THERAPY
	Rotenone	Several products	Vomiting, nausea, diarrhea, respiratory stimulation, convulsions, followed by respiratory failure	Emesis or gastric lavage before convulsive stage. Activated charcoal. Warmth, quietness. Assist respiration as needed. Control the seizures
	Chlorinated hydrocarbons	Several products	Hyperexcitability, anorexia, muscle weakness, tremors; advanced stages are paralysis, tonic and clonic convulsions, unconsciousness	If ingested, induce vomiting. Activated charcoal. Oil laxatives are contraindicated because they assist absorption. Control the seizures
	Nicotine sulfate	Black Leaf 40	Salivation, excitement, tachypnea, tachycardia, vomiting, diarrhea, ataxia, tremors, seizures	Emesis or gastric lavage with 1:10,000 potassium permanganate. Activated charcoal. Control the seizures. Supportive treatment otherwise
Miticide	Amitraz	Mitaban (19.6% liquid concentrate), Taktic (12.5% liquid concentrate), several amitraz-impregnated collar products for tick control	Not recommended for cats or dogs younger than 3 mo of age; weakness, salivation, ataxia, tremors, dyspnea, coma	Wash skin with soap and water. Administer yohimbine. Supportive treatment otherwise
Insect repellent	Diethyltoluamide (also known as DEET)	Deep Woods Off, Cutter Insect Repellent, OFF, Jungle Plus, Muskol, 6-12 Plus, Blockade, DMT-50	Emesis, lethargy, ataxia, tremors, seizures, excessive salivation	Emesis or gastric lavage. Activated charcoal. Control the seizures
Rodenticides	Strychnine		Nervousness, stiffness, violent tetanic seizures, respiratory failure	Emesis or gastric lavage with 1%–2% tannic acid or 1:2000 potassium permanganate, followed by activated charcoal. Control the seizures
	Sodium fluoroacetate	Compound 1080	Hyperirritability, emesis, repeated eliminations (micturition and defecation), tenesmus, dyspnea, seizures, running fits, respiratory failure. Few, if any, survive once signs begin	Emesis or gastric lavage with milk or limewater. Administer orally glyceryl monoacetate (monoacetin) 0.55 g/ kg IM or 8 ml/kg 50% ethanol and 8 ml/kg 5% acetic acid. Control the seizures
	Phosphide derivatives, zinc phosphide, aluminum phosphide		Emesis, anorexia, abdominal pain, lethargy, ataxia, respiratory failure, seizures, running fits	Emesis or gastric lavage. Activated charcoal. Control the seizures. Supportive treatment otherwise
	α-Naphthylthiourea	ANTU	Emesis, salivation, dyspnea, restlessness, coughing, cyanosis, respiratory failure	Emesis or gastric lavage. Activated charcoal. Supportive treatment otherwise

Table 22-1 **Major Toxic Components, Synonyms or Trade Names, Clinical Effects, and Therapy for Common Toxic Agents** *Continued*

AGENTS	MAJOR TOXIC COMPONENTS	SYNONYMS OR TRADE NAMES	CLINICAL EFFECTS	THERAPY
	Thallium		Severe vomiting and diarrhea, ataxia, convulsions, renal failure, brick-red mucous membranes, skin lesions (erythema, crusts, alopecia, ulceration). Hair loss with minimal skin alteration may be seen	Emesis or gastric lavage. Administer diphenylthiocarbazone. Control the seizures. Supportive treatment otherwise
	α-Chloralose		Ataxia, hyperexcitability, weakness, prostration, shallow breathing, weak pulse, hypothermia	Emesis or gastric lavage. Activated charcoal. Supportive treatment otherwise
	Crimidine	Castrix	Seizures	Control the seizures. Administer pyridoxine hydrochloride 20 mg/kg IV. Activated charcoal
	Red squill		Emesis, incoordination, hyperesthesia, convulsions, cardiac (digitalis effect) failure	Emesis or gastric lavage. Activated charcoal. Control the seizures. Treat as for digitalis overdose
	Pyriminil	Vacor (withdrawn from commercial availability)	Vomiting, depression, abdominal pain, anorexia, dilated pupils, weakness, tremors, visual problems	Emesis or gastric lavage. Activated charcoal. Administer nicotinamide 50–100 mg IM q4h 8 times, follow with oral administration 3–5 times daily for 7–10 days
	Warfarin, coumafene, zoocoumarin	Warf 42, Rax, Dethmor, Coumafene, Rodex, Tox-Hid, Prolin, Ratron	Repeated exposures lead to presentation of bleeding diatheses, altered coagulation profile (OSPT, APIT, ACT, clotting time tests)	Emesis. Activated charcoal. Remove animal from source. Administer vitamin K_1 for 7 days or longer. Supportive treatment otherwise
	Coumafuryl, fumarin, tomarin	Ratafin, Lurat, Rat-a-way, Krumkil, Fumisol	See Warfarin	Emesis. Activated charcoal. Remove animal from source. Administer vitamin K_1 for 7 days or longer. Supportive treatment otherwise
	Brodifacoum, volak, BFC	Talon, Havoc, Weather Block, De-Mice, D-Con 2	Single exposure leads to presentation of bleeding diatheses, altered coagulation profile as for warfarin	Emesis. Activated charcoal. Remove animal from source. Administer vitamin K_1 (5 mg/kg/day divided into 3 doses) for up to 30 d. Supportive treatment otherwise
	Bromadiolone, bromone	Maki, Contrac, Super Caid, Ratimus	See Brodifacoum	See Brodifacoum
	Diphacinone, diphenadione, diphenacin	Promar, Ramik, Diphacin	See Brodifacoum	See Brodifacoum

Table continued on following page

Table 22–1 Major Toxic Components, Synonyms or Trade Names, Clinical Effects, and Therapy for Common Toxic Agents *Continued*

AGENTS	MAJOR TOXIC COMPONENTS	SYNONYMS OR TRADE NAMES	CLINICAL EFFECTS	THERAPY
	Chlorophacinone, chlorodiphacinone, chlorphenacone, chlorphacinone, liphadione	Afnor, Caid, Drat, Quick, Raticide-Caid, Ramucide, Ratomet, Raviac, Rozol, Redentin, Topitox, Ratindan 3	See Brodifacoum	See Brodifacoum
	Pindone, pivalyl valone, pivaldione	Pival, Pivalyn	See Brodifacoum	See Brodifacoum
	Valone, indanedione, isovaleryl, isoval	PMP, Motomco tracking powder	See Brodifacoum	See Brodifacoum
	Cholecalciferol (vitamin D_3)	Quintox, Rampage, Rat-B-Gone, Mouse-B-Gone	Polyuria, muscular weakness, anorexia, vomiting, seizures, polydipsia, hypercalcemia, depression, cardiac and renal dysfunction	Emesis or gastric lavage. Activated charcoal. Administer treatment for hypercalcemia. Monitor cardiac and renal function. Supportive treatment otherwise
	Bromethalin	Assault, Vengeance, Trounce	Tremors, clonic convulsions, prostration, lethargy, hind leg weakness, loss of muscle tone, paralysis, death (repeated small exposures far below LD_{50} will induce CNS signs)	Emesis or gastric lavage. Activated charcoal. Control the seizures. Must treat cerebral edema and increased cerebrospinal fluid pressure. Supportive treatment otherwise
Molluscacide	Metaldehyde	Snarol	Tremors, seizures, ataxia, hyperthermia, nystagmus in cats, salivation, respiratory failure	Emesis or gastric lavage with milk or limewater. Activated charcoal. Control the seizures. Supportive treatment otherwise
Herbicides	Arsenic trioxide, lead arsenate, dimethylarsenate, monosodium methane arsenate, disodium methane arsenate, octyldodecyl ammonium, salts of methyl arsenic acid	Several products	Anorexia, vomiting, abdominal pain, diarrhea, ataxia, paresis of hind legs, renal failure	Emesis or gastric lavage. Activated charcoal. Administer dimercaprol (BAL). Supportive treatment otherwise
	Diquat, paraquat	Ortho Paraquat	Hyperexcitability, oral lesions, incoordination, seizures, respiratory and renal failure, progressive pulmonary fibrosis	Emesis or gastric lavage. Activated charcoal. Control the seizures. Supportive treatment otherwise. Oxygen contraindicated
	Phenoxyacetic acids	2,4-D, MCPP, Mecoprop, MCPA, Weedone, Silvex	Emesis, diarrhea, anorexia, salivation, weakness, ataxia, tremors, myotonia in dogs	Emesis or gastric lavage. Activated charcoal. Supportive treatment otherwise
	Triazines, prometon atrazine	Triox, Aatrex	Generally nontoxic; may cause lethargy, depression, ataxia, tremors	Emesis or gastric lavage. Activated charcoal. Supportive treatment otherwise

AGENTS	**MAJOR TOXIC COMPONENTS**	**SYNONYMS OR TRADE NAMES**	**CLINICAL EFFECTS**	**THERAPY**
	Alachlor, benefin, bensulide, DCPA, dicamba, glyphosate, oxadiazon, proachlor, trifluralin	Lasso, Balan, Betasan, Dacthal, Banvel, Roundup, Kleenup, Ronstar, Ramrod, Treflan	Generally nontoxic; may cause lethargy, depression, vomiting, muscular weakness, salivation	Emesis or gastric lavage. Activated charcoal. Supportive treatment otherwise
Fertilizers	Urea and/or ammonium salts. Nitrates, phosphates	Several products	Vomiting, diarrhea, possible polyuria	Emesis or gastric lavage. Activated charcoal. Supportive treatment otherwise
Glues and adhesives	Aliphatic or aromatic hydrocarbons (acetone, toluol, toluene, methyl acetone, naphtha), cyanoacrylate, starchy wallpaper pastes	Several products	Mucosal/skin irritation, depression, vomiting, adhered tissues, abdominal pain and gas formation (wallpaper pastes)	Supportive treatment
Insulation	Styrofoam, fiberglass, vermiculite	Several products	Irritation of digestive tract, possibly act as foreign object	Oily or saline cathartic. Supportive treatment otherwise
Furniture polishes	Petroleum distillates, mineral seal oil, petroleum naphthas, turpentine, waxes, pine oils	Several products	Eye/skin/mucosal irritation, depression, disorientation, vomiting, aspiration or hydrocarbon pneumonia, hepatorenal damage	Prevent aspiration pneumonia. *Avoid gastric lavage or proceed cautiously to prevent aspiration.* Monitor and treat for pneumonia. Supportive treatment otherwise
Paint and varnish removers	Benzene, methanol, acetone, toluene	Several products	Skin irritation, depression, pneumonia, disorientation, hepatorenal damage	See Furniture polishes
Solvents	Methanol (methyl alcohol, wood alcohol, wood spirits, carbinol, methyl hydrate)	Several products	Emesis, dyspnea, ataxia, restlessness, abdominal pain, cold extremities, hypothermia, coma	Emesis or gastric lavage. Activated charcoal. Administer ethanol. Supportive treatment otherwise
	Methylene chloride (methylene dichloride, methylene bichloride)	Several products	Reddened mucous membranes, salivation, vomiting, dyspnea, increased respiratory rate	Oxygen therapy. Supportive treatment otherwise
	Toluene (toluol, methylbenzene, phenylmethane), xylene (dimethylbenzene), benzene	Several products	Emesis, ataxia, tremors, restlessness, seizures, cardiac arrhythmias, pneumonia, hepatorenal damage	Emesis or gastric lavage. Activated charcoal. Control the seizures and monitor cardiac function. Supportive treatment otherwise
	Turpentine (spirits of turpentine, gum turpentine, oil of turpentine)	Several products	Eye/skin irritation, emesis, congested mucous membranes, salivation, diarrhea, ataxia, depression, dyspnea, cardiac arrhythmias, renal damage	See Toluene, xylene, benzene

Table continued on following page

Table 22–1 Major Toxic Components, Synonyms or Trade Names, Clinical Effects, and Therapy for Common Toxic Agents *Continued*

AGENTS	MAJOR TOXIC COMPONENTS	SYNONYMS OR TRADE NAMES	CLINICAL EFFECTS	THERAPY
	Petroleum hydrocarbons (mineral, white and petroleum spirits; Stoddard solvent; thinners Nos. 40–80)	Several products	See Toluene, xylene, benzene	See Toluene, xylene, benzene
Kerosene	Kerosene, coal oil; in the British Isles known as paraffin	Several fuels, water-white kerosene and insect repellent products	Eye/skin/mouth irritation, emesis, salivation, diarrhea, ataxia, dyspnea, coughing, tremors, depression, seizures, cardiac arrhythmias, coma, pneumonia if aspirated	See Furniture polishes
Gasoline, motor fuels, heating oils	Aliphatic, alicyclic, aromatic hydrocarbons	Several products	See Kerosene	See Furniture polishes
Lubricants	Motor oils (new or used), gear oils, greases, tractor transmission fluid, hydraulic brake fluid, automatic transmission fluids (toxicity due to antifoaming agents, detergents, antioxidants, lithium, and lead in products)	Several products	Emesis, depression, ataxia, circling, seizures, posterior paralysis, coma	Emesis or gastric lavage. Bathe with mild detergent. Control the seizures. Supportive treatment otherwise
Animal repellents, mace-type products	Chloroacetophenone, capsicum ketone, methylnonyl ketone	Several products	Eye/skin/mouth irritation, salivation, emesis	Supportive treatment
Antifreeze, photographic film processing solution	Ethylene glycol and isopropanol, propylene glycol	Several products	Disorientation, depression, ataxia, vomiting, weakness, polydipsia and polyuria, seizures, oliguric renal failure (later sign) (renal failure is not associated with propylene intoxication)	Emesis or gastric lavage. Correct dehydration and promote diuresis. Administer ethanol or 4-methylpyrazole early. 4-Methylpyrazole is not effective in cats. Supportive treatment otherwise
Denture cleaners	Sodium perborate	Several products	Eye/skin/mucosal irritation, salivation, lacrimation, vomiting, depression	Flush liberally with water. Supportive treatment otherwise
Deodorants	Aluminum chloride, aluminum chlorohydrate	Several products	Eye/skin/mucosal irritation, vomiting, diarrhea, renal damage, incoordination	Emesis or gastric lavage. Supportive treatment otherwise
Detergents (anionic/nonionic)	Sulfonated or phosphorylated hydrocarbons	Several products (hand dishwashing liquids, soaps, laundry compounds, hair shampoos)	Emesis, lethargy, dyspnea, diarrhea	Lavage with milk or water

Table 22–1	Major Toxic Components, Synonyms or Trade Names, Clinical Effects, and Therapy for Common Toxic Agents *Continued*			
AGENTS	MAJOR TOXIC COMPONENTS	SYNONYMS OR TRADE NAMES	CLINICAL EFFECTS	THERAPY
Detergents (cationic)	Quaternary ammonium with alkyl or aryl substituent groups	Several products	Eye/skin/mucosal irritation, vomiting, diarrhea, weakness, abdominal pain, skin burn when exposed to concentrated solution	Milk soap, or activated charcoal orally. Supportive treatment otherwise
Drain cleaners	Sodium hydroxide, sometimes sodium hypochlorite	Several products	Eye/skin/mucosal irritation and inflammation, results in necrosis and scarring	Flush with water or milk. *Do not use emetics or lavage.* Supportive treatment otherwise
Dry-cleaning fluids	1,1,1-Trichloroethane, tetrachloroethylene	Several products	Eye/skin/mucosal irritation, depression, disorientation, vomiting, aspiration or hydrocarbon pneumonia, cardiac arrhythmias, hepatorenal damage	*Do not use emetics or lavage.* Administer activated charcoal. Supportive treatment otherwise
Fireworks	Oxidizing agents (nitrates, chlorates), metals (mercury, antimony, copper, strontium, barium, phosphorus)	Several products	Emesis, diarrhea, abdominal pain. Chlorates may cause methemoglobinemia	Emesis or gastric lavage. Treat for methemoglobinemia. Treat for specific metal(s) if known. Administer activated charcoal. Supportive treatment otherwise
Fire extinguisher (liquid)	Chlorobromomethane, methyl bromide	Several products	Eye/skin/mucosal irritation, salivation, vomiting, coma, disorientation, paresis, pulmonary edema, hepatorenal damage (metabolized to methanol)	Flush with soap and water. *Do not use emetics or lavage.* Supportive treatment otherwise
Fireplace colors	Heavy metal salts (copper, rubidium, cesium, lead, zinc, arsenic, selenium, barium, antimony)	Several products	Emesis, diarrhea, toxicity and signs vary with metal involved, renal damage	Supportive treatment. Activated charcoal. Specific metal antidotes if possible
Fluxes (solder)	Acids (hydrochloric, glutamic, salicylic, boric)	Several products	Eye/skin/mucosal irritation, vomiting diarrhea, hyperthermia	Supportive treatment
Household bleach	Sodium hypochlorite	Several products	Eye/skin/mucosal irritation, vomiting, diarrhea	Flush skin and eyes with water. *Do not use emetics or lavage.* Administer oral milk of magnesia or aluminum hydroxide. Oral sodium thiosulfate detoxifies hypochlorite
Matches	Potassium chlorate, red phosphorus	Several products	Emesis, diarrhea (chlorates may induce methemoglobinemia)	Symptomatic treatment
Mothballs and moth crystals or flakes	Naphthalene, paradichlorobenzene	Several products	Emesis, diarrhea, hemolysis, ataxia, tremors, seizures	Emesis or gastric lavage. Control the seizures. Supportive treatment otherwise

Table continued on following page

Table 22–1

Major Toxic Components, Synonyms or Trade Names, Clinical Effects, and Therapy for Common Toxic Agents *Continued*

AGENTS	MAJOR TOXIC COMPONENTS	SYNONYMS OR TRADE NAMES	CLINICAL EFFECTS	THERAPY
Perfumes	Perfume essence comprising various volatile oils (savin, rue, tansy, juniper, cedar)	Several products	Eye/skin/mucosal irritation, vomiting, diarrhea, salivation, hepatorenal damage, restlessness, ataxia, coma, volatile odor of oils on breath	Emesis or gastric lavage. Supportive treatment otherwise
Photographic developers	*p*-Methylaminophenol	Several products	Eye/skin/mucosal irritation, vomiting, diarrhea, ataxia, disorientation, seizures, coma, methemoglobinemia	Emesis or gastric lavage. Treat methemoglobinemia. Control the seizures. Supportive treatment otherwise
Phenol-containing cleansers	Phenols, cresol, hexachlorophene	Lysol, Pine-Sol	Eye/skin/mucosal irritation, vomiting, diarrhea, ataxia, depression, seizures, hepatorenal damage, methemoglobinemia	Emesis or gastric lavage. Treat methemoglobinemia. Control the seizures. Supportive treatment otherwise
Radiator cleaners	Oxalic acid (40%–100%)	Several products	Eye/skin/mucosal irritation, vomiting, diarrhea, hypocalcemic seizures, renal damage	Oral calcium salts. Control the seizures. Supportive treatment otherwise
Household alcohols	Ethanol, isopropyl alcohol	Several products	Emesis, dyspnea, ataxia, restlessness, abdominal pain, cold extremities, hypothermia, coma, hepatorenal damage	Emesis or gastric lavage. Supportive treatment otherwise
Shampoo	Lauryl sulfates, triethanolamine dodecyl sulfate, wide variety of surfactants	Several products	Eye/mucosal irritation, emesis, diarrhea	Emesis or gastric lavage. Administer activated charcoal and saline cathartic. Supportive treatment otherwise
Sunscreen lotion	Alcohol	Several products	See Household alcohols	See Household alcohols
Lead	Lead	Numerous lead-containing products (household, construction, automotive, and sporting goods items)	Emesis, diarrhea, abdominal pain, aggression, restlessness, ataxia, tremors, seizures, blindness, dementia, weight loss, anemia with inappropriate numbers of nucleated RBCs and basophilic stippling, blood lead levels > 0.35 ppm (35 µg/dl)	Emesis or gastric lavage and enemas. Administer specific antidote for lead. Supportive treatment otherwise
Analgesic drugs	Acetaminophen	Tylenol, Excedrin, Anacin-3, Datril, and others	Facial/paw edema, depression, weakness, anorexia, vomiting, tachypnea, tachycardia, cyanosis, methemoglobinemia, hemolytic anemia, Heinz bodies, liver damage	Emesis or gastric lavage. Administer activated charcoal and acetylcysteine. *Do not administer activated charcoal and oral acetylcysteine together.* Treat methemoglobinemia. Supportive treatment otherwise

Table 22–1	**Major Toxic Components, Synonyms or Trade Names, Clinical Effects, and Therapy for Common Toxic Agents** *Continued*			
AGENTS	**MAJOR TOXIC COMPONENTS**	**SYNONYMS OR TRADE NAMES**	**CLINICAL EFFECTS**	**THERAPY**
	Aspirin (salicylates)	Several products	Emesis (often blood tinged), anorexia, hemorrhage, depression, hyperthermia, tachypnea, ataxia, coma, Heinz bodies, renal damage	Emesis or gastric lavage. Administer activated charcoal. Supportive treatment otherwise
	Ibuprofen	Several products	Emesis (often blood tinged), anorexia, hemorrhage, depression, hyperthermia, tachypnea, ataxia, coma, renal damage	Emesis or gastric lavage. Administer activated charcoal. Supportive treatment otherwise
Oxidant agents	Phenazopyridine, methylene blue, allyl propyl disulfide (onions, raw and cooked), naphthalene (mothballs), benzocaine	Several products	See Acetaminophen	See Acetaminophen (acetylcysteine is not administered)
Methylxanthine compounds	Caffeine (in coffee, tea, chocolate, colas, stimulant drugs), theobromine (chocolate, cocoa beans, cola, tea), theophylline (tea)	Several products	Restlessness, hyperesthesia, hyperirritability, tachycardia, cardiac arrhythmias, vomiting, diarrhea, polyuria, hyperthermia, seizures, ataxia, tremors, abdominal pain, coma	Emesis or gastric lavage. Administer activated charcoal and sodium or magnesium sulfate. Control the seizures. Supportive treatment otherwise
Cigarettes and cigars	Nicotine	Several products	Salivation, excitement, tachypnea, tachycardia, vomiting, diarrhea, ataxia, tremors, seizures	Emesis or gastric lavage with 1:10,000 potassium permanganate. Control the seizures. Administer activated charcoal. Supportive treatment otherwise
Marijuana	Tetrahydrocannabinol (from the hemp plant *Cannabis sativa*)	Hashish, cannabis, "hash brownies"	Drowsiness, depression, hypothermia, ataxia, salivation, vomiting, mydriasis, bradycardia	Emesis or gastric lavage and enemas. Administer activated charcoal. Supportive treatment otherwise
Amphetamines	Amphetamine sulfate, dextroamphetamine, methamphetamine, phenyliso-propylamine	Several over-the-counter products, "speed," "uppers," "dexies," "bennies"	Hyperexcitability, hyperesthesia, tachycardia, hyperthermia, panting, mydriasis, vomiting, diarrhea, tremors, seizures	Emesis or gastric lavage. Administer activated charcoal and sodium sulfate. Control the seizures and hyperthermia. Supportive treatment otherwise
Phencyclidine	[1-(1-Phenyl-cyclohexyl piperidine)]	Angel dust, PCP, variety of other ever-changing street names	Drowsiness or hyperexcitability, muscle contractions, hyperthermia, nystagmus, mydriasis, vomiting, seizures, coma	Emesis or gastric lavage. Administer activated charcoal. Control the seizures and muscle contractions and hyperthermia. Supportive treatment otherwise

Table continued on following page

| Table 22–1 | Major Toxic Components, Synonyms or Trade Names, Clinical Effects, and Therapy for Common Toxic Agents *Continued* |

AGENTS	MAJOR TOXIC COMPONENTS	SYNONYMS OR TRADE NAMES	CLINICAL EFFECTS	THERAPY
Phenyl-propanolamine	Chemically related to amphetamine and ephedrine	"Black beauties," "white crosses," several over-the-counter products containing phenylpropanolamine with caffeine	See Amphetamines	See Amphetamines
Cocaine	Alkaloid extracted from South American shrub *Erythroxylon coca*	Cocaine hydrochloride, topical solution, "coke," "snow," "blow," "toot," "crack"	Hyperexcitability, tachycardia, hyperthermia, panting, mydriasis, vomiting, tremors, seizures, cardiac arrhythmias	See Amphetamines
Opioids	Morphine-like compounds	Heroin, "Persian brown," "China white"	Depression, depressed respiration, miosis, hypothermia, muscular flaccidity, vomiting, pulmonary edema. *Withdrawal effects:* Restlessness, mydriasis, abdominal pain, vomiting, diarrhea, salivation, oculonasal discharge, muscle spasms	Emesis or gastric lavage. Administer activated charcoal and specific antidote. Supportive treatment otherwise
Psilocybin mushrooms	Psilocybin and psilocin	Similar to effects of lysergic acid diethylamide (LSD)	Drowsiness, ataxia, tremors, inconsistent pupillary changes, muscle hypertonicity, hyperthermia, convulsions and respiratory arrest	See Phencyclidine
Lysergic acid diethylamide	LSD	LSD	Drowsiness, ataxia, tremors, inconsistent pupillary changes, muscle hypertonicity, hyperthermia, convulsions and respiratory arrest	See Phencyclidine

CNS = Central nervous system; RBCs = red blood cells; IV = intravenous administration; IM = intramuscular administration.

Table 22–2	Plants Producing Systemic Poisoning and Contact Irritation		
NAME	**POISONOUS PART OF PLANT (ACTIVE PRINCIPLE, IF KNOWN)**	**CLINICAL EFFECTS**	**THERAPY**
Calla lily (*Zantedeschia aethiopica*)	Leaves (raphides of calcium oxalate and unidentified protein)	Mouth/skin/mucosal irritation, stomatitis, irritant dermatitis	Flush the skin, eyes, or mouth with cool liquids or demulcents
Elephant's ear (*Alocasia* spp)	Leaves and stems (calcium oxalate raphides)	Mouth/skin/mucosal irritation, stomatitis, irritant dermatitis	Flush the skin, eyes, or mouth with cool liquids or demulcents
(*Caladium* spp)	Whole plant (calcium oxalate raphides)	Mouth/skin/mucosal irritation, stomatitis, irritant dermatitis	Flush the skin, eyes, or mouth with cool liquids or demulcents
(*Colocasia* spp)	Leaves (calcium oxalate raphides)	Mouth/skin/mucosal irritation, stomatitis, irritant dermatitis	Flush the skin, eyes, or mouth with cool liquids or demulcents
Dumbcane (*Dieffenbachia* spp)	Leaves (calcium oxalate raphides and unidentified protein)	Mouth/skin/mucosal irritation, stomatitis, irritant dermatitis	Flush the skin, eyes, or mouth with cool liquids or demulcents
Philodendron (*Philodendron* spp)	Leaves (calcium oxalate raphides and unidentified protein)	Mouth/skin/mucosal irritation, stomatitis, irritant dermatitis	Flush the skin, eyes, or mouth with cool liquids or demulcents
Pothos, devil's ivy (*Epipremnum aureum*)	Whole plant (calcium oxalate raphides and unidentified protein)	Mouth/skin/mucosal irritation, stomatitis, irritant dermatitis	Flush the skin, eyes, or mouth with cool liquids or demulcents
Oleander (*Nerium oleander*)	Whole plant, including smoke from burning and water in which the flowers have been placed (cardioactive glycosides similar to digitalis)	Emesis, abdominal pain, diarrhea, cardiac arrhythmias	Emesis or gastric lavage, administer activated charcoal, saline cathartics useful, control cardiac arrhythmias
Yew, ground hemlock (*Taxus* spp)	Most of the plant, including the seeds but not the red aril (taxine alkaloids)	Incoordination, dry mouth initially, mydriasis, abdominal pain, emesis, salivation, cyanosis, weakness, coma, cardiac arrhythmias, cardiac or respiratory failure	Emesis or gastric lavage, administer activated charcoal, monitor cardiac and respiratory function, supportive treatment otherwise
Bird of paradise, Barbados pride, dwarf poinciana (*Caesalpinia* spp)	Seeds (tannins)	Emesis, diarrhea, recovery usually in 24 h	Treat as for gastroenteritis, supportive treatment otherwise
Buckeye, horse chestnut (*Aesculus* spp)	Nuts and twigs (mixture of saponins known as aescin)	Severe emesis and diarrhea	Treat as for gastroenteritis, supportive treatment otherwise
Apricot, cherry, choke cherry, peach, plum, sloe (*Prunus* spp)	Kernel in the pit (cyanogenetic glycosides, amygdalin, liberate hydrocyanic acid on hydrolysis)	Emesis, abdominal pain, lethargy, cyanosis, convulsions, muscle flaccidity, incontinence, coma	Emesis or gastric lavage, administer activated charcoal and cyanide antidote, supportive treatment otherwise
Chrysanthemum, feverfew, marguerite, daisy (*Chrysanthemum* spp)	Sap (sesquiterpene lactones in all plant parts except the pollen)	Contact dermatitis (sequentially—immediate erythema, rash, pruritus, crusting, and scaling)	Prompt removal of irritant with running water, topical steroids
Buttercup, crowfoot (*Ranunculus* spp)	Sap (protoanemonin)	Mouth/skin/mucosal irritation, emesis, diarrhea, abdominal pain, renal failure, incoordination, convulsions	Emesis or gastric lavage, monitor renal function, supportive treatment otherwise
Azalea, rhododendron (*Rhododendron* spp)	Leaves and honey made from flower nectar (grayanotoxins also referred to as andromedotoxins)	Mouth/mucosal irritation, salivation, marked emesis, diarrhea, weakness, altered vision, bradycardia, convulsions, coma	Emesis or gastric lavage, monitor cardiac function, supportive treatment otherwise

Table continued on following page

Table 22-2 Plants Producing Systemic Poisoning and Contact Irritation *Continued*

NAME	POISONOUS PART OF PLANT (ACTIVE PRINCIPLE, IF KNOWN)	CLINICAL EFFECTS	THERAPY
Holly, American holly, English holly, yaupon (*Ilex* spp)	Fruit (saponins)	Emesis, diarrhea	Treat as for gastroenteritis, supportive treatment otherwise
Hydrangea (*Hydrangea macrophylla*)	Flower bud (cyanogenetic glycoside, hydrangin, liberates hydrocyanic acid on hydrolysis)	Emesis, abdominal pain, lethargy, cyanosis, convulsions, muscle flaccidity, incontinence, coma	Emesis or gastric lavage, administer activated charcoal and cyanide antidote, supportive treatment otherwise
Indian tobacco, blue cardinal flower, cardinal flower, (*Lobelia* spp)	Whole plant (lobeline and related alkaloids, similar to nicotine)	Emesis, excitement, weakness, ataxia, tremors, seizures	Emesis or gastric lavage with 1:10,000 potassium permanganate, control seizures, supportive treatment otherwise
Iris, flag (*Iris* spp)	Rootstock (unidentified)	Emesis, diarrhea, abdominal pain	Treat as for gastroenteritis, supportive treatment otherwise
Yellow jessamine (*Gelsemium sempervirens*)	Whole plant (gelsemicine and related alkaloids)	Incoordination, altered vision, dry mouth, difficulty in swallowing, muscular weakness, seizures, respiratory failure	Emesis or gastric lavage, administer activated charcoal, control seizures, support respiratory function, supportive treatment otherwise
Mountain laurel (*Kalmia* spp)	Leaves and nectar (grayanotoxins, also referred to as andromedotoxins)	Mouth/mucosal irritation, salivation, emesis, diarrhea, weakness, altered vision, bradycardia, convulsions, coma	Emesis or gastric lavage, monitor cardiac function, supportive treatment otherwise
Lupin, lupine (*Lupinus* spp)	Whole plant, especially seeds (lupinine and related alkaloids)	Muscular weakness, paralysis, depressed breathing, convulsions	Emesis or gastric lavage, control convulsions, supportive treatment otherwise
Manchineel (*Hippomane mancinella*)	Sap (diterpenes)	Mouth/mucosal irritation, emesis, bloody diarrhea, contact and allergic dermatitis, keratoconjunctivitis	Emesis or gastric lavage, wash skin with soap and water, supportive treatment otherwise
Mistletoe (*Phoradendron* spp)	Whole plant; berries if consumed in large amounts (phoratoxin)	Emesis, abdominal pain, diarrhea	Emesis or gastric lavage, treat as for gastroenteritis
European mistletoe (*Viscum album*)	Leaves and stems (viscumin)	Emesis, abdominal pain, diarrhea	Emesis or gastric lavage, treat as for gastroenteritis
Poinsettia (*Euphorbia pulcherrima*)	Leaves and stems (complex terpenes)	Mild emesis, diarrhea	Emesis or gastric lavage, treat as for gastroenteritis
Birdseye primrose, German primrose, primula (*Primula* spp)	Leaves and stems	Mouth/mucosal irritation, emesis, diarrhea, contact dermatitis	Emesis or gastric lavage, wash skin with soap and water, supportive treatment otherwise
Privet, hedge plant, lovage, prim (*Ligustrum vulgare*)	Whole plant including the berries (syringin, also referred to as ligustrin, an irritant glycoside; nuzhenids, secoiridoid glucosides)	Emesis, abdominal pain, diarrhea	Emesis or gastric lavage, treat as for gastroenteritis
Glory lily, climbing lily, gloriosa lily (*Gloriosa* spp)	Whole plant, particularly the tubers (colchicine)	Mouth/mucosal irritation, emesis, abdominal pain, diarrhea, renal failure	Emesis or gastric lavage, monitor renal function, supportive treatment otherwise

Table 22-2	Plants Producing Systemic Poisoning and Contact Irritation *Continued*		
NAME	POISONOUS PART OF PLANT (ACTIVE PRINCIPLE, IF KNOWN)	CLINICAL EFFECTS	THERAPY
Wisteria, wistaria, kidney bean tree (*Wisteria* spp)	Whole plant (uncharacterized glycoside, wistarine, and lectin)	Emesis, abdominal pain, diarrhea	Emesis or gastric lavage, treat as for gastroenteritis
Pokeweed, poke, American nightshade (*Phytolacca americana*)	Leaves and roots (phytolaccatoxin and related triterpenes)	Emesis, abdominal pain, diarrhea	Emesis or gastric lavage, treat as for gastroenteritis
Aloe (*Aloe* spp)	Sap (barbaloin, an anthraquinone glycoside)	Diarrhea	Emesis or gastric lavage, treat as for enteritis
Poison ivy, poison oak, poison sumac (*Toxicodendron* spp)	Whole plant (various unsaturated, long-chain, substituted catechols)	Allergic contact dermatitis (sequentially—erythema, edematous swelling, rash, blisters, pruritus, crusting, and scaling)	Prompt removal of allergen with running water, topical steroids
Monkshood, aconite wolfsbane (*Aconitum* spp)	Whole plant, especially leaves and roots (aconitine and related alkaloids)	Mouth/mucosal irritation, emesis, salivation, altered vision, mydriasis, weakness, incoordination, cardiac arrhythmias	Emesis or gastric lavage, monitor cardiac function, supportive treatment otherwise
Jerusalem cherry, nightshade, love apple, bittersweet, nipplefruit, Carolina horse nettle, star-potato vine, apple of Sodom, potato (*Solanum* spp)	Immature fruit (solanine glycoalkaloids)	Emesis, diarrhea	Emesis or gastric lavage, treat as for gastroenteritis
Elderberry (*Sambucus* spp)	Whole plant (cyanogenetic glycosides, primarily in the roots, stems, and leaves; and unidentified cathartic, primarily in the bark and roots)	Emesis, abdominal pain, diarrhea	Emesis or gastric lavage, treat as for enteritis
Crocus (*Colchicum* spp)	Whole plant (colchicine)	Emesis, abdominal pain, diarrhea, renal failure	Emesis or gastric lavage, monitor renal function, supportive treatment otherwise
Onion, garlic, field garlic (*Allium* spp)	Bulbs, bulblets, flowers, stems (*N*-propyl sulfide, methyl disulfide, and allyl disulfide)	Emesis, diarrhea, weakness, anorexia, methemoglobinemia, hemolytic anemia, Heinz bodies, liver damage	Emesis or gastric lavage, administer activated charcoal, supportive treatment otherwise
Rosary pea, crab's eyes (*Abrus precatorius*)	Chewed or broken seed (abrin)	Emesis, diarrhea (ingestion of one well-chewed seed may be fatal)	Emesis or gastric lavage, supportive treatment otherwise
Carolina allspice (*Calycanthus* spp)	Seeds (calycanthin and related alkaloids)	Emesis, incoordination, depression, convulsions, cardiac dysfunction	Emesis or gastric lavage, monitor cardiac function, control convulsions, supportive treatment otherwise

Table 22-3 Toxins: Clinical Effects from and Therapy for Bites of Venomous Animals

NAME	ENVENOMATION TOXIN	CLINICAL EFFECTS	THERAPY*
Spiders (*Latrodectus* spp), black widow spider, Australian red-back spider, katipo	Neurotoxin produced by females	Highly variable—no effects or local inflammation at bite site, regional lymphadenopathy, abdominal pain, vomiting, salivation, ataxia, seizures, coma, respiratory failure	*Local effects:* Cold compresses, parenteral steroids, and analgesics. *Systemic effects:* 10% calcium gluconate 5–10 ml IV slowly or methocarbamol or narcotic analgesics; as last resort consider antivenin
Atrax (Sydney funnel-web spider)	Neurotoxin (atraxotoxin) produced by males	*Minor effects:* Transient cardiovascular signs	Treatment of local bite site only
Spiders (*Loxosceles* spp), brown recluse spiders, fiddleback spiders	Complex of necrotizing enzymes and other proteins	*Minor local effects:* Swelling progresses to blister, then to black scab, then to ulcer	Treatment of local bite site only; if deep ulcer—surgical excision
Scorpion *Centuroides sculpturatus*	Neurotoxin	Local inflammation at sting site, restlessness, vomiting, difficulty in breathing, salivation, mydriasis, seizures, respiratory failure	*Local effects:* Cold compresses, parenteral steroids, and analgesics (narcotic analgesics are contraindicated). *Systemic effects:* Induce barbiturate anesthesia, administer specific antivenin
Bees (wild bees are more likely to attack than are the tame bees), wasps, hornets, ants	Toxins in saliva and/or stingers	Highly variable—no effects or local inflammation at sting site, restlessness, vomiting, difficulty in breathing, salivation, mydriasis, seizures, respiratory failure, hemolysis	*Local effects:* Treatment of local bite site only; if deep ulcer—surgical excision. *Systemic effects:* Cold compresses, parenteral steroids, and analgesics. Monitor packed cell volume for hemolysis
Ticks: *Dermacentor andersoni, Dermacentor variabilis, Ixodes holocyclus* (Australian tick), *Rhipicephalus* spp	Neurotoxin that affects neuromuscular junctions	Symmetric ascending paresis or paralysis (weakness, hypotonicity, ataxia, hyporeflexia), ticks present, dysphagia, regurgitation, respiratory failure	Removal of ticks, supportive treatment otherwise
Venomous snakes, North American pit vipers, eastern and western diamondback rattlesnakes, cottonmouth, water moccasin, copperhead, northern massasauga, southern pygmy rattlesnake	Toxins are hemotoxic, vasculotoxic, and necrogenic	*Mild effects:* Fang marks and mild pain, local swelling and hemorrhage that are not progressing in 1 h, no systemic signs. *Moderate effects:* Fang marks and pain, progressive local swelling, mild hypovolemic shock, bleeding from bite wound and venipunctures. *Severe effects:* Fang marks and pain, severe progressive swelling, severe hypovolemic shock, bleeding from multiple sites, muscle fasciculations, cardiac arrhythmias, renal failure	Wash wound thoroughly. *Mild effects:* Administer balanced electrolyte solution, supportive treatment otherwise. *Moderate effects:* Administer balanced electrolyte solution, administer 3–5 vials of antivenin IV slowly, monitor for anaphylaxis and progression of signs and cardiac function; treat shock if present, supportive treatment otherwise. *Severe effects:* Administer balanced electrolyte solution, administer 5–8 vials of antivenin IV slowly, monitor for anaphylaxis and progression of signs for 24 h (fails to respond—administer more antivenin to total dose of 15–20 vials) and cardiac function, treat shock if present, administer whole fresh blood and antibiotics, supportive treatment otherwise

Table 22–3	Toxins: Clinical Effects from and Therapy for Bites of Venomous Animals		
NAME	**ENVENOMATION TOXIN**	**CLINICAL EFFECTS**	**THERAPY***
Coral snake *Micrurus fulvius*	Neurotoxin and cardiotoxin	*Minor local effects:* Fang marks and pain. *Systemic effects:* Restlessness, ptosis, dysphagia, salivation, muscular weakness, paralysis	*Local effects:* Wash wound thoroughly. *Systemic effects:* Administer balanced electrolyte solution, administer 1–2 vials of antivenin IV or IM initially, if systemic signs worsen administer 5–7 vials IV slowly, monitor for anaphylaxis and cardiac and respiratory function, supportive treatment otherwise
Australian venomous snakes—most likely elapids; common brown snake (*Pseudonaja textilis*), western brown snake (*Pseudonaja nuchalis*, spotted brown snake or dugite (*Pseudonaja affinis*), king brown snake (*Pseudechis australis*), red-bellied black snake (*Pseudechis porphyriacus*), copperhead (*Austrelaps* spp), tiger snakes (*Notechis* spp), death adder (*Acanthopis antarcticus*), Taipan (*Oxyuranus scutellatus*)	Neurotoxins, coagulants, hemolysins, cytotoxins	*Local effects:* Fang marks are usually not seen. *Systemic effects:* Collapse, ataxia, ascending paralysis, mydriasis, salivation, vomiting, diarrhea, hematuria, myoglobinuria, bleeding from bite wound or multiple sites, respiratory failure	*Local effects:* Wash wound thoroughly. *Systemic effects:* Administer balanced electrolyte solution; administer antivenin IV slowly†; monitor for anaphylaxis, shock, cardiac and respiratory function; supportive treatment otherwise
Toads, *Bufo* spp	Toxins in their skin and parotid glands	Mouthing or ingestion of toads causes mouth irritation, salivation, vomiting	Emesis or gastric lavage, flush mouth with water, supportive treatment otherwise
Bufo marinus	Digitalis-like factor	Salivation, mouth irritation, cyanosis, collapse, cardiac arrhythmias, seizure, cardiac arrest	Emesis or gastric lavage, flush mouth with water, administer propranolol, control seizures, monitor cardiac function, supportive treatment otherwise

IM = intramuscular; IV = intravenous.

*Sources for antivenins:

1. *Latrodectus mactans* (black widow spider) antivenin, equine origin, Merck & Co, West Point, PA 19486; 215-699-5311.

2. Atrax (Sydney funnel-web spider) antivenin, Commonwealth Serum Laboratories, 212 Willoughby Road, Naremburn, NSW, Australia 2065; Tel. 4397011.

3. *Loxosceles* (brown recluse spider) antivenin—none available.

4. *Centuroides* (scorpions) antivenin, Iatrics Laboratory, Arizona State University, Tempe, AZ 85282; 602-966-3116.

5. Canine hyperimmune serum for Australian tick paralysis, Commonwealth Serum Laboratories (see entry 9 for addresses).

6. North American pit vipers (*Crotalidae*) polyvalent antivenin, equine origin, Wyeth Laboratories, Philadelphia, PA 19101; 215-688-4400.

7. North American pit vipers (*Crotalidae*) polyvalent antivenin, equine origin, Fort Dodge Laboratories, Fort Dodge, IA 50501; 515-955-4600.

8. *Micrurus fulvius* (North American coral snake) antivenin, equine origin, Wyeth Laboratories, Philadelphia, PA 19101; 215-688-4400.

9. Australian snake antivenins, Commonwealth Serum Laboratories, Australia Victoria—45 Poplar Road, Parkville 3052; Tel. 3891385. New South Wales—212 Willoughby Road, Naremburn 2065; Tel. 4397011. Queensland—86 Brookes Street, Fortitude Valley 4006; Tel. 524392. South Australia—282–284 Gilbert Street, Adelaide 5000; Tel. 516556. West Australia—416 Newcastle Street, Perth 6000; Tel. 328281.

†Choice of antivenin and initial antivenin dosage when the Australian snake has been identified:
Tiger snake (tiger snake antivenin)—3000 units
Tasmanian tiger snake (tiger snake antivenin)—6000 units
Chappell Island black tiger snake (tiger snake antivenin)—12,000 units
Death adder (death adder antivenin)—6000 units
Taipan (Taipan snake antivenin)—12,000 units
Copperhead (tiger snake antivenin)—3000 units
Brown snake dugite (brown snake antivenin)—1000 units
Black snake (tiger snake antivenin)—3000 units
King brown or mulga snake (tiger snake antivenin)—9000 units

Table 22–4 General Treatment of Poisoning

I. Preliminary instructions to owner
  A. Prevent further exposure to toxicant
  B. Topical exposure—cleanse the animal's skin or eyes with large amounts of clean, fresh water
  C. Induce vomiting—best if done within 2 h of ingestion
    1. Contraindications—ingestion of petroleum distillates, acids, alkali, and tranquilizers; CNS depression or hyperactivity; loss of postural or gag reflex
    2. Household remedies—syrup of ipecac (1–2 ml/kg PO), hydrogen peroxide (1–5 ml/kg PO)—these are generally ineffective and sometimes dangerous
  D. Allow the animal to drink as much water as it wants
  E. Owner should be instructed to bring vomitus or suspected toxic materials or their containers (labels) with the animal for possible analysis
II. Prevention of further absorption of toxicant
  A. Induction of vomiting
    1. Make sure stomach contains food material or liquid before inducing vomiting
    2. Apomorphine is most effective emetic in dogs; however, it may aggravate CNS depression Dose—0.04 mg/kg IV or 0.08 mg/kg IM or SC
    3. Antagonists to apomorphine
      a. Naloxone hydrochloride 0.04 mg/kg IV, IM, SC
      b. Levallorphan tartrate 0.02–0.2 mg/kg IV, IM, SC
      c. Nalorphine hydrochloride 0.1 mg/kg IV, IM, SC
    4. Xylazine is more effective in cats; however, it may aggravate CNS or respiratory depression Dose—1.1 mg/kg IM
    5. Antagonists to xylazine—yohimbine 0.1 mg/kg IV
  B. Gastric lavage—best if done within 2 h of ingestion
    1. Animal should be unconscious or under light anesthesia
    2. Cuffed endotracheal tube placed in trachea—tube tip should extend 2 inches (5 cm) beyond incisor teeth to prevent laryngotracheal aspiration and pneumonia
    3. Use large-bore stomach tube, at least as large as endotracheal tube
    4. Lower the head and thorax slightly below rest of the body
    5. Premeasure stomach tube from tip of nose to the last rib and mark the tube
    6. Pass lubricated stomach tube to 75% of premeasured mark; do not force the stomach tube
    7. Use 5–10 ml of water or lavage solution (normal saline solution or half-strength saline solution) per kilogram of body weight for each washing; use low pressure
    8. Aspirate with large aspirator bulb or 60-ml syringe
    9. Infusion and aspiration cycle should be repeated 10–15 times
  C. Gastrointestinal absorbents
    1. Activated charcoal of vegetable origin is best. Activated charcoal tablets (5 g) are easiest to handle
    2. Slurry of charcoal with water—1 g activated charcoal/5 ml water
    3. Dose—10 ml slurry of charcoal with water per kilogram of body weight
    4. Allow last slurry lavage to sit in stomach for 30 min; then administer a cathartic
  D. Cathartics
    1. Sodium sulfate (Glauber's salt). Dose—1 g/kg body weight PO
    2. Sorbitol (70%). Dose—3 ml/kg body weight PO
    3. Mineral oil. Dose—5–15 ml (dog) or 2–6 ml (cat) PO
  E. Enemas—use tepid water; avoid hexachlorophene soaps and hypertonic sodium phosphate enema solutions
III. Specific systemic antidotes and dosages for toxicant: See Table 22–5
IV. Hasten elimination of absorbed toxicant
  A. Maintain renal function and urine output
    1. Insert an IV catheter and infuse a multiple electrolyte solution or normal saline solution
    2. Diuretics—be sure animal is well hydrated first
      a. 10% dextrose/water 20 ml/kg alternated with 20 ml/kg normal saline solution or lactated Ringer's solution IV over 6–8 h
      b. 20% mannitol 5–10 ml/kg IV over 30 min—single dose only
      c. Furosemide—initial dose 2–4 mg/kg IV, if no response (second and third doses) 4–8 mg/kg IV
  B. Ion trapping—ionized compounds traverse cell membranes less readily than do nonionized compounds; therefore, ionized compounds are poorly resorbed by renal tubules
    1. Alkaline urine facilitates ionization of acid compounds, i.e., aspirin, barbiturates
    2. Acidic urine tends to ionize basic compounds, i.e., amphetamines, strychnine. To acidify the urine, give ammonium chloride 100–200 mg/kg/d orally in 3–4 divided doses
  C. Peritoneal dialysis may be tried for dialyzable toxins, e.g., ethylene glycol

Table 22-4	**General Treatment of Poisoning** *Continued*

V. Supportive measures for animal experiencing toxicant
  A. Respiratory support
    1. Adequate, patent airway
    2. Oxygen and positive-pressure ventilatory support
  B. Cardiovascular support
    1. Maintain adequate tissue perfusion; treat shock if present
    2. Identify and treat cardiac arrhythmias
    3. Correct electrolyte and acid-base imbalances
    4. Maintain normal hydration and adequate blood volume.
  C. Body temperature control
    1. Hypothermia—blankets, heat lamps, circulating water pads
    2. Hyperthermia—ice bags, cold water baths, alcohol baths
  D. Central nervous system support
    1. Depression—oxygen and respiratory support is best
    2. Hyperactivity and/or seizures
       a. Diazepam (dog: 5–40 mg IV to effect; cat: 2.5–5 mg or phenobarbital, 2–10 mg/kg IV, IM to effect)
       b. Seizures may cause cerebral edema; therapy with 20% mannitol and/or dexamethasone may be appropriate
       c. CNS hyperactivity—the animal should be placed in a quiet, dark room to prevent additional auditory or visual stimulation
VI. Owner education on toxicant
  A. Proper management of the animal and proper dosing of medications favor a positive outcome for the animal. Lack of owner compliance in following home treatments may result in an apparent therapeutic failure
  B. Animal frequently will poison itself repeatedly unless the owner makes sure that access to the source of the toxicant is removed

CNS = Central nervous system; IV = intravenous administration; IM = intramuscular administration; SC = subcutaneous administration; PO = oral administration.
Adapted from Bailey EM Jr: Emergency and general treatment of poisonings. *In* Kirk RW (ed): Current Veterinary Therapy IX. Philadelphia, WB Saunders Co, 1986, p 135.

functions. Immediate intervention may include establishment of a patent airway, artificial respiration, cardiac massage, and perhaps the application of defibrillation techniques. Following stabilization of the vital signs, the veterinarian may proceed with subsequent therapeutic measures as outlined in Table 22–4.

Administration of Systemically Acting Antidotes. There are a few specific systemically acting antidotal agents available for some of the known animal toxicants. A list of recommended antidotal procedures is presented in Table 22–5.

Plant-Induced Poisonings. Treatment of plant-induced poisonings may differ slightly from that of other toxicants. Whenever possible, the plant should be identified by direct examination. The common name of the plant, although useful as a starting point, may be inaccurate and is subject to a wide geographic variation (Hoskins, 1989).

Observation is usually recommended for asymptomatic animals who have ingested an un-identified plant. When it is known that a potentially dangerous plant has been eaten, however, vomiting should be induced immediately. Vomiting is generally more effective for removing plant material from the stomach than is gastric lavage. If vomiting is not induced or there is inadequate recovery of material from the stomach, lavage should be performed. Activated charcoal with water should be administered after vomiting has ceased or can be instilled at completion of lavage before the stomach tube is removed. When the delay following ingestion makes evacuation of the stomach contents of doubtful practicality, the administration of activated charcoal and water is advised.

If spontaneous vomiting occurred after plant ingestion with adequate return of stomach contents, induction of vomiting or gastric lavage usually is unnecessary. The animal should be monitored for fluid and electrolyte disturbances after profuse and protracted vomiting and diarrhea because hypovolemic shock can develop rapidly.

Table 22–5 Specific Systemic Antidotes and Dosages

TOXIC AGENT	SYSTEMIC ANTIDOTE	DOSAGE AND METHOD FOR TREATMENT
Acetaminophen	Acetylcysteine (Mucomyst)	140 mg/kg loading dose, orally or IV, then 70 mg/kg q6h for 3–5 treatments
Amphetamines	Chlorpromazine or acepromazine	0.05–1.0 mg/kg IM, IV, SC; administer only half dose if barbiturates have been given
Arsenic, mercury	Dimercaprol (BAL)	10% solution in oil; give 2.5–5.0 mg/kg IM (0.025–0.05 ml/kg) q4–6h for 2 d; bid for the next 2 d or until recovery
Atropine, belladonna alkaloids	Physostigmine salicylate	0.1–0.6 mg/kg (do not use neostigmine)
Bromides	Chlorides (sodium or ammonium salts)	0.5–1.0 g daily until recovery; hasten excretion
Carbon monoxide	Oxygen	Pure oxygen at normal or high pressure
Cholinergic agents, cholinesterase inhibitors	Atropine sulfate	0.2–2.0 mg/kg q4–6h IV, SC, IM; give 1/4 dose IV and remainder IM or SC as needed. Blocks only muscarinic effects. Atropine in oil may be injected for prolonged effect during the night. Avoid atropine intoxication
	Pralidoxime chloride 2-PAM (Protopam Chloride)	5% solution; 20–50 mg/kg IM or slow IV (0.2–1.0 mg/kg) injection (maximum dose is 500 mg/min), given bid for 24–36 h. 2-PAM alleviates nicotinic effect and regenerates cholinesterase. Morphine, succinylcholine, and phenothiazine tranquilizers are contraindicated
	Diphenhydramine	4 mg/kg q8h IV, SC, IM; alleviates nicotinic effects
Copper	D-penicillamine	10–15 mg/kg q12h
Coumarin-derivative anticoagulants	Vitamin K$_1$	2.5 mg/kg SC, IM, or IV (slowly in 10 ml 5% dextrose/water) q12h until normal coagulation times. Follow with oral dosage 1.0–2.5 mg/kg divided tid or bid for 5–7 d
Cyanide	Methemoglobin (amyl nitrite and sodium nitrite are used to form methemoglobin)	Crush 1 ampule amyl nitrite in gauze pad and hold 1 inch from nostrils for 15–30 s/min inhalation; prepare sodium nitrite for IV; then stop amyl nitrite and slowly inject 16 mg/kg (0.5 ml/kg) of 3% sodium nitrite solution
	Sodium thiosulfate	Follow with 25% solution at dosage of 30–40 mg/kg (0.12–0.16 ml/kg) IV. If treatment is repeated, use only sodium thiosulfate
Diphacinone and other long-acting anticoagulants	Vitamin K$_1$	5 mg/kg SC or IM as a loading dose. Follow within 6–12 h with oral dosage of 5 mg/kg given divided tid or bid for 21 d
Fluoride	Calcium gluconate (10% solution)	3–15 ml IV (slowly)
Fluoroacetate (Compound 1080)	Glyceral monoacetin	0.1–0.5 mg/kg IM hourly for several hours (total 2–4 mg/kg); or diluted (0.5%–1.0%) IV (danger of hemolysis). Monoacetin is available only from chemical supply houses
Lead	Calcium disodium vensenate (CaEDTA)	100 mg/kg divided into 4 daily doses given SC after dilution to 10 mg CaEDTA/ml of 5% dextrose/water for 5 d. Daily dose should not exceed 2 g and should not be continued for more than 5 consecutive days. May need to be repeated for an additional 5 d
	D-Penicillamine	110 mg/kg daily for 1- to 2-week courses separated by 1-week intervals. Daily dose should be divided and given at 6- to 8-hour intervals
	Succimer or mesodimercaptosuccinic acid (Chemet, McNeil)	10 mg/kg orally tid for 5 days, followed by 10 mg/kg orally bid for 14 d

Table 22–5	**Specific Systemic Antidotes and Dosages** *Continued*	
TOXIC AGENT	**SYSTEMIC ANTIDOTE**	**DOSAGE AND METHOD FOR TREATMENT**
Metaldehyde	Diazepam	2.5–20 mg IV as needed
	Pentobarbital	To effect
Methanol and ethylene glycol	Ethanol	Treatment within 24 h of ingestion. Dog: 5.5 ml/kg 20% solution IV q4h for 5 treatments and then q6h for 4 more treatments. Cat: 5.0 ml/kg 20% solution IV q6h for 5 treatments and then q8h for 4 more treatments. Treatment after 24 h of ingestion: ethanol treatment is not indicated
	4-Methylpyrazole (Antizol-Vet; Orphan Medical, Minnetonka, MN)	Treatment within 24 h of ingestion. Dog: 20 mg/kg initially, followed by 15 mg/kg IV at 12 and 24 h and 5 mg/kg IV 36 h after first dose. Treatment after 24 h of ingestion: 4-methylpyrazole treatment is not indicated. Methylpyrazole is not effective in cats
Morphine and related drugs	Naloxone hydrochloride	0.04 mg/kg IV, IM, SC
	Levallorphan tartrate	0.02–0.2 mg/kg IV, IM, SC
	Nalorphine hydrochloride	0.1 mg/kg IV, IM, SC. Dog: max 5 mg; cat: max 1 mg
Oxalates	Calcium gluconate (10% solution)	3–15 ml IV (slowly)
Phenothiazine	Methylamphetamine	0.1–0.2 mg/kg IV. Available only in tablet form
	Diphenhydramine hydrochloride	For CNS depression: 2–5 mg/kg IV for extrapyramidal symptoms
Thallium	Diphenylthiocarbazone (Dithizone)	Treatment within 36 h of ingestion: dogs only—70 mg/kg orally tid for 5 d
	Prussian blue	100 mg/kg orally tid for 5 d
	Potassium chloride	Give simultaneously with Dithizone or Prussian blue, 2–6 ml KCl orally/d in divided doses or 20–30 mEq/L IV fluids
Zinc	Calcium disodium vensenate (CaEDTA)	100 mg/kg divided into daily doses given SC after dilution to 10 mg CaEDTA/ml of 5% dextrose/water for 5 d. Daily dose should not exceed 2 g and should not be continued for more than 5 consecutive days. May need to be repeated for an additional 5 d
	D-Penicillamine	110 mg/kg daily for 1- to 2-week courses separated by 1-week intervals. Daily dose should be divided and given at 6- to 8-hour intervals

CNS = Central nervous system; IV = intravenous administration; IM = intramuscular administration; SC = subcutaneous administration; bid = twice daily; tid = three times daily.

Adapted from Bailey EM Jr: Emergency and general treatment of poisonings. *In* Kirk RW: Current Veterinary Therapy IX. Philadelphia, WB Saunders, 1986, p 139.

There are relatively few specific antidotes for plant poisonings. In general, the recommended management depends on the course and severity of the intoxication in the particular animal. The amount and nature of the toxins in any plant species may vary widely with geographic location, growing condition, maturity, and the plant part ingested (see Table 22–2). Good clinical judgment must prevail.

Bites from Venomous Animals. Treatment of envenomations produced by the bites or stings of spiders, scorpions, ticks, bees, and snakes differs according to the venomous animal involved. Whenever possible, the venomous animal should be identified by direct examination. The signs produced by envenomation vary greatly depending on the venomous animal involved. Not every exposure to a venomous animal results in significant envenomation. Because of protection provided by the haircoat of dogs and cats and, in some cases, because of inherent resistance to the toxins, envenomation by spiders and scorpions is probably much less common among dogs and cats than among humans. General treatment for envenomations produced by the bites or stings of the more common spiders, scorpions, bees, and ticks is presented in Table 22–3.

On the other hand, envenomation by snakes commonly occurs among dogs and cats that wander into areas inhabited by snakes. Snake venoms are complex, lethal animal toxins containing enzymes and nonenzymatic proteins. The severity of snakebite varies greatly depending on the snake species, size and age of the snake, volume of venom injected, amount of toxins in the venom, and the size of the animal bitten. Some of the most lethal venomous snakes reside in Australia. Early administration of antivenin and supportive treatment are the basis for successful management of snake envenomation. Because of the high cost and limited availability of antivenin and the possibility of serious adverse reactions to it, every effort should be made to confirm severity of envenomation before the administration of antivenin.

Extreme caution is advised in the use of first aid or in-hospital surgical procedures in cases of snakebite. Owners should be instructed to present the bitten animal as quickly as possible without attempting first aid measures. Immobilization of a bitten extremity and immediate cooling in ice may prevent venom spread. Ice should not, however, be used if it takes more than 30 minutes to get the bitten animal to a veterinary hospital. On arrival at the hospital, a thorough physical examination should be performed to look for fang marks, assess the severity of envenomation, evaluate systemic changes, and examine for cardiac arrhythmias, bleeding diatheses, and shock. General treatment for snakebite according to snake species is presented in Table 22–3.

Toad Poisoning. Many members of the toad genus *Bufo* contain toxins in their skin and parotid glands. Mouthing or ingestion of toads by dogs and cats may cause profuse salivation and irritation of mucous membranes. Only the large toad *Bufo marinus*, when mouthed or ingested, may cause a potentially fatal poisoning. The treatment of toad poisoning is presented in Table 22–3.

References and Supplemental Reading

Bailey EM Jr: Emergency and general treatment of poisonings. *In* Kirk RW, Bonagura JD (eds): Current Veterinary Therapy X. Philadelphia, WB Saunders, 1989, p 116.

Carothers M, Chew DJ: Management of cholecalciferol rodenticide toxicity. Compend Contin Educ Pract Vet 13:1058, 1991.

Dumonceaux GA, Beasley VR: Emergency treatments for police dogs used for illicit drug detection. J Am Vet Med Assoc 197:185, 1990.

Hoskins JD: Plants and their clinical importance. Vet Technician 10:93, 1989.

Lampe KF, McCann MA: AMA Handbook of Poisonous and Injurious Plants. Chicago, American Medical Association, 1985.

Lewis PF: Snakebite in animals in Australia. Twelfth Annu Rep Postgrad Found Vet Sci 36:287, 1977.

Lockey RF: The imported fire ant: Immunopathologic significance. Hosp Pract 15:109, 1990.

Oehme FW: Emergency kit for treatment of small animal poisoning (antidotes, drugs, equipment). *In* Kirk RW (ed): Current Veterinary Therapy VIII. Philadelphia, WB Saunders, 1983, p 92.

Osweiler GD, Carson TL, Buck WB, eds: Clinical and Diagnostic Veterinary Toxicology, 3rd ed. Dubuque, IA, Kendall-Hunt Publishing, 1985.

Environmental Injuries

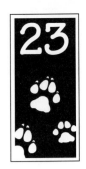

Teresa M. Rieser and Lesley G. King

ELECTRICAL SHOCK

Although animals of any age are susceptible to environmental injuries, puppies and kittens are especially at risk because of their immature internal regulatory mechanisms that predispose them to hypothermia and make them ill-equipped to deal with hyperthermia. In addition, their native curiosity puts them at risk as they explore their environment for the first time.

In puppies and kittens, most injuries associated with electrical shock are from chewing on household electrical cords rather than from high-voltage or lightening strike injuries. As young animals become ambulatory and begin to explore their environment, injuries from electrical cords become a risk. One study found the average age of affected animals to be 3.5 months (Kolata and Burrows, 1981). Clinical experience suggests a higher incidence in puppies than in kittens. There appears to be a seasonal distribution, with most cases occurring between March and August. The distribution may correspond to increased use of electrical devices in the household but may also be related to increased purchase of new puppies and kittens in the springtime.

Pathophysiology

The severity of an electrical injury depends on the type (alternating current is more dangerous than direct current) and the intensity of the current (amperage). Most households have 60 Hz alternating current. Injuries occur because of the heat generated locally in tissue by the current and by depolarization of excitable cell membranes due to the electrical charge.

Alternating current has been found to cause seizures and paralysis of the respiratory center in puppies. In addition to tonic-clonic seizures, the lips, tongue, and oral cavity of the animal are frequently burned. These burns, which may later be accompanied by considerable edema, result from heat that is generated by the flow of electrical current both through tissue and across an air gap between the electric cord and the animal's mouth (arc burns). This heat can result in coagulation of tissue proteins, thrombosis of small vessels, and degenerative changes in the walls of small arteries. When current passes through cardiac muscle it can induce ventricular fibrillation.

Finally, chewing on electrical cords is associated with the development of noncardiogenic pulmonary edema. This type of pulmonary edema results from an increase in vascular endothelial permeability and is quite different from the pulmonary edema associated with left-sided congestive heart failure. The exact mechanism behind the change in permeability is not fully understood but may involve an increase in sympathetic nervous stimulation. Shock may occur because of fluid loss, decreased cardiac output, and hypoxia.

Clinical Findings

Most animals stiffen immediately upon biting an electrical cord. They may then exhibit tonic-clonic seizure activity that may include urination or defecation. Upon regaining consciousness, they may be weak and ataxic. Some

511

animals stop breathing immediately and die because of ventricular fibrillation.

Burns are commonly seen at the commissures of the lips, gums, tongue, and hard palate and may be accompanied by edema of the oral soft tissues. Animals may present a few days after the injury with the complaint of dysphagia as a result of oral burns.

Acute respiratory distress can develop as early as 30 minutes after the insult but may not be seen until as long as 24 to 36 hours after the injury. Auscultation commonly reveals harsh lung sounds, and crackles may be present. The degree of dyspnea is variable. It may be mild enough to be clinically inapparent or severe enough to result in cyanosis. Signs of hypovolemic shock or cardiac arrhythmias may be recognized, including pale mucous membranes, tachycardia, cool extremities, and weak pulses or the presence of pulse deficits.

Diagnosis

Frequently the diagnosis is made based on a history of the owner seeing the animal bite the electrical cord or finding a frayed electrical cord in the environment. The presence of oral lesions is consistent with electrical cord injury but not diagnostic because many other injuries, including thermal and chemical burns, may result in the same oral lesions. Hematology and serum chemistries are usually within normal limits.

If the history is unknown and oral lesions are equivocal, survey thoracic radiographs may assist in diagnosis, especially if the animal develops respiratory signs. If noncardiogenic pulmonary edema occurs, there is classically an interstitial/alveolar pattern with a caudodorsal distribution (Fig. 23–1) as compared with the perihilar distribution of cardiogenic pulmonary edema or the cranioventral distribution of aspiration pneumonia. It is important to rule out congenital cardiac disease before making the diagnosis of noncardiogenic pulmonary edema secondary to electrical shock injury. If there is a question about the presence of cardiac disease, echocardiography or placement of a pulmonary artery catheter to measure pulmonary capillary wedge pressures may be helpful, although rarely needed. In addition to cardiac disease, other causes of noncardiogenic pulmonary edema such as head trauma, seizures, and episodes of airway obstruction should be ruled out. Arterial blood gases may show hypoxemia, the severity of which corresponds with the degree of pulmonary injury. Most animals with hypoxemia also have hypocarbia, as low blood oxygen levels drive the hyperventilation. If the pulmonary insult is extremely severe, hypercarbia may occur. Pulse oximetry can be used to evaluate oxygen saturation (SaO_2) noninvasively and is a useful technique for real-time monitoring of critical animals.

Therapy

Obviously, the first priority is removing the animal from the source of current. The electric cord must be unplugged or turned off before attempts are made to help the animal. Next, the ABCs of emergency medicine should be followed. Of first importance is to determine whether the animal has a patent airway. Upper airway obstruction may occur due to edema following the electrical burns and can be diag-

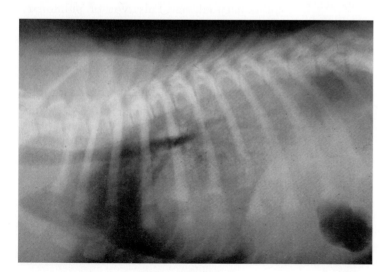

Figure 23–1. Lateral radiograph of a dog with noncardiogenic pulmonary edema. Noncardiogenic pulmonary edema has a caudodorsal distribution. (Courtesy of Dr. Kenneth Drobatz, University of Pennsylvania.)

nosed by the presence of inspiratory distress or stridor. If the airway is not patent or the animal is unconscious, endotracheal intubation should be attempted. It may be necessary to use a small endotracheal tube, and animals with severe airway obstruction may require short-term anesthesia before an airway can be obtained. If the oral approach of tracheal intubation is not possible, an emergency tracheostomy can be performed and a cuffed tracheostomy tube placed.

If the animal is not spontaneously breathing, manual mechanical ventilation should be initiated, with an AMBU bag attached to an oxygen supply line. If the animal is breathing on its own but is in respiratory distress, supplemental flow-by or mask oxygen can be provided until a full assessment can be completed. An intravenous catheter should be placed, and, if the animal is cardiovascularly unstable, therapy should be aimed at achieving cardiovascular stability by treating hypovolemic shock with cautious fluid administration. If the animal is stable but requires ongoing oxygen supplementation, an oxygen cage, mask, or nasal cannula can provide it.

Treatment of noncardiogenic pulmonary edema is supportive, providing time for resolution of the pulmonary changes. Supplemental oxygen should be provided to maintain the partial pressure of oxygen (PaO_2) above 70 mmHg or SaO_2 greater than 92%. Usually, oxygen supplementation is started at a FIO_2 of 40% and increased until the animal has reached an acceptable SaO_2 or PaO_2. Because of the risk of oxygen toxicity, it is always preferable to use the minimal amount of oxygen supplementation needed to maintain adequate oxygenation. If supplemental oxygen alone is inadequate to maintain oxygenation in the animal, mechanical ventilation with the use of positive end-expiratory pressure (PEEP) is indicated. Diuretics such as furosemide can be used (0.5 to 1 mg/kg intravenously or intramuscularly) but have not been proved to be of benefit because the edema is caused by vascular permeability rather than increased venous hydrostatic pressure. If diuretics are used, it is important that they do not create hypovolemia as any compromise of cardiac output can be detrimental. There is no evidence that the use of corticosteroids is of any benefit in noncardiogenic pulmonary edema, and they may be detrimental by causing immunosuppression and predisposing to secondary bacterial pneumonia. Clinical evaluation, serial arterial blood gases, and thoracic radiographs can determine response to therapy.

Burns of the face and oral cavity are usually treated with conservative debridement. Even if there is no evidence of respiratory difficulty, the animal should be hospitalized for at least 24 hours after the injury, as pulmonary edema may develop later. The wounds should be kept clean, and broad-spectrum antimicrobial agents can be used if needed. If burns are severe, reconstructive surgery may be required, but this is usually delayed until 3 to 4 weeks after the injury. Burns may take a few weeks to heal, and serial debridements should be performed as dead tissue demarcates and sloughs. While oral burns are healing it may be necessary to feed soft foods, or, if the animal is unwilling to eat, alternate routes of enteral feeding, such as a nasoesophageal or percutaneous endoscopic gastrostomy tube can be considered.

Long-Term Prognosis and Owner Education

When animals present with noncardiogenic pulmonary edema secondary to an electrical shock injury there is a significant mortality rate (38.5% in one study). The first 24 to 48 hours are critical. If the animal responds to supplemental oxygen and pulmonary edema begins to resolve, the prognosis is good for long-term survival. In most cases, there is no permanent pulmonary damage and no risk of spontaneous recurrence of edema. If the pulmonary edema is severe and nonresponsive to therapy, the prognosis is guarded at best. Most oral burns heal well with conservative therapy and do not require reconstructive surgery. Owners should be instructed about the risks of electrical cords, and any damaged cords should be discarded.

THERMAL AND CHEMICAL BURNS

Burns occur for a variety of reasons. In young puppies and kittens, heating pads or heat lamps are frequently implicated. These types of burn may not become apparent until days after the insult. Other causes of burns include chemical agents, scalds, and direct flame burns from house and industrial fires. In the case of house fires, the veterinarian should consider not only the burns but also the possibility of carbon monoxide toxicity and significant pulmonary damage from smoke inhalation.

Classification

The severity of a burn is determined by both the depth of the burn and the percentage of affected total body surface area (TBSA). A superficial burn involves only the epidermis with minimal tissue damage. Partial thickness burns may be either superficial or deep. A superficial partial thickness burn involves the epidermis and the superficial dermis, whereas a deep partial thickness burn is associated with damage that extends into the mid to deep dermis. A total thickness burn damages the entire epidermis and dermis. The percentage of affected TBSA can be estimated using the rule of nines. According to this scheme, each forelimb represents 9% of TBSA, each hindlimb is 18%, the head and neck is 9%, and the dorsal and ventral thorax/abdomen are each 18%.

Pathophysiology

At the site of the burn, the insult results in vascular damage and the release of a variety of vasoactive substances. This causes a local increase in capillary permeability and movement of albumin and plasma water into the interstitium. When large portions of the TBSA are burned, the loss of fluid and protein may result in profound hypovolemia and hypoproteinemia. By 48 hours after the burn injury, the integrity of the microvasculature returns to normal, and edema fluid is gradually resorbed. At this point, there is considerable resorption of solute from the burned tissue, causing an increase in urine output, which can be attributed to an obligate solute diuresis. At the site of burn injuries, there is usually a rim of ischemia, where cells have been damaged by the burn but are potentially still viable. Over time, these cells may die, changing a partial thickness burn to a full thickness injury. The presence of necrotic tissue represents a route of invasion for bacteria, of which *Staphylococcus intermedius* and *Streptococcus* spp are usually the first to colonize a burn. Within a few days coliforms and *Pseudomonas* spp may also be present. These animals are at high risk of infection with nosocomial gram-negative pathogens, which predisposes to sepsis and the systemic inflammatory response syndrome. Because the most common route for the spread of nosocomial infection is on the hands of hospital personnel, it is imperative that medical staff wash their hands before and after handling these fragile animals.

After a serious burn injury, cardiac output is markedly decreased, attributable at least in part to hypovolemia from the massive fluid shifts that are occurring. Also contributing to the decrease in cardiac output are increases in both systemic vascular resistance and pulmonary vascular resistance, caused by high levels of circulating catecholamines. Myocardial function may be compromised by the release of myocardial depressant factors. Once hypovolemia has been corrected, a hyperdynamic state can be expected, with an increased heart rate, increased cardiac output, and decreased systemic vascular resistance. Even a week after the insult, cardiac output and heart rate may still be increased, and systemic vascular resistance may still be low. Generalized edema may accumulate because of the decreased plasma oncotic pressure.

In animals with burns of more than 20% TBSA, impairment of humoral and cell-mediated immunity occurs, placing the animal at special risk of infection and sepsis. Hemolysis can occur because of direct thermal injury as well as damaged microcirculation.

Immediately after a thermal injury, the metabolic rate is decreased. Within a few days, the animal becomes hypermetabolic. The elevation in metabolic rate is variable but may approach 50% above resting metabolic rate. The hypermetabolic state continues until wound closure.

Damage to the pulmonary system can occur from the inhalation of heated particles, which results in direct damage to the respiratory tract mucosa. Severe laryngospasm caused by direct heat can lead to an effective upper airway obstruction. In the trachea and lower airways, thermal damage from inhaled particles can result in congestion, hemorrhage, ulceration, mucosal sloughing, and increased bronchial secretions. Edema and swelling of the airway mucosa can lead to obstruction of the small bronchioles. Damage to the mucociliary escalator leads to loss of the normal protective barrier in the lung, leaving the animal open to secondary bacterial infection. This, coupled with the effects of thermal injuries on the immune system, makes the animal especially susceptible to superimposed pneumonia and sepsis.

In addition to the direct respiratory system injury, damage also occurs from inhaled water and lipid-soluble gases. The most important of these is carbon monoxide, which binds with great affinity to hemoglobin, thus decreasing the amount of hemoglobin available to bind oxygen and deliver it to the tissues. Other inhaled gases such as hydrogen cyanide interfere with cellular metabolism. Increased amounts of inhaled carbon dioxide contribute to hypoxemia as well as increase the toxicity of the other inhaled gases.

Because of hypoproteinemia, the potential for the systemic inflammatory response syndrome, and the requirement for high rates of

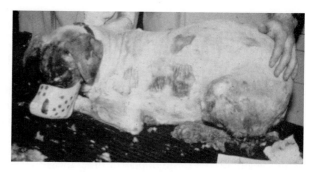

Figure 23–2. Thermal burn injuries in a dog. (Courtesy of Dr. Kenneth Drobatz, University of Pennsylvania.)

fluid supplementation, animals with severe burns are at a high risk of developing pulmonary edema. The local damage to the respiratory system, coupled with the systemic changes, increases the risk for development of acute respiratory distress syndrome (ARDS). The risk period for development of ARDS is greatest 2 to 4 days after the thermal injury.

Clinical Findings

The clinical appearance of burns varies with the degree. Superficial burns are typically hyperemic and painful, and desquamation may be present. Partial thickness burns have decreased sensitivity and are typically exudative, and there is normally some resistance to pulling hair. Full-thickness burns are classically associated with the formation of brown to black eschar that feels leathery and may be accompanied by subcutaneous edema. Hair is usually missing, but, if it is present, it epilates easily. Full-thickness burns are not painful.

When animals have suffered severe thermal injuries, they commonly exhibit signs of hypovolemic shock, such as pale mucous membranes, tachycardia, and weak pulses. Smoke inhalation and direct thermal injury can result in respiratory distress from laryngeal edema, which is manifested by signs of airway obstruction such as an increase in upper airway noise or inspiratory stridor. In addition, animals may be hypoxic from damage to the bronchial mucosa or pulmonary edema. Auscultation may reveal harsh lung sounds or crackles. Animals that have been in house fires commonly present with burns on the extremities, such as the paws and ear pinnae, and also often have corneal ulceration.

Diagnosis

Diagnosis is usually based on historical and physical examination findings (Figs. 23–2 and 23–3). Veterinarians can employ the rule of nines to determine the extent of the injuries. Smoke inhalation and the severity of pulmonary damage can be assessed with survey thoracic radiographs, pulse oximetry, and arterial blood gases. In addition, carboxyhemoglobin measurements may be considered if carbon monoxide poisoning is a concern. Complete blood count and chemistry profiles are of use in assessing the hematologic and electrolyte disturbances,

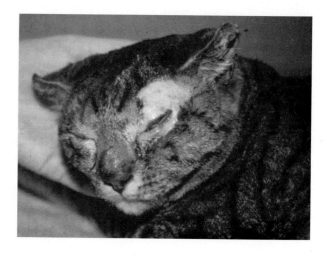

Figure 23–3. Thermal burn injuries in a cat. (Courtesy of Dr. Kenneth Drobatz, University of Pennsylvania.)

including serum magnesium concentration. Hypomagnesemia frequently occurs in animals with severe burn injuries and can cause ventricular arrhythmias, neurologic signs, and refractory hypokalemia. Cultures from burns, blood, and transtracheal washes may also be indicated to guide antibiotic therapy.

Because the animal is at risk for the development of disseminated intravascular coagulation (DIC), coagulation profiles including prothrombin time and partial thromboplastin time, measurement of fibrin degradation products, and platelet count should be performed. If these tests are not available, an activated clotting time can provide some information, and a blood smear allows estimation of platelet numbers and evaluation of red and white blood cell morphology.

Treatment of Thermal Burns

The first goals of treatment are to ensure that the airway is patent and that the animal can breathe without distress. Animals with laryngeal obstruction may require temporary intubation or tracheostomy. If carbon monoxide toxicity is a concern, a high concentration (80% to 100%) of inspired oxygen should be administered for at least 30 minutes. This aids in the rapid clearance of carbon monoxide by displacing it from hemoglobin. Later, a lower inspired oxygen concentration can be used, if necessary.

If shock is present, crystalloid fluids should be used to stabilize the animal. If a peripheral intravenous catheter cannot be placed because all of the animal's legs have suffered burn injuries, an intraosseous catheter can be used. Intraosseous catheters are especially effective for the very young animal because they are well tolerated and relatively easily placed. Alternatively, a central venous catheter can be considered, but these have been associated with an increased risk of thromboembolism and sepsis in humans. Because of the increased microvascular permeability and potential loss of colloid into the interstitium, if possible colloids should be avoided in the first 6 to 8 hours after the injury. After 8 hours, colloid therapy can be instituted. Plasma can be administered at 6 to 12 ml/kg intravenously three times a day, or synthetic colloids such as hetastarch can be used at up to 20 to 40 ml/kg per day. Fresh or fresh frozen plasma has the advantage of supplying albumin, acute phase proteins, and clotting factors. Whole blood or packed red blood cells may also be indicated if the packed cell volume decreases. If needed, pressors (dopamine 3 to 10 μg/kg per minute constant rate of infusion [CRI]) can be used to maintain cardiac output; however, they should not be used in lieu of adequate fluid resuscitation.

After initial resuscitation, the rate of fluid therapy should be guided by clinical cardiovascular parameters and urine output. The minimum acceptable rate of urine production is 1 to 2 ml/kg per hour, but urine output may be higher than expected because of the obligate solute diuresis that occurs after burn injuries. If the urine output is high, increased fluid replacement may be required to avoid hypovolemia. Because of the massive fluid shifts and loss of electrolyte and protein-rich fluid, serial electrolyte, albumin, and colloid osmotic pressure monitoring are all important for guiding fluid therapy. Serum magnesium concentration should be monitored, and, if hypomagnesemia occurs, it should be supplemented (magnesium sulfate 1 mEq/kg per 24 hours CRI). Neither steroids nor antimicrobial agents are used prophylactically in burn injuries.

For animals with smoke inhalation, systemic antimicrobial agents are not indicated unless there is evidence of pneumonia or sepsis. If respiratory distress is present, all medications should be administered parenterally, and oral medications should be avoided. To help support the respiratory musculature and dilate the small airways, bronchodilators such as aminophylline (puppies: 10 mg/kg orally or intravenously every 8 hours; kittens: 5 mg/kg orally every 8 to 12 hours or 4 mg/kg intramuscularly or intravenously every 12 hours) or terbutaline (puppies: 0.03 mg/kg orally every 8 hours; kittens: 1.25 mg orally every 8 hours or 0.01 mg/kg subcutaneously every 4 hours) can be used. Serial thoracic radiographs are of value to monitor pulmonary changes, and serial arterial blood gas measurements can be used to guide oxygen therapy. Saline nebulization and chest wall coupage should be used to optimize clearance of pulmonary secretions. If the degree of respiratory impairment is severe, positive-pressure ventilation with PEEP may be indicated.

Animals suffering severe burns exist in a hypermetabolic state for an extended period of time as their wounds heal. It is essential that they receive nutritional support, and, when possible, enteral feeding is the preferred method. Caloric requirements should be calculated to ensure that food intake is adequate. Caloric requirements can be calculated as $M = 132 \times (WT_{KG})^{0.75}$ for puppies and $M = 60 \times WT_{KG}$ for cats. If the animal is unable or unwilling to eat, a nasoesophageal or pharyngostomy tube can be placed. If the animal has suffered severe burns to the face or neck, a gastrostomy tube can be placed endoscopically. If the animal cannot tolerate enteral feeding, total parenteral nutrition can be administered. Total parenteral nutrition cannot be administered through a peripheral catheter because of the hyperosmolarity of the solution and should only be given through a central line. Partial parenteral nutrition, which is less hyperosmolar, can be administered through a peripheral line but will not meet all of the animal's nutritional requirements.

Once the animal has been stabilized, the local burns should be clipped and flushed with cold saline or water. Ice packs should be avoided, as excessive cold may result in further ischemic insult to the already damaged tissues. Wounds should be flushed or immersed for at least 30 minutes. Care should be taken to prevent systemic hypothermia if the surface area of the wound is large. Water-soluble topical ointments should be applied after wound debridement. The ointment of choice is silver sulfadiazine. Sterile occlusive dressing should then be applied to protect the wound and prevent dessication. Wounds should be cleaned, debrided, and redressed at least once daily. Purulent exudates and wound biopsy specimens should be cultured if infection is suspected either locally or systemically. Large full-thickness burns may require aggressive surgical excision. Sepsis is a major complication of burn injuries, so an aseptic technique cannot be overemphasized. Hospital staff treating burn animals should wash their hands before handling the animal, and every effort should be made to keep bandages clean and dry.

Pain management is an important issue in the treatment of burn injuries. Narcotics such as oxymorphone (0.04 to 0.2 mg/kg intravenously or intramuscularly every 4 to 6 hours as needed) or butorphanol (0.2 to 0.4 mg/kg intravenously or intramuscularly every 4 to 6 hours as needed) provide good pain control that is sparing of the cardiovascular system. Alternatively, transdermal fentanyl patches provide an excellent option for more long-term control. Fentanyl patches are supplied in 25-, 50-, 75-, and 100-μg/h sizes (Table 23–1).

Treatment of Chemical Burns

The severity of burns caused by exposure to chemicals depends on the chemical, its concentration, duration of contact, mechanism of action, and the depth of penetration. Most chemi-

Table 23–1	Fentanyl Patch Dosages for the Dog	
WEIGHT (kg)	PATCH SIZE (μg/h)
<10	25
10–20	50
20–30	75
>30	100

cal burns should initially be treated in the same way as a thermal burn, with copious lavage. After lavage, the appropriate neutralizing agent can be applied (Table 23–2). Hot tar injuries require emulsification to facilitate tar removal. Neosporin ointment is a good emulsifying agent (commonly available in veterinary clinics) because it contains the emulsificant polyoxyethylene sorbitan (Tween-80). Other emulsifying agents can also be used.

Long-Term Prognosis and Survival

Prognosis and survival for animals with burn wounds depend on the severity and extent of the burns. Animals with burns greater than 50% of TBSA have a guarded to poor prognosis. Pulmonary damage from smoke inhalation is a life-threatening condition and should also carry a guarded prognosis. In addition, complications of pneumonia and sepsis lead to further worsening of the prognosis. Owners should be aware that animals with severe burn injuries might require multiple reconstructive surgeries. If the injuries have occurred in puppies and kittens because of heating pads or hot lamps, owners should be educated about the dangers of these devices, and alternatives such as well-wrapped hot water bottles can be suggested.

HYPERTHERMIA

Hyperthermia is an excessive elevation in body temperature. With hyperthermia, the internal hypothalamic thermoregulatory set point does not change. In contrast, with fever, the internal set point of the body is moved upward. Hyperthermia results from the inability of the body's heat-dissipating mechanisms to keep up with heat production. Mechanisms of heat dissipation include panting, increased respiratory rate, anorexia, postural changes, and cutaneous vasodilation. One of the most common causes of hyperthermia is the confinement of animals in

Table 23–2 Injurious Chemical Agents

AGENT	CLINICAL PRESENTATION	MECHANISM OF SYSTEMIC TOXICITY	IMMEDIATE CLEANSING	NEUTRALIZATION
Common acids				
Sulfuric, nitric, hydrochloric, trichloroacetic	Yellow, brown, gray, or black eschar	Vapor	Water and soap	Magnesium hydroxide or sodium bicarbonate solution
Hydrofluoric	Erythema with central necrosis	None	Water	Calcium gluconate (10%) subcutaneously
Oxalic	Chalky white indolent ulcers	Ingestion only	Water	Calcium gluconate (10%)
Phenol (carbolic) and analogues	Painless, white or brown skin burn	Skin absorption	Water	Ethyl alcohol (10%) or glycerol
Chromic	Ulceration, blisters	Vapor	Water	Sodium hyposulfite
Hypochlorous (Clorox)	Second-degree burn	None	Water	Sodium thiosulfate (1%)
Other acids				
Tungstic, picric, tannic, cresylic, formic	Hard eschar	Skin absorption	Water	Cover with oil
Lyes (alkali)				
Sodium hydroxide, potassium hydroxide, calcium hydroxide, barium hydroxide, lithium hydroxide	Bullous erythema or slimy or slick eschar	Ingestion only	Water	Weak (0.5% to 5.0%) acetic acid; lemon juice
Ammonia	Bullous erythema or slimy or slick eschar	Vapor	Water	Weak (0.5% to 5.0%) acetic acid; lemon juice
Lime	Bullous erythema or slimy or slick eschar	Ingestion only	Brush off lime in water	Weak (0.5% to 5.0%) acetic acid; lemon juice
Alkyl mercury salts	Erythema, blisters	Skin absorption from blisters	Water and remove blisters	Copious irrigation
Sodium metal	Painful deep burns	None	Cover with oil	None except excision
Vesicants				
Mustard gas	Painful bullae	Vapor	Water; open vesicles during copious lavage	British antilewisite (BAL)
Tear gas	Erythema, ulcers	Vapor	Water	No specific agent
Phosphorus	Erythema to third-degree burn	Tissue absorption	Water; cold water packs	Copper sulfate for identification only
Ethylene oxide	Erythema to third-degree burn	None	Allow to vaporize; then water lavage	No specific agent

From Lee-Paritz DE, Pavletic MM: Physical and chemical injuries: Heatstroke, hypothermia, burns, and frostbite. *In* Murtaugh RM, Kaplan PM (eds): Veterinary Emergency and Critical Care Medicine. St Louis, Mosby, 1992, p 201.

cars during warm weather. Hyperthermia is also common in animals with compromised ability to thermoregulate, for example, in animals with upper airway obstruction such as brachycephalic airway syndrome.

Thermoregulation in neonates is not fully developed, but usually they are at more risk from hypothermia than from hyperthermia. The average rectal temperature of a 1-day-old puppy is 96° F. By 4 weeks of age, the normal temperature has increased to 100° F. Young puppies may not have a fully developed panting response to increases in temperature.

Pathophysiology

Hyperthermia results in direct thermal injury and cellular necrosis in a variety of body tissues. The severity of the damage depends on the maximum temperature that the body reaches and on the duration of the hyperthermia. Hyperthermia (heat stroke) is present when the body temperature exceeds 106° F and there is a history of environmental overheating or airway obstruction, with no obvious evidence of infection. Temperatures between 107° and 109° F are critical and can result in enzyme alterations and multiple organ damage.

Hyperthermia frequently results in damage to the central nervous system. It is believed that cerebral ischemia and neuronal cell death occur as a result of decreased mean arterial pressure and increased intracranial pressure from cerebral edema. Together these two factors result in a decrease in cerebral perfusion pressure, which leads to cerebral ischemia and cell death.

In moderate hyperthermia, a decrease in systemic vascular resistance occurs as a result of cutaneous vasodilation, and systemic arterial pressure and cardiac output are maintained by elevations in heart rate. As hyperthermia becomes severe, increases in heart rate can no longer maintain mean arterial pressure, and cardiac output, central venous pressure, and systemic vascular resistance all decline. Dehydration from vomiting or diarrhea can also contribute to hypovolemia in the severely hyperthermic animal. In addition, direct thermal damage to the myocardium can result in the development of tachyarrhythmias.

Decreased perfusion of the gastrointestinal tract can result in mucosal cell death, ulceration, and development of profuse, bloody diarrhea. Loss of the gastrointestinal mucosal barrier permits translocation of bacteria and subsequent endotoxemia and sepsis. Both thermal damage and ischemia can contribute to liver damage, which may result in decreased production of coagulation factors and contribute to the development of coagulopathies.

The kidney is at special risk for damage. In addition to the direct thermal insult and the ischemia that occur secondary to decreased perfusion and hypoxia, the renal tubules may also suffer a toxic insult from myoglobin liberated from heat-damaged muscle tissue. In cases of heat stroke, acute renal failure is a common sequela.

A number of hematologic abnormalities are seen after hyperthermia. Hemoconcentration occurs secondary to dehydration, or anemia may be seen because of blood loss through the gastrointestinal tract or due to coagulopathies. Thermal insults have a profound effect on the clotting proteins and platelets. Hyperthermia may result in direct destruction of clotting proteins, and liver damage can result in decreased coagulation factor production. Thrombocytopenia may occur secondary to consumption when hemorrhage is present or to activation in response to systemic endothelial injury. In addition, insults to the megakaryocytic line can be manifested as thrombocytopenia, which becomes evident a few days after the initial insult. Hyperthermia can also result in thrombocytopathia. Disruption of vascular endothelium, vascular stasis, and coagulation factor consumption all contribute to the development of DIC, which may be apparent on initial presentation or may develop a few days after the insult. Excessive panting causes respiratory alkalosis as carbon dioxide declines, whereas shock may result in profound metabolic acidosis.

Clinical Findings

The clinical findings vary depending on the severity of the insult (determined by the highest temperature and the duration of the hyperthermia) and the organs affected. Animals frequently pant excessively and have brick-red mucous membranes. The capillary refill time may be very rapid, or, if perfusion is severely impaired, it may be prolonged. Examination of the mucous membranes may reveal petechiae. Pulses are rapid and may be poor in quality. If the animal is extremely tachycardic or if ventricular premature beats are present, there may be pulse deficits. Neurologic signs may include ataxia, seizures, stupor, and coma. Oliguria or anuria may be present on presentation, and pigmenturia may be evident. Insults to the gut may be manifested as vomiting or diarrhea, and hypersalivation may also be seen.

Diagnosis

The diagnosis of hyperthermia is based on the physical finding of increased temperature without an obvious source of infection. Hyperthermia may be readily explained with a history of even short-duration confinement to an enclosed space such as a car on a hot day. Animals may also develop hyperthermia when exercised. This may be the case when animals and their owners go out on the first warm day of the spring or summer before they have acclimated to the change in ambient temperature. An in-depth history may reveal signs of a predisposing condition such as laryngeal paralysis, cardiac disease, upper airway disease, or neurologic disease.

If the owners have already instituted cooling measures, the animal may have a normal or even decreased rectal temperature by the time it reaches the veterinarian. Packed cell volume, total solids, and physical findings may provide evidence of dehydration. A blood smear should be used to evaluate platelet numbers and to look for red cell fragments, which may be seen with DIC. Chemistry profiles may show increases in liver enzymes if liver damage has occurred. In addition, creatinine and blood urea nitrogen (BUN) levels can be used to assess renal function, although the BUN may be increased with gastrointestinal bleeding. When interpreting these values in the neonate, it is important to remember that the reference range is different, as both BUN and creatinine are lower in puppies and kittens than in adults. Blood urea nitrogen is considered to be a more accurate measure of renal function than creatinine in young puppies. In puppies, renal function is subnormal until at least 3 months of age. Urine specific gravity is lower in puppies, with a specific gravity of 1.006 to 1.017 considered normal even in the presence of dehydration. The urinalysis can provide evidence of renal tubular damage if casts are seen. A coagulation profile, including prothrombin and partial thromboplastin times and measurement of fibrin degradation products, and a manual platelet count aid greatly in the diagnosis of DIC or underlying coagulopathy. Because of the concomitant thrombocytopathia that can be seen in hyperthermia, petechiae and other evidence of spontaneous bleeding may be seen at higher platelet counts than expected. Arterial blood gases may be of value in guiding acid-base therapy as well as providing information on ventilation and oxygenation. If there is a suspicion of underlying disease, a thorough upper airway examination, thoracic radiography, and electrocardiography may be helpful.

Therapy

Minimizing the duration of hyperthermia is a crucial part of successful treatment. If possible, owners should initiate cooling by spraying the animal with cool water before taking it to the veterinary clinic. Upon presentation, the animal should be sprayed or immersed in cool water. Ice packs can be placed around the animal to further facilitate cooling, but ice baths are not recommended as they may result in peripheral vasoconstriction and shivering. Cold water enemas are an aggressive method of cooling, but they destroy the ability to evaluate temperature using a rectal thermometer. Once a rectal temperature of 103° F has been reached, active

efforts at cooling should be stopped to avoid the development of hypothermia.

Initially, the animal should be assessed for patency of the airway, which may be a problem if the animal has laryngeal paralysis or laryngeal edema. If the airway is completely obstructed, orotracheal intubation or emergency tracheostomy should be performed. Intubation is also indicated if the animal is comatose. If the animal is hyperthermic because of partial airway obstruction such as laryngeal paralysis or brachycephalic airway syndrome, sedation with acepromazine (0.01 to 0.05 mg/kg intravenously) may be helpful. Anti-inflammatory doses of corticosteroids are also indicated for animals with presumed inflammation or edema of the airway. If sedation is used, care should be taken to avoid compromising the cardiovascular stability of the animal.

If the animal is in shock, crystalloid fluids should be administered at shock rates (up to 60 to 90 ml/kg bolus intravenously) to improve perfusion. Blood pressures can be monitored by Doppler, oscillometric, or direct methods. Mean arterial pressures below 70 mmHg are associated with decreased renal perfusion. If there is evidence of cerebral edema (coma, neurologic signs), mannitol can be administered as a 0.5-g/kg slow intravenous bolus over 20 minutes. Elevating the head of the animal and avoiding compression of the jugular veins and hyperventilation may help decrease intracranial pressure and prevent further cerebral edema formation.

Anemia should be treated with transfusions of either packed red blood cells or whole blood. Fresh frozen plasma is indicated if there is evidence of coagulopathy and can be combined with heparin (75 to 100 IU/kg subcutaneously every 4 to 6 hours or 10 to 20 IU/kg CRI per hour intravenously) if DIC is suspected. If synthetic colloids are being used for cardiovascular support, the veterinarian should keep in mind that they could cause or exacerbate coagulopathies.

The minimum acceptable rate of urine production is 1 to 2 ml/kg per hour. An indwelling urinary catheter with a closed collection system should be considered if there is concern about the development of oliguric or anuric renal failure. Serial urine sediment examinations can be performed to look for the presence of casts or evidence of myoglobinuria. If the animal is oliguric or anuric, immediate steps should be taken. Decreased urine production because of hypovolemia or low systemic blood pressure should be differentiated from true oliguria and anuria. If the mean arterial pressure is below 70 mmHg, this should be corrected before concluding that the animal is in acute anuric renal failure.

If arterial blood pressure is adequate for renal perfusion, the next step is to confirm that intravascular volume is adequate. Boluses of 10 to 20 ml/kg of crystalloid fluids can be administered as a fluid challenge. Central venous pressure can be monitored to determine whether fluid therapy has been adequate and to detect fluid overload. If urine output is still unacceptable, attempts should be made to increase urine production with furosemide (boluses 2 to 4 mg/kg intravenously or 1 mg/kg per hour CRI intravenously). Boluses of mannitol (0.5 g/kg slowly intravenously) can also be used but should not be repeated if an increase in urine output does not occur. Dopamine infusion (1 to 3 μg/kg per minute) can be used to increase renal blood flow in puppies. Studies have shown that kittens lack dopamine receptors in their kidneys. If systemic arterial pressures are low, higher doses of dopamine (5 to 15 μg/kg per minute) can be used to increase systemic arterial pressure and thus increase renal blood flow in both puppies and kittens. Should all of these measures fail to increase urine output, the next alternative is peritoneal dialysis or hemodialysis. If severe renal damage is present, serum creatinine and BUN may rise despite aggressive fluid therapy. Given enough time, however, kidneys can recover from acute renal failure due to ischemic insults.

Systemic antimicrobial agents can be administered if there is concern about sepsis from translocation of gut bacteria. Nonsteroidal antiinflammatory drugs, corticosteroids, and antipyretics such as dipyrone are contraindicated in hyperthermia. Both nonsteroidal antiinflammatory drugs and corticosteroids can exacerbate damage in the ischemic kidney and gut. Antipyretics are of no value because the thermal set point of the animal is normal, and they may even cause hypothermia, which can be detrimental to the animal.

After the initial stabilization, hyperthermic animals should receive close monitoring and supportive care for several days. Some of the complications of hyperthermia, such as DIC and shock gut, may not be evident until a few days after the insult. Animals should be monitored with serial blood work to monitor changes in their renal parameters, liver enzymes, electrolytes, and coagulation profiles. Continuous electrocardiographic monitoring is helpful in detecting arrhythmias. Ventricular premature beats and ventricular tachycardia should not be treated unless they are adversely affecting the perfusion of the animal. Should this be the case, lidocaine boluses 2 to 4 mg/kg intravenously can be given and, if effective, a lidocaine infusion should be started (30 to 75 μg/kg per minute). Animals should be monitored closely for signs of lidocaine toxicity.

For most animals with metabolic acidosis from hyperthermia, fluid therapy will improve perfusion and correct the acidosis. If severe metabolic acidosis is refractory to fluid therapy, sodium bicarbonate (mEq total deficit = 0.3 × body weight [kg] × base excess) can be administered. One-third of the total calculated dose can be given as a slow intravenous bolus and the response to therapy monitored with serial blood gases. If the response is not adequate, the bolus can be repeated, or the remainder of the dose can be added to the intravenous fluids and given over 12 to 18 hours.

Prognosis and Client Education

The prognosis in hyperthermia depends on the systems affected and on the severity of the damage. Most cases carry a guarded prognosis. The development of DIC is always a poor prognostic indicator. Acute renal failure carries a guarded prognosis if polyuria is present and a poor to grave prognosis if oliguria or anuria is present. Animals may suffer permanent renal, liver, or neurologic damage from hyperthermia. Owners should be instructed to avoid further situations that may result in hyperthermia. Animals should always have access to water and shade. If the animal has a predisposing factor such as brachycephalic airway syndrome, that animal should be kept in a cool environment as much as possible.

HYPOTHERMIA AND FROSTBITE

Hypothermia refers to a drop in body temperature below normal and may result in the impairment of multiple body systems. Frostbite is the actual freezing of tissue and results in ischemia and necrosis of that tissue. Young animals are at especial risk for developing hypothermia for a number of reasons. Puppies and kittens rapidly lose heat by conduction, convection, radiation, and evaporation. Because thermogenesis and vasoconstrictive responses are not fully developed in newborns, they are frequently unable to generate enough heat to compensate for their losses. The shivering reflex does not develop until the sixth day of life, and newborns rely on warmth from the body of their mother. If puppies or kittens are separated from the mother, it is essential that they be housed in an ambient temperature to avoid hypothermia.

Pathophysiology

Hypothermia is classified as mild, moderate, or severe. Generally, mild hypothermia is not harmful to the animal. The normal responses to hypothermia are increased shivering thermogenesis and nonshivering thermogenesis primarily from brown adipose tissue. Severe hypothermia exists at temperatures less than 86° F.

As hypothermia worsens, hemodynamics are affected because of the hypometabolism induced by the lowered core temperature. Initially, with mild hypothermia, heart rate and blood pressure increase. As the animal becomes moderately to severely hypothermic, cardiac output, heart rate, blood pressure, and oxygen consumption all decrease. Moderate to severe hypothermia decreases renal blood flow and glomerular filtration rate (GFR). Tubular resorption is also impaired, resulting in increased urine output. This is referred to as cold diuresis and can contribute to dehydration and hemoconcentration in the hypothermic animal. As temperatures are increased, renal blood flow and GFR return to normal.

Cerebral metabolism also decreases in the hypothermic animal. As metabolism slows, the brain becomes more tolerant of decreased perfusion. The protective effects of hypothermia against cerebral ischemia are used to good effect in human neurosurgery. Animals that are severely hypothermic and in asystole or ventricular fibrillation can sometimes be successfully resuscitated after a prolonged period of time and suffer little if any neurologic damage.

As hypothermia becomes moderate to severe, multiple electrocardiographic abnormalities and arrhythmias can occur. Cold-induced electrocardiographic changes include prolonged PR intervals, widened QRS complexes, prolonged QT segments, and inversion of T waves. In humans, the presence of J waves, which are extra deflections at the QRS-ST junction, are pathognomonic for hypothermia; however, this electrocardiographic change has rarely been reported in veterinary medicine. Hypothermia is associated with increased myocardial irritability, and ventricular ectopic beats can occur. In addition, atrial arrhythmias are also possible. When temperatures drop below 72° to 74° F, ventricular fibrillation can occur, and below 68° F asystole is seen.

Low body temperatures decrease the partial pressure of oxygen, increase oxygen solubility, and shift the oxygen-hemoglobin dissociation curve to the left. These changes result in decreased tissue oxygenation; however, this is offset by the decrease in oxygen demands at the level of the hypothermic tissue. Vasoconstriction further decreases oxygen delivery to tissues. With time, oxygen requirements exceed oxygen delivery, and metabolic acidosis develops due to lactic acid formation from anaerobic metabolism.

Frostbite results when tissue is frozen. Ice crystals form both intracellularly and extracellularly and result in cell membrane damage. As water is drawn osmotically out of cells, intracellular dehydration and cell death occur. A third mechanism of tissue damage with frostbite is endothelial damage with hypoxia and local thrombosis. Peripheral vasoconstriction leads to hypoxia and contributes to cell death in frostbite. Local release of inflammatory mediators worsens the endothelial damage and contributes to further cell death.

Clinical Signs

Except in puppies and kittens, animals suffering from mild hypothermia are often shivering. They may have an increased heart rate and respiratory rate. As hypothermia worsens, they exhibit cerebral obtundation, shivering ceases, and heart and respiratory rate decrease. As the hypothermia becomes severe, reflexes and response to noxious stimuli such as pain are lost. Finally, some severely hypothermic animals may present apneic with ventricular fibrillation or asystole.

Clinically, frostbite is usually seen at peripheral sites such as the ears, tail, and digits of hypothermic animals. Areas of frostbite may not be evident for several days. After rewarming, first-degree frostbite injuries are numb, have a central white plaque, and are surrounded by erythema. Second-degree injuries result in blisters filled with clear or whitish fluid that develop during the first 24 hours after rewarming. The blisters are surrounded by edema and erythema. Third-degree injuries result in hemorrhagic blister formation with indications of deeper tissue injury. Within a few weeks a black eschar will form at the site. Fourth-degree injuries have complete necrosis and loss of tissue.

Diagnosis

Diagnosis is based on the finding of a decreased rectal temperature. Historical findings may reveal a small puppy or kitten that has been exposed to a cold environment or immersed in very cold water. In puppies and kittens, the ambient temperature does not have to be particularly low for hypothermia to develop.

Temperatures can be determined by rectal thermometer or esophageal temperature probe. Tympanic membrane temperature readings can also be taken, but may be less accurate than those obtained by other methods. A complete blood count or packed cell volume may be useful, as hemoconcentration can be seen with hypothermia. In addition, thyroxine and thyroid-stimulating hormone testing may also be valuable. A screening electrocardiogram should be obtained to determine whether cardiac arrhythmias are occurring. Serial blood gas analysis can be used to guide oxygen supplementation and acid-base therapy. Blood gas machines automatically run samples at 37° C and then perform corrections for the animal's temperature. When possible, the uncorrected values from the blood gas machine should be used to guide therapy. Chemistry and coagulation profiles are also of value as coagulopathies have been associated with hypothermia.

Therapy

The main goal of therapy is to rewarm the animal, and various methods can be employed to achieve this. If the animal is suffering from mild hypothermia, passive external warming can be used. This consists of drying the animal if it is wet and placing it in a warm environment with blankets for insulation. If the animal is moderately hypothermic, more aggressive measures may be taken in the form of active external rewarming. This consists of the application of hot water bottles and heating pads. If the animal is wet, a hair dryer can be used for drying. Care should be taken with active external rewarming to avoid the phenomenon of afterdrop. Afterdrop occurs when peripheral vasodilation results in the rapid return of cold and toxic blood from the periphery to the core. It results in a further drop in core temperature and may worsen hemodynamic instability.

If the animal is severely hypothermic (less than 86° F), methods of active central rewarming should be employed. In veterinary medicine, warm peritoneal lavage can be used to good effect. Dialysate that has been warmed to about 55° C should be infused through a catheter into the peritoneal cavity. By the time it has passed through the intravenous line into the animal, it should have cooled to about 45° C. Warm gas-

tric lavage can also be used but necessitates tracheal intubation to protect the airway. If possible, peritoneal lavage is preferred over gastric lavage. Ventilation with warm, humidified air can be added to these therapies and may help to decrease heat loss from the respiratory system. Warm intravenous fluids can be administered, but care should be taken to avoid volume overload. The use of active central warming techniques minimizes the adverse effects of active surface rewarming.

If the animal is in ventricular fibrillation or asystole, cardiac compressions should be started while steps are taken to rewarm the animal. Care should be used in the administration of resuscitative drugs, as there may be decreased drug clearance in the hypothermic animal. Animals are generally refractory to defibrillation until they have been rewarmed to a core temperature above 28° C.

In the puppy or kitten, hypothermia is usually concomitant with hypoglycemia. Puppies and kittens can receive a bolus of dextrose (0.5 g/kg intravenous or intraosseous, diluted to 25%) while steps are taken to rewarm them. One must keep in mind that the normal temperature of the puppy or kitten during the first week of life is 96° F, and after 3 to 4 weeks of age it increases to 99° to 100° F. Puppies and kittens should not be fed enterally if their temperature is below 96° F, as gastrointestinal ileus is likely to be present.

Frostbite injuries should be rewarmed rapidly in an environment where refreezing will not occur. The affected area can be immersed in warm water to maintain a temperature of 104° to 108° F for 20 minutes or until thawing is complete. The damaged tissue should not be rubbed or massaged. Soft bandages should be applied to protect the affected areas, and the animals should receive analgesics for pain control. If areas on the feet are frostbitten, cage rest is indicated. The affected area should be watched closely and necrotic tissue débrided as needed. If the affected area has suffered a severe insult, amputation may be indicated.

Prognosis and Owner Education

Owners should be advised of the risks of exposing their animals to inclement weather. This is especially true in the case of small puppies and kittens that have a larger surface area to mass ratio. Puppies and kittens should be kept in a warm ambient environment, and owners should ensure that orphaned or rejected puppies and kittens are being fed frequently enough to meet their energy requirements.

References and Supplemental Reading

Beasley VR: Smoke inhalation. Vet Clin North Am Small Anim Pract 20:545, 1990.

Broman M, Kallskog O: The effects of hypothermia on renal function and haemodynamics in the rat. Acta Physiol Scand 153:179, 1995.

Carter LJ, Wingfield WE, Allen TA: Clinical experience with peritoneal dialysis in small animals. Compend Contin Educ Pract Vet 11:1335, 1989.

Crisp MS, Chew DJ, DiBartola SP, et al: Peritoneal dialysis in dogs and cats: 27 cases (1976–1987). J Am Vet Med Assoc 195:1262, 1989.

Delaney KA, Howland MA, Vassallo S, et al: Assessment of acid-base disturbances in hypothermia and their physiologic consequences. Ann Emerg Med 18:72, 1989.

Dhupa N: Burns and smoke inhalation—An overview. Proc IVECCS 4:50, 1994.

Dieterich RA: Cold injury (hypothermia, frostbite, freezing). In Kirk RW (ed): Current Veterinary Therapy VI. Philadelphia, WB Saunders, 1977, p 205.

Drobatz KJ: Smoke inhalation in dogs and cats. Proc 14th ACVIM Forum, 1996, p 195.

Drobatz KJ, Concannon K: Noncardiogenic pulmonary edema. Compend Contin Educ Pract Vet 16:333, 1994.

Drobatz KJ, Macintire DK: Heat-induced illness in dogs: 42 cases (1976–1993). J Am Vet Med Assoc 209:1894, 1996.

Drobatz KJ, Saunders HM, Pugh CR, et al: Noncardiogenic pulmonary edema in dogs and cats: 26 cases (1987–1993). J Am Vet Med Assoc 206:1732, 1995.

Farrow CS: Thermal injuries. In Kirk RW (ed): Current Veterinary Therapy VI. Philadelphia, WB Saunders, 1977, p 195.

Fish R: Electric shock part I: Physics and pathophysiology. J Emerg Med 11:309, 1993a.

Fish R: Electric shock part II: Nature and mechanisms of injury. J Emerg Med 11:457, 1993b.

Gautier H, Gaudy JH: Ventilatory recovery from hypothermia in anesthetized cats. Respir Physiol 64:329, 1986.

Giesbrecht GGR, Bristow GK: Recent advances in hypothermia research. Ann NY Acad Sci 813:663, 1997.

Gregory NG, Constantine E: Hyperthermia in dogs left in cars. Vet Rec 139:349, 1996.

Gubler KD, Gentilello LM, Hassantash SA, et al: The impact of hypothermia on dilutional coagulopathy. J Trauma 36:847, 1994.

Johnston DE, Bojrab MJ: Thermal burns. In Bojrab MJ (ed): Current Techniques in Small Animal Surgery, 3rd ed. Philadelphia, Lea and Febiger, 1990, p 494.

Kern MR, Stockham SL, Coates JR: Analysis of serum protein concentrations after severe thermal injury in a dog. Vet Clin Pathol 21:19, 1992.

Klein GL, Nicolai M, Langman CB, et al: Dysregulation of calcium homeostasis after severe burn injury in children: Possible role of magnesium depletion. J Pediatr 131:246, 1997.

Kolata RJ, Burrows CF: The clinical features of injury by chewing electrical cords in dogs and cats. J Am Anim Hosp Assoc 17:219, 1981.

Larach MG: Accidental hypothermia. Lancet 345:493, 1995.

Lauri T: Cardiovascular responses to an acute volume load in deep hypothermia. Eur Heart J 17:606, 1996.

Lee-Paritz DE, Pavletic MM: Physical and chemical: Heatstroke, hypothermia, burns, and frostbite. In Murtaugh RJ, Kaplan PM (eds): Veterinary Emergency and Critical Care Medicine. St. Louis, Mosby-Year Book, 1992, p 199.

Lin M: Heatstroke-induced cerebral ischemia and neuronal damage: Involvement of cytokines and monoamines. Ann NY Acad Sci 813:572, 1997.

Lord PF: Neurogenic pulmonary edema in the dog. J Am Anim Hosp Assoc 11:778, 1975.

Miki K, Morimoto T, Nose H, et al: Circulatory failure during severe hyperthermia in dog. Jpn J Physiol 33:269, 1983.

Nemoto EM, Klementavicius R, Melick JA, et al: Effect of mild hypothermia on active and basal cerebral oxygen metabolism and blood flow. Adv Exp Med Biol 361:469, 1994.

Pickoff AS, Stolfi A, Campbell P: Temperature dependency of the vagal chronotropic response in the young puppy: An environmental-autonomic interaction. J Auton Nerv Syst 64:107, 1997.

Poffenbarger EM, Chandler ML, Ralston SL, et al: Canine neonatology. Part I. Physiologic differences between puppies and adults. Compend Contin Educ Pract Vet 12:1601, 1990.

Reamy BV: Frostbite: Review and current concepts. J Am Board Fam Pract 11:34, 1998.

Remedios AM, Fowler JD: Axial pattern flaps in the cutaneous reconstruction of lower limb wounds. Compend Contin Educ Pract Vet 17:1356, 1995.

Saxon WD, Kirby R: Treatment of acute burn injury and smoke inhalation. In Kirk RW, Bonagura JD (eds): Current Veterinary Therapy XI. Philadelphia, WB Saunders, 1992, p 146.

Scardino MS, Henderson RA, Wilson ER, et al: Enhancing wound closure on the limbs. Compend Contin Educ Pract Vet 18:919, 1996.

Schall WD: Heat stroke (heat stress, hyperpyrexia). In Kirk RW (ed): Current Veterinary Therapy VI. Philadelphia, WB Saunders, 1977, p 202.

Smith M: Hypothermia. Compend Contin Educ Pract Vet 7:321, 1985.

Swaim SF: Management and bandaging of soft tissue injuries of dog and cat feet. J Am Anim Hosp Assoc 21:329, 1985.

van den Broek AHM: Treatment of burns in dogs. Vet Annu 31:204, 1991.

Anesthesia and Surgery

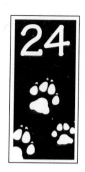

Giselle Hosgood

Surgery in puppies and kittens is often necessary for correction of life-threatening congenital anomalies and other problems and for institution of an early spay and neuter program. Compared with the physiology of adult dogs and cats, most body systems in puppies and kittens are immature, especially during the first few weeks of life. Hence, despite the obvious challenge of performing surgery on a sometimes very small animal, the preoperative, anesthetic, and postoperative management also requires careful consideration for age-related physiologic differences.

PREOPERATIVE CONSIDERATIONS

Physical Examination

Before surgery, all animals should have a thorough physical examination, with particular attention to the cardiovascular and respiratory systems. The normal heart rate of puppies and kittens is 200 or more beats per minute (Finley and Kelly, 1986), and the normal respiratory rate is 15 to 35 breaths per minute (Mosier, 1978). Normal body temperature for animals younger than 2 weeks is 35.5° to 36° C (96° to 97° F), which increases to 37.7° C (100° F) by 4 weeks of age (Mosier, 1978). Auscultation and localization of the heart sounds may be difficult; use of a pediatric chest piece (2-cm bell and 3-cm diaphragm) over the left cardiac apex (left fifth or sixth intercostal space in the ventral third of the thorax) may be helpful. Heart rate and rhythm and the presence or absence of a murmur are important phenomena to determine on auscultation (Hoskins, 1990).

The respiratory system is best evaluated by observation of the rate, rhythm, and character of breathing. Upper airway obstruction most often produces an increased inspiratory effort, whereas lower respiratory obstruction produces an increased expiratory effort (Turnwald, 1995). Restrictive respiratory diseases are characterized by respiratory distress and restricted expansion of the lungs, which are often compensated for by a rapid, shallow breathing pattern (Turnwald, 1995).

Dehydration occurs very quickly in puppies and kittens, and the determination of degree is probably irrelevant. Hydration status can be assessed based on historical information of fluid intake and loss, moistness of mucous membranes, position of eyes in their orbits, heart rate, character of peripheral pulses, and capillary refill time. The assessment of skin turgor is not useful for puppies and kittens younger than 6 weeks of age. The color of the urine may be used as an indicator of dehydration in puppies and kittens younger than 6 weeks of age. The urine is normally clear or colorless, and any color tint indicates dehydration.

Laboratory Evaluation

Veterinarians may be restricted to in-house laboratory tests because of the difficulty in obtaining adequate blood samples from puppies and kittens for commercial laboratory assessment. In-house tests are, however, sufficient to identify the presence of illness. Tests should be performed to determine packed cell volume and total solids (with a microhematocrit tube), erythrocyte and leukocyte morphology (with

525

blood film examination), blood glucose and blood urea nitrogen levels (with reagent strips for whole blood), urine specific gravity (with a refractometer), and urine glucose, ketone, protein, and bilirubin levels (with reagent strips). In addition, microscopic evaluation of urine sediment is indicated. High packed cell volumes are common during the first few days of life. These levels decrease to 27% by 7 weeks of age and thereafter increase to normal adult levels (Meyers-Wallen et al, 1984; Shifine et al, 1973).

Compared with adults, puppies and kittens have higher white blood cell counts in the first few days of life; however, by 3 weeks of age white blood cell counts decrease to their lowest level but then peak again at 7 weeks of age (Meyers-Wallen et al, 1984; Shifine et al, 1973). Blood urea nitrogen and urine specific gravity levels are lower in puppies and kittens than they are in adults because renal function is undeveloped (Horster and Valtin, 1971; Hoskins et al, 1991).

Coagulation disorders can be screened by determining platelet counts, activated clotting time, and buccal mucosal bleeding time. Common manifestations associated with coagulopathy include stillbirth, neonatal death, hematoma formation, and prolonged bleeding after tail docking and dewclaw removal. Further evaluation of clotting disorders may require determination of prothrombin times, activated partial thromboplastin times, fibrinogen levels, or specific coagulation factor levels. Normal values for these parameters have not been reported for puppies and kittens but are comparable to adult values by 8 weeks of age (Center et al, 1995).

PHYSIOLOGIC DIFFERENCES RELEVANT TO ANESTHESIA AND SURGERY

Major functional differences in the cardiovascular, respiratory, hepatorenal, metabolic, and thermoregulatory systems of puppies and kittens compared with adult animals must be considered in the selection of anesthetic agents and the management of the animal before and after surgery (Dale et al, 1968; Donovan, 1985; Grandy and Dunlop, 1991; Hosgood and Hoskins, 1998a; Poffenbarger et al, 1990; Robinson, 1983).

Cardiovascular System

Puppies and kittens have lower blood pressures, stroke volumes, and peripheral vascular resistance but higher heart rates, cardiac outputs, plasma volumes, and central venous pressures than in adult cats and dogs (Driscoll et al, 1979). Mean arterial blood pressure increases after 6 weeks of age and approaches adult values after several months (Arango and Rowe, 1971). As a result, the pediatric heart is less able to increase the force of contraction (stroke volume), and cardiac output depends primarily on heart rate.

The autonomic innervation of the pediatric heart involves a mature parasympathetic innervation but immature sympathetic innervation (Friedman, 1972). The dominant parasympathetic innervation may cause severe bradycardia (less than 150 beats per minute) (Grandy and Dunlop, 1991). Subsequently, hypotension can be a problem, particularly because cardiac output depends on heart rate (Grandy and Dunlop, 1991).

Puppies and kittens are less able than adult animals to compensate for blood loss. Intravenous fluid administration may correct hypotension in adult dogs and cats, but in puppies and kittens the ventricles are less compliant and have a limited ability to increase cardiac output in response to volume loading (Grandy and Dunlop, 1991).

Hemoglobin concentrations are lower in puppies and kittens than in adult animals because of a lower rate of erythrocyte production, shorter erythrocyte life span, and hemodilution by an expanding blood volume (Meyers-Wallen et al, 1984). During surgery, small volumes of blood loss in puppies and kittens may result in clinically notable anemia. This is particularly apparent in animals between 2 and 8 weeks of age (Grandy and Dunlop, 1991) as hematopoiesis does not begin until 6 to 12 weeks of age, at which time low levels of hemoglobin stimulate erythrocyte production (Donovan, 1985).

Respiratory System

The oxygen demand of puppies and kittens is two to three times that of adult animals. After 4 weeks of age, the tidal volume is similar to that in adult animals; therefore, the respiratory rate must be two to three times greater than the adult rate to meet the minute ventilation necessary for the greater oxygen demand (Grandy and Dunlop, 1991; Parot et al, 1984; Poffenbarger et al, 1990). Because most anesthetic agents depress respiration, a high respiratory rate during anesthesia must be maintained. High alveolar ventilation increases the exchange of gases in the lungs, causing a more rapid induction and recovery from inhalation anesthesia.

Compared with adult animals, puppies and kittens have smaller and less rigid airways, smaller alveoli, and a more compliant chest wall (Donovan, 1985; Grandy and Dunlop, 1991). The smaller, less rigid airways make intubation difficult. The compliant chest wall causes the end-expiratory pressure to be zero rather than negative; therefore, the force maintaining open alveoli is lower than that in adult animals. Unlike that in adult animals, the thoracic wall in puppies and kittens tends to collapse rather than expand on inspiration, again limiting the degree of negative pleural pressure developed and subsequent alveolar ventilation. The consequence is that puppies and kittens may encounter some difficulty in overcoming the critical opening pressure (12 to 20 cm H_2O) necessary to expand collapsed alveoli. This may be compounded by a reduction in the tone of the intercostal muscles and diaphragm during anesthesia. Hypoventilation and atelectasis may develop but can be alleviated by the use of intermittent positive-pressure ventilation. Extreme care is required during intermittent positive-pressure ventilation to prevent lung trauma and pneumothorax. Animals older than 4 weeks can be allowed to ventilate spontaneously (Grandy and Dunlop, 1991).

Hepatorenal System

The hepatic enzyme systems for biotransformation of compounds are immature in puppies and kittens. At least 4 weeks are necessary for these systems to develop (Short, 1980). Consequently, drugs that undergo phase I hepatic metabolism should be avoided, if possible, in puppies and kittens. If such drugs are used, dosages should be modified taking into consideration that the drugs will have a longer half-life (Jones, 1987). Albumin levels in puppies younger than 4 weeks are lower than albumin levels in adult animals; adult levels are attained by 8 weeks of age (Center et al, 1995). Because of this fact, if a drug is administered intravenously, there will be a greater unbound fraction of the drug circulating. Consequently, puppies and kittens have a greater sensitivity than adult animals to highly protein-bound drugs (Grandy and Dunlop, 1991).

Nephrogenesis is incomplete in neonates until 3 weeks of age (Horster and Valtin, 1971) and the renal concentrating and diluting ability is less than that of adult animals. In puppies, renal excretion of drugs is affected by the facts that glomerular filtration matures between 2 to 3 weeks of age and that tubular secretion matures between 4 to 8 weeks of age (Horster et al, 1971; Kleinman and Lubbe, 1972). Urine protein and glucose levels are higher in puppies and kittens than in adult animals; urine specific gravity is lower (Poffenbarger et al, 1990).

Puppies and kittens have greater fluid requirements relative to body mass than those of adult animals. They also have greater insensible water losses, and, because they are less able to concentrate urine, they are more likely to become dehydrated after water restriction. Although puppies and kittens have a high requirement for fluids, they cannot accommodate large volumes of fluid administered within a short period. For this reason and because of an impaired ability to excrete a solute load, fluid therapy should be administered carefully. Puppies up to 3 weeks of age excreted only 10% compared with 50% in adults of an isotonic sodium load within 2 hours of administration (Kleinman, 1979; Steichen and Kleinman, 1975).

Metabolic System

Normal blood glucose levels can be maintained in healthy, fasted puppies and kittens by hepatic glycogenolysis (Kleigman et al, 1983). The hepatic store of glycogen in puppies and kittens is minimal, however, and rapidly declines during fasting. In newborn puppies, hepatic glycogen levels dropped to 31% of birth levels after 24 hours of fasting (Kleigman et al, 1983). Once hepatic glycogen stores are depleted, hepatic gluconeogenesis will take over to maintain normal blood glucose levels (Aschinberg et al, 1975). Subsequently, factors other than fasting (e.g., chilling, septicemia) may contribute to hypoglycemia in puppies and kittens. Hypoglycemia can contribute to a reduction in mean arterial blood pressure.

Fluid compartments in puppies and kittens are different in size and distribution from those in adult animals. The body of a human infant at birth is approximately 80% water, half of which is extracellular. The total water content then decreases to 60% (one third is extracellular) over the first year of life (Fomon, 1967). Compared with adult animals, puppies and kittens have a smaller reserve of intracellular water, a higher surface area to body weight ratio, and a higher relative energy and fluid requirement (McIntyre and Ederstrom, 1958). The larger surface area results in a greater heat loss by radiation and evaporation, thereby necessitating more heat generation and a larger consumption of water relative to body mass (Fettman and Allen, 1991). Increased body temperature from fever or heat stress can impose a proportionately greater burden on water balance.

Thermoregulatory System

Puppies and kittens have a tendency to develop hypothermia, which can cause bradycardia, low cardiac output, and hypotension. These effects, in turn, may prolong drug elimination and recovery from anesthesia. Factors that contribute to the development of hypothermia in puppies and kittens include a large surface area to body weight ratio with high radiation and evaporative heat losses, an inability to shiver, a small amount of subcutaneous fat, and an immature thermoregulatory system (Fettman and Allen, 1991; Grandy and Dunlop, 1991; McIntyre and Ederstrom, 1958).

Other factors exacerbate heat loss during anesthesia and surgery. During anesthesia, heat production is lowered as a result of depressed thermoregulation and metabolic and muscle activity decreases. Heat loss by evaporation can be exacerbated by the use of surgical antiseptic solutions on the skin. Alcohol or alcohol-containing antiseptic solutions, in particular, should be avoided. Other solutions can be warmed before use on the skin. Evaporative losses also occur from exposed body cavities and by the inhalation of dry gases (Shanks, 1974). Heat loss by conduction can result from contact with cool surfaces. Radiation losses from the body can also occur into a cool environment (Dale et al, 1968).

Drug Distribution

Compared with adults, puppies and kittens have a lower albumin level, larger percentage of total body water, higher distribution of cardiac output to vessel-rich organs, lower body fat, and reduced hepatorenal function. All of these factors affect drug distribution (Short, 1980, 1984). Lower albumin levels result in higher unbound fractions of intravenous drugs. The high percentage of total body water results in a larger volume of distribution of nonprotein-bound, water-soluble drugs, which may result in resistance to the initial intravenous bolus of a drug. Lipid-soluble drugs are not stored in large quantities because puppies and kittens have small amounts of body fat. Consequently, drugs that require redistribution to fat will have prolonged effects after repeated administration. Drugs that require redistribution to muscle will also have a prolonged effect after repeated administration because puppies and kittens have a small muscle mass. Reduced hepatorenal function prolongs drug metabolism and excretion.

ANESTHETIC SELECTION AND MANAGEMENT

Preanesthetic Fasting

It is usually unnecessary to withhold food from nursing puppies and kittens before anesthesia. Blood glucose is difficult to regulate in puppies and kittens because of a lack of adequate feedback mechanisms between hepatic gluconeogenesis and blood glucose concentrations. Therefore, in weaned puppies and kittens, fasting should not be for more than 1 or 2 hours, and intravenous fluids containing glucose in a balanced electrolyte solution should be administered during anesthesia (Table 24–1). Access to water should not be restricted (Hosgood and Hoskins, 1998a). An exception to these recommendations for fasting would be animals that have delayed gastric emptying or a similar ailment. Such animals may require preoperative fluid support.

Table 24–1	Fluid Therapy Guidelines for Puppies and Kittens		
FLUID THERAPY	**DOSE**	**COMMENTS**	
2.5% dextrose in 0.45% saline solution or 5% dextrose in Ringer's solution	4–10 ml/kg/h intraoperative	Administer via syringe pump or with use of an inline reservoir or fluid regulator with a minidrip set (60 drops/ml)	
Avoid boluses	44 ml/kg/24 h maintenance	Maintain blood glucose between 80 and 220 mg/dl	
50% dextrose solution	Administer orally to effect if blood glucose is <80 mg/dl	Risk of cerebral edema with profound hyperglycemia	

Preanesthetic Agents

The preanesthetic agents used for puppies and kittens depend on the age of the animal, overall condition of the animal, the surgical procedure to be performed, amount of sedation and analgesia required, and experience and preference of the veterinarian. Administration of premedications to animals younger than 12 weeks may not be indicated (Hosgood and Hoskins, 1998a). Administration of a tranquilizer or analgesic preoperatively will reduce stress and allow a smooth induction, maintenance, and recovery from anesthesia, as well as reducing the dose of the more hemodynamically depressing induction and maintenance anesthetic agents. Preanesthetics may include anticholinergics, tranquilizers/sedatives, analgesics, and/or dissociatives (Table 24–2).

Anticholinergic Agents

Because the cardiac output of puppies and kittens is highly dependent on heart rate and the dominant parasympathetic nervous system results in strong vagal tone, administration of an anticholinergic agent is necessary before induction of general anesthesia (Grandy and Dunlop, 1991). Atropine or glycopyrrolate can be used (Grandy and Dunlop, 1991). These drugs have the additional benefit of decreasing respiratory tract secretions, which reduces the potential for airway obstruction and/or laryngotracheal aspiration (Grandy and Dunlop, 1991). Anticholinergic agents may not be effective in animals younger than 2 weeks because of their immature autonomic nervous system (Robinson, 1983). Glycopyrrolate takes longer to exert its effects but lasts longer than atropine (2 to 3 hours as opposed to 1 to 1.5 hours) and is less likely to produce sinus tachycardia. Either agent can be given to effect intraoperatively if sinus bradycardia (less than 150 beats per minute) develops.

Tranquilizers/Sedatives

Benzodiazepines (diazepam and midazolam) are the sedatives of choice for puppies and kittens (Hosgood and Hoskins, 1998a). The benzodiazepines are mild, nonanalgesic, short-acting sedatives; however, they require hepatic metabolism, and hence their duration of action may be

Table 24–2	Anesthetic and Analgesic Agents and Suggested Doses for Use in Puppies and Kittens	
AGENT	**DOSAGE**	**COMMENTS**
ANTICHOLINERGICS		
Atropine	0.02–0.04 mg/kg IV, IM, SC	Recommended to offset dominant parasympathetic effects and maintain heart rate, cardiac output, and blood pressure. Also decreases airway secretions
Glycopyrrolate	0.01 mg/kg IV, IM	Glycopyrrolate does not cross the blood-brain barrier, takes longer to onset of action, and has increased duration compared with atropine
TRANQUILIZERS/SEDATIVES		
Diazepam	0.2–0.4 mg/kg IV, IM	Propylene glycol carrier makes uptake unpredictable from IM site. Will not mix in same syringe with any drug except ketamine
Midazolam	0.1–0.2 mg/kg IV, IM, SC	Water soluble. More potent and shorter acting than diazepam. Mixes with other agents. May cause excitement on recovery in some cats
Acepromazine	0.025–0.05 mg/kg IM, SC	2 mg maximum. Avoid in animals younger than 8 weeks of age. Requires hepatic degradation. Potentiates hypotension and hypothermia. Does not provide analgesia and is not reversible. Best to dilute to 1 mg/ml solution
α_2-AGONISTS		
Xylazine	1–2 mg/kg IM	Avoid in animals younger than 12 weeks of age. Requires hepatic degradation and causes marked bradycardia and decreased cardiac output. Reversible
Medetomidine	20–30 μg/kg IM	May cause vomiting. Always use with an anticholinergic. Medetomidine is more potent and longer acting than xylazine

Table continued on following page

Table 24–2	Anesthetic and Analgesic Agents and Suggested Doses for Use in Puppies and Kittens *Continued*	
AGENT	**DOSAGE**	**COMMENTS**
OPIOIDS		
Meperidine	1–2 mg/kg IM Epidural: 0.5–1.5 mg/kg	Mild analgesia. May cause histamine release if injected IV. Reversible
Morphine	0.2–1.0 mg/kg IM, SC Epidural: 0.1 mg/kg in 0.5 ml/kg volume of NaCl	Analgesia with sedation and cardiopulmonary depression. Administer with an anticholinergic. Potentiates hypothermia. Most common agent used for epidural analgesia. Reversible
Oxymorphone	0.05–0.2 mg/kg IV, IM, SC Epidural: 0.1 mg/kg in 0.5 ml/kg volume of NaCl	4 mg maximum. Analgesia with sedation. Causes panting. Administer with an anticholinergic. Commonly combined with acepromazine in animals older than 12 weeks of age for neuroleptanalgesia. Can be used for epidural analgesia. Reversible

Fentanyl	2–4 μg/kg IV
	CRI: 2–4 μg/kg/h IV
	Transdermal patch:
	  2.5–10 kg, use 25-μg patch (all or part)
	  10–20 kg, use 50-μg patch
	  20–30 kg, use 75-μg patch
	Epidural: 1–10 μg/kg in 0.5 ml/kg volume of NaCl
		Very potent analgesic. Rapid onset and short duration of action. Minimal cardiopulmonary effects. Can be delivered by a variety of routes, including epidural. Reversible

Buprenorphine	0.01–0.02 mg/kg IV, IM, SC	30–45 min to onset; long duration due to slow rate of dissociation from receptor, unpredictable reversal with opioid antagonists
Butorphanol	0.2–0.4 mg/kg IV, IM, SC CRI: 0.2–0.4 mg/kg/h IV	Agonist-antagonist. Minimal cardiopulmonary depression. Good visceral analgesia. Used to reverse agonist adverse effects and preserve analgesia
INTRAVENOUS ANESTHETICS		
Thiopental	4–6 mg/kg IV, to effect	Ultrashort-acting thiobarbiturate. Termination of action depends on redistribution and hepatic degradation. May be dysrhythmogenic. Respiratory depression common; be prepared to intubate and ventilate
Methohexital	4–6 mg/kg IV, to effect	Ultrashort-acting oxybarbiturate. Terminated by redistribution with minimal hepatic metabolism. May cause excitement on induction and recovery. Be prepared to intubate and ventilate
Propofol	2–6 mg/kg IV, to effect CRI: 10–12 mg/kg/h IV	Alkyl phenol. Do not give in a bolus—give slowly, over several minutes. Ultrashort-acting, rapid onset, rapid recovery. Noncumulative; can be used as constant rate infusion without prolonged recovery. Be prepared to intubate and ventilate
Etomidate	1–2 mg/kg IV CRI: 2–4 mg/kg/h IV	Nonbarbiturate. No cardiopulmonary effects. May cause nausea, vomiting, myoclonus, and excitement on induction and recovery. Noncumulative; can be used as constant rate infusion
Ketamine	1–2 mg/kg IV 11–22 mg/kg IM	Dissociative anesthetic. Excessive salivation controlled with anticholinergics. Increases intracranial and intraocular pressures. May cause seizures. Elimination depends on renal and hepatic function
Telazol	1–2 mg/kg IV 5–13 mg/kg IM	Contains 50:50 tiletamine, a dissociative anesthetic, and zolazepam, a benzodiazepine. Tiletamine is more potent and longer lasting than ketamine. Zolazepam effects may be prolonged in some cats and cause rough recovery

CRI = continuous rate infusion; IM = intramuscular; IV, intravenous; SC = subcutaneous.

Data from Hosgood G, Hoskins JD: Anaesthesia and pain management. *In* Hosgood G, Hoskins JD (eds): Small Animal Paediatric Medicine and Surgery. Oxford, Butterworth Heinemann, 1998, p 18.

prolonged in animals younger than 8 weeks. The benzodiazepines characteristically produce good muscle relaxation with minimal central nervous system and cardiovascular depression. Midazolam is more potent yet shorter acting than diazepam. Both diazepam and midazolam have dose-dependent respiratory depressant effects and may cause hypoventilation or apnea (Hosgood and Hoskins, 1998a). Careful monitoring of the respiratory system is recommended, especially if the benzodiazepines are administered with other respiratory depressant agents. Due to its propylene glycol carrier, diazepam cannot be mixed in the same syringe with any other agents except ketamine. Diazepam has unpredictable absorption from intramuscular sites. In contrast, midazolam is water soluble and readily combines with other agents. Midazolam is well absorbed from subcutaneous or intramuscular sites. Both agents are commonly used in combination with narcotics or dissociative agents for premedication, induction to anesthesia, or alone for short and nonpainful procedures (Fagella and Arohnson, 1993) (Table 24–3). Zolazepam is a benzodiazepine that is combined with the dissociative anesthetic tiletamine in Telazol. Both midazolam and zolazepam have been reported to cause prolonged excitement in adult cats. This excitement can be alleviated by administration of the specific benzodiazepine antagonist flumazenil (Table 24–4) or the administration of another tranquilizer.

Acepromazine, a commonly used tranquilizer in adult animals, can be used safely in puppies and kittens older than 8 weeks if reduced doses are used (see Table 24–2). The availability of less depressing, reversible tranquilizers/sedatives, however, makes acepromazine a less desirable choice for any puppy or kitten younger than 6 months (Hosgood and Hoskins, 1998a). Acepromazine does not provide analgesia and can cause pronounced and prolonged central nervous system depression in young animals with immature hepatic function. A peripheral vasodilator, acepromazine causes hypotension and potentiates hypothermia. The commercially prepared concentration (10 mg/ml) makes it difficult to accurately measure small doses; therefore, a dilute solution (1 mg/ml) can be made by combining nine parts of sterile water with one part of acepromazine (Hosgood and Hoskins, 1998a).

Alpha$_2$-agonists (xylazine and medetomidine) provide sedation, analgesia, and muscle relaxation while profoundly depressing both heart rate and respiration, even at low doses (Haskins et al, 1986). These agents undergo extensive hepatic degradation and are not recommended for animals that are severely liver compromised or younger than 8 weeks. Concurrent use of an anticholinergic is imperative (Hosgood and Hoskins, 1998a). Specific antagonists are available (see Table 24–4).

Opioids

Opioids provide analgesia and sedation and are well tolerated even by critically ill pediatric animals (Hosgood and Hoskins, 1998a). Their effects are due to activation of one or more endogenous opioid receptors. The degree of analgesia and potential for side effects are related to their individual receptor affinities (Table 24–5).

Bradycardia, a potentially serious, dose-related side effect of opioids, can be avoided by co-administration of an anticholinergic (Hosgood and Hoskins, 1998a). Any reduction in heart rate, with the resultant drop in cardiac output, is poorly tolerated by neonatal and pediatric animals. Respiratory depression is another potentially serious dose-related effect due to the limited respiratory reserve of pediatric animals. Concurrent administration of other anesthetic agents may potentiate the cardiopulmonary depressant effects. Agents classified as partial agonists or agonist-antagonists provide moderate analgesia with the least cardiopulmonary depression (see Table 24–5). Premedication with an opioid can decrease the amount of inhalation agent necessary. Thus, the use of a well-balanced anesthetic regimen can provide the desired level of anesthesia and analgesia without significantly depressing the myocardium yet maintaining hemodynamics. Whenever opioids are used, careful cardiopulmonary monitoring is prudent.

Antagonists are available if reversal is desired (see Table 24–4). Although a pure antagonist (naloxone, naltrexone) will reverse any adverse effects, it will also reverse any analgesia. To preserve analgesia, reversal with a partial antagonist such as butorphanol is indicated. Opioids can be effectively administered by a variety of routes: parenteral, oral, nasal, rectal, transdermal, epidural, spinal, and intraarticular. Short-acting, highly potent opioid agonists, like fentanyl, can be delivered through a transdermal patch or as a continuous infusion intravenously or epidurally. Local application of these agents (epidurally or intraarticularly) provides prolonged analgesia without systemic side effects.

Table 24–3	Combination Anesthetic Protocols for Use in Puppies and Kittens	
AGENT(S)	DOSE	COMMENTS
KITTENS		
Midazolam Ketamine	0.22 mg/kg IM 11–22 mg/kg IM	Most effective combination for ovariohyster-ectomy in kittens when followed by inhalation anesthesia. Provides insufficient analgesia as sole protocol for castration of kittens
Atropine Midazolam Ketamine Butorphanol	0.04 mg/kg IM 0.22 mg/kg IM 11 mg/kg IM 0.44 mg/kg IM	Not recommended as sole protocol. Supplement with inhalation anesthesia
Atropine Midazolam Ketamine Oxymorphone	0.04 mg/kg IM 0.11 mg/kg IM 11 mg/kg IM 0.07 mg/kg IM	Not recommended as sole protocol. Supplement with inhalation anesthesia. May cause hyperexcitement during recovery
Telazol	11 mg/kg IM	Most effective protocol for castration of kittens. Provides most analgesia of all protocols. May be necessary to supplement with inhalation anesthesia
PUPPIES		
Atropine Midazolam Butorphanol Xylazine	0.04 mg/kg IM 0.22 mg/kg IM 0.44 mg/kg IM 1.1 mg/kg IM	Not recommended. Unsatisfactory protocol for castration of puppies. Significant respiratory depression
Atropine Midazolam Oxymorphone Xylazine	0.04 mg/kg IM 0.22 mg/kg IM 0.22 mg/kg IM 1.1 mg/kg IM	Not recommended. Unsatisfactory protocol for castration of puppies. Significant respiratory depression
Atropine Oxymorphone followed by propofol	0.04 mg/kg IM 0.22 mg/kg IM followed by 3.5 mg/kg IV	Provides best-quality anesthesia for castration of puppies. Provides best-quality anesthesia for ovariohysterectomy in puppies when followed by inhalation anesthesia. Transient apnea after propofol administration
Midazolam Butorphanol followed by propofol	0.22 mg/kg IM 0.44 mg/kg IM followed by 3.5 mg/kg IV	Provides little sedation before propofol injection, but provides good operative analgesia. Transient apnea after propofol administration. Administer propofol over 1–2 min to effect to avoid apnea
Atropine Midazolam Oxymorphone	0.04 mg/kg IM 0.22 mg/kg IM 0.22 mg/kg IM	
Midazolam Butorphanol	0.22 mg/kg IM 0.44 mg/kg IM	Suitable premedication before inhalation induction of anesthesia
Telazol	13.2 mg/kg IM	Unsatisfactory protocol for castration of puppies. Causes hypersalivation

IM = Intramuscular; IV = intravenous.

Data from Fagella AM, Arohnson MG: Anesthesia techniques for neutering 6- to 14-week-old kittens. J Am Vet Med Assoc 202:56, 1993; Fagella AM, Aronsohn MG: Evaluation of anesthetic protocols for neutering 6- to 14-week-old pups. J Am Vet Med Assoc 205:308, 1994.

Table 24–4 Tranquilizer/Sedative Antagonist Agents and Suggested Doses for Puppies and Kittens

AGENT	ANTAGONISTIC EFFECTS	DOSE	COMMENTS
Flumazenil	Benzodiazepines	0.1 mg/kg IV to effect	Duration short: 1 h in adults. May have agonist effects at high dose
Yohimbine	α_2-Receptors	0.25–0.5 mg/kg IM 0.15 mg/kg IV to effect	May cause excitement after IV administration
Atipamazole	α_2-Receptors	0.2 to 0.4 mg/kg IM	Most effective reversal agent
Tolazoline	α_1- and α_2-Receptors	0.3 mg/kg IV to effect	
Naloxone	Pure narcotic antagonist	0.04–0.4 mg IV to effect	Short duration: 0.5–1.5 h. Animals may renarcotize
Naltrexone	Pure narcotic antagonist	0.04 mg/kg IV	8–12 h duration. Most effective for reversal of central effects relative to epidural opioid administration
Nalmefene	Pure narcotic antagonist	0.1–0.2 mg/kg IV or IM	8–10 h duration. New agent
Butorphanol	Narcotic agonist-antagonist	0.2 mg/kg IV, IM, SC	Used to reverse bradycardia and respiratory depression of agonists, while maintaining analgesia
Nalbuphine	Narcotic agonist-antagonist	0.5–2.0 mg/kg IV, IM, SC	Lasts 2–4 h. Less potent analgesic than butorphanol

IM = Intramuscular; IV = intravenous; SC = subcutaneous.
Data from Hosgood G, Hoskins JD: Anaesthesia and pain management. *In* Hosgood G, Hoskins JD: Small Animal Paediatric Medicine and Surgery. Oxford, Butterworth-Heinemann, 1998, p 18.

Table 24–5 Relative Activity and Potency of Opioids

AGENT	SCHEDULE	RECEPTOR ACTIVITY*		RELATIVE POTENCY	DURATION
		Mu	Kappa		
Morphine	II	+ +	+	1.0	4 h
Meperidine	II	+	+	0.5	1–2 h
Oxymorphone	II	+ +	+	5–10	4–6 h
Fentanyl	II	+ + +	+	100	15–30 min
Buprenorphine	V	P	Unknown	5	8–12 h
Butorphanol	Not controlled (IV)†	−	+ +	3–5	4–6 h

*+ = Agonist; − = antagonist; P = partial agonist; Mu effects = supraspinal analgesia, respiratory depression, bradycardia, sedation, miosis, hypothermia, euphoria, physical dependence; Kappa effects = spinal analgesia, mild respiratory depression, sedation.
†Some states in the United States have begun to schedule butorphanol as a Class IV agent.
Data from Hosgood G, Hoskins JD: Anaesthesia and pain management. *In* Hosgood G, Hoskins JD (eds): Small Animal Paediatric Medicine and Surgery. Oxford, Butterworth-Heinemann, 1998, p 14.

Anesthesia Induction
INJECTABLE ANESTHETICS

Several injectable anesthetic agents produce rapid and reliable induction to general anesthesia. Young animals have a higher percentage of total body water than do adults and a larger volume of distribution, which may necessitate higher doses of water-soluble agents to achieve desired effects. Duration of action and side effects may, however, then be prolonged due to decreased muscle and fat for redistribution, immature hepatic enzyme systems, and delayed excretion. Several of the intravenous induction agents cause respiratory depression and apnea after injection, of particular concern in puppies and kittens with little or no respiratory reserve. It is imperative to be prepared to intubate and provide oxygen to these animals after the administration of such agents.

Thiopental. Thiopental is an ultrashort-acting barbiturate that can be used for intravenous induction to general anesthesia in healthy puppies and kittens older than 8 weeks. Thiopental is highly protein bound in plasma. Because puppies and kittens have lower albumin concentrations than adult animals, a greater percentage of active circulating drug is available to cross the blood-brain barrier, resulting in a lower dose requirement for induction. Dose-dependent respiratory depression makes it important to obtain an accurate weight in order to ensure proper dosing. The use of a dilute 1% to 2% solution will increase the total volume injected and facilitate titration of small dosages (Grandy and Dunlop, 1991). Termination of the anesthetic effect of thiopental is due to redistribution of the agent to fat and muscle as well as hepatic degradation. Hence, for puppies and kittens, additional doses of thiopental after induction should be avoided because the limited fat and muscle deposits will be readily saturated and the immature hepatic enzyme systems will be overwhelmed, leading to a prolonged recovery. Thiopental may precipitate cardiac arrhythmias and does not provide analgesia. It is extremely irritating to tissues if injected perivascularly.

Methohexital. Methohexital is also an ultrashort-acting barbiturate. It has similar effects to those of thiopental, but, because of a shorter elimination half-life, its use is associated with a faster recovery. Methohexital may cause seizures, and dysphoria is often seen on induction and recovery in unpremedicated animals.

Propofol. Propofol is an ultrashort-acting intravenous anesthetic agent that can be used for induction or maintenance of general anesthesia in puppies and kittens. Two serious dose-related side effects of propofol administration are respiratory depression and hypotension (Smith et al, 1993). Propofol should be used with care in puppies and kittens younger than 8 weeks due to their lack of respiratory reserve and unreliable baroreceptor reflexes. Rapid intravenous injection will increase the likelihood and severity of depressant effects (Smith et al, 1993). Propofol should be administered as a slow bolus over 1 to 2 minutes until the desired effect is achieved. A slow injection rate allows the use of a lower total induction dose and offsets cardiopulmonary depression. Termination of effects is due to redistribution and hepatic metabolism. Although not completely understood, extrahepatic mechanisms appear to be responsible for metabolism of the drug. Therefore, repeat doses or continuous infusion of propofol can be administered without accumulation and prolonging recovery.

Propofol does not provide analgesia and should not be used as the sole anesthetic for painful procedures. It is formulated in a 1% emulsion similar to parenteral lipid formulations and packaged in vials intended for a single (human) dose. Because the vials do not contain any preservatives or bacteriostatic agents, to prevent waste, any remaining propofol should be carefully transferred into empty, sterile multiuse vials. The lipid emulsion is a perfect culture medium, so great care must be taken to avoid contamination during transfer to and withdrawal from the multiuse vial.

Etomidate. Etomidate is an ultrashort-acting nonbarbiturate intravenous anesthetic agent that can be used for induction or maintenance of general anesthesia. Etomidate does not depress respiratory or cardiac function. Duration is determined by rate of redistribution to well-perfused tissues and hepatic metabolism. Etomidate's anesthetic effects are noncumulative, and anesthesia can be maintained by continuous infusion. Etomidate does not provide analgesia, and administration is associated with several adverse effects, including pain on injection, vomiting, and dysphoria during induction and recovery (Muir and Mason, 1989). These effects can be eliminated by premedication. Although this drug has been proved safe for adult animals, its suitability for puppies and kittens has not been documented.

Ketamine. Ketamine is a dissociative anesthetic that can be safely used alone, or in combination with a tranquilizer/sedative, for induction or maintenance of general anesthesia in puppies and kittens (Fagella and Arohnson, 1993, 1994) (see Tables 24–2 and 24–3). At recommended dosages, ketamine does not compromise cardiopulmonary function. Because termination of effects depends on renal elimination in cats and hepatic degradation in dogs, dissociative agents must be used with caution in animals younger than 8 weeks old due to their reduced hepatic metabolism and renal clearance abilities. Additional doses should be avoided due to accumulation and prolonged recovery. The level of analgesia provided by ketamine is a matter of controversy. Ketamine interferes with the perception of pain by depressing spinal cord transmission of pain impulses and functionally disorganizing specific midbrain and thalamic pathways. There may also be some activity at opioid receptors. The degree of analgesia provided by ketamine alone is sufficient for some minor procedures, but supplementation with opioids and/or inhalation agents is necessary for invasive surgical procedures (Hosgood and Hoskins, 1998a). Copious salivation is a common side effect that can be controlled by the co-administration of atropine or glycopyrrolate. Pharyngeal reflexes remain intact during dissociative anesthesia, but aspiration can still occur. Endotracheal intubation is highly recommended after the administration of ketamine. Both intraocular and intracranial pressures are increased by ketamine; therefore, it is contraindicated for animals with head trauma or injury to the globe. Seizures have also been reported after its administration. There is not an antagonist available for ketamine.

Telazol. Telazol is a commercial preparation composed of a dissociative anesthetic, tiletamine, and a benzodiazepine, zolazepam. Tiletamine is similar in activity to ketamine but is more potent and has a longer duration of action. Telazol provides smooth anesthetic induction and recovery; however, the same precautions should be taken as with ketamine. The zolazepam component may contribute to an excitable, prolonged recovery, particularly in cats. Telazol, alone, is ideal for castration of 8- to 12-week-old kittens but requires supplementation with an inhalation anesthetic for castration of puppies and ovariohysterectomy in kittens and puppies (see Table 24–3).

INHALATION AGENTS

Anesthetic induction with inhalation agents occurs quickly in pediatric animals because of their decreased functional residual capacity, increased alveolar ventilation, and centralized circulation. These factors make it easier to rapidly reach an excessive depth of anesthesia in puppies and kittens; however, they also make an overdose easier to reverse. The speed of induction is also affected by the hydration status of the animal, type of breathing circuit used, and oxygen flow rate. All inhalation agents depress cardiopulmonary function in a dose-dependent manner. Premedication will decrease the amount of inhalation agent required and reduce depressant effects.

Isoflurane and halothane are the agents of choice. Although isoflurane is as hypotensive as halothane, it is less of a cardiac depressant, undergoes minimal hepatic metabolism, and lowers cerebral oxygen need. Halothane is less irritating to airways but is dysrhythmogenic and undergoes greater hepatic metabolism. Sevoflurane, a new inhalation agent similar to isoflurane, is gaining popularity for use in human infants because it provides an even faster induction and recovery, without airway irritation. Nitrous oxide can be used at a 50:50 ratio with oxygen to invoke the second-gas effect and speed induction. Animals younger than 12 weeks are particularly sensitive to apnea and hypoxia, and nitrous oxide should not be used during maintenance without the support of an oxygen analyzer to ensure adequate oxygen delivery. Waste anesthetic gases from anesthetic machines must be scavenged and removed from the workplace to eliminate danger to personnel.

Mask Induction and Intubation

Mask induction is usually easily accomplished in animals younger than 10 weeks. Nitrous oxide can be added to oxygen at a ratio of 2:1 or 3:1 to invoke the second-gas effect and minimize the excitement phase during induction (Meyer, 1987); however, nitrous oxide should be discontinued after tracheal intubation (Hosgood and Hoskins, 1998a). Animals 10 to 16 weeks old and those difficult to restrain can be induced in a chamber infused with the gases. Sedation can be used before chamber induction. Selection of a preanesthetic agent that provides analgesia reduces the requirement of the volatile agent and subsequently reduces the degree of cardiovascular depression.

If possible, intubation of puppies and kittens should be performed with a cuffed Magill endotracheal tube or a noncuffed Cole endotracheal tube. Care should be taken to avoid laryngeal trauma, which may induce swelling. The noncuffed endotracheal tube allows use of a maximum diameter tube. This is important for very small animals because the resistance to airflow is inversely proportional to the radius of the airway. The Cole tube is, however, more rigid and more easily dislodged from the airway than is the cuffed Magill tube (Robinson, 1983). Endotracheal tubes as small as 2.4 mm in diameter are available; however, tubes smaller than 3.0 mm in diameter are easily obstructed by secretions and should be suctioned every 20 to 30 minutes. Soft silicone tubing can be used to make an endotracheal tube if appropriate sizes are not available.

If intubation cannot be performed, a tight-fitting mask can be used to minimize dead space and anesthetic gas leakage into the environment (Haskins et al, 1986). Clear plastic masks allow visualization of mucous membrane color and nares; an accumulation of secretions in the nares may cause mechanical obstruction of airflow.

Ventilation

Neonatal and pediatric animals have a high metabolic need and oxygen consumption. Their respiratory rate is two to three times that of adults in order to supply this need. Most anesthetic agents will depress respiratory function. This is particularly critical in puppies and kittens, which have little or no respiratory reserve and are subsequently prone to hypoventilation and hypoxemia. To guarantee adequate ventilation and oxygenation during anesthesia, ventilation should be assisted or controlled. Ventilation can be assisted manually or with a mechanical ventilator. The tidal volume for animals less than 12 weeks of age is 2.5 to 3 ml/ kg; older animals have a tidal volume of 5 ml/ kg. Airway pressures should not exceed 15 to 20 cm H_2O. Specific pediatric ventilators are available, or adult ventilators can be fitted with a pediatric bellows system.

Anesthesia Breathing Circuits

The selection of an anesthetic delivery circuit depends on body weight. Non-rebreathing systems (Ayre's T-piece, Norman elbow, Bain circuit) are used in animals weighing less than 4.5 kg to reduce resistance and work of breathing. The fresh gas flow should be 200 ml/kg per minute to prevent rebreathing of exhaled gases (Dunlop, 1992). The fresh gas enters directly at the airway in these systems, and response to vaporizer adjustments is much faster. The high gas flows of non-rebreathing systems contribute

to hypothermia and insensible fluid loss, as well as using more oxygen and agent. For animals weighing 4.5 to 10 kg, either a non-rebreathing or pediatric circle system can be used. A pediatric circle system is similar to the adult version except that the delivery hoses are shorter and smaller in diameter (15 vs. 22 mm). Some systems are equipped with smaller carbon dioxide absorber canisters. These systems should be used with oxygen flow rates of 30 ml/kg per minute (Dunlop, 1992; Grandy and Dunlop, 1991). An adult circle system can be used for animals weighing more than 10 kg (Hosgood and Hoskins, 1998a).

INTRAOPERATIVE CONSIDERATIONS

Fluid and Metabolic Support

During anesthesia, an intravenous fluid rate of 4 to 10 ml/kg per hour should be maintained to replace insensible water losses and limited blood loss and to offset hypotension (see Table 24–1). Careful determination of body weight is important for calculation of rate, and administration should be precisely controlled with a pediatric minidrip fluid administration set (60 drops/ml), an inexpensive, inline fluid regulator, an inline reservoir, or a syringe infusion pump. If none of these control devices is available, the hourly requirement can be divided, and microboluses can be given every 5 to 10 minutes (Hosgood and Hoskins, 1998b).

The maintenance fluid of choice for young animals is 2.5% to 5% dextrose in a balanced electrolyte solution. In the case of a septic or hypoglycemic animal, 10% dextrose or higher may be indicated. During prolonged anesthetic periods, glucose should be checked periodically and the dextrose concentration of the fluid adjusted as necessary. Continuous glucose administration is preferred over bolus administration to avoid development of profound hyperglycemia. Because the blood-brain barrier in the pediatric animal is less functional than in the adult, profound hyperglycemia may cause glucose to cross the blood-brain barrier, resulting in the development of cerebral edema. When there is measurable blood loss during surgery, replacement is 3 ml for every 1 ml of blood of the balanced electrolyte maintenance fluid being used. If blood loss exceeds 15% to 20% of blood volume, however, it should be replaced with an equal volume of a blood product.

Intravenous catheterization of the jugular or cephalic vein is best for administration of intraoperative fluids, electrolytes, drugs, or blood products. All air should be carefully purged from the administration set before connection, as even a small amount may be significant in an animal weighing less than 5 kg (Hosgood and Hoskins, 1998b). Drugs administered intravenously during fluid administration should be given as closely to the catheter as possible to avoid having to give a fluid bolus.

When intravenous catheterization cannot be performed, fluids can be administered by intraosseous or subcutaneous routes. Intraosseous cannulation of the humerus, femur or tibia can be performed readily without any special equipment or training (Otto et al, 1989). This route can be used for rapid administration of fluids, blood, and drugs. Fluid flow rates of up to 11 ml/min can be achieved with gravity (Otto et al, 1989).

Subcutaneous fluid administration is less reliable than intravenous or intraosseous administration, and the amount of fluid that can be given is limited by the animal's size. Small volumes should be administered through multiple sites. Only isotonic fluids with less than 5% dextrose fluids should be used.

Blood transfusion or blood component therapy is best administered intravenously; however, intraosseous administration is possible (Otto et al, 1989). Absorption of blood components by the intraosseous route is rapid; absorption is 95% complete within 5 minutes (Hodge et al, 1987; Spivey et al, 1985). Whole blood can be infused at rates up to 22 ml/kg per day, especially to compensate for hypovolemia. Care should be taken, however, not to induce circulatory overload. Plasma (for clotting factor deficiencies) can be administered at rates up to 6 to 10 ml/kg two or three times a day for 3 to 5 days or until bleeding has stopped (Authement et al, 1987).

Thermal Support

Puppies and kittens tend to develop hypothermia, which prolongs anesthetic recovery and cardiovascular depression. Continuous monitoring of body temperature is very important. Precautions can be taken to avoid the development of profound hypothermia (Table 24–6).

Intraoperative Monitoring

The level of monitoring for pediatric animals should be consistent with the severity of the underlying disease and the surgical procedure. Pediatric animals, especially those younger than

Table 24–6 Precautions to Prevent Profound Hypothermia During Anesthesia and Surgery

Maintain a warm ambient temperature in the surgical suite
Place a circulating warm-water blanket underneath the animal during surgery and recovery
Warm the intravenous and lavage fluids
Keep the animal dry
Minimize the amount of hair clipped
Avoid use of alcohol or alcohol-containing skin disinfectants
Warm the skin disinfectants
Humidify the inhaled gases
Keep the animal covered when possible
Minimize the surgery time, especially if a body cavity is open

12 weeks of age, decompensate rapidly due to minimal cardiopulmonary reserves, and diligent monitoring of all systems is imperative to their well-being. Physiologic monitoring can be accomplished by invasive or noninvasive methods (Table 24–7) (Hosgood and Hoskins, 1998b).

Noninvasive methods are generally easy to perform and inexpensive and can provide accurate and reliable information, or at least indicate trends, depending on the method used (Hosgood and Hoskins, 1998b). Direct observation during surgery is facilitated by the use of a clear plastic drape. Invasive methods require the placement of instrumentation inside the body. Invasive monitoring is more accurate but often requires expensive equipment and special techniques. Puppies and kittens weighing less than 2.5 kg are difficult to monitor because of their small size. It is imperative that instrumentation be placed quickly to avoid development of profound hypothermia before the surgical procedure has even started. Monitoring methods that provide the most information with the least difficulty are preferred. Accurate interpretation and integration of information obtained by individual monitoring methods are imperative if it is to be of value.

Cardiovascular System

Basic cardiac monitoring includes the constant evaluation of heart rate and rhythm, pulse quality, capillary refill time, and mucous membrane color, all of which can be determined by simple auscultation and palpation. Direct contact with a small puppy or kitten that is undergoing surgery, however, may be difficult.

Table 24–7	Available Physiologic Monitors and Their Applications for Puppies and Kittens		
MONITOR	COST ($US)	PARAMETERS	COMMENTS
Esophageal Stethoscope	$17–$300	Heart and respiratory rate and rhythm	Inexpensive, user friendly, accurate; can be used with earpieces or an amplifier
Respiratory Monitor	$115–$300	Respiratory air movement and apnea monitor	Inexpensive; sensitivity depends on monitor; can be used with mask; pressure on thorax can produce false respiratory sounds; adapter adds dead space
Ultrasonic Doppler Unit	$500–$700	Pulse rate, rhythm, and quality; estimates systolic blood pressure	Relatively inexpensive, versatile, accurate, small probes available, use with cuff and manometer to measure systolic blood pressure, inaccurate at low blood pressures
Oscillometric Blood Pressure	$2500	Heart rate; systolic, diastolic, and mean blood pressures	Easy to use, accuracy depends on cuff size, inaccurate at low blood pressures and in small animals, useful reflection of trends
Pulse Oximeter	$1200–$2000	Pulse rate and functional oxygen saturation of hemoglobin	Noninvasive, various style probes available, valuable for animals younger than 8 wk of age due to rapid desaturation, accuracy affected by hypotension and hypothermia
Electrocardiograph	$2700–$5995	Heart rate; identification of rhythm	Expensive, various style leads available, electrical activity can continue without mechanical activity
Capnometer/ Capnograph	$2695	Inspired or expired carbon dioxide concentration; respiratory rate	Noninvasive, assesses ventilation and rebreathing, adds dead space and may be less accurate with non-rebreathing circuits
Invasive Blood Pressure Monitor	$2700–$5995	Heart rate; direct arterial systolic, diastolic, and mean blood pressures; pulse pressure wave	Requires placement of arterial catheter; most accurate; pulse wave reflects inotropic function, stroke volume, volume status, and peripheral vascular resistance; need transducer between catheter and monitor; samples from arterial catheter source for blood gas determination

The esophageal stethoscope provides a remote, noninvasive, and simple way to continuously monitor both cardiac and respiratory sounds (see Table 24–7). An ultrasonic Doppler crystal, placed over a peripheral artery, detects blood flow and provides an audible signal that allows continuous evaluation of pulse rate, rhythm, and strength (see Table 24–7). In small puppies or kittens, the crystal can be placed on the thorax, directly over the heart. The Doppler can be used to measure systolic blood pressure by placement of an occlusive cuff connected to an aneroid manometer proximal to the Doppler crystal on a limb or at the base of the tail. The cuff is inflated until the pulse is no longer detected. The pressure is then released slowly until the pulse can be detected again. The pressure at which the first sound is detected is systolic blood pressure.

Systolic, diastolic, and mean arterial blood pressure as well as heart rate can be obtained intermittently with an automatic oscillometric blood pressure monitor (see Table 24–7). The oscillations caused by varying pulse pressures are measured during gradual deflation of an air-filled cuff. The measurements are then interpreted and electronically displayed. Accuracy, for both Doppler and oscillometric methods, depends on the use of the appropriate sized cuff. The width of the cuff should be approximately 40% of the circumference of that part of the limb to which it is applied. Indirect blood pressure determinations are difficult to obtain consistently in animals less than 4.5 kg, and accuracy is decreased at low blood pressures. Knowledge of blood pressure trends, however, provides important information about cardiovascular status.

The electrocardiogram (ECG) provides a noninvasive, continuous evaluation of heart rate and rhythm (see Table 24–7). The ECG, however, records only myocardial electrical activity and provides no information about myocardial function. Lead placement is not critical for monitoring intraoperatively. What is important is the recognition of any changes in the appearance of the complexes or rhythm during the anesthetic period.

Direct measurement of arterial blood pressure requires catheterization of a peripheral artery. The arterial catheter is then connected to a measuring device. Fluid-filled extension tubing connected to an aneroid manometer is an inexpensive way to determine mean arterial blood pressure. Connection of the arterial catheter to a commercially available transducer and recording system provides a continuous, accurate, quantitative measurement of heart rate and systolic, diastolic, and mean blood pressures (see Table 24–7). A pulse pressure wave display is also generated and provides insight with regard to myocardial inotropic function, stroke volume, volume status, and peripheral vascular resistance.

The arteries most accessible for catheterization in puppies and kittens are the dorsal pedal, femoral, and lingual. The area over the artery is surgically prepared, and the appropriate-sized catheter is inserted. Complications associated with arterial catheterization include hematoma formation, air embolization, infection, and arterial thrombosis.

Respiratory System

Basic monitoring of the respiratory system consists of constant evaluation of respiratory rate, pattern, effort of breathing, changes in tidal volume, and mucous membrane color through simple observation and auscultation. Observation of thoracic excursions or movement of the rebreathing bag is a reliable method for determination of rate and rhythm. In animals less than 4.5 kg, however, it may be difficult to visualize chest movement once they are draped for surgery, and movement of the reservoir bag in a non-rebreathing system is often hard to detect and less reliable than that of a circle system.

The esophageal stethoscope provides a remote, noninvasive, and simple way to continuously monitor both respiratory and cardiac sounds. Simple breath monitors attach to the end of the endotracheal tube and beep with each breath or sound an alarm if there are no breaths detected within a specified time (see Table 24–7). The movement of air or change in temperature is detected by a sensor located within the connector on the end of the endotracheal tube.

The high sensitivity of these monitors may, however, result in false breaths being registered during surgical manipulation of viscera, whenever the thorax is touched, or when the animal is moved. False breath sounds may also be heard when the esophagus is mistakenly intubated, delaying recognition of a problem. The endotracheal tube connector increases dead space in the breathing circuit that could be significant in animals weighing less than 2 kg.

Respiratory frequency and rhythm do not, however, reflect ventilatory effectiveness. Direct measurement of arterial partial pressure of carbon dioxide ($PaCO_2$) is the most accurate and representative way to determine if ventilation is normal. This requires the collection of an arterial blood sample. The measurement of expired or end-tidal carbon dioxide concentration (E_TCO_2) is an easy and reliable method to approximate $PaCO_2$. A capnometer or capnograph uses infrared technology to continuously measure the partial pressure of CO_2 in expired respiratory gases, as well as respiratory rate (see Table 24–7). Two types of sample analysis are available: mainstream and sidestream. With mainstream evaluation, the sensor is located on a connector attached to the endotracheal tube and readings are instantaneous. In sidestream analysis, gases are aspirated from the breathing system via a sampling line attached to a T-connector placed at the end of the endotracheal tube. Samples are drawn into the monitor for evaluation, and there is a slight delay. The E_TCO_2 is typically less than the actual $PaCO_2$, with a 1 to 10 mmHg gradient being normal in small animals. The endotracheal tube connector increases dead space and rebreathing of expired gases, which may be significant in animals weighing less than 2 kg. Capnography is an important tool that can be used for detection of airway obstruction or disconnection, bronchospasm, severe cardiovascular disturbances, increased metabolic rate, malignant hyperthermia, and hypothermia.

Oxygenating efficiency of the lungs is best determined by analysis of the arterial partial pressure of oxygen (PaO_2), requiring an arterial blood sample. Use of a pulse oximeter is a noninvasive method of continuously monitoring pulse rate and functional hemoglobin oxygen saturation (see Table 24–7). Hemoglobin saturation is related to the PaO_2 by a sigmoid curve. A specially designed probe transmits red and near-infrared light through tissues, senses the movement of a pulsating arteriolar bed, interprets color absorption in the moving tissue, and relates it to oxygen saturation (SaO_2 or SpO_2). A variety of probe configurations are available.

The most useful sites for probe placement include tongue, cheek, gums, pinna, toe or toe web, and skinfolds. Hair and highly pigmented skin will interfere with the ability to obtain an accurate and consistent reading. A reflectance-type probe for esophageal or rectal placement is also available. Accuracy is affected by changes in cardiopulmonary status, peripheral vasoconstriction, hypothermia, dyshemoglobinemias, shivering, and interference from fluorescent or red-light heat lamps. Puppies and kittens are highly susceptible to the development of hypoxemia, and pulse oximetry is a valuable tool for early detection of hemoglobin desaturation and hypoxemia.

As stated earlier, the most accurate way to evaluate ventilation and oxygenation is by the analysis of carbon dioxide and oxygen concentrations in an arterial blood sample. This requires the collection of an arterial blood sample and the availability of a blood gas analyzer. There are several portable blood analyzers currently available that make determination of arterial blood gas concentrations more affordable and practical. Arterial samples may, however, be difficult to obtain in pediatric animals, and analysis can be done only intermittently rather than on a continuous basis.

Temperature

Temperature monitoring can be done continuously with an esophageal or rectal probe attached to a temperature monitor or intermittently with a thermometer. Some esophageal temperature probes are also esophageal stethoscopes and can be used to monitor heart and lung sounds. Aural temperatures are used if other sites are inaccessible. Aural temperatures are usually about 1° F less than rectal temperatures.

Instrumentation and Tissue Handling

The delicate tissue of puppies and kittens must be handled with great care. During preoperative clipping of the hair, appropriate-size clipper blades should be used to avoid laceration of the skin. The use of special pediatric instruments facilitates proper tissue handling. Addition of these instruments to a surgical pack may be warranted if surgery is performed on puppies and kittens frequently (Table 24–8). Meticulous hemostasis is imperative because even a small volume of blood loss can represent a relatively large total blood volume loss. Radiosurgery may facilitate hemostasis but should be kept to a minimum because of its potential deleterious effect on wound healing (Fucci and Elkins, 1991). In addition, use of the appropriate setting (cut versus coagulation versus cut/coagulation) and wattage is important. Use of a fine-tipped, bipolar handpiece allows precise placement of the current and avoids excessive tissue damage. Bleeding vessels should be ligated with a fine, absorbable suture material; 4–0 or 5–0 poliglecaprone 25, glycomer 631, polyglactin 910, or chromic catgut is appropriate (Table 24–9). Hemostatic clips may be useful on small, fragile vessels to avoid tearing during ligation (Arohnson and Fagella, 1993).

Magnification

The use of magnification will facilitate pediatric surgery. Head loupes constitute the most practical and versatile magnification equipment. These can be mounted to the frame of eyeglasses or on a headband and are usually hinged such that they can be lifted up out of the line of sight. Some companies can fit prescription lenses to the eyeglasses. Most models come with a halogen or fiberoptic light that can be clipped to the loupe or to the headband if using the glasses-mounted loupe (Surgitel, General Scientific Corporation, Ann Arbor, MI; Orascoptic

Table 24–8   Selected Pediatric Surgical Instruments for Addition to a General Surgery Pack

INSTRUMENT	USE AND COMMENTS
3 1/2-inch Backhaus towel clamps	Less traumatic and bulky than standard-size towel clamps
5-inch Hartmann mosquito forceps (straight and curved)	
5-inch Micro mosquito forceps (curved, delicate)	
5-inch Metzenbaum scissors (straight, delicate)	Easier to use than standard-size Metzenbaum scissors
5-inch Adson microtissue forceps (delicate)	Very fine-tipped atraumatic thumb forceps; grasps tissue more firmly than plain tissue forceps
5-inch Plain tissue forceps (delicate)	Fine-tipped atraumatic thumb forceps
6-inch DeBakey tissue forceps	Although long, they are very easy to use and cause minimal trauma associated with grasping tissue
3 3/8-inch Bishop-Harmann thumb forceps (1 × 2 teeth, 0.5 mm)	Fine, rat-toothed forceps useful for delicate tissue
6 1/4-inch Mixter gall duct forceps or 7 1/2-inch Kantrowitz thoracic forceps	Excellent for blunt dissection around delicate structures (e.g., patent ductus venosus, portosystemic shunt)
5 3/4-inch Babcock forceps (pediatric)	Essential for any gastrointestinal surgery or urogenital surgery; considered atraumatic in their use for grasping viscera
Bard-Parker tonsil scalpel handle, No. 7	Long handled, allows finer control than standard-size scalpel handle
Derf needle holder	Smaller than standard-size needle holders; useful for suturing with 3–0 to 5–0 suture
Iris scissors	Very small, usually sharp-pointed scissors; useful for controlled cutting of delicate tissue (e.g., vessels after ligation, ureters, urethra)
Castroviejo needle holder (5 1/2 inches)	Ophthalmic-type needle holder essential for use of suture material 5–0 and smaller
3 1/2-inch spread pediatric Gosset abdominal retractor	Similar to a Balfour abdominal retractor but smaller size for animals less than 6 kg
1 3/4-inch Barraquer eye speculum (10- or 15-mm blades)	Can be used as an abdominal retractor in very small animals less than 4 kg
Finochietto-DeBakey infant rib spreader	Essential for thoracic surgery

Data from Hosgood G, Hoskins JD: General surgical principles. *In* Hosgood G, Hoskins JD (eds): Small Animal Paediatric Medicine and Surgery. Oxford, Butterworth-Heinemann, 1998, p 58.

Table 24–9   Characteristics of and Indications for Different Suture Material Suitable for Puppies and Kittens

SUTURE MATERIAL	ABSORPTION	RETENTION OF TENSILE STRENGTH	COMMENTS
MONOFILAMENT ABSORBABLE WITHOUT PROLONGED ABSORPTION			
Poliglecaprone 25	90–120 d	67% retained by 7 d 33% retained by 14 d 0% retained by 21 d	Soft, pliable suture with good knot security. Moderately rapid rate of loss of tensile strength. Suitable for ligatures and subcutaneous closure. Possibly useful for gastrointestinal or urogenital closure in the healthy animal. Suitable for oral cavity. Use caution in the linea alba or gastrointestinal or urogenital tract in debilitated animals because of moderately rapid loss of tensile strength
Glycomer 631	90–110 d	66% retained by 7 d 41% retained by 14 d 23% retained by 21 d 11% retained by 28 d	As for poliglecaprone

Table continued on following page

Table 24–9 Characteristics of and Indications for Different Suture Material Suitable for Puppies and Kittens *Continued*

SUTURE MATERIAL	ABSORPTION	RETENTION OF TENSILE STRENGTH	COMMENTS
MULTIFILAMENT ABSORBABLE WITHOUT PROLONGED ABSORPTION			
Catgut (chromic)	>90 d	50% retained by 7 d 17% retained by 14 d 0% retained by 21 d	Incites variable degree of inflammatory reaction; unpredictable strength and absorption Probably better absorbable suture material now available
Polyglycolic acid	60–90 d	65% retained by 14 d 35% retained by 21 d	Substantial tissue drag and poor knot security Suitable for ligatures and gastrointestinal, linea alba, and subcutaneous closure. Suitable for oral cavity Prefer monofilament suture over multifilament
Polyglactin 910	56–70 d	83% retained at 7 d 75% retained by 14 d 50% retained by 21 d 0% retained by 28 d	As for polyglycolic acid
MONOFILAMENT ABSORBABLE WITH PROLONGED ABSORPTION			
Polydioxanone	186 d	80% retained at 7 d 70% retained at 14 d 50% retained at 28 d 25% retained at 42 d	Stiff suture with good knot security but some handling difficulties Suitable for ligatures and gastrointestinal and linea alba closures. Suitable for use in the oral cavity but may require removal Unsuitable for subcutaneous closure due to prolonged absorption Prolonged tensile strength probably unnecessary in healthy animal. Calcinosis circumscripta reported with use in young dogs
Polyglyconate	180 d	80% retained by 7 d 75% retained by 14 d 65% retained by 21 d 50% retained by 28 d 25% retained by 42 d	As for polydioxanone except slightly softer and easier to use. Calcinosis circumscripta not reported
MONOFILAMENT NONABSORBABLE			
Polypropylene			Moderate tensile strength with fair to good knot security. Considered inert Suitable for ligation and linea alba closure in debilitated animal; suitable for skin sutures; suitable for use in infected wounds No advantage to use in the linea alba in healthy animals
Polybutester			As for polypropylene but improved handling and slight elastic properties
Nylon			High tensile strength but poor knot security. Considered inert Also available in multifilament form. Indications as for polypropylene Suitable for use in infected wounds in monofilament form
Stainless steel			Monofilament and multifilament forms available Difficult to handle. Extreme tensile strength and permanency probably unnecessary and use not recommended May cut through delicate tissue
MULTIFILAMENT NONABSORBABLE			
Polyester, silk, caprolactam			Use not recommended. Unsuitable for implantation into tissue. Use restricted to skin sutures only

Suture Selection

Before a suture material is selected, the strength of the tissue, the rate of healing of the tissue, and the physical condition of the animal should be considered. In the otherwise healthy animal, a rapid gain in wound strength is observed at 7 to 10 days after surgery. Most absorbable suture materials provide adequate tensile strength for this period (see Table 24–9). Soft, nonirritating suture material, such as poliglecaprone 25, glycomer 631, or polyglactin 910, is preferred. Generally, a monofilament is preferable to a multifilament suture material. Polydioxanone has a prolonged rate of absorption and has been reported to cause calcinosis circumscripta in young dogs (Kirby et al, 1989). In severely debilitated animals when wound healing is delayed, the use of polydioxanone may be more appropriate than the more rapidly absorbed suture materials, or even the use of an inert, nonabsorbable suture material such as polypropylene or nylon may be indicated. Multifilament or coated nonabsorbable suture material such as polyester or caprolactam should not be used in deep tissue.

Suture material of the smallest possible diameter should be used—that is, 4–0 to 5–0 suture material for most tissues of very young animals, increasing to 3–0 to 4–0 suture material for older animals.

The skin of puppies and kittens is thin and delicate. Skin sutures made with very fine nonabsorbable suture material such as 4–0 or 5–0 nylon should be placed loosely. Skin tension should be alleviated with a subcutaneous or subcuticular closure (5–0 poliglecaprone 25, glycomer 631, polyglactin 910); if this is not done, the skin sutures may tear out. Tight skin sutures may cause skin necrosis, especially if swelling occurs. A subcuticular closure may alleviate the need for skin sutures. This is desirable to avoid the dam or queen's inadvertently chewing the sutures.

Needles

Appropriate selection of surgical needles is critical because the needle can induce the most trauma associated with suturing (Hosgood and Hoskins, 1998b). Use of swaged needles is essential. Selection of the smallest needle possible will minimize tissue trauma. A needle appropriate to the size of the suture should be used; some small-gauge suture materials come on many different needles. Use of a cutting needle in dense tissue will minimize trauma associated with passing the needle through the tissue. If a cutting needle is selected, use of a reverse cutting needle, with the cutting edge on the convex or outer edge of the needle, will reduce the likelihood of tearing through the tissue. These needles are stronger than the conventional cutting needle, which has the cutting edge on the concave or inside edge of the needle. Reverse cutting needles are applicable for use in the dermis and fascia and in oral surgery and some intestinal surgeries. Tapered cutting needles also minimize tissue trauma because they have a cutting point, either reverse or conventional, but a tapered body. These are useful in tissue that may have a dense and delicate component, such as the gastrointestinal tract.

Tissue Adhesives

Tissue adhesives are cyanoacrylate polymers that are catalyzed by minute amounts of water on the wound surface. Shorter chain derivatives (methyl-cyanoacrylate and ethyl-cyanoacrylate) have proven histotoxicity. These compounds are often the components of household "super glues." Longer chain derivatives (butyl-cyanoacrylate and isobutyl-cyanoacrylate) are much less histotoxic and are preferred (Hampel, 1991). The cyanoacrylate polymer is self-sterilizing with a setting time between 2 and 60 seconds.

The cyanoacrylates may offer an alternative to skin sutures in the young animal. Note that the healing tissue cannot penetrate the cyanoacrylate and must advance around the polymer. Hence, meticulous use is required. The cut surfaces should be dry and free of blood; the cyanoacrylate should be "spot welded" along the top of the cut edges and not placed directly on the cut surface. The amount of adhesive used should be minimized. Although the adhesive is relatively inert, granulomas, wound infection, and delayed healing have been reported, particularly if the adhesive is placed on the cut surface. Other reported uses of cyanoacrylate have been in oral surgery, intestinal anastomoses, the control of hemorrhage from parenchymatous organs, microvascular anastomoses, fracture repair, prosthetic implant maintenance, and skin graft placement.

Dimension-3, Orascoptic Acuity, Orascoptic Research Inc., Madison, WI; Perisphere Prism Loupes, Perisphere Industries Inc., Torrance, CA). Generally, magnification between $2.0\times$ and $2.5\times$ is adequate. Models are available in different working distances; for example, the Perisphere loupe is available in 300 or 420 mm. Generally, the shorter working distance is more suitable.

Fibrin-based glues may provide additional mechanical strength in wounds in the lag phase of healing, that is, at 0 to 3 to 5 days. These glues, as opposed to cyanoacrylate glues, are used as an adjunct to sutured or stapled closures, for example, to reduce the incidence of early leakage from anastomoses. Experimental and clinical evidence is still equivocal to date, and this, along with their expense, may limit their application.

Skin Staples

Skin staples substantially reduce the time required for skin closure and tend to discourage the animal or its mother from licking the wound. Although there are two sizes available (regular, with a 9.9-mm span before closure and 4.8 mm wide and 3.4 mm high when closed; and wide, with an 11.98-mm span before closure and 6.5 mm wide and 3.6 mm high when closed), even the regular may be too large for some puppies or kittens, and the staples will rotate in the skin or fall out. Skin staples are usually available in different cartridges containing 12, 25, or 35 staples. Partially used cartridges can be resterilized with ethylene oxide. Note that staples are most easily removed with a special yet inexpensive staple remover.

POSTOPERATIVE CONSIDERATIONS
Recovery and Body System Support

Continuous monitoring of vital signs (temperature, pulse, and respiration) and blood glucose is important in the first few hours after surgery. Fluid therapy can be discontinued after the animal has recovered sufficiently to eat or drink. In the awake animal, 50% dextrose solution can be administered orally if profound hypoglycemia is present. When the animal is eating normally, glucose determinations are no longer required. Respiratory depression is not uncommon, and, if narcotics have been used, reversal of their action is usually indicated. Untoward effects of other preanesthetic agents can also be reversed if an antagonist is available (see Table 24–3).

A quiet, warm environment is required for recovery. Careful, slow rewarming after surgery is accomplished most effectively by wrapping the animal in a circulating warm-water blanket or placing the animal on a circulating warm-water blanket under a 250-watt infrared heat lamp (Haskins, 1981). Care must be taken when heat lamps or hot water bottles are used as thermal injury can result (Dunlop et al, 1989).

Analgesic Therapy

Postoperative pain management in puppies and kittens younger than 8 weeks can be difficult because of the concerns about inducing or exacerbating bradycardia and respiratory depression. Ideally, analgesics should be administered before the painful event. This preemptive approach to pain management reduces the analgesic dose necessary and alleviates the stress on the animal. Analgesics can be administered as preanesthetics or intraoperatively. Parenterally administered agents, like butorphanol or buprenorphine, that cause minimal cardiopulmonary depression are recommended (see Table 24–3). Fentanyl is a potent analgesic that has minimal sedative and cardiopulmonary effects when delivered via transdermal patch at the appropriate dose (see Table 24–2). It takes at least 12 hours for effective drug levels to be reached, however, and the patch configuration makes it difficult to dose and regulate in animals that weigh less than 2 kg. Fentanyl can also be administered by continuous rate infusion, providing excellent analgesia with minimal side effects. This may require an additional intravenous catheter and is best done with the aid of a syringe infusion pump. Due to fentanyl's short duration of action, effects are terminated within 15 minutes of stopping the infusion.

Regional techniques provide postoperative analgesia without the potentially serious cardiopulmonary side effects of parenterally administered medications (Skarda, 1996). Most local techniques used for adults can be successfully used for puppies and kittens (Table 24–10).

Close attention to dose and technique is essential to avoid complications. Use of a lumbosacral epidural or spinal (subarachnoid) route with a local anesthetic, an opioid, or both is an acceptable technique for providing intraoperative and postoperative analgesia for many procedures (see Table 24–10). Epidural administration is associated with less risk of spinal cord damage and fewer side effects than is spinal administration. The selection of an agent or combination of agents depends on the condition of the animal, the type of surgery, and the desired effect (Krechel, 1990). Local anesthetics provide a total sensory and motor blockade for 1 to 6 hours, depending on the agent used (Table 24–11).

The epidural route can be used in a sedated or anesthetized animal. When part of the anes-

Table 24–10	Indications for and Application of Epidural Anesthesia and Analgesia	
INDICATION	**PROCEDURE(S)**	**COMPLICATION(S)**
Postoperative analgesia (opioids) without cardiopulmonary depression	Hindlimb fractures, amputation, other procedures	Hypovolemia (use local block)
	Abdominal surgery	Hypotension (use local blocks)
	Surgery of the perineum, tail	Coagulopathy
Total regional anesthesia (locals)	Cesarean section	Pyoderma at site of needle placement
	Thoracotomy	Septicemia
Decreased requirement for general anesthesia		Neurologic disorder
		Anatomic abnormalities
		Clipping hair on dorsum undesirable to owner

Data from Hosgood G, Hoskins JD: General surgical principles. *In* Hosgood G, Hoskins JD (eds): Small Animal Paediatric Medicine and Surgery. Oxford, Butterworth-Heinemann, 1998, p 58.

thetic protocol, epidural administration is best done immediately after induction, before the surgical procedure, but may be done at the termination of the surgery before recovery. A 22- to 20-gauge, 1.5- to 2.5-inch spinal needle is inserted with sterile technique into the lumbosacral space, between L7 and S1, on midline, parallel to the spine, at a 90° angle with the skin. The subarachnoid space of cats normally extends to or beyond the lumbosacral area, but in adult dogs it ends before L7. In young and small dogs, however, the subarachnoid space is often found to be further caudal, making the risk of dural puncture high in puppies and kittens younger than 6 months.

Intraarticular injection of local anesthetics and opioids has been shown to provide effective postoperative analgesia in adult dogs. For best results, the joint capsule should be closed before drugs are introduced into the joint space. Either 0.5% bupivacaine at 0.5 ml/kg or morphine at 0.1 mg/kg diluted in saline to a volume of 0.5 ml/kg will reduce pain related to intraarticular surgery (Sammarco et al, 1996). These agents can be combined, with bupivacaine as the diluent for the morphine.

Table 24–11	Comparison of Agents for Epidural Anesthesia and Analgesia	
AGENT	**EFFECTS**	**COMPLICATIONS**
LOCAL ANESTHETICS*		
Lidocaine 2%	Sensory blockade	Hypotension
Procaine 2%	Motor blockade	Hypothermia
Carbocaine 2%	Sympathetic tone blockade	Respiratory depression
Bupivacaine 0.5%		Respiratory arrest
Etidocaine 1%		Accidental intravenous or subarachnoid injection
		Incomplete block
		Sepsis due to nonsterile technique
OPIOIDS (ANALGESIA)		
Morphine	Long-duration visceral and somatic analgesia without systemic effects	Pruritus
Oxymorphone		Delayed-onset respiratory depression
Meperidine		Delayed-onset sedation
Fentanyl	Not a block	Delayed-onset bradycardia
		Urinary retention
		Reduced gastrointestinal motility
		Accidental intravenous or subarachnoid injection
		Sepsis due to nonsterile technique

*With or without epinephrine.
Data from Hosgood G, Hoskins JD: Anaesthesia and pain management. *In* Hosgood G, Hoskins JD: Small Animal Paediatric Medicine and Surgery. Oxford, Butterworth-Heinemann, 1998, p 18.

A thoracotomy is a common surgical approach for correction of congenital cardiac anomalies and is associated with significant postoperative pain. Intercostal nerve blocks provide analgesia during and after thoracotomy. Local anesthetic is deposited on the nerves of two adjacent intercostal spaces both cranial and caudal to the incision. A long-acting local anesthetic is injected caudal to the dorsal angle of the rib. A dose of 0.25 to 1.0 ml of 0.25% or 0.5% bupivacaine, with or without epinephrine, will provide 3 to 6 hours of analgesia without respiratory compromise. Care should be taken not to exceed a total dose of 3 mg/kg.

Wound Protection

Protection of the surgical incision from self-mutilation is imperative to avoid wound breakdown. For animals that are not weaned, protection of the surgical incision from licking by the bitch or queen is extremely important. Keeping the incision site covered with a bandage or separating the young from the dam, except for feeding, is necessary. In weaned animals, protection of the incision through the use of an Elizabethan collar, either commercial or fashioned from cardboard or plastic, is preferred to bandaging to avoid bandaging complications. Inadvertent compression of the thorax or abdomen can occur easily with circumferential bandages. Tight bandages or bandages that do not extend far enough beyond the incision cause swelling proximal and distal to the bandaged area. If a limb requires bandaging, the entire limb should be covered by the bandage. Application of a surgical skin spray to the surgical incision will protect the uncovered wound from moisture and contamination. In contrast to surgical incisions, open wounds obviously require bandage protection.

Suture Removal

Suture removal from healthy puppies and kittens can be performed 7 days after surgery. For debilitated animals or when radiosurgery has been used on the surgical wound margins, suture removal should be delayed to 10 to 14 days after surgery (Fucci and Elkins, 1991).

References and Supplemental Reading

Arango A, Rowe MI: The neonatal puppy as an experimental subject. Bio Neonat 18:173, 1971.

Arohnson MG, Fagella AM: Surgical techniques for neutering 6- to 14-week-old kittens. J Am Vet Med Assoc 202:53, 1993.

Aschinberg LC, Goldsmith DI, Olbing H, et al: Neonatal changes in renal blood flow distribution in puppies. Am J Physiol 228:1453, 1975.

Authement JM, Wolfsheimer KJ, Catchings S: Canine blood component therapy: Product preparation, storage, and administration. J Am Anim Hosp Assoc 23:483, 1987.

Center SA, Hornbuckle WE, Hoskins JD: The liver and pancreas. In Hoskins JD (ed): Veterinary Pediatrics: Dogs and Cats from Birth to Six Months, 2nd ed. Philadelphia, WB Saunders, 1995, p 189.

Dale HE, Elefson EE, Neimeyer KH: Influence of environmental temperature on recovery of dogs from pentobarbital anesthesia. Am J Vet Res 29:1339, 1968.

Donovan EF: Perioperative care of the surgical neonate. Surg Clin North Am 65:1061, 1985.

Driscoll DJ, Gillette PC, Lewis RM, et al: Comparative hemodynamic effects of isoproterenol, dopamine, and dobutamine in the newborn dog. Pediatr Res 13:1006, 1979.

Dunlop CI: The case for rebreathing circuits for very small animals. Vet Clin North Am Small Anim Pract 22:400, 1992.

Dunlop CI, Daunt DA, Haskins SC: Thermal burns in four dogs during anesthesia. Vet Surg 18:242, 1989.

Fagella AM, Arohnson MG: Anesthesia techniques for neutering 6- to 14-week-old kittens. J Am Vet Med Assoc 202:56, 1993.

Fagella AM, Aronsohn MG: Evaluation of anesthetic protocols for neutering 6- to 14-week-old pups. J Am Vet Med Assoc 205:308, 1994.

Fettman MJ, Allen TA: Developmental aspects of fluid and electrolyte metabolism and renal function in neonates. Compend Contin Educ Pract Vet 13:392, 1991.

Finley JP, Kelly C: Heart rate and respiratory patterns in mild hypoxia in unanesthetized newborn mammals. Can J Pharmacol 64:122, 1986.

Fomon SJ: Body composition of the male reference infant during the first year of life. Pediatrics 40:863, 1967.

Friedman WF: The intrinsic physiologic properties of the developing heart. Prog Cardiovasc Dis 15:87, 1972.

Fucci V, Elkins AD: Electrosurgery: Principles and guidelines in veterinary medicine. Compend Contin Educ Pract Vet 13:407, 1991.

Grandy JL, Dunlop CI: Anesthesia of pups and kittens. J Am Vet Med Assoc 198:1244, 1991.

Hampel N: Effects of isobutyl-2-cyanoacrylate on skin healing. Compend Contin Educ Pract Vet 13:80, 1991.

Haskins SC: Hypothermia and its prevention during general anesthesia in cats. Am J Vet Res 42:856, 1981.

Haskins SC, Patz JD, Farver TB: Xylazine and xylazine-ketamine in dogs. Am J Vet Res 47:636, 1986.

Hodge D, Delgado-Paredes C, Fleisher G: Intraosseous infusion flow rates in hypovolemic "pediatric" dogs. Ann Emerg Med 16:305, 1987.

Horster M, Kember B, Valtin H: Intracortical distribution of number and volume of glomeruli during postnatal maturation in the dog. J Clin Invest 50:796, 1971.

Horster M, Valtin H: Postnatal development of renal function: Micropuncture and clearance studies in the dog. J Clin Invest 50:779, 1971.

Hosgood G, Hoskins JD: Anaesthesia and pain management. In Hosgood G, Hoskins JD (eds): Small Animal Paediatric Medicine and Surgery. Oxford, Butterworth-Heinemann, 1998a, p 18.

Hosgood G, Hoskins JD: General surgical principles. In Hosgood G, Hoskins JD (eds): Small Animal Paediatric Medicine and Surgery. Oxford, Butterworth-Heinemann, 1998b, p 58.

Hoskins JD: Clinical evaluation of the kitten: From birth to eight weeks of age. Compend Contin Educ Pract Vet 12:1215, 1990.

Hoskins JD, Turnwald GH, Kearney MT, et al: Quantitative urinalysis in kittens from four to thirty weeks after birth. Am J Vet Res 52:1295, 1991.

Jones RL: Special considerations for appropriate antimicrobial therapy in neonates. Vet Clin North Am Small Anim Pract 17:577, 1987.

Kirby BM, Knoll JS, Manley PA, et al: Calcinosis circumscripta associated with polydioxanone suture in two young dogs. Vet Surg 18:216, 1989.

Kleigman RM, Miettinen EL, Morton SK: Hepatic and cerebral energy metabolism after neonatal canine alimentation. Pediatr Res 17:285, 1983.

Kleinman LI: Renal sodium reabsorption during saline loading and distal blockade in newborn dogs. Am J Physiol 237:F392, 1979.

Kleinman LI, Lubbe RJ: Factors affecting the maturation of glomerular filtration rate and renal plasma flow in the newborn dog. J Physiol 223:395, 1972.

Krechel SW: Spinal opiates in pediatric anesthesia practice. Prog Anesth IV:78, 1990.

McIntyre DG, Ederstrom HE: Metabolic factors in the development of homeothermy in dogs. Am J Physiol 194:293, 1958.

Meyer RE: Anesthesia for neonatal and geriatric patients. In Short CE (ed): Principles and Practice of Veterinary Anesthesia. Baltimore, Williams & Wilkins, 1987, p 330.

Meyers-Wallen VN, Haskins ME, Patterson DF: Hematologic values in healthy neonatal, weanling, and juvenile kittens. Am J Vet Res 45:1322, 1984.

Mosier JE: The puppy from birth to six weeks. Vet Clin North Am Small Anim Pract 8:79, 1978.

Muir WW, Mason DE: Side effects of etomidate. J Am Vet Med Assoc 194:1430, 1989.

Otto CM, Kaufman GM, Crowe DT: Intraosseous infusion of fluids and therapeutics. Compend Contin Educ Pract Vet 11:421, 1989.

Parot S, Bonora M, Gautier H, et al: Developmental changes in ventilation and breathing patterns in unanesthetized kittens. Respir Physiol 58:253, 1984.

Poffenbarger EM, Ralston SL, Chandler ML, et al: Canine neonatology. Part I. Physiologic differences between puppies and adults. Compend Contin Educ Pract Vet 12:1601, 1990.

Robinson EP: Anesthesia of pediatric patients. Compend Contin Educ Pract Vet 12:1004, 1983.

Sammarco JL, Conzemius MG, Perkowski SZ, et al: Postoperative analgesia for stifle surgery: A comparison of intra-articular bupivacaine, morphine, or saline. Vet Surg 25:59, 1996.

Shanks CA: Humidification and loss of body heat during anesthesia. I. Quantification and correlation in the dog. Br J Anaesth 46:859, 1974.

Shifine M, Munn SL, Rosenblatt LS, et al: Hematologic changes to 60 days of age in clinically normal beagles. Lab Anim Sc 23:894, 1973.

Short CR: Drug elimination in the newborn animal. Proc Symp Vet Pharmacol Ther 2:81, 1980.

Short CR: Drug disposition in neonatal animals. J Am Vet Med Assoc 184:1161, 1984.

Skarda RT: Local and regional anesthetic and analgesic techniques A: Dogs. In Thurmon JC, Tranquilli WJ, Benson GJ (eds): Lumb and Jones Veterinary Anesthesia, 3rd ed. Baltimore, Williams & Wilkins, 1996, p 426.

Smith JA, Gaynor JS, Bednarski RM, et al: Adverse effects of administration of propofol with various preanesthetic regimens in dogs. J Am Vet Med Assoc 202:1111, 1993.

Spivey WH, Lathers CM, Malone D, et al: Comparison of intraosseous, central and peripheral routes of administration of sodium bicarbonate during CPR in pigs. Ann Emerg Med 14:1135, 1985.

Steichen JJ, Kleinman LI: Influence of dietary sodium intake on renal maturation in unanesthetized canine puppies. Proc Soc Exp Biol Med 148:748, 1975.

Turnwald GH: The respiratory system. In Hoskins JD (ed): Veterinary Pediatrics: Dogs and Cats from Birth to Six Months. Philadelphia, WB Saunders, 1995, p 71.

Index

Note: Page numbers in *italics* refer to illustrations; page numbers followed by t refer to tables.

Fungal infection(s) *(Continued)*
  upper respiratory, 85
Furniture polish(es), toxicity of, 495t
Furosemide, for respiratory disorders, 87t
Furunculosis, with canine demodicosis, 238
Fusobacterium spp., in bite wound abscess, 231

β-Galactocerebrosidase deficiency, 441t
Galactose-1-phosphate uridyltransferase deficiency, 360t, 364
Galactosemia, 360t, 364, 365, 366–367
  management of, 368
β-Galactosidase deficiency, 441t
Gallbladder, accessory, 201
  cleft (diverticular), 200–201, *201*
  congenital disorders of, 200–201
Gamma globulin, plasma/serum levels of, age-related changes in, 303
Gamma glutamyltransferase activity, in puppies/kittens, 200, 201t
Gangliosidosis, 211
  GM₁, 441t
    breeds predisposed to, 428t, 429t, 430t
    feline, corneal abnormalities in, 279
      fundic lesions in, 292–293
  GM₂, 441t
    breeds predisposed to, 430t
Garbage raiding, 28
Garlic, 503t
Gas anesthesia restraint, 8
Gasoline toxicity, 496t
Gastric acid reflux-induced esophagitis, 158
Gastric decompression, 177
Gastric dilation-volvulus, 175–177
  diagnosis of, *175*, 175–177, *176*
  prevention of, 177
  treatment of, 177
Gastric emptying, 174
Gastric pH, drug absorption and, 36
Gastric protectant(s), for bacterial infections, 68t
Gastric retention disorder(s), 171–174
  causes of, 171–174
  diagnosis of, 174
Gastrin, 174
Gastritis, 167–171
  bacterial, 170
  causes of, 170
  chlamydial, 170
  diagnosis of, 170
  endoparasitic, 170
  fungal, 170
  signs of, 167–168
  treatment of, 170–171
  viral, 170
Gastrocolopexy, in prevention of gastric dilation-volvulus, 177
Gastroesophageal intussusception, 166–167, *169*
Gastroesophageal junction, disorders of, 166–167
Gastrointestinal tract, bleeding in, 168
  hyperthermia and, 519, 520
  in thiamine deficiency, 485
Gastropexy, in prevention of gastric dilation-volvulus, 177
Gastrostomy, tube, in prevention of gastric dilation-volvulus, 177
Gauze-tie extender(s), for restraint, 7, *8*
Gear oil toxicity, 496t
Gelsemium sempervirens, 502t
Gene, 78
Genetic laboratory, commercial, 212

Genetic marker(s), 78
Genetics, 78–79
Genitals, from four weeks to six months, 7
Genome, 78
Gentamicin, excretion of, 39–40
  Fanconi's syndrome caused by, 381
  for bacterial infections, 68t
  for canine parvovirus-2 enteritis, 71
  for gastrointestinal disorders, 172t
  for pneumonia, 93
  for respiratory disorders, 86t
  for skin infection, 232t
  for urinary tract infections, 394t
German primrose, 502t
German shepherd, amylo-1,6-glucosidase deficiency in, 364
  bacterial folliculitis, furunculosis, and cellulitis of, 231
  bone cysts in, 419
  cataracts in, *288*, 289t
  cervical vertebral instability in, 437
  cleft palate-cleft lip complex and, 150
  congenital heart disease in, 108t, 113, 117, 122
  congenital pancreatic hypoplasia in, 219
  congenital renal disease in, 374t
  congenital vestibular disease in, 428t, 435
  degenerative myelopathy in, 439
  dermatoses in, 226t, 227t, 229t
  dermoid in, 279
  diabetes in, 353
  dystrophic calcification of flexor tendon origin in, 408
  epilepsy in, 442
  fragmented coronoid process in, 405
  giant axonal neuropathy in, 428t
  glycogen storage disorder in, 360t, 448
  glycogen storage disorder with hepatomegaly in, 211
  mandibular brachygnathism in, 138
  megaesophagus in, 162
  nictitating membrane of, eversion of cartilage of, 277
  oligodontia in, 139
  optic nerve hypoplasia in, 293
  osteochondritis dissecans in, 402
  Pelger-Huet anomaly in, 311
  pituitary dwarfism in, 347, *348*
  primary parathyroid hyperplasia in, 357
  serum IGF-1 level in, in pituitary dwarfism, 347
    normal, 347
  spinal muscular atrophy in, 428t
  ununited anconeal process in, 407
  vascular ring anomaly in, 158
  ventricular arrhythmias in, 126
German short-haired pointer, congenital heart defects in, 108t
  dermatoses in, 226t, 228t
  GM₁ gangliosidosis in, 428t
  nictitating membrane of, eversion of cartilage of, 277
  standard, factor XII deficiency in, 323, 324t
  tail docking guidelines for, 254t
  X-linked muscular dystrophy in, 446
German wire-haired pointer, follicular dysplasia in, 228t
  tail docking guidelines for, 254t
Giant axonal neuropathy, breeds predisposed to, 428t
Giant cell tumor(s), feline, 250
Giardiasis (*Giardia* infection), 76
  diarrhea in, 65
  drug therapy for, 181t, 182t, 183t, 184t
Gingiva, 136
Gingival sulcus, 136
Gingivitis, 136
Glanzmann's thrombasthenia, 330t, 331